AF777998

Tumors of the Liver

AFIP Atlas of Tumor Pathology

AMERICAN REGISTRY OF PATHOLOGY

1976

ARP PRESS

Washington, DC

Senior Editorial Director: Mirlinda Q. Caton
Production Editor: Dian S. Thomas
Technical Editor and Subscription Manager: Magdalena C. Silva
Copyeditor: Audrey Kahn
Editorial Assistant: Elizabeth Tomlinson

Available from the American Registry of Pathology
Washington, DC 20006
www.arppress.org
ISBN 1-933477-41-5
978-1-933477-41-1

Copyright © 2018 The American Registry of Pathology

All rights reserved. No part of this publication may be reproduced or transmitted in any form or by any means: electronic, mechanical, photocopy, recording, or any other information storage and retrieval system without the written permission of the publisher.

Printed in South Korea

AFIP ATLAS OF TUMOR PATHOLOGY

Fourth Series
Fascicle 27

TUMORS OF THE LIVER

by

Michael Torbenson, MD
Professor of Pathology
Mayo Cinic
Rochester, Minnesota

Yoh Zen, MD, PhD, FRCPath
Professor of Pathology
Department of Diagnostic Pathology
Kobe University Graduate School of Medicine
Kobe, Japan

Matthew M. Yeh, MD, PhD
Professor of Pathology
Adjunct Professor of Medicine
Director, Gastrointestinal and Hepatic Pathology Fellowship Program
University of Washington School of Medicine
Seattle, Washington

Published by the
American Registry of Pathology
Washington, DC
2018

AFIP ATLAS OF TUMOR PATHOLOGY

EDITOR
Steven G. Silverberg, MD
Department of Pathology
University of Maryland School of Medicine
Baltimore, Maryland

ASSOCIATE EDITOR
Ronald A. DeLellis, MD
Warren Alpert Medical School
of Brown University
Providence, Rhode Island

ASSOCIATE EDITOR
Leslie H. Sobin, MD
Armed Forces Institute of Pathology
Washington, DC

EDITORIAL ADVISORY BOARD

Jorge Albores-Saavedra, MD	Médica Sur Clinic and Foundation Mexico City, Mexico
William J. Frable, MD	Virginia Commonwealth University Richmond, Virginia
Kim R. Geisinger, MD	Wake Forest University School of Medicine Winston-Salem, North Carolina
Leonard B. Kahn, MD	Long Island Jewish Medical Center New Hyde Park, New York
Donald West King, MD	National Library of Medicine Bethesda, Maryland
James Linder, MD	University of Nebraska Medical Center Omaha, Nebraska
Virginia A. LiVolsi, MD	University of Pennsylvania Medical Center Philadelphia, Pennsylvania
Elizabeth A. Montgomery, MD	Johns Hopkins University School of Medicine Baltimore, Maryland
Juan Rosai, MD	Istituto Nazionale Tumori Milan, Italy
Mark H. Stoler, MD	University of Virginia Health System Charlottesville, Virginia
William D. Travis, MD	Memorial Sloan Kettering Cancer Center New York, New York
Mark R. Wick, MD	University of Virginia Medical Center Charlottesville, Virginia

Manuscript reviewed by:
Ronald A. DeLellis, MD
Elizabeth A. Montgomery, MD

EDITORS' NOTE

The Atlas of Tumor Pathology has a long and distinguished history. It was first conceived at a cancer research meeting held in St. Louis in September 1947, as an attempt to standardize the nomenclature of neoplastic diseases. The first series was sponsored by the National Academy of Sciences-National Research Council. The organization of this formidable effort was entrusted to the Subcommittee on Oncology of the Committee on Pathology, and Dr. Arthur Purdy Stout was the first editor-in-chief. Many of the illustrations were provided by the Medical Illustration Service of the Armed Forces Institute of Pathology (AFIP), the type was set by the Government Printing Office, and the final printing was done at the Armed Forces Institute of Pathology. The American Registry of Pathology (ARP) purchased the Fascicles from the Government Printing Office and sold them virtually at cost. Over a period of 20 years, approximately 15,000 copies each of nearly 40 Fascicles were produced. The worldwide impact of these publications over the years has largely surpassed the original goal. They quickly became among the most influential publications on tumor pathology, primarily because of their overall high quality, but also because their low cost made them easily accessible the world over to pathologists and other students of oncology.

Upon completion of the first series, the National Academy of Sciences-National Research Council handed further pursuit of the project over to the newly created Universities Associated for Research and Education in Pathology (UAREP). A second series was started, generously supported by grants from the AFIP, the National Cancer Institute, and the American Cancer Society. Dr. Harlan I. Firminger became the editor-in-chief and was succeeded by Dr. William H. Hartmann. The second series' Fascicles were produced as bound volumes instead of loose leaflets. They featured a more comprehensive coverage of the subjects, to the extent that the Fascicles could no longer be regarded as "atlases" but rather as monographs describing and illustrating in detail the tumors and tumor-like conditions of the various organs and systems.

Once the second series was completed, with a success that matched that of the first, ARP, UAREP, and AFIP decided to embark on a third series. Dr. Juan Rosai was appointed as editor-in-chief, and Dr. Leslie Sobin became associate editor. A distinguished Editorial Advisory Board was also convened, and these outstanding pathologists and educators played a major role in the success of this series, the first publication of which appeared in 1991 and the last (number 32) in 2003.

The same organizational framework applies to the current fourth series, but with UAREP and AFIP no longer functioning, ARP is now the responsible organization. New features include a hardbound cover and illustrations almost exclusively in color. There is also an increased emphasis on the cytopathologic (intraoperative, exfoliative, or fine needle aspiration) and molecular features that are important in diagnosis and prognosis. What does not change from the three previous series, however, is the goal of providing the practicing pathologist with thorough, concise, and up-to-date information on the nomenclature and classification; epidemiologic, clinical, and pathogenetic features; and, most importantly, guidance in the diagnosis of the tumors and tumorlike lesions of all major organ systems and body sites.

As in the third series, a continuous attempt is made to correlate, whenever possible, the nomenclature used in the Fascicles with that proposed by the World Health Organization's Classification of Tumors, as well as to ensure a consistency of style. Close cooperation between the various authors and their respective liaisons from the Editorial Board will continue to be emphasized in order to minimize unnecessary repetition and discrepancies in the text and illustrations.

Particular thanks are due to the members of the Editorial Advisory Board, the reviewers, the editorial and production staff, and the individual Fascicle authors for their ongoing efforts to ensure that this series is a worthy successor to the previous three.

Steven G. Silverberg, MD
Ronald A. DeLellis, MD
Leslie H. Sobin, MD

PREFACE AND ACKNOWLEDGMENTS

Numerous advances in our understanding of the pathology and molecular features of liver tumors have been made since the publication of the Third Series Fascicle, Tumors of the Liver and Intrahepatic Bile Ducts, nearly two decades ago. Examples of recent advances include the identification of novel entities, including their precursor lesions, the discovery of key molecular changes, including the fusion transcript between the DNAJB1 gene and the PRKACA gene in fibrolamellar carcinoma, the use of glutamine synthetase in the diagnosis of focal nodular hyperplasia, and the subtyping of hepatocellular adenomas using molecular and immunohistochemical methods. Together with the more unified classification and terminology of intrahepatic bile duct tumors and their precursors, these advances call for updated information that is presented in this volume.

A handful of invaluable figures from the previous series (Fascicle 31) are included in this new Fascicle. We are grateful to Drs. Kamal Ishak, Zachary Goodman, and Thomas Stocker for their contribution to our understanding of these tumors, and for providing the foundations of the previous and current Fascicles.

We thank Dr. Steven Silverberg for inviting us to take on this project and Drs. Elizabeth Montgomery and Ronald DeLellis for critically reviewing the manuscript. Their comments were invaluable. We also thank Mirlinda Caton and her team including Dian Thomas, Magdalena Silva, Audrey Kahn, and Elizabeth Tomlinson, at the American Registry of Pathology for their efforts to bring this book to fruition.

Michael Torbenson, MD
Yoh Zen, MD, PhD, FRCPath
Matthew M. Yeh, MD, PhD

Permission to use copyrighted illustrations has been granted by:

Nature
Mod Pathol 207;20:701-9. For table 7-11.

Springer
Aloia T, Pawlik TM, Taouli B, Rubbia-Brandt L, Vauthey JN. Intrahepatic bile ducts. In: Amin MB, Edge SB, Greene FL, et al., eds. AJCC cancer staging manual, 8th ed. Switzerland: Springer; 2017:295-302. For tables 7-7, 7-8, 12-1, 12-2, 12-3, and 12-4.

CONTENTS

1 EMBRYOLOGY, HISTOLOGY, AND ANATOMY

EMBRYOLOGY

At the beginning of fetal development (toward the latter part of the third week of gestation), the hepatic diverticulum buds from the ventral foregut. The hepatic diverticulum then gives rise to the transverse septum (septum transversum), a structure situated between the pericardial and peritoneal cavities (1,2). Mesenchymal elements of the transverse septum, which already exist, are invested by liver parenchyma formed from hepatic endodermal cells (also known as hepatoblasts) of the hepatic diverticulum to give rise to the liver buds (3). During fetal development the liver buds function as a hematopoietic organ, which is composed of hepatocytic cords, venous-sinusoidal plexus, and hematopoietic precursor cells, including Kupffer cells (macrophages residing in liver). The umbilical vein supplies most of the blood during development of the liver. The remaining smaller amount of blood is supplied by the portal vein and hepatic artery.

During fetal development, the placenta executes the major functions performed by the adult liver, including the absorption of nutrients and the excretion of bile containing waste products; bile secretion by fetal liver is negligible before birth. Nonetheless, the fetal liver produces alpha-fetoprotein and other plasma proteins, synthesizes bile acids, and stores fat, glycogen, iron, and copper.

The anterior portion of the hepatic diverticulum forms the liver and intrahepatic bile ducts, while the posterior portion gives rise to the gallbladder and extrahepatic bile ducts (2,4–6). The ultimate formation of intrahepatic bile ducts occurs late during development, and is completed after birth, during the first year of life. The development of small intrahepatic bile ducts begins when the ductal plate is formed, which is a single-layered sheath of small flat epithelial cells assembled by the periportal hepatoblasts in intimate contact with the portal mesenchyme surrounding a portal vein branch (2). In the weeks that follow, certain parts of the ductal plates are duplicated by a second layer of cells, to become double-layered ductal plates, which then dilate to form cylindrical structures to be integrated into the mesenchyme of the newly formed portal region (fig. 1-1). When they are integrated into the portal space, the immature tubules evolve into bile ducts that are embraced by connective tissue and gradually situated in their usual location in the portal tracts as the portal tracts increase in size (2,7–9).

GROSS ANATOMY

The liver can be divided into the right and left lobes by the middle hepatic vein and a plane between the inferior vena cava and the gallbladder fossa. Anteriorly, this division is visible by the falciform ligament. Viewed from the under surface, there are also the quadrate lobe in the vicinity of the gallbladder fossa and the caudate lobe which in part encases the vena cava.

There are dual afferent blood supplies in the liver: hepatic artery and portal vein. The hepatic artery (branches from the celiac artery) transports 30 to 40 percent and the portal vein (drains the intestine) transports up to 70 percent of the oxygenated blood to the liver. The sinusoids then carry blood from hepatic arteries and portal veins to the terminal hepatic venules, and subsequently through the hepatic vein to the inferior vena cava.

Functionally, the liver is better divided into eight segments based on the blood supply, known as the Couinaud classification, or Couinaud scheme (fig. 1-2). The segments are numbered in Roman numerals I to VIII. Segment I essentially represents the caudate lobe, which drains directly into the inferior vena cava. Segments II to VIII are then numbered in a clockwise manner in a frontal plane beginning superiorly

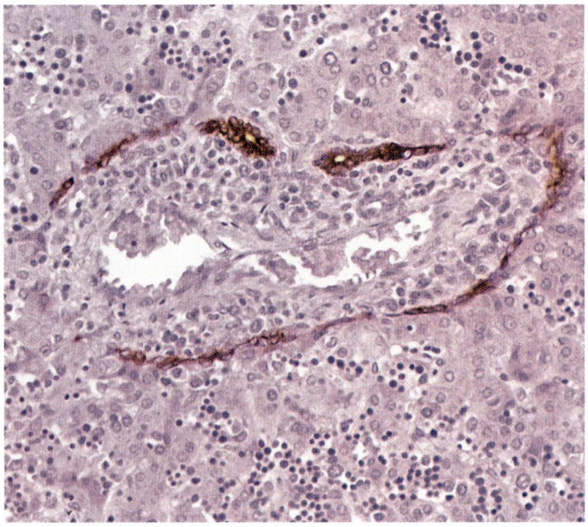

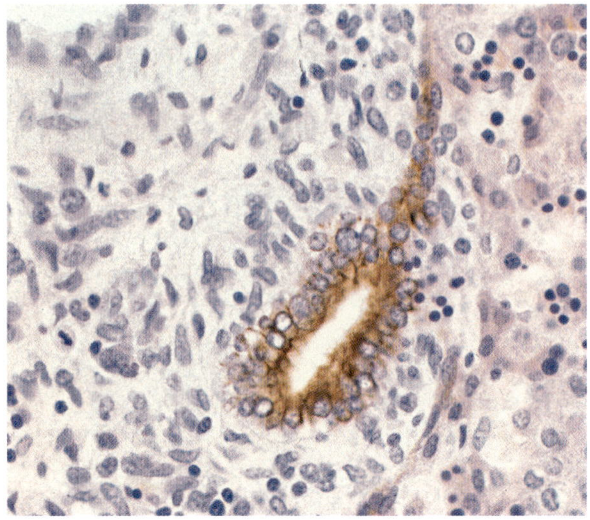

Figure 1-1

FETAL LIVER

Left: The embryonic ductal plate, composed of cytokeratin-rich cells, forms a layer that surrounds the portal area. This immunostain for cytokeratin (CK) 18 shows that the ductal plate is discontinuous and in a few places forms a double layer of cells with small lumina.

Right: Higher magnification of another portal area shows the bile duct forming from the ductal plate, which will eventually disappear as the liver grows.

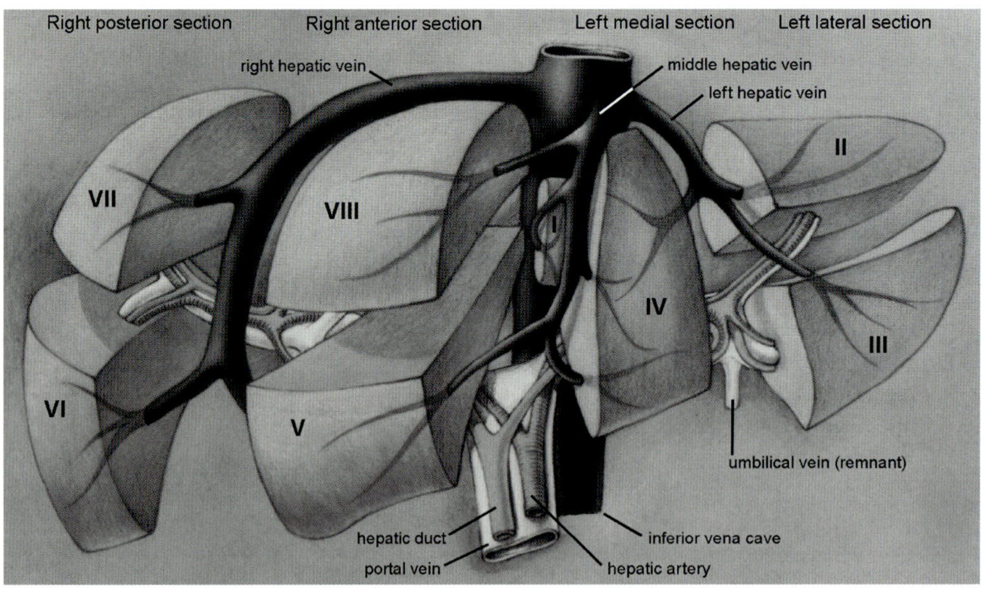

Figure 1-2

SEGMENTAL ANATOMY OF THE LIVER

The segments, designated by Roman numerals, can be resected surgically because each is supplied by a major branch of the hepatic artery and portal vein and drained by a major tributary of the hepatic vein.

from the left lobe. These segments are bounded by the three main branches of the hepatic veins: the left, middle, and right hepatic veins. Each segment drains into branches of the hepatic veins and then into the inferior vena cava. Overall, segments I to IV represent the functional left lobe, whereas segments V to VIII are considered the functional right lobe. Division of the liver according to the Couinaud scheme allows the surgical removal of a single segment, or two or more adjacent segments en bloc, in such a fashion to avoid damaging the remaining segments. The Couinaud scheme also serves as a common terminology for communicating among physicians of different disciplines: surgeons, hepatologists, oncologists, radiologists, and pathologists (10).

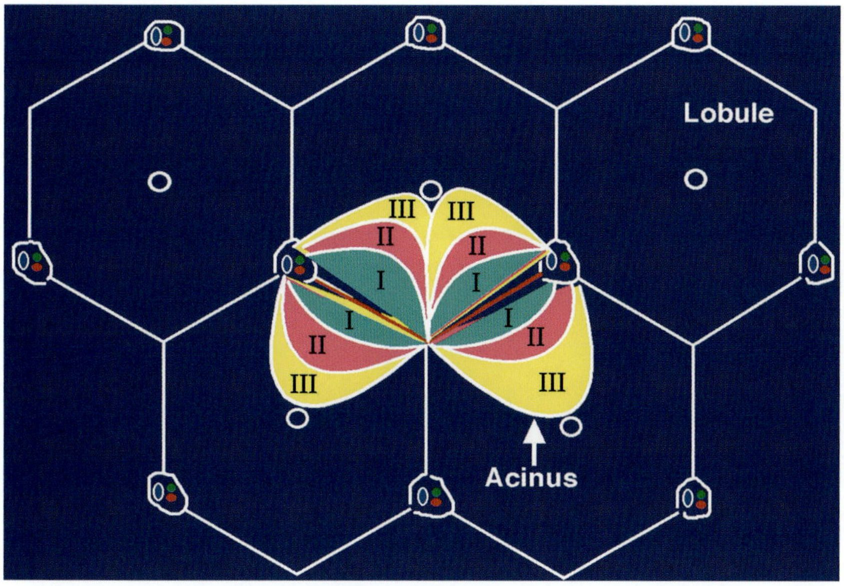

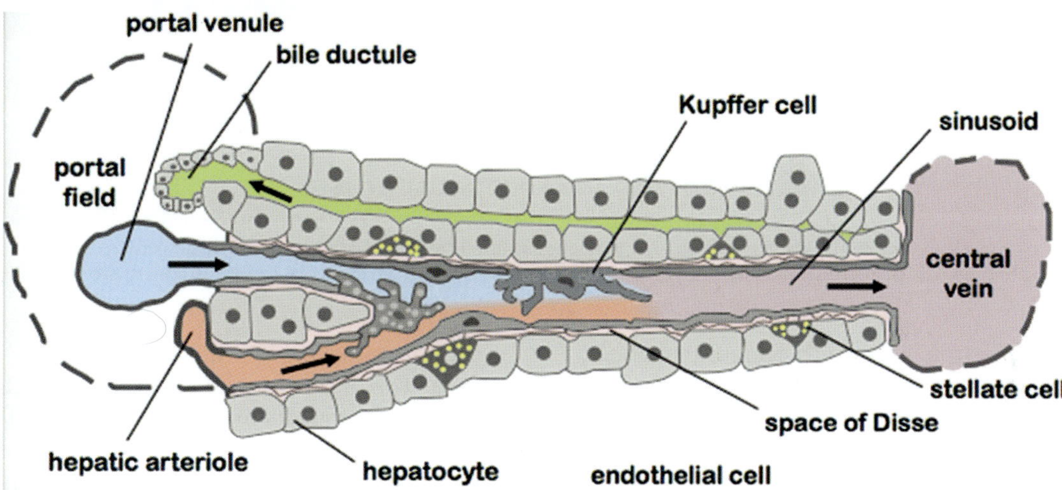

Figure 1-3

HISTOLOGIC ORGANIZATION OF THE LIVER

Left: *Hepatic Architecture.* Two views of the architecture of the liver as seen in microscopic sections. The lobules have a central vein at the center and portal spaces at the corners. A cross section of an acinus superimposed on two lobules shows that zone 3 tends to be centrilobular, zone 2 midzonal, and zone 1 periportal, but all three are crescent shaped and may extend into other parts of the classic lobule.

Bottom: *Liver Blood Flow.* Figure from "Gastrointestinal Tract—Liver Development" from embryology.med.unsw.edu.au.

HISTOLOGIC ORGANIZATION

The liver is structurally organized into parenchymal, vascular, bile ductal, and interstitial components (11). Traditionally, the smallest functional unit has been conceptualized as the hepatic lobule or three dimensionally as the hepatic acinus, as defined by Rappaport (12). Most oxygenated blood flows from the terminal branches of portal veins and hepatic arteries in the portal tracts, via the sinusoids to supply the hepatocytes, and finally draining into the terminal branches of the hepatic (central) veins at the peripheral part of the acinus (11). The acinus can also be conceptualized as a three-dimensional spherical structure with portal tracts at the center. The spherical area of those hepatocytes surrounding the portal tract is referred to as zone 1, which has the richest oxygenated blood. The area outside of zone 1 is referred to as zone 2. Zone 3 is further out, corresponding to the region surrounding the terminal hepatic vein, where the oxygen content in blood is the lowest (fig. 1-3).

The two-dimensional concept of the lobule, as seen on slides, serves the purpose of histologic visualization, but zonal subdivision of the acinus incorporates the physiologic concept into histologic organization and facilitates the recognition of certain liver injury patterns. These patterns include the gradual increasing vulnerability to ischemic and toxic/metabolic

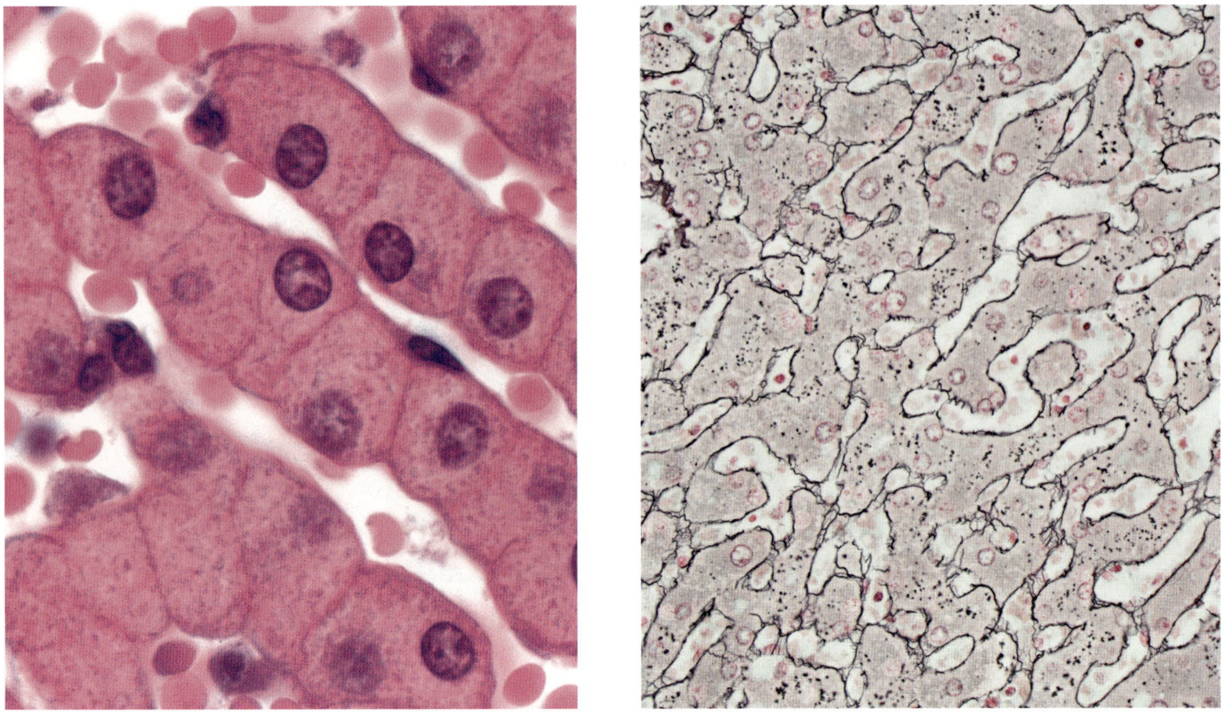

Figure 1-4

HEPATOCYTES AND ENDOTHELIAL CELLS

Left: Normal hepatocytes are polyhedral cells arranged in plates that are one cell thick. They have granular, eosinophilic cytoplasm and usually one nucleus. The sinusoids between the hepatocytes are lined by inconspicuous endothelial cells.

Right: The hepatocytic plates are normally one cell layer in thickness and are separated by the sinusoidal space (reticulin stain).

injuries from zone 1 through zone 2 to zone 3, as well as the distinction between adult nonalcoholic steatohepatitis (zone 3 accentuated) and pediatric nonalcoholic steatohepatitis (zone 1 accentuated) (13–15).

Hepatocytes are formed in plates of one cell in thickness, which can be highlighted by a reticulin stain (fig. 1-4, right). The hepatocytic plates are organized in a radial fashion between the portal tracts and terminal hepatic venules (fig. 1-5), and are separated by sinusoids lined by endothelial cells, with oxygenated blood flowing from the portal tracts to the terminal hepatic venules. The radial alignment is most pronounced in the hepatocyte plates surrounding the terminal hepatic venules. In normal liver, the portal tracts are composed of at least one hepatic artery branch, one portal vein branch, and one interlobular bile duct (fig. 1-6). The boundary between the portal tracts and the first layer of hepatocytes in the parenchyma is termed the limiting plate.

Bile ductules and canals of Hering are structures at the periphery of the portal tracts and are not conspicuous by hematoxylin and eosin (H&E) stain in normal liver. They are the conduits between the biliary tree and hepatocyte canaliculi. The canals of Hering drain bile from bile canaliculi into bile ductules, and then into the interlobular bile ducts. Canals of Hering are important for liver regeneration since the hepatic progenitor cells reside here (16,17).

HISTOLOGY

Cells of the Liver

Hepatocytes. Hepatocytes, which originate from endoderm, comprise the primary cell population in liver, accounting for 75 to 80 percent of the liver volume (18). They are hexagonal or polyhedral in cross section, and have an eosinophilic cytoplasm containing a centrally placed round nucleus; occasional hepatocytes may be binucleatic. In the adult liver, hepatocytes are

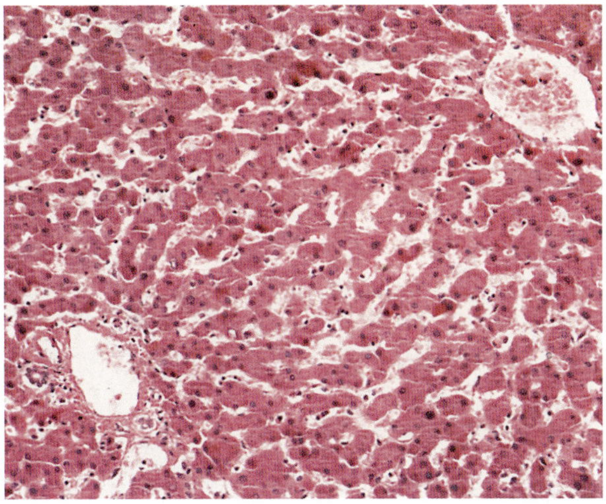

Figure 1-5

HEPATIC ARCHITECTURE

Plates of hepatocytes extend from the portal area (lower left) to the terminal hepatic venule or central vein (upper right). Blood that enters the liver through branches of the portal vein and hepatic artery perfuses the sinusoids and exits through tributaries of the hepatic vein.

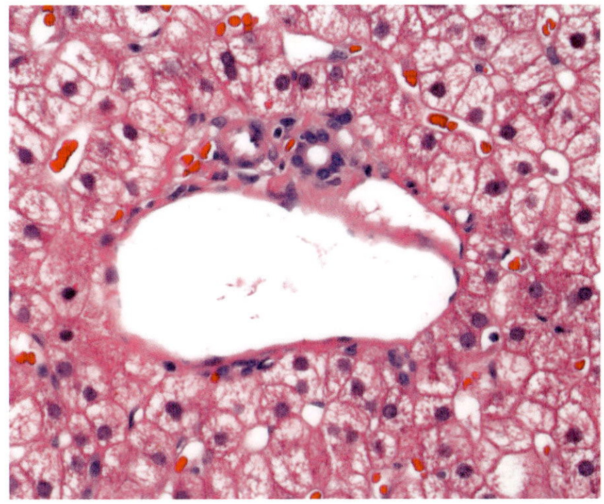

Figure 1-6

PORTAL TRACT

A normal portal tract has at least one portal vein, one hepatic artery, and one bile duct. The interlobular bile duct is approximately the same diameter as the hepatic artery and is approximately the same distance as its own diameter away from it.

aligned as anastomosing plates, normally one cell layer in thickness (fig. 1-4). The hepatocytic plates are separated by sinusoids, in which the oxygenated blood flows from the portal tracts to the terminal hepatic venules.

Bile is produced exclusively by hepatocytes and secreted into the bile canaliculi, which are gutter-like structures between two or three adjacent hepatocytes in the hepatocytic plates (11). The canalicular surface is lined by glycoprotein I, which cross reacts with polyclonal carcinoembryonic antigen (CEA), an immunohistochemical marker specific for hepatocytic differentiation (fig. 1-7), although its sensitivity is not optimal and its interpretation requires experience. Canalicular staining is also observed using a CD10 immunostain (19). Immunohistochemical stains for cytokeratin (CK) 8 and 18 are positive in hepatocytes, as is CAM5.2 (20). Since the hepatocytes are rich in urea cycle proteins, antibodies against some urea cycle enzymes have been used widely as hepatocytic markers, such as hepatocyte paraffin-1 (HepPar1) (21) and arginase-1 (22). Various cytoplasmic contents, pigments, and materials are also present within the hepatocytes, including fat, glycogen, bile, lipofuscin, and hemosiderin. However, they are not always seen nor are they absolutely specific for hepatocytic differentiation.

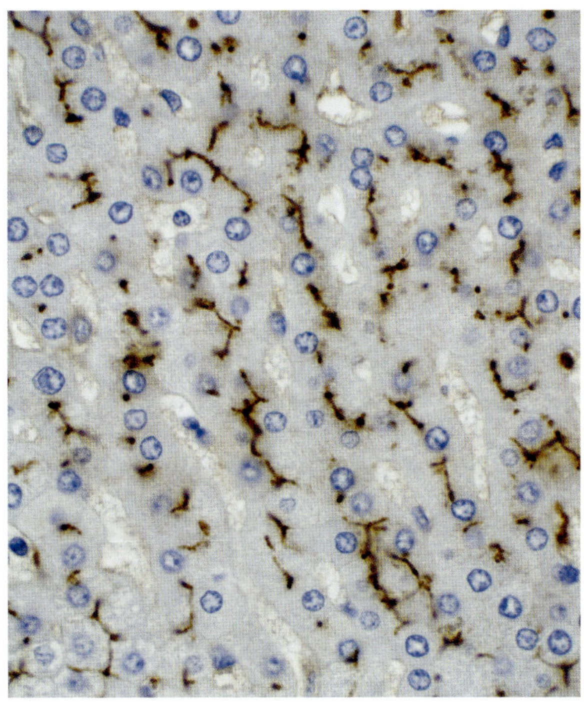

Figure 1-7

HEPATOCYTES

Canalicular structures between the hepatocytes are highlighted by polyclonal carcinoembryonic antigen (CEA) due to cross reaction with the glycoprotein on the canalicular surface.

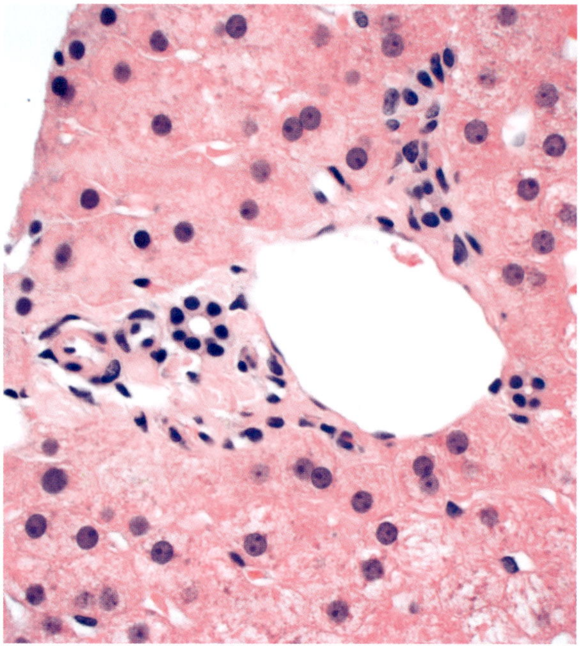

Figure 1-8

INTERLOBULAR BILE DUCTS

Lining cells of the interlobular bile ducts are cuboidal and form a circular structure in cross section. Their nuclei are round and regular, without prominent nucleoli.

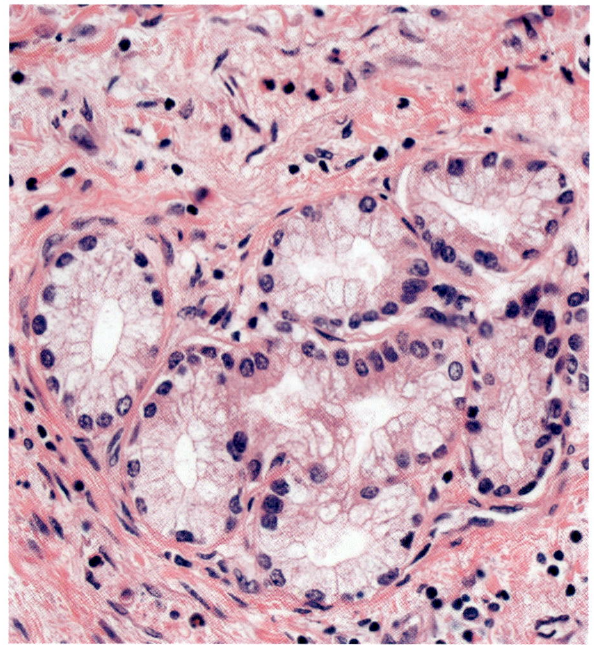

Figure 1-9

PERIBILIARY GLANDS

Small glands in the walls of large bile ducts are composed of small acini of cuboidal cells with clear cytoplasm.

Biliary Epithelial Cells. The lining epithelial cells of the septal or larger intrahepatic bile ducts are tall columnar to cuboidal, while those of the interlobular bile ducts are typically cuboidal (fig. 1-8). These cells are encased by a layer of periodic acid–Schiff (PAS)-positive basement membrane and are further surrounded by connective tissue of variable amount, depending on the size of the bile ducts. The interlobular bile duct and hepatic artery are typically adjacent to each other, with a similar diameter and a distance apart approximately the same as their own diameters. The bile ducts are connected to the bile canaliculi via the canals of Hering. On cross section, the configuration of the bile duct appears as a chain of pearls (fig. 1-8). Bile ductal cells express CK7 and CK19, reflected by immunohistochemical staining. Like the hepatocytes, they also express CK8 and CK18.

Peribiliary Gland Cells. Peribiliary glands are small accessory glands of the bile ducts in liver. They communicate with the lumens of the intrahepatic and extrahepatic large bile ducts via specialized conduits (7,23,24), densely populated in the hilar bile ducts, cystic duct, and periampullary areas (24–28). Peribiliary glands are composed of glandular and branched tubuloalveolar structures that form small acini that surround the intrahepatic and extrahepatic large bile ducts. The glandular cells are cuboidal, clear (fig. 1-9), and seromucinous in nature, secreting lactoferrin and lysozyme (26).

Ductular Cells. Bile ductules are also known as cholangioles. The terms bile ductules and canals of Hering are sometimes used interchangeably, however, they represent two different physiologic and histologic structures. The canals of Hering are the physiologic link between the biliary tree and hepatocyte canaliculi (29). They are lined partially by cholangiocytes and partially by hepatocytes. They continue into bile ductules, which represent the conduits between canals of Hering and the interlobular bile ducts. Bile ducts are lined entirely by cholangiocytes.

The bile ductules are situated at the edge of the portal tracts. They may also penetrate the limiting plate so they not only have an intraportal segment, but also have an intralobular

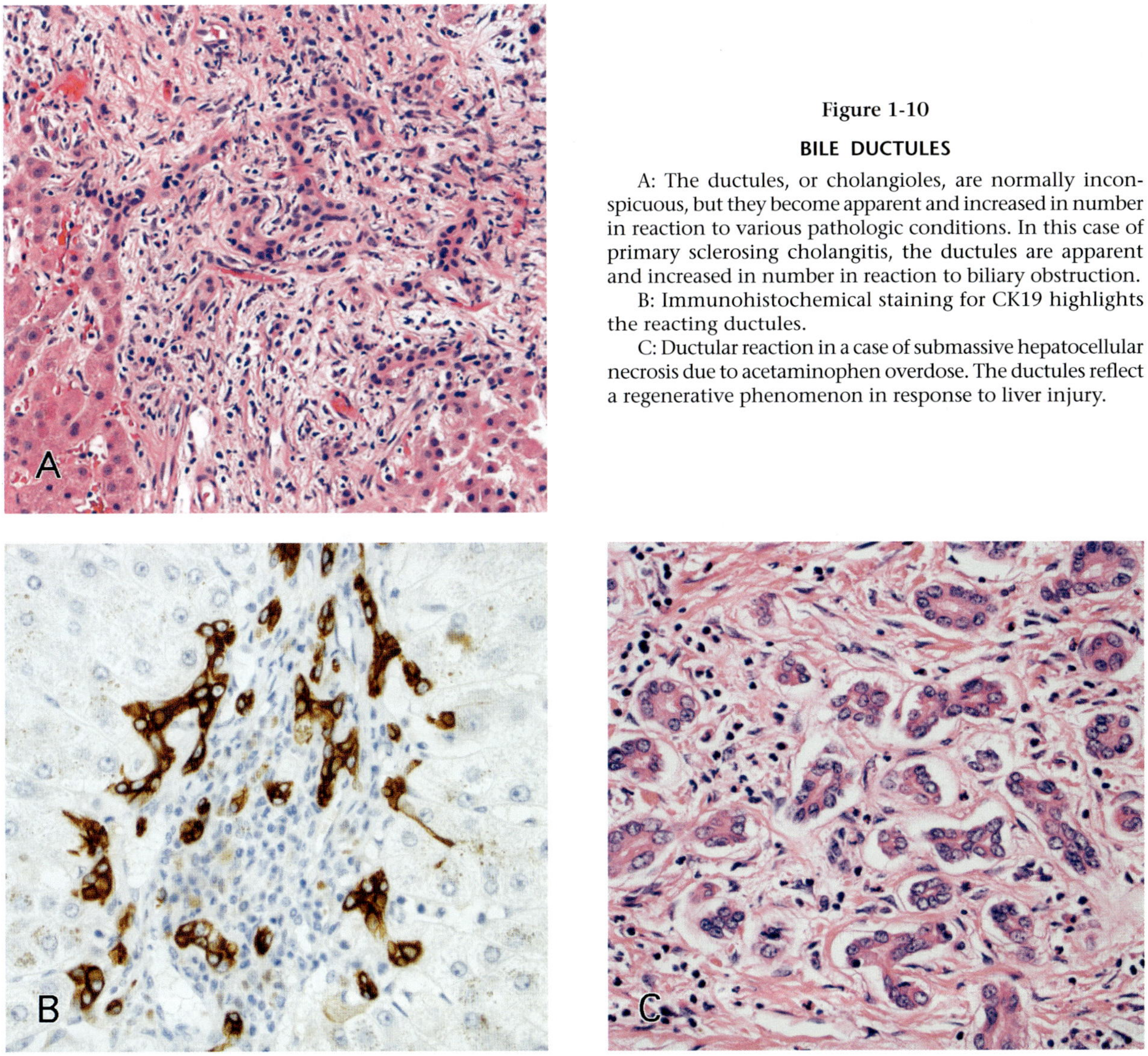

Figure 1-10

BILE DUCTULES

A: The ductules, or cholangioles, are normally inconspicuous, but they become apparent and increased in number in reaction to various pathologic conditions. In this case of primary sclerosing cholangitis, the ductules are apparent and increased in number in reaction to biliary obstruction.

B: Immunohistochemical staining for CK19 highlights the reacting ductules.

C: Ductular reaction in a case of submassive hepatocellular necrosis due to acetaminophen overdose. The ductules reflect a regenerative phenomenon in response to liver injury.

segment (11,29). Unlike the interlobular bile duct, the bile ductules are not accompanied by a hepatic artery branch (11). Their lumens are also smaller than those of interlobular bile ducts (29). The lining cells of the canals of Hering stain for CK7, CK19, and the hepatic stem cell marker NCAM/CD56, demonstrating the scattered presence of hepatic progenitor cells in these structures (16,17).

Ductular reaction is a phenomenon seen in diseased liver, either acute or chronic disease (fig. 1-10). It is a reaction of ductular phenotype, but not necessarily of ductular origin (29), as it may arise from proliferation of preexisting cholangiocytes, progenitor cells (either local and/or circulating cells such as bone marrow-derived), or biliary metaplasia of hepatocytes (rare) (29).

Endothelial Cells. The endothelial cells lining the portal veins, hepatic arteries, and terminal hepatic venules share the same properties and immunophenotype as the endothelial cells lining the arteries, veins, and capillaries in other organs. Their single layer of flattened endothelial cells is attached above a basement membrane and lines the vascular spaces of these vessels. They are immunoreactive to antibodies against CD31, CD34, and factor VIII-related antigen (von Willebrand factor).

In contrast, endothelial cells lining the sinusoidal spaces do not have a basement membrane

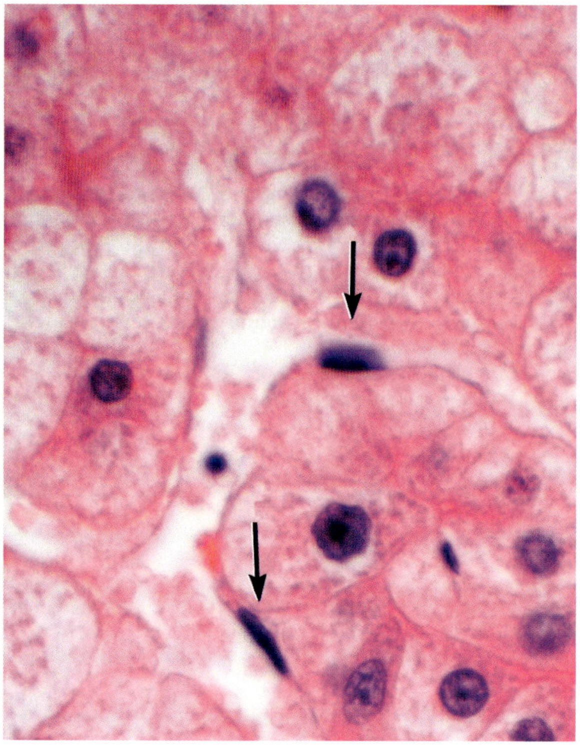

Figure 1-11

SINUSOIDAL ENDOTHELIAL CELLS

The endothelial cells lining the sinusoidal spaces are inconspicuous (arrows).

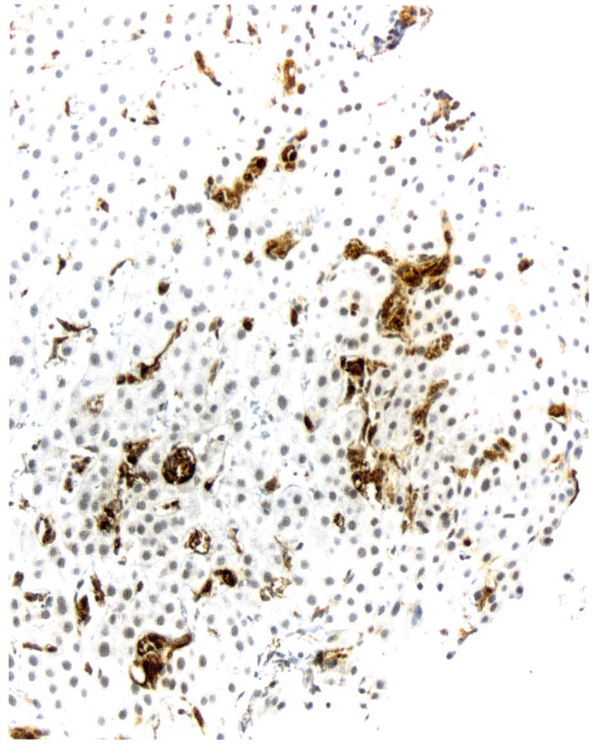

Figure 1-12

KUPFFER CELLS

Kupffer cells enlarge and become apparent when they engulf and phagocytose debris resulting from liver injury. They are highlighted by a CD68 immunostain.

(fig. 1-11). In normal liver, the sinusoidal spaces are fenestrated and are lined by endothelial cells that are immunohistochemically nonreactive to CD31 or CD34. The fenestration allows plasma to be transported between the sinusoidal spaces and the hepatocytes underneath the subendothelial space of Disse. When there is neoplastic change of the hepatocytes, the fenestration is decreased, and the sinusoidal endothelial cells become reactive to CD31 or CD34, a phenomenon known as capillarization of the sinusoids. These changes are also observed in preneoplastic lesions, i.e., dysplastic nodules (30–32). Capillarization also occurs in livers with chronic injury or cirrhosis, beginning at the periportal region and extending to the hepatic lobules, although the changes are not as significant as in neoplasia.

Kupffer Cells. Kupffer cells are specialized macrophages of the mononuclear phagocyte system that line the walls of the sinusoidal spaces. Normally they are not prominent, but enlarge and become noticeable when they engulf and phagocytose debris resulting from liver injury (fig. 1-12). Hemosiderin pigments may be deposited in Kupffer cells, due to secondary iron overload, or more rarely, hereditary hemochromatosis due to mutation in the *SLC40A1/ferroportin 1* gene (33). Lipofuscin pigment may also appear in Kupffer cells.

Kupffer cells are variably PAS positive and diastase resistant since they contain many lysosomes. They are also positive for macrophage markers such as CD68 (KP1).

Hepatic Stellate Cells. The compartment between the hepatocyte cytoplasmic membrane and the sinusoidal space, underneath the fenestrated sinusoidal endothelial cells, is the space of Disse, where hepatic stellate cells reside. A number of synonyms were previously used for these cells, such as Ito cells, fat-storing cells, perisinusoidal cell lipocytes, and parasinusoidal cells, but the preferred nomenclature by the

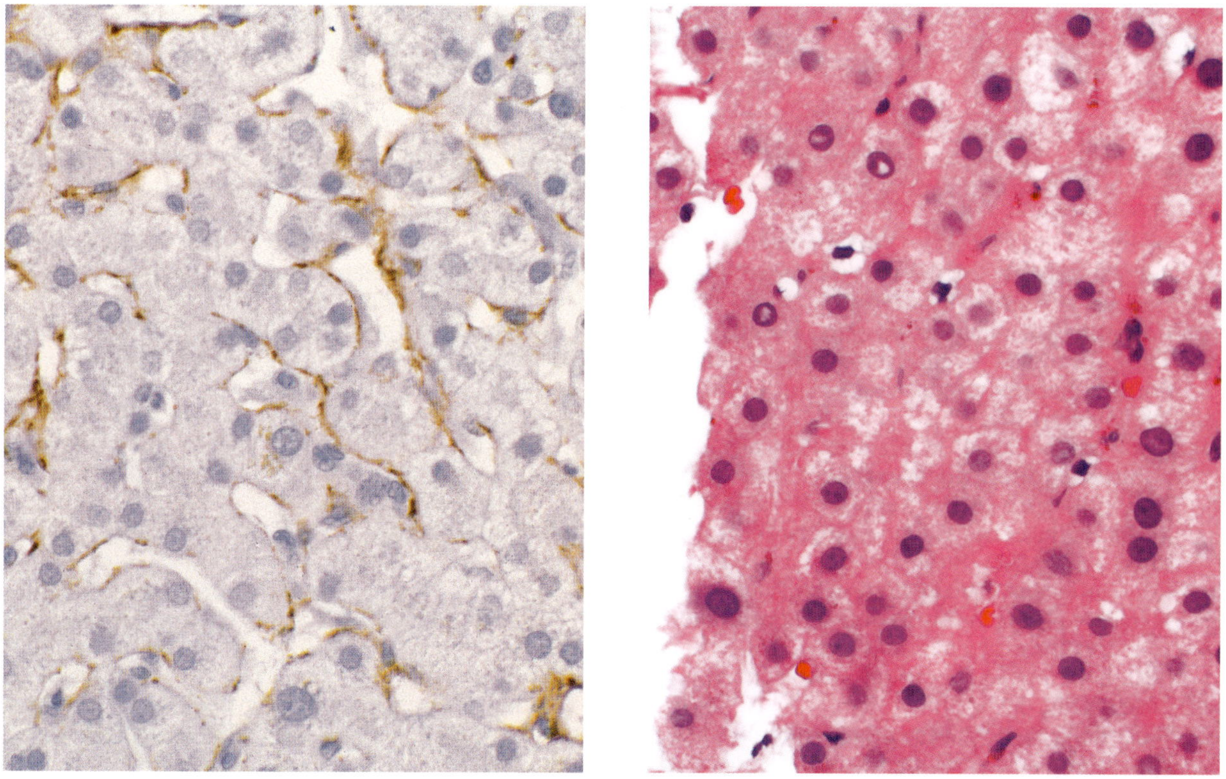

Figure 1-13

HEPATIC STELLATE CELLS

Left: Hepatic stellate cells are identified with an immunostain for smooth muscle actin.

Right: The hepatic stellate cells become conspicuous in hepatotoxicity due to hypervitaminosis A, which shows bubbly cells due to the deposition of fat in the cytoplasm, with hyperchromatic and scalloped nuclei.

consensus of investigators studying this cell is hepatic stellate cell (34).

Within the subendothelial spaces of normal liver, these cells store vitamin A (retinoid) droplets in their cytoplasm (35). In their quiescent phase, they are not conspicuous in formalin-fixed normal liver, but may become discernible by immunohistochemistry using anti-smooth muscle actin (fig. 1-13, left) or anti-desmin antibodies. Hepatic stellate cells are also prominent during hepatotoxicity associated with hypervitaminosis A, becoming bubbly cells due to the deposition of fat in the cytoplasm, with hyperchromatic and scalloped nuclei (fig. 1-13, right).

Hepatic stellate cells are responsible for hepatic fibrogenesis. They can transform into myofibroblasts when they are activated in response to chronic liver disease with activated TGF-β and other signaling pathways. This phenotypic change triggers a series of accumulation as well as inhibition of the breakdown of matrix proteins, hence leading to liver fibrosis (36).

Pit Cells. Another cell residing in the space of Disse is the pit cell. Pit cells are large granule-containing lymphoid cells possessing natural killer cell properties that are liver specific (37). Pit cells are not readily identifiable under light microscopy, but have been characterized by electron microscopy as cells containing multivesicular body-related dense granules and rod-cored vesicles (38).

Inflammatory Cells. In normal liver, inflammatory cells are inconspicuous, except for occasional lymphocytes, Kupffer cells, and neutrophils in the sinusoids. The portal tracts have few lymphocytes and macrophages, and their number appears to correlate with age, likely reflecting a remnant response to previous injuries in the liver.

REFERENCES

1. Tremblay KD, Zaret KS. Distinct populations of endoderm cells converge to generate the embryonic liver bud and ventral foregut tissues. Dev Biol 2005;280:87-99.
2. Strazzabosco M, Fabris L. Development of the bile ducts: essentials for the clinical hepatologist. J Hepatol 2012;56:1159-1170.
3. Houssaint E. Differentiation of the mouse hepatic primordium. I. An analysis of tissue interactions in hepatocyte differentiation. Cell Differ 1980;9:269-279.
4. Tan J, Hytiroglou P, Wieczorek R, et al. Immunohistochemical evidence for hepatic progenitor cells in liver diseases. Liver 2002;22:365-373.
5. Roskams T, Desmet V. Embryology of extra- and intrahepatic bile ducts, the ductal plate. Anat Rec (Hoboken) 2008;291:628-635.
6. Lemaigre FP. Mechanisms of liver development: concepts for understanding liver disorders and design of novel therapies. Gastroenterology 2009;137:62-79.
7. Nakanuma Y, Hoso M, Sanzen T, Sasaki M. Microstructure and development of the normal and pathologic biliary tract in humans, including blood supply. Microsc Res Tech 1997;38:552-570.
8. Libbrecht L, Cassiman D, Desmet V, Roskams T. Expression of neural cell adhesion molecule in human liver development and in congenital and acquired liver diseases. Histochem Cell Biol 2001;116:233-239.
9. Fabris L, Cadamuro M, Libbrecht L, et al. Epithelial expression of angiogenic growth factors modulate arterial vasculogenesis in human liver development. Hepatology 2008;47:719-728.
10. Majno P, Mentha G, Toso C, Morel P, Peitgen HO, Fasel JH. Anatomy of the liver: an outline with three levels of complexity—a further step towards tailored territorial liver resections. J Hepatol 2014;60:654-662. 10. Zhou Z, Xu MJ, Gao B. Hepatocytes: a key cell type for innate immunity. Cell Mol Immunol 2016;13:301-315.
11. Suriawinata A, Thung S. Liver. In: Mills SE, ed. Histology for pathologists, 4th ed. Philadelphia: Lippincott Williams & Wilkins; 2012:733-758.
12. Rappaport AM. The structural and functional unit in the human liver (liver acinus). Anat Rec 1958;130:673-689.
13. Kleiner DE, Brunt EM, Van Natta M, et al. Design and validation of a histological scoring system for nonalcoholic fatty liver disease. Hepatology 2005;41:1313-1321.
14. Schwimmer JB, Behling C, Newbury R, et al. Histopathology of pediatric nonalcoholic fatty liver disease. Hepatology 2005;42:641-649.
15. Yeh MM, Brunt EM. Pathological features of fatty liver disease. Gastroenterology 2014;147:754-764.
16. Theise ND, Saxena R, Portmann BC, et al. The canals of Hering and hepatic stem cells in humans. Hepatology 1999;30:1425-1433.
17. Turner R, Lozoya O, Wang Y, et al. Human hepatic stem cell and maturational liver lineage biology. Hepatology 2011;53:1035-1045.
18. Zhou Z, Xu MJ, Gao B. Hepatocytes: a key cell type for innate immunity. Cell Mol Immunol 2016;13:301-315.
19. Loke SL, Leung CY, Chiu KY, Yau WL, Cheung KN, Ma L. Localisation of CD10 to biliary canaliculi by immunoelectron microscopical examination. J Clin Pathol 1990;43:654-656.
20. van Eyken P, Sciot R, van Damme B, de Wolf-Peeters C, Desmet VJ. Keratin immunohistochemistry in normal human liver. Cytokeratin pattern of hepatocytes, bile ducts and acinar gradient. Virchows Arch A Pathol Anat Histopathol 1987;412:63-72.
21. Butler SL, Dong H, Cardona D, et al. The antigen for Hep Par 1 antibody is the urea cycle enzyme carbamoyl phosphate synthetase 1. Lab Invest 2008;88:78-88.
22. Yan BC, Gong C, Song J, et al. Arginase-1: a new immunohistochemical marker of hepatocytes and hepatocellular neoplasms. Am J Surg Pathol 2010;34:1147-1154.
23. Terada T, Nakanuma Y, Ohta G. Glandular elements around the intrahepatic bile ducts in man; their morphology and distribution in normal livers. Liver 1987;7:1-8.
24. Igarashi S, Sato Y, Ren XS, Harada K, Sasaki M, Nakanuma Y. Participation of peribiliary glands in biliary tract pathophysiologies. World J Hepatol 2013;5:425-432.
25. Tsuneyama K, Kono N, Yamashiro M, et al. Aberrant expression of stem cell factor on biliary epithelial cells and peribiliary infiltration of c-kit-expressing mast cells in hepatolithiasis and primary sclerosing cholangitis: a possible contribution to bile duct fibrosis. J Pathol 1999;189:609-614.
26. Nakanuma Y, Zen Y, Portman B. Diseases of the bile ducts. In: MacSween RN, Burt AD, Portman B, Ferrell LE, eds. MacSween's pathology of the liver. Edinburg: Churchill Livingstone/Elsevier; 2012:491-562.

27. Terada T, Nakanuma Y, Ohta G. Glandular elements around the intrahepatic bile ducts in man; their morphology and distribution in normal livers. Liver1987;7:1-8.
28. Lim JH, Zen Y, Jang KT, Kim YK, Nakanuma Y. Cyst-forming intraductal papillary neoplasm of the bile ducts: description of imaging and pathologic aspects. AJR Am J Roentgenol 2011;197:1111-1120.
29. Roskams TA, Theise ND, Balabaud C, et al. Nomenclature of the finer branches of the biliary tree: canals, ductules, and ductular reactions in human livers. Hepatology 2004;39:1739-1745.
30. Ruck P, Xiao JC, Kaiserling E. Immunoreactivity of sinusoids in hepatocellular carcinoma. An immunohistochemical study using lectin UEA-1 and antibodies against endothelial markers, including CD34. Arch Pathol Lab Med 1995;119:173-178.
31. Park YN, Yang CP, Fernandez GJ, Cubukcu O, Thung SN, Theise ND. Neoangiogenesis and sinusoidal "capillarization" in dysplastic nodules of the liver. Am J Surg Pathol 1998;22:656-662.
32. Bedossa P, Hytiroglou P, Yeh M. Vascular Disorders. In: Burt A, Ferrell LD, Hubscher S, eds. MacSween's pathology of the liver, 7th ed: Philadelphia: Elsvier; 2018:636-672.
33. Pietrangelo A. The ferroportin disease. Blood Cells Mol Dis 2004;32:131-138.
34. Friedman SL. Hepatic stellate cells: protean, multifunctional, and enigmatic cells of the liver. Physiol Rev 2008;88:125-172.
35. Wake K. "Sternzellen" in the liver: perisinusoidal cells with special reference to storage of vitamin A. Am J Anat 1971;132:429-462.
36. Hernandez-Gea V, Friedman SL. Pathogenesis of liver fibrosis. Annu Rev Pathol 2011;6:425-456.
37. Wisse E, Luo D, Vermijlen D, Kanellopoulou C, De Zanger R, Braet F. On the function of pit cells, the liver-specific natural killer cells. Semin Liver Di. 1997;17:265-286.
38. Nakatani K, Kaneda K, Seki S, Nakajima Y. Pit cells as liver-associated natural killer cells: morphology and function. Med Electron Microsc 2004;37:29-36.

2 BENIGN HEPATOCELLULAR TUMORS AND TUMOR-LIKE LESIONS

This chapter discusses benign lesions and tumors that are the result of the proliferation of hepatocytes. These lesions mainly include nodular regenerative hyperplasia, focal nodular hyperplasia, and hepatocellular adenoma. Most of the time they occur in a noncirrhotic liver. Nodular regenerative hyperplasia is a diffuse and generalized process involving the entire liver, whereas focal nodular hyperplasia and hepatocellular adenoma are frequently solitary and distinct, but can also be multiple.

NODULAR REGENERATIVE HYPERPLASIA

Definition. *Nodular regenerative hyperplasia* is a benign entity characterized by diffuse, small regenerative and hyperplastic nodules that alternate with parenchymal atrophy, evenly throughout the entire liver, but without cirrhosis, bridging fibrosis, or significant fibrosis (1,2). It is thought to be a generalized hyperplasia of the liver parenchyma in response to vascular injuries due to a variety of etiologies, which may cause noncirrhotic portal hypertension.

Clinical Features. The clinical presentation of nodular regenerative hyperplasia varies. Many patients have no symptoms or abnormal liver tests. Other patients have elevated alkaline phosphatase and γ-glutamyl-transferase, whereas transaminases are usually normal (3,4). The clinical manifestations of nodular regenerative hyperplasia, if present, include the features of noncirrhotic portal hypertension, such as splenomegaly, thrombocytopenia, and esophageal varices (3,5).

The incidence of nodular regenerative hyperplasia ranges from 0.72 to 2.6 percent in autopsy series (2,4,7,8). It is rare in the Western world, but is gaining increasing recognition. Nodular regenerative hyperplasia occurs in all ages, but is more common in older individuals. This may be attributed to more underlying diseases occurring in the elderly. There is no gender predilection.

Etiology. The underlying pathogenesis of nodular regenerative hyperplasia is generally thought to be vascular injuries in the liver due to various causes and involving small portal veins and hepatic arteries. The consequence of obliteration of these vessels results in atrophy of the hepatic acini fed by these vessels; the unaffected acini respond with compensatory nodular hyperplasia (6,7). An array of disorders is etiologically associated with nodular regenerative hyperplasia (Table 2-1). These include various systemic and autoimmune disorders underlying vascular diseases, hematologic diseases such as myeloproliferative and lymphoproliferative disorders, thrombophilic status, and infectious diseases. Medications, such as steroids, oral contraceptives, immunosuppressive agents, and toxic and chemotherapeutic agents (notably oxaliplatin, a chemotherapeutic agent in the treatment of colorectal liver metastases) (3,6,7, 9–15) are also associated with the disease (16). Rare occurrence within family members has also been described (17).

Although the exact underlying mechanisms are not clearly delineated, recent data have demonstrated downregulation of the endothelial signaling pathways Dll4/Notch1 and ephrinB2/EphB4 in nodular regenerative hyperplasia, suggesting an etiologic role for sinusoidal injury in this lesion (18).

Gross Findings. Nodular regenerative hyperplasia is grossly characterized by numerous small nodules that are diffusely and evenly distributed throughout the entire liver. These nodules range from 1 to 3 mm in diameter and may resemble cirrhosis on the liver surface due to the nodularity (2). Occasionally, the nodules coalesce to become a larger tumor nodule. The nodules typically appear paler than the surrounding liver parenchyma (figs. 2-1, 2-2).

Microscopic Findings. The diagnosis of nodular regenerative hyperplasia relies on the

Table 2-1

DISEASES ASSOCIATED WITH NODULAR REGENERATIVE HYPERPLASIA

Hematologic disorders	Myeloproliferative diseases Lymphoproliferative diseases
Systemic disorders	Systemic lupus erythematosus Systemic sclerosis CREST syndrome Antiphospholipid syndrome Rheumatoid arthritis Felty syndrome Polyarteritis nodosa
Liver disorders	Primary sclerosing cholangitis Primary biliary cholangitis Vascular disorders Hepatoportal sclerosis Budd-Chiari syndrome Hereditary hemorrhagic telangiectasia Liver allograft after liver transplantation
Liver harboring metastatic neoplasms	
Kidney disorders	End-stage kidney diseases Glomerulonephritides Renal allograft after renal transplantation
Prothrombotic states	
Medications	Corticosteroids Contraceptives Immunosuppressive agent (azathioprine) Androgens Chemotherapeutic agents (oxaliplatin) AIDS therapy (didanosine)
Other disorders	Common variable immunodeficiency Chronic granulomatous disease Cystinosis

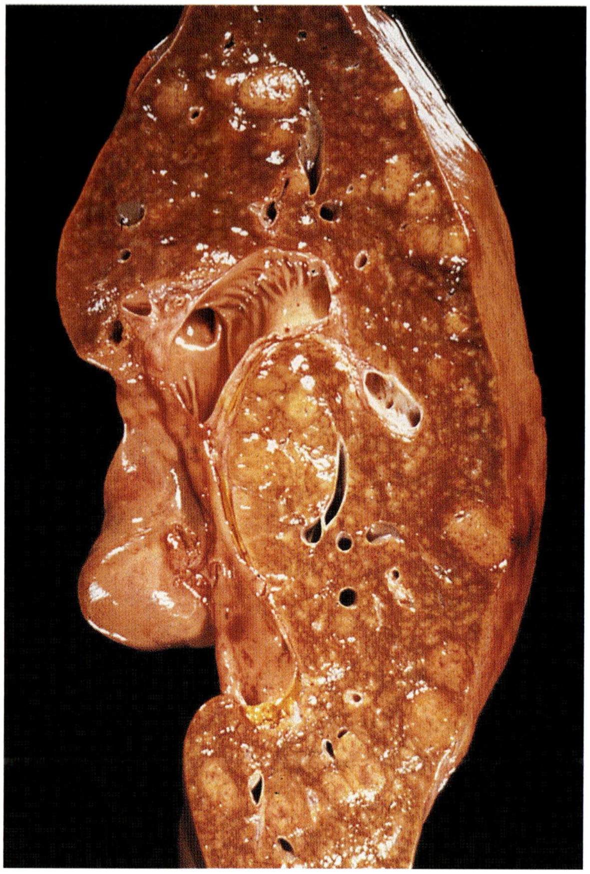

Figure 2-1

NODULAR REGENERATIVE HYPERPLASIA

Pale nodules of varied size are dispersed throughout the liver.

histologic findings of hyperplastic and regenerative nodules containing portal tracts at the center and centrizonal areas at the periphery (19). A characteristic finding is the intervening compression atrophy (manifested by thinning of hepatocytic plates) alternating with hypertrophy (manifested by thickened hepatocytic plates) within the nodules (fig. 2-3). These architectural changes and nodularity may be challenging to recognize in needle biopsy specimens, where diagnostic features are not readily apparent on hematoxylin and eosin (H&E)-stained slides. It is helpful to note two distinct populations of hepatocytes of different sizes: one that is small and thin because of the compression atrophy, which may also be accompanied by dilatation of the sinusoidal spaces; another that is thick and large due to the compensatory hypertrophy of hepatocytic cords. A reticulin stain is particularly useful in highlighting the thick and hypertrophic nodules, with compression atrophy of reticulin fibers of the adjacent hepatocytic plates at the periphery of the nodules (fig. 2-4, left). A Masson trichrome stain, however, does not show significant fibrosis (fig. 2-4, right).

Other histologic findings include thrombi, either old or fresh, in the portal veins or hepatic arteries with underlying portal venopathy or arteriopathy. Thrombophlebitis or sclerosis with concentric or eccentric occlusion of the portal

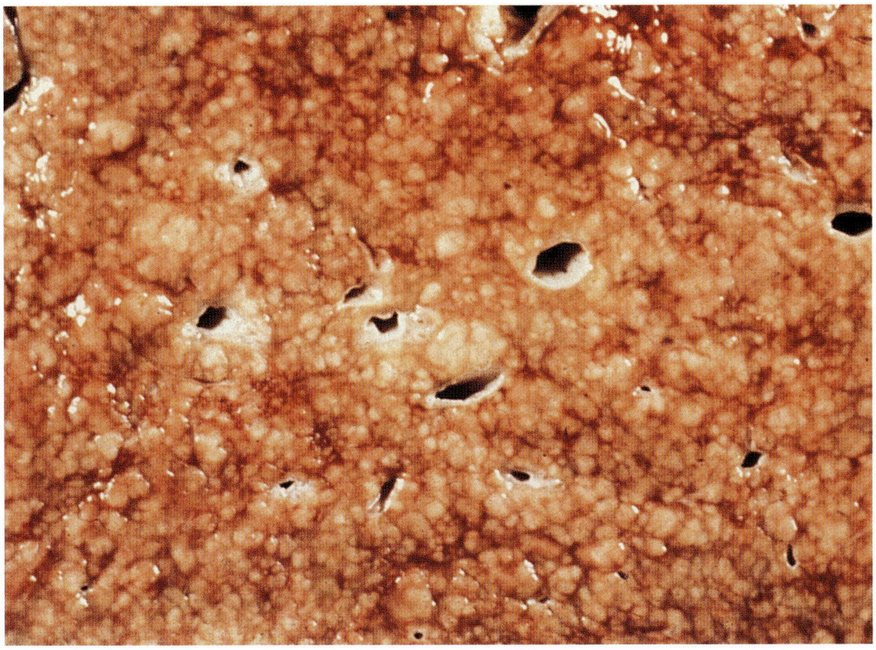

Figure 2-2

NODULAR REGENERATIVE HYPERPLASIA

Multiple, small, light tan nodules with no associated fibrosis are present.

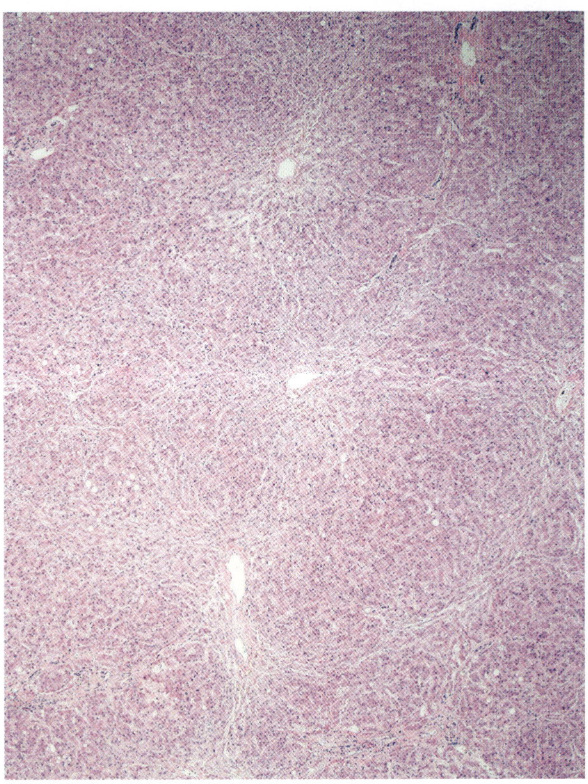

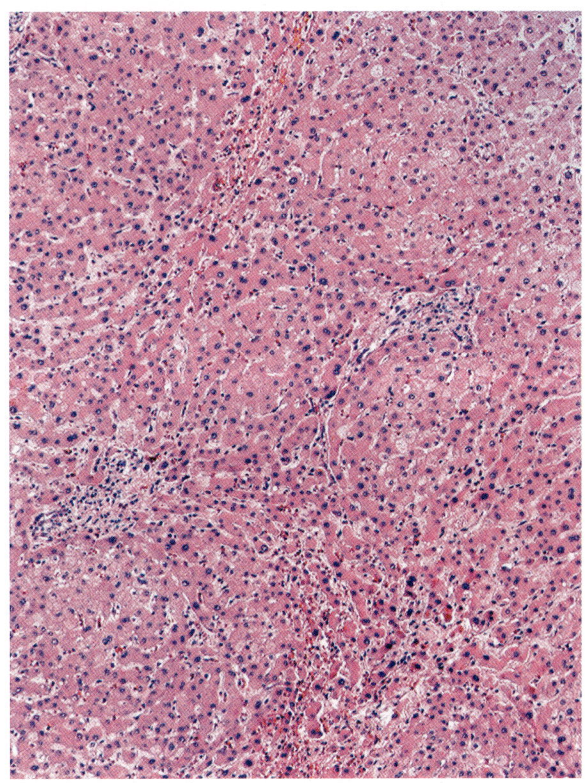

Figure 2-3

NODULAR REGENERATIVE HYPERPLASIA

Left: Low-power magnification shows generalized nodular-appearing hepatic parenchyma.

Right: Higher magnification shows hyperplastic and regenerative nodules with intervening compression atrophy alternating with hypertrophy within the nodules.

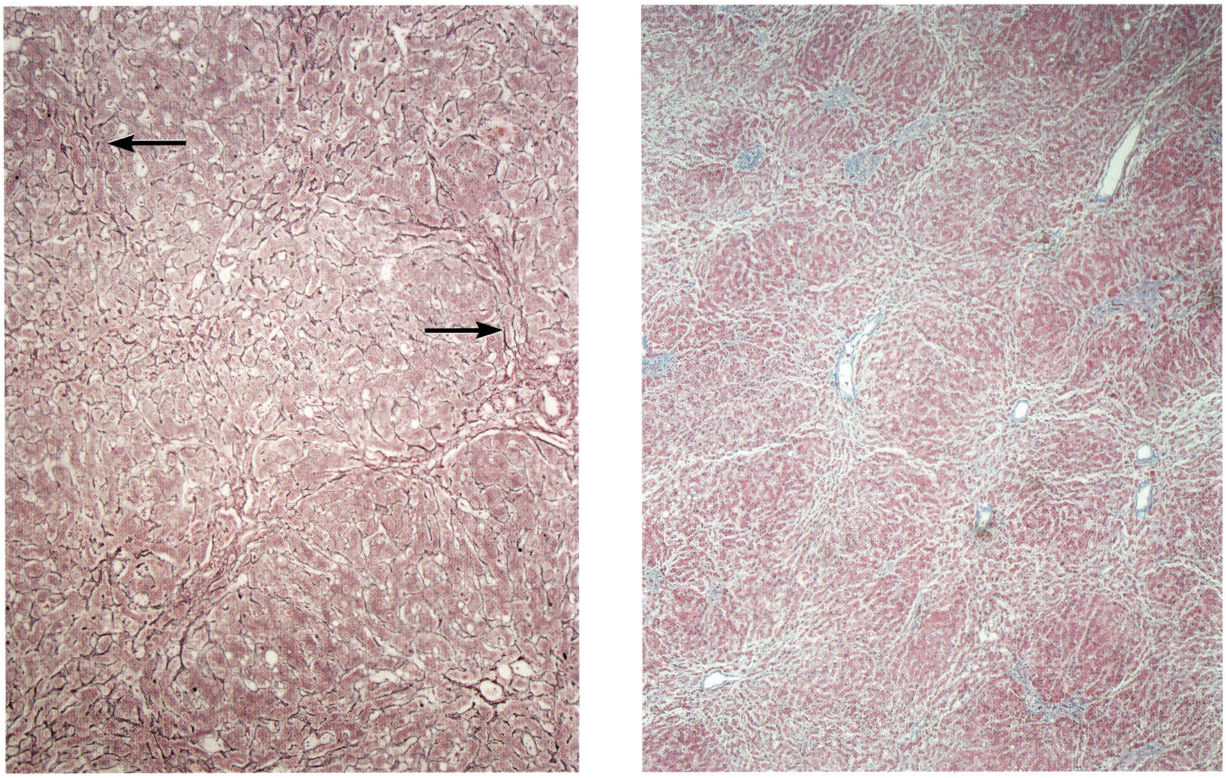

Figure 2-4

NODULAR REGENERATIVE HYPERPLASIA

Left: A reticulin stain highlights the thick and hypertrophic nodules, with compression atrophy of the adjacent hepatocytic plates at the periphery of the nodules (arrows).

Right: A Masson trichrome stain does not show bridging fibrosis or cirrhosis.

vein branches may also be present. If these vascular changes are not present, the portal tracts may appear entirely normal.

Immunohistochemical Findings. There have not been useful immunohistochemical stains for the diagnosis of nodular regenerative hyperplasia. Sato et al. (20) have described the lack of perivenular staining in hepatocytes in nodular regenerative hyperplasia using glutamine synthetase.

Cytologic Findings. Nodular regenerative hyperplasia is a very diffuse lesion; accordingly, fine needle aspirations are usually not performed.

Differential Diagnosis. *Cirrhosis.* Nodular regenerative hyperplasia needs to be distinguished from cirrhosis. Both are manifested as diffuse regenerative nodules throughout the liver; however, the Masson trichrome stain shows no or only minimal fibrosis in nodular regenerative hyperplasia, whereas prominent fibrous septa surrounding the regenerative nodules is the hallmark of cirrhosis. The intervening compression atrophy, with alternating hyperplasia of the hepatocellular plates, is characteristic of nodular regenerative hyperplasia. The clinical history of chronic liver disease in cirrhosis and various underlying medical conditions in nodular regenerative hyperplasia may help to distinguish these two entities.

Hepatocellular Adenoma. The small nodules of nodular regenerative hyperplasia may merge into a large tumor nodule that resembles hepatocellular adenoma, as both show benign hepatocytes. Nodules of sinusoidal dilatation and hepatocellular atrophy in nodular regenerative hyperplasia may also mimic hepatocellular adenoma, especially the inflammatory subtype, which is characterized by telangiectatic changes (21). Imaging findings of diffuse and generalized nodules favor nodular regenerative hyperplasia.

On computerized tomography (CT), regenerative nodules of nodular regenerative hyperplasia remain isodense or hypodense in both arterial and portal venous phases, distinguishing them from hepatocellular adenoma (2,22). The clinical histories of female gender, high body mass index, alcohol use, and diabetes in hepatocellular adenoma, and various medical and systemic conditions or medication history in nodular regenerative hyperplasia may also facilitate the distinction.

Focal Nodular Hyperplasia. Both focal nodular hyperplasia and nodular regenerative hyperplasia are composed of nodules of benign hepatocytes. The small, generalized and evenly distributed nature of nodular regenerative hyperplasia is distinguished from the typically distinct and isolated nodular mass in focal nodular hyperplasia. In addition, dense fibrous septa (central scar), containing thick-walled arteries, inflammatory infiltrates, and ductular reaction in focal nodular hyperplasia are distinguishing features. Immunohistochemical staining using glutamine synthetase in nodular regenerative hyperplasia does not show the typical map-like pattern seen in focal nodular hyperplasia.

Treatment and Prognosis. Treating identifiable underlying diseases and the resulting portal hypertension and its complications is considered the management of choice for nodular regenerative hyperplasia (4). Severe complications due to portal hypertension may occur, but the prognosis is generally associated with the underlying condition. Overall, the prognosis is much worse in patients with malignancies than in those with prothrombotic conditions (3). Rare association with the development of hepatocellular carcinoma has been reported (23).

FOCAL NODULAR HYPERPLASIA

Definition. *Focal nodular hyperplasia* is a frequently encountered benign hepatocellular lesion. It is the second most common benign hepatic lesion (only after hemangioma) and the most frequent benign hepatocellular lesion, with an incidence ranging from 0.6 to 3.0 percent (24,25). It is not a neoplasm, but thought to be a regenerative and hyperplastic process in response to vascular anomalies (26). The lesion is defined by typical pathologic findings: histologically characterized by a well-circumscribed nodule composed of a central scar that contains inflammatory cells, thick-walled arteries and proliferating ductules, and benign hepatocytes within the nodular parenchyma. The H&E findings are diagnostic. Immunohistochemistry using glutamine synthetase is not necessary in all cases, but may be helpful for a confirmatory diagnosis (27), especially when the histologic findings are equivocal.

Clinical Features. Most patients with focal nodular hyperplasia have no symptoms and the lesion is often found incidentally by imaging or during surgery or autopsy (28). In most cases, focal nodular hyperplasia presents as a single lesion, but multiple lesions in a single patient are also common. Large areas of focal nodular hyperplasia may cause compression of adjacent organs or abdominal pain. Lesions do not bleed, nor do they undergo malignant transformation. Patients often present with other lesions, which are often vascular in nature, such as hepatic hemangioma; meningioma, astrocytoma, berry aneurysm, and brain telangiectasia; dysplastic systemic arteries; and portal vein atresia (29). Notably, many of these cases with associated lesions occur in patients with multifocal nodular hyperplasia. Wanless et al. (29) have reported a patient with several of these lesions, including multiple focal nodular hyperplasia, meningioma, astrocytoma, vascular malformation of the brain stem, and hemangioma of the liver. Patients with focal nodular hyperplasia typically do not have any underlying liver diseases.

Focal nodular hyperplasia is typically found in women in the third or fourth decade of life. While it may be observed at any age and in both genders, elderly individuals with focal nodular hyperplasia are rarely reported (25).

Etiology. The exact etiology of focal nodular hyperplasia is still unclear (26). It has been hypothesized that the lesion is a compensatory response of the hepatic parenchyma to vascular injury, especially of the portal vein, which leads to subsequent shunting between the arteries and portal veins (30–32). The background liver is typically normal.

Focal nodular hyperplasia has been shown to be polyclonal (33). Molecular studies have revealed an increase in the gene expression ratio of angiopoietin-1/angiopoietin-2 in focal nodular hyperplasia (30,34), suggesting an underlying vascular mechanism. Additionally,

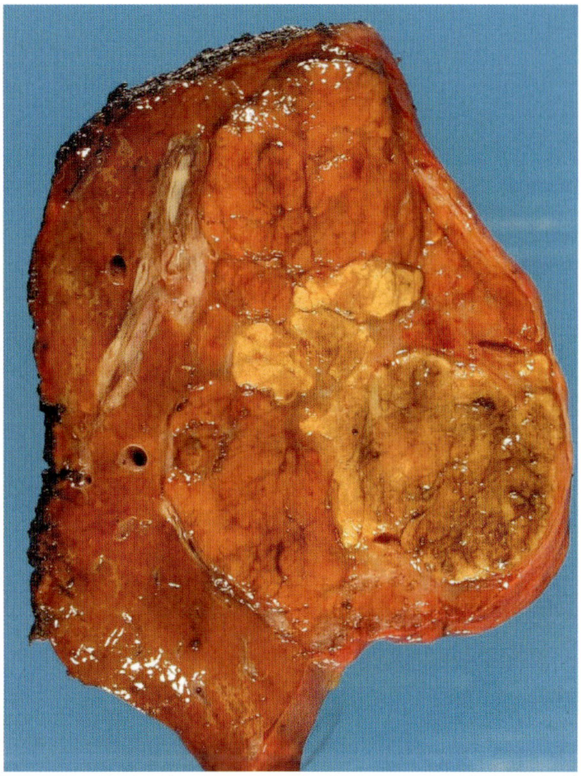

Figure 2-5

FOCAL NODULAR HYPERPLASIA

An oval, well-defined, lobulated, and unencapsulated lesion, with partial necrosis.

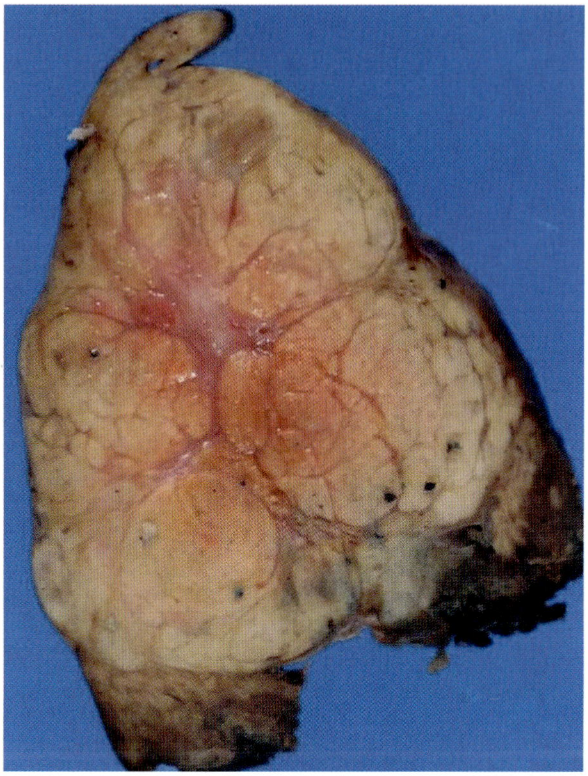

Figure 2-6

FOCAL NODULAR HYPERPLASIA

A round, well-circumscribed, and lobulated mass with a central whitish scar.

the β-catenin pathway is activated but without *β-catenin* mutation (35). The activation of this pathway is suggested to be attributed to the result of increased blood flow. This phenomenon provides the foundation of the "map-like" immunohistochemical staining pattern of glutamine synthesis in focal nodular hyperplasia (see Immunohistochemical Findings) (24).

Gross Findings. Focal nodular hyperplasia may be single (two thirds of the cases) or multiple. On cut surface, it appears firm and pale. The lesions are round, well defined, lobulated, and unencapsulated (fig. 2-5), and may range from several millimeters to greater than 10 cm in dimension. A central scar with radiating septa within the lesion is a classic finding (fig. 2-6); a central scar may be absent in some cases (fig. 2-7).

Microscopic Findings. The classic histologic features of focal nodular hyperplasia are clear and well-demarcated benign hepatocellular nodules with a central scar composed of thick and radiating fibrous septa (fig. 2-8), containing ductular reaction, abnormal thick-walled arteries, and lymphocytic or mixed inflammatory cells (fig. 2-9). These diagnostic features may not always be present, especially in a biopsy specimen. Ductular reactions are common at the periphery of the fibrous stroma, bordering the hepatic parenchyma (fig. 2-10). Although the fibrous septa may resemble portal tracts, there is a paucity of portal veins and bile ducts, corresponding to the dystrophic arteries. The dystrophic arteries in the fibrous septa are large and fibrotic, with eccentric thickening of the intima (fig. 2-9). Disrupted and reduplicated internal elastic lamina may be seen. Other vascular abnormalities, such as numerous small arterioles and veins in the fibrous septa, are often present. Focal nodular hyperplasia contains hepatocellular plates that are two to three cells in thickness and separated by sinusoidal spaces lined by inconspicuous endothelial cells (36).

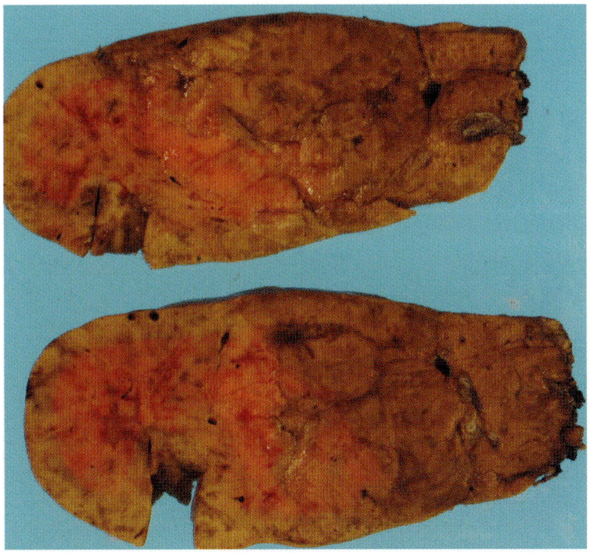

Figure 2-7

FOCAL NODULAR HYPERPLASIA

An oval, lobulated, and unencapsulated lesion without an obvious central scar.

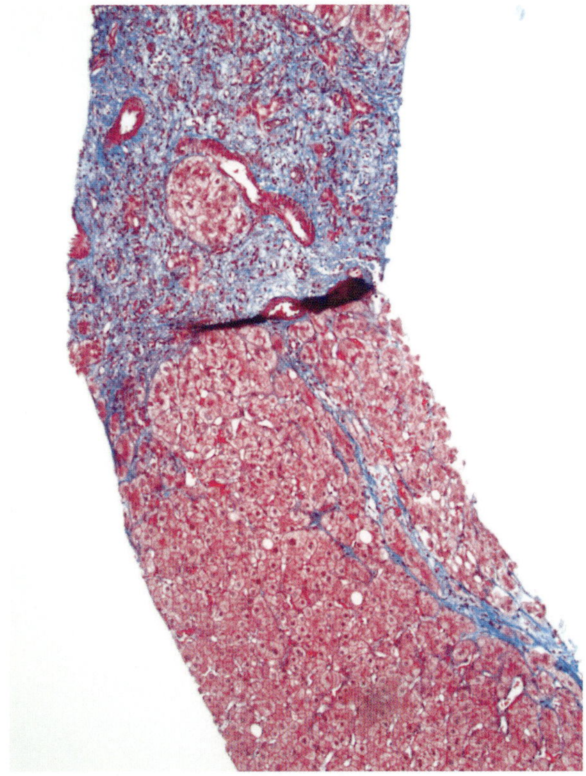

Figure 2-8

FOCAL NODULAR HYPERPLASIA

A liver biopsy shows nodular hepatocellular parenchyma with thick radiating fibrous septa highlighted by a Masson trichrome stain.

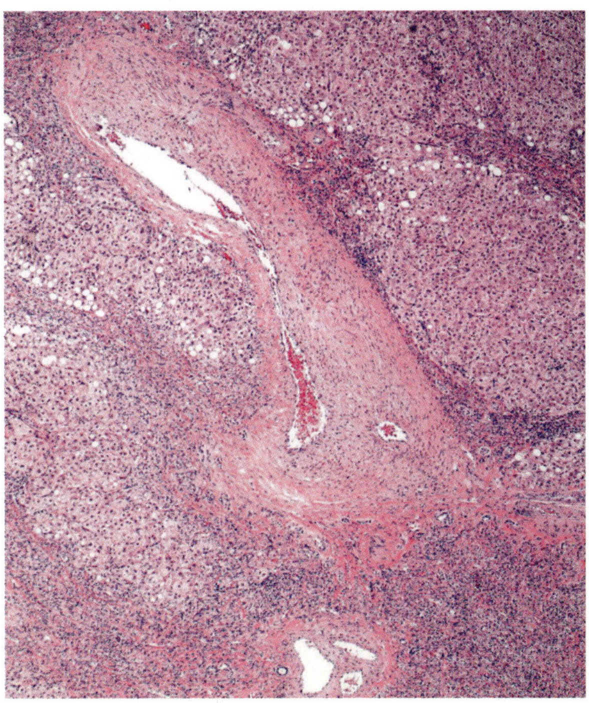

Figure 2-9

FOCAL NODULAR HYPERPLASIA

Nodular benign hepatocellular parenchyma with thick central radiating fibrous septa containing ductular reaction, thick-walled arteries with eccentric thickening in the intima, and inflammatory cells.

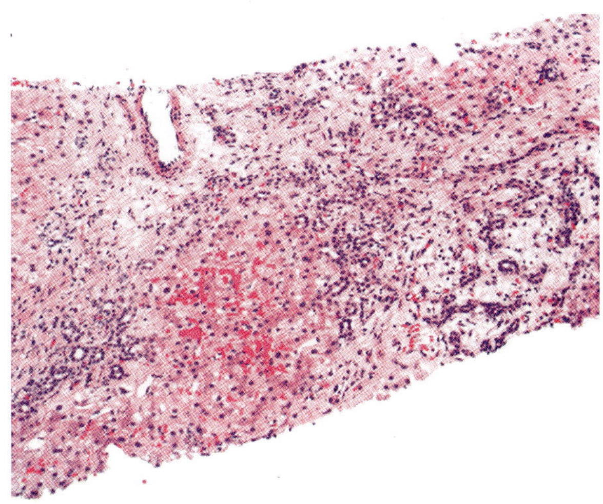

Figure 2-10

FOCAL NODULAR HYPERPLASIA

Ductular reaction is seen at the periphery of the fibrous septa bordering hepatic parenchyma.

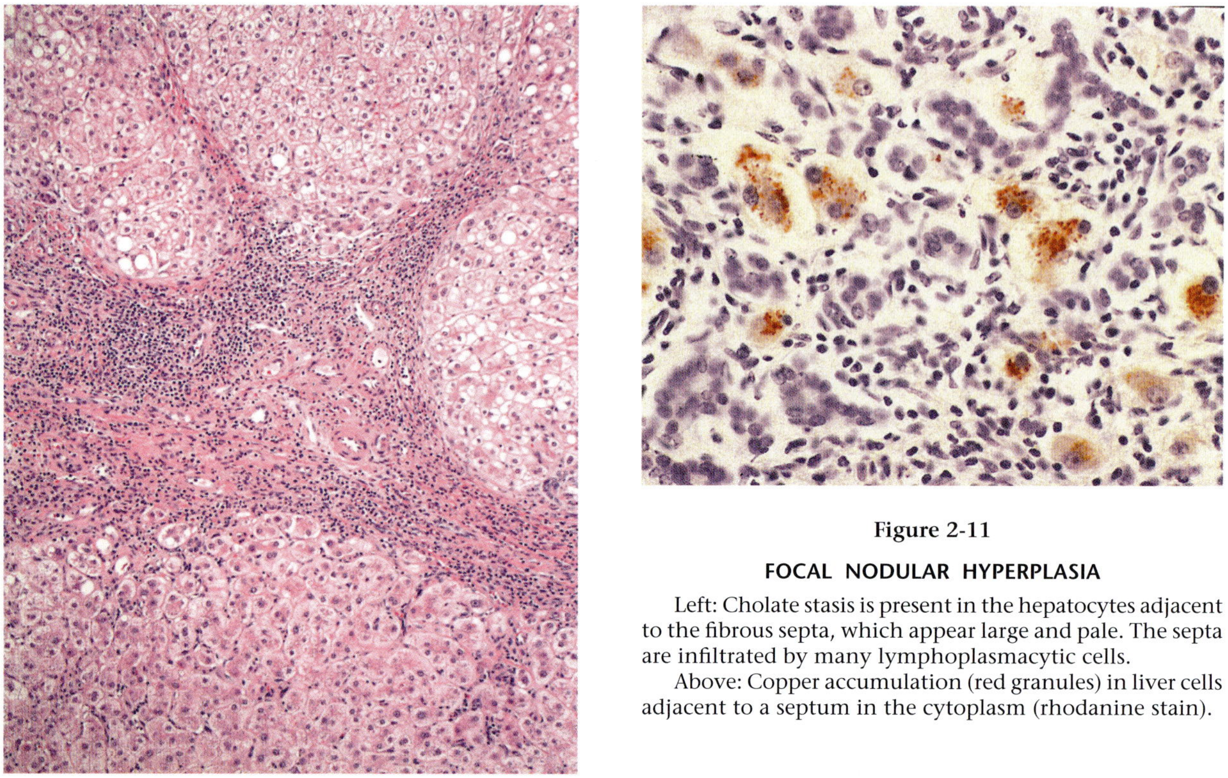

Figure 2-11

FOCAL NODULAR HYPERPLASIA

Left: Cholate stasis is present in the hepatocytes adjacent to the fibrous septa, which appear large and pale. The septa are infiltrated by many lymphoplasmacytic cells.

Above: Copper accumulation (red granules) in liver cells adjacent to a septum in the cytoplasm (rhodanine stain).

Cholate stasis is a common finding in the hepatocytes adjacent to the fibrous septa (fig. 2-11) (36). These hepatocytes appear large and pale and can be demonstrated by a rhodanine copper stain showing copper granules or a Victoria blue stain showing copper binding protein in the cytoplasm (36). A variable degree of steatosis (fig. 2-12), or even features of steatohepatitis, may also be present within focal nodular hyperplasia and need to be distinguished from fatty hepatocellular adenoma/carcinoma or the steatohepatitic variant of hepatocellular carcinoma (36,37).

Immunohistochemical Findings. A definitive diagnosis of focal nodular hyperplasia is facilitated by immunohistochemical staining for glutamine synthetase, which is a downstream target gene of the Wnt/β-catenin pathway. Glutamine synthetase is only expressed in the perivenular hepatocytes in normal liver (30,35). In focal nodular hyperplasia, the Wnt/β-catenin pathway is activated but not mutated (35), leading to expansion of the hepatocytes expressing glutamine synthesis and forming the characteristic anastomosing "map-like" staining pattern (fig. 2-13) (27).

Cytologic Findings. Fine-needle aspiration cytology of focal nodular hyperplasia shows abundant, bland-appearing hepatocytes forming loosely cohesive sheets and clusters and benign epithelial cells in ductal formations or tightly packed groups, sometimes accompanied by fibrous tissue (38).

Differential Diagnosis. *Hepatocellular Adenoma.* Both focal nodular hyperplasia and hepatocellular adenoma consist of well-demarcated nodules composed of benign hepatocytes, however, the characteristic fibrous central scars and broad bands typically seen in focal nodular hyperplasia are not common in hepatocellular adenoma. Unpaired arteries in the lesional parenchyma are increased in hepatocellular adenoma, whereas thick-walled arteries are typically seen within the dense collagen fibrous septa in focal nodular hyperplasia, but not in the lesional hepatic parenchyma. In addition, portal tracts are not present within hepatocellular adenoma. Although a ductular reaction at the periphery of fibrous septa is a characteristic feature of focal nodular hyperplasia, a cytokeratin (CK)7-positive ductular reaction may also be present surrounding the unpaired

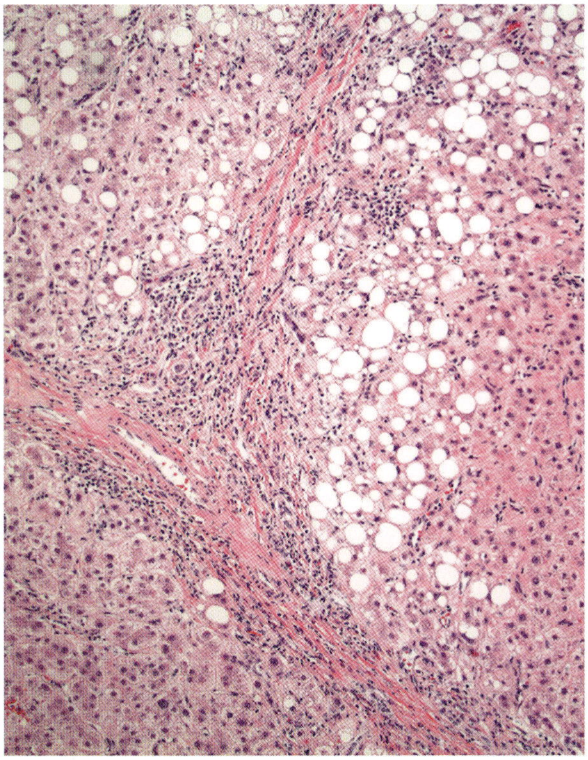

Figure 2-12

FOCAL NODULAR HYPERPLASIA

Steatosis can be seen within focal nodular hyperplasia.

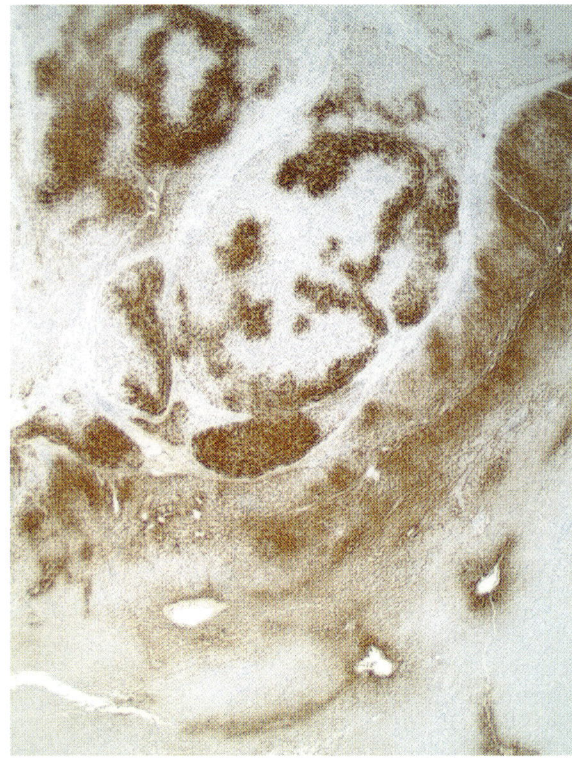

Figure 2-13

FOCAL NODULAR HYPERPLASIA

The characteristic anastomosing "map-like" staining pattern with glutamine synthetase is seen (top left) whereas normal liver shows perivenular staining pattern (lower right).

arteries in the parenchyma of the inflammatory subtype of hepatocellular adenoma, where they may be mistaken as a ductular reaction in portal tracts, sometimes referred to as pseudo-portal tracts (fig. 2-14). This pitfall may be overcome by performing an immunohistochemical stain for glutamine synthetase, which shows the characteristic map-like staining pattern in focal nodular hyperplasia, and the usually negative or only perivenular staining in hepatocellular adenoma (unless in the *β-catenin* mutated subtype, which shows diffuse staining) (25,39).

Cirrhosis. The fibrous septa with hepatocellular nodular lesions in focal nodular hyperplasia can be confused with cirrhotic nodules, typically in a needle biopsy specimen. The clinical history of chronic liver disease and portal hypertension, as well as imaging studies showing the generalized nodular appearance, favor cirrhosis over focal nodular hyperplasia.

Hepatocellular Carcinoma. Focal nodular hyperplasia and well-differentiated hepatocellular carcinoma are both composed of low-grade appearing hepatocytes. Additionally, ductular reaction and inflammation, features of focal nodular hyperplasia, are also common in hepatocellular carcinoma. The distinction becomes even more challenging if the patient is cirrhotic, where fibrous septa are also present. Nevertheless, the lack of portal tracts in hepatocellular carcinoma helps distinguish hepatocellular carcinoma from focal nodular hyperplasia. Nuclear atypia and pleomorphism, increased nucleus to cytoplasmic ratio, mitotic figures, thickened trabecula, and pseudoacini support a diagnosis of hepatocellular carcinoma.

The steatohepatitis-like changes common in fatty focal nodular hyperplasia may mimic the steatohepatitic variant of hepatocellular carcinoma, which tends to appear better differentiated (40). Both lesions have steatosis and ballooned cells, and may show pericellular fibrosis; the steatohepatitic variant of hepatocellular carcinoma is established if the clinical

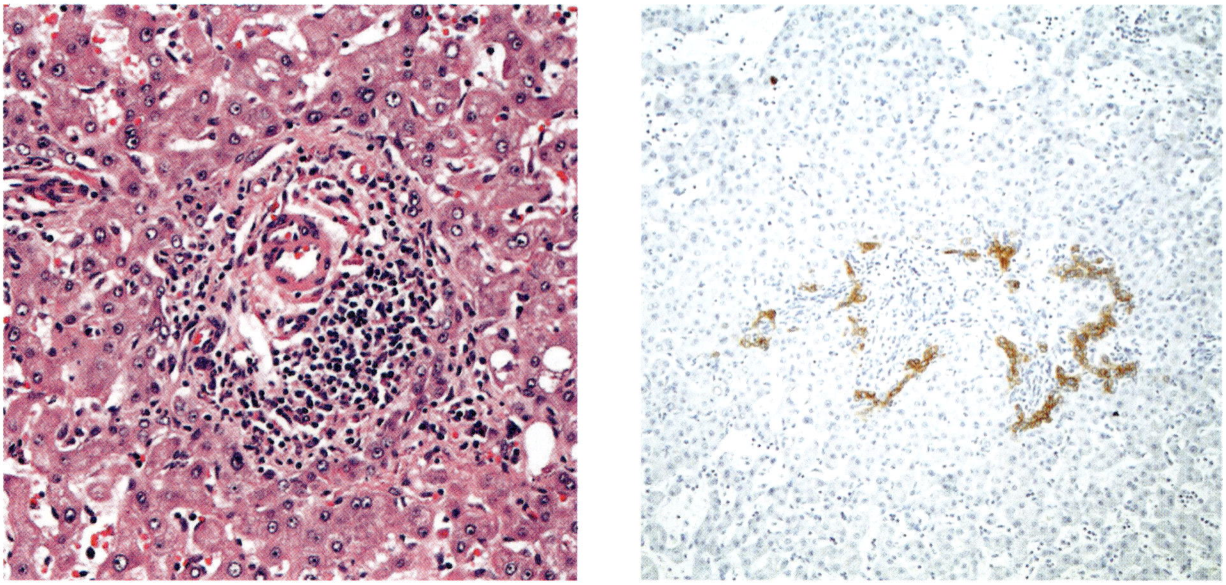

Figure 2-14

HEPATOCELLULAR ADENOMA, INFLAMMATORY SUBTYPE

Left: Ductular reaction, along with inflammatory infiltrates, surround the unpaired arteries. Referred to as pseudo-portal tracts, they can be highlighted by CK7 immunohistochemical stain.

Right: Telangiectatic changes are present, which show dilatation of the sinusoidal spaces.

history of chronic liver disease or cirrhosis is known (37). Deniz et al. (37) found ductular reaction in fibrous septa present in all steatotic focal nodular hyperplasia cases, whereas steatotic-hepatocellular carcinomas usually lack ductular reaction and thick bands of fibrosis.

Treatment and Prognosis. As focal nodular hyperplasia does not expand or cause complications such as hemorrhage, rupture, or malignant transformation (41,42), therapy is not required unless there are symptoms due to the subcapsular location in the liver (43).

HEPATOCELLULAR ADENOMA

Definition. *Hepatocellular adenomas* are uncommon benign hepatocellular liver neoplasms. These neoplastic clonal proliferations are most commonly seen in women of child-bearing age, but are also increasingly noted in men, especially those with metabolic syndromes. The tumor is defined by its characteristic histologic findings and immunohistochemistry. Histologically, the tumor is composed of bland-appearing hepatocytes with no malignant features. Immunohistochemical or histochemical (such as reticulin) stains exclude other neoplasms or malignancies.

Clinical Features. The known risk factors for hepatocellular adenoma include female gender, oral contraceptive use, anabolic steroid use, maturity onset diabetes of the young type 3 (MODY 3), and glycogen storage disease (types I and III) (Table 2-2) (44). Recently recognized risk factors include obesity and excessive alcohol use (45). Hepatocellular adenomas are often detected incidentally upon imaging or when there is abdominal pain. Liver tests are usually normal. Liver tumor markers, including alpha-fetoprotein (AFP), are also normal. Bleeding, rupture (fig. 2-15), and malignant transformation are severe complications of hepatocellular adenoma.

Hepatocellular adenoma occurs in 2 to 4 individuals per 100,000 (26,46). Most patients are women. The classic scenario for the occurrence of hepatocellular adenoma is a woman taking oral contraceptives. There is a striking difference in the prevalence of hepatocellular adenoma between Western and Asian countries. Most series have been described in the West, whereas only rare cases have been observed in Asia. This discrepancy may in part be attributed to different methods of contraception used. Most women take oral contraceptives in the West; this is not

Table 2-2

RISK FACTORS OF HEPATOCELLULAR ADENOMA

Oral contraceptives use
Anabolic androgenic steroid use
Excessive endogenous androgens or estrogens
Excessive ethanol use
High body mass index
Diabetes
Dyslipidemia
Hypertension
Glycogen storage disease (types I and III)
Maturity-onset diabetes of the young type 3 (MODY-3)
McCune-Albright syndrome
Klinefelter syndrome
Familial adenomatosis coli

a common contraceptive practice in Asia (25). It has been estimated that the annual incidence in women who have never used oral contraceptives is nearly 1/1,000,000 (46). Hepatocellular adenomas are much rarer in men than in women, and they are often associated with alcohol use and high body mass index (45).

Etiology. Recent studies have revealed that hepatocellular adenomas arise due to a variety of etiologies. High levels of estrogen or androgen increase the risk of developing hepatocellular adenomas in both men and women. While oral contraceptive use is the most common cause of hepatocellular adenoma in women, anabolic steroid use also contributes to its development; hepatocellular adenomas may regress after stopping the use of anabolic steroids and oral contraceptives.

Excessive ethanol use has also been linked to hepatocellular adenoma, especially in men (45). Hepatocellular adenomas are also frequently observed in patients with glycogen storage diseases, especially type I, and rarely, type III (25), and malignant transformation may occur (47). Recently, metabolic syndromes, such as obesity, diabetes, dyslipidemia, and hypertension have been increasingly recognized as risk factors for the development of hepatocellular adenoma (48). While these risk factors are attributed to insulin resistance, the exact mechanisms are still undergoing investigation.

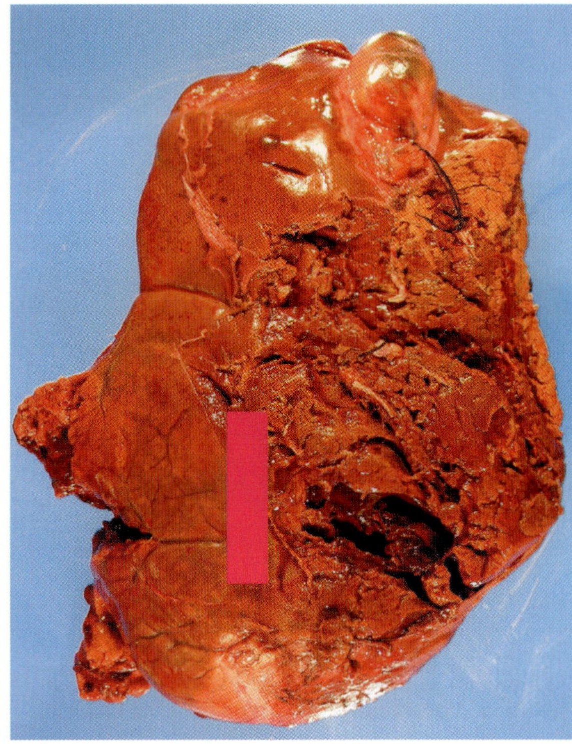

Figure 2-15

RUPTURED HEPATOCELLULAR ADENOMA

A ruptured hepatocellular adenoma was surgically resected.

Gross Findings. Hepatocellular adenomas are single or multiple and range in size from several millimeters to up to 30 cm in diameter (most are 5 to 15 cm). The term *adenomatosis* is applied when the number of tumors exceeds 10, and numerous ill-defined nodules are present throughout the liver. Glycogen storage disease-associated hepatocellular adenomas are often multiple. In many instances, hepatocellular adenoma is present immediately underneath the liver surface, which bulges out and commonly shows prominent blood vessels (fig. 2-16). Some hepatocellular adenomas may be pedunculated.

On cut section, the masses are generally soft and tan, brown, yellow, or green (fig. 2-17). They can be well (fig. 2-18) or ill defined. Hepatocellular adenoma can be a homogenous mass or a partially hemorrhagic and necrotic mass (fig. 2-19) with occasional fibrous bands, but without an apparent fibrous capsule. Fatty change, peliosis, and congestion are common. Infarction can

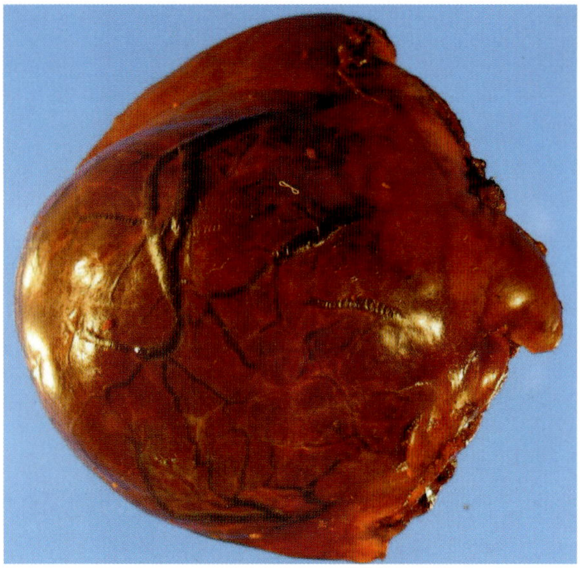

Figure 2-16

HEPATOCELLULAR ADENOMA

This tumor is underneath the liver surface and bulges out. There are prominent blood vessels on the external surface.

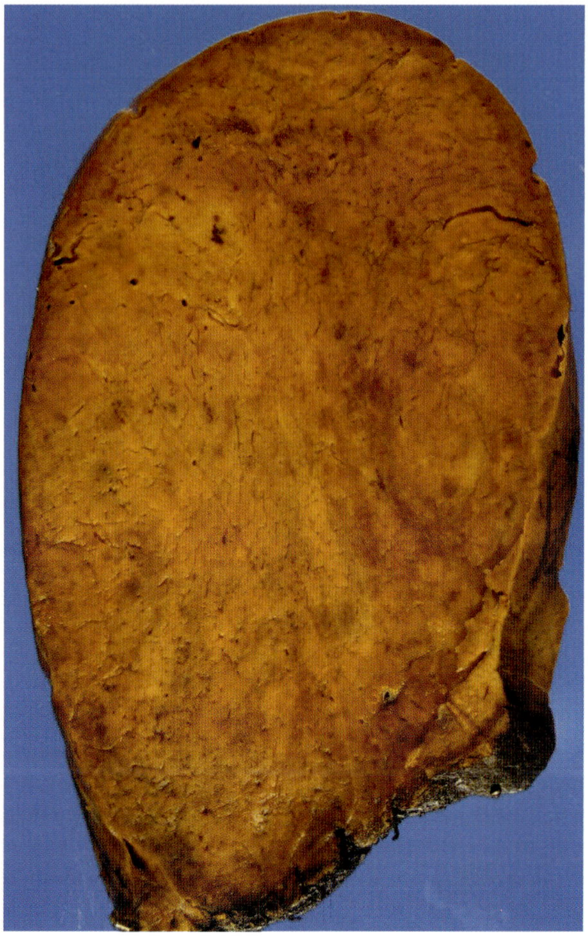

Figure 2-17

HEPATOCELLULAR ADENOMA

The cut surface shows a soft and yellow mass, without a fibrous capsule.

also be seen (fig. 2-20). The surrounding liver parenchyma typically does not show cirrhosis.

Microscopic Findings. The background liver typically is not cirrhotic in hepatocellular adenoma. There may be some degree of fibrosis due to underlying fatty liver disease or glycogen storage disease. Hepatocellular adenomas consist of benign hepatocytes arranged in plates, cords, and sheets, that are typically one or at most two layers in thickness (fig. 2-21). Portal tracts and interlobular bile ducts are absent (figs. 2-21,left; 2-22). There are increased unpaired arteries (fig. 2-22). Capillarization of the sinusoids, with CD34-positive sinusoidal endothelial cells, can also be seen, but its extent may not be as much as is seen in hepatocellular carcinoma. Bile may be present in the cytoplasm or canaliculi. Fat within the tumor is a common finding (fig. 2-23).

The tumor cells may appear larger, clearer, and paler (fig. 2-24) than nontumor hepatocytes in the surrounding parenchyma due to the accumulation of fat or glycogen. The nuclei are regular and uniform, with a normal nuclear/cytoplasmic ratio (fig. 2-25). Nuclear atypia, pleomorphism, and mitoses are rare; if present, the possibility of hepatocellular carcinoma needs to be excluded (Table 2-3).

Immunohistochemical and Molecular Genetic Findings. Recent advances in molecular classification of hepatocellular adenoma have led to the immunohistochemical distinction between hepatocellular adenoma and focal nodular hyperplasia, as well as the subclassification of hepatocellular adenoma (27). Currently, four subtypes of hepatocellular adenoma exist based on genotypic and immunohistochemical classification, endorsed by the World Health Organization (WHO) (26,44): 1) hepatocyte nuclear factor (HNF)-1α inactivated hepatocellular adenoma (H-HCA), 2) β-catenin activated (β-HCA), 3) inflammatory (I-HCA), and 4) unclassified (I-HCA or U-HCA), which can also be β-catenin activated (Tables 2-4, 2-5).

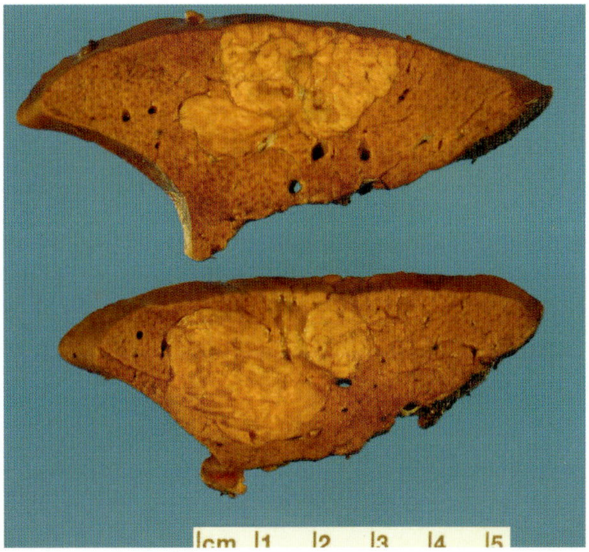

Figure 2-18

HEPATOCELLULAR ADENOMA

The cut surface shows a well-defined, soft, tan-yellow lobulated mass.

Hepatocyte Nuclear Factor (HNF)-1α Inactivated Hepatocellular Adenoma (H-HCA). Somatic inactivation of the *HNF-1α* gene defines this group, which accounts for approximately 30 percent of hepatocellular adenomas. This subtype carries the lowest risk for malignant transformation (49,50), although rare cases of malignant transformation have been reported (51). HNF-1α is a transcription factor that controls the metabolism of hepatocytes. Most H-HCAs (85 percent) are caused by somatic mutation of the *HNF-1α* gene in both alleles, while the remaining 15 percent carry a germline mutation in *HNF-1α* gene in one allele and a somatic mutation in the other allele (50,52), which is associated with maturity onset of diabetes of the young type 3 (MODY-3). H-HCAs are not seen in patients with glycogen storage disease. They also are not associated with *IL6ST*, *GNAS*, and *STAT3*, or *CTNNB1* mutations, which are seen in I-HCA or β-HCA, respectively (53).

H-HCA may be single or multiple. Moderate to severe macrovesicular steatosis (fig. 2-26), typically with diffuse distribution but sparing the arterialized zone within the tumor is a common finding (25). There are rare cases without steatosis. The tumor cells typically appear bland, without cytologic atypia or inflammatory infiltrates.

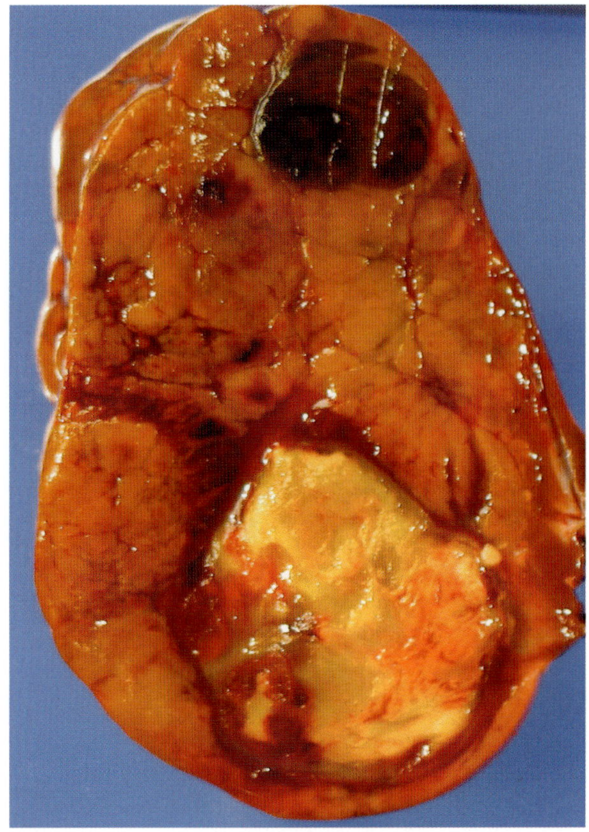

Figure 2-19

HEPATOCELLULAR ADENOMA

The tumor is partially hemorrhagic and necrotic.

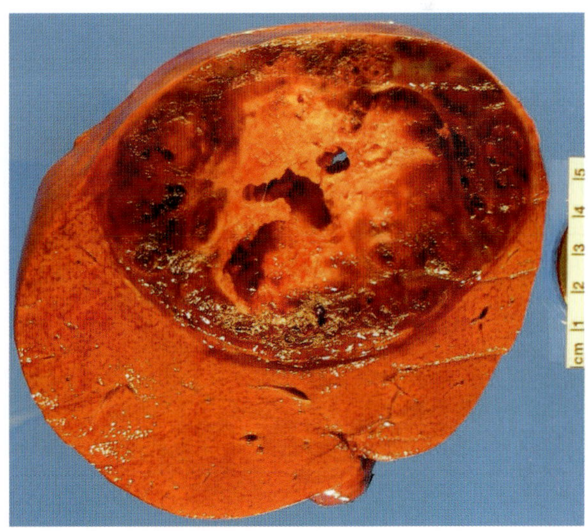

Figure 2-20

HEPATOCELLULAR ADENOMA

A well-defined mass has hemorrhage and infarction.

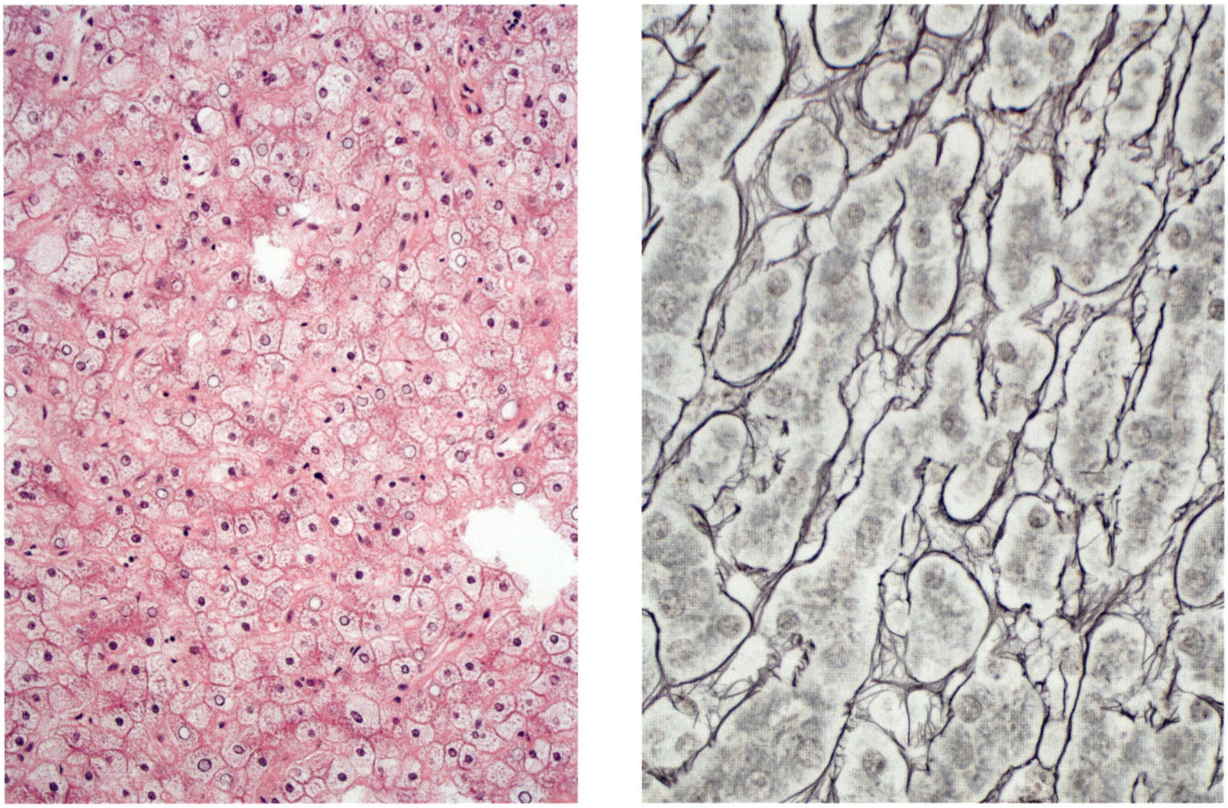

Figure 2-21

HEPATOCELLULAR ADENOMA

Left: Benign hepatocytes are arranged in plates, cords, and sheets, without portal tracts. Right: A reticulin stain shows the plates are one, or at most two, layers in thickness.

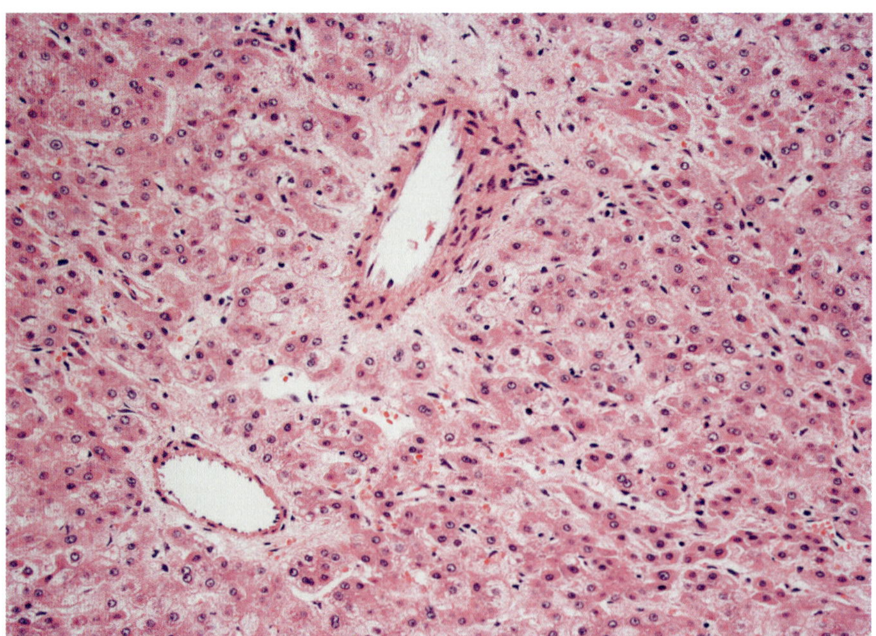

Figure 2-22

HEPATOCELLULAR ADENOMA

Unpaired arteries are increased, while portal tracts and interlobular bile ducts are absent. The adenoma cells are arranged in sheets or cords. There is no nuclear atypia or pleomorphism.

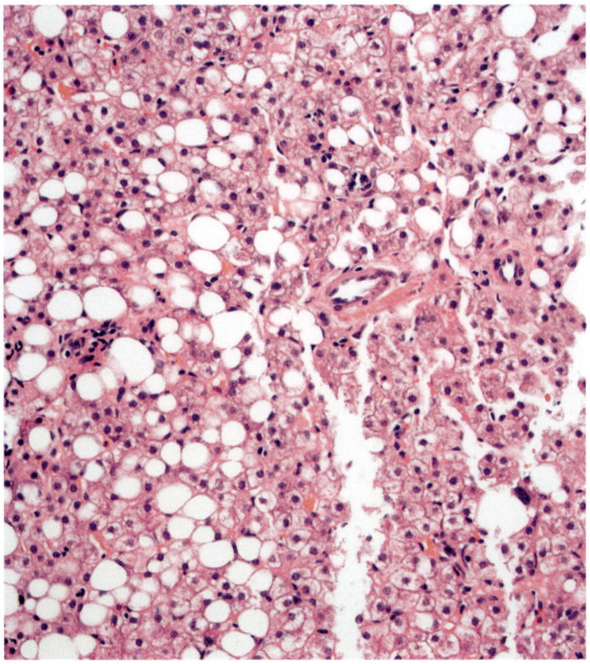

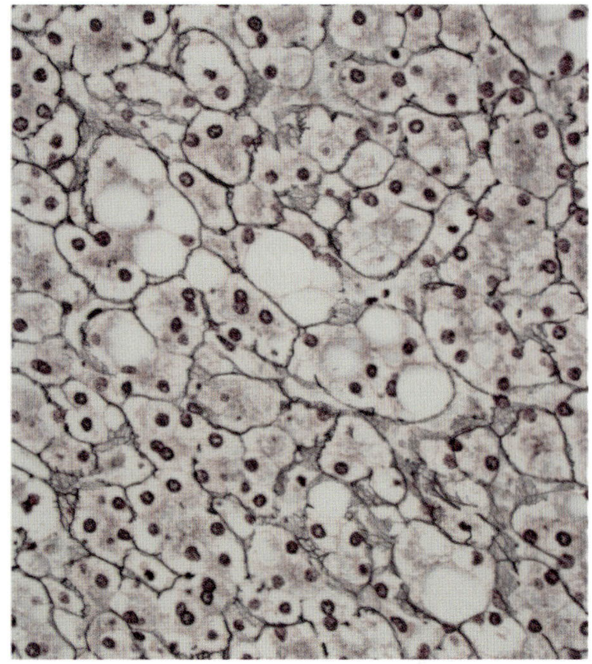

Figure 2-23

HEPATOCELLULAR ADENOMA

Left: Fat within the tumor is a common finding. There are unpaired arteries.

Right: Reticulin loss on reticulin stain within the fatty area is also common in fatty hepatocellular adenoma, a diagnostic pitfall that may result in an overdiagnosis of hepatocellular carcinoma.

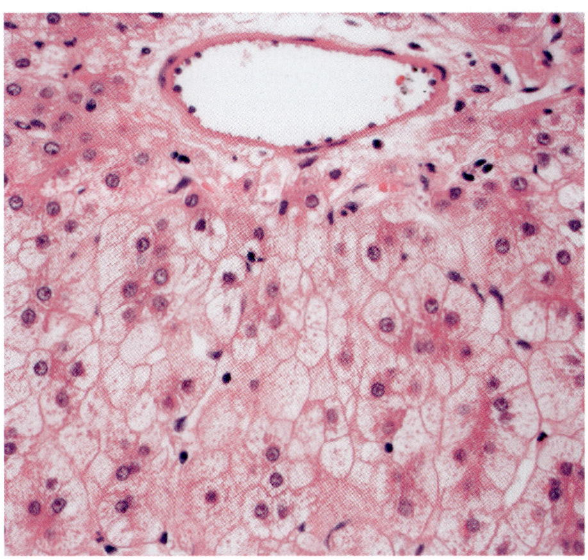

Figure 2-24

HEPATOCELLULAR ADENOMA

The tumor cells are large, clear, and pale due to accumulation of glycogen. There is an unpaired artery at the top.

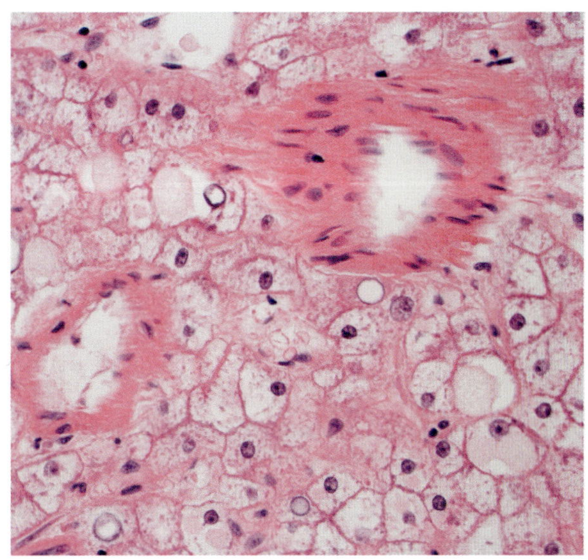

Figure 2-25

HEPATOCELLULAR ADENOMA

The tumor cells have abundant cytoplasm and show normal nucleus to cytoplasm ratio. The nuclei are regular and round, without atypia or mitotic figures. Unpaired arteries are present.

Table 2-3

HISTOLOGIC FEATURES OF HEPATOCELLULAR ADENOMA AND HEPATOCELLULAR CARCINOMA[a]

Features	Hepatocellular Adenoma	Hepatocellular Carcinoma
Nuclei	Regular, no atypia	Atypia, pleomorphism present
Nucleoli	Not prominent	Prominent
Mitoses	Absent	Common
Nuclear/cytoplasmic ratio	Normal	Increased
Trabecula	One to two hepatocytes in thickness	More than two hepatocytes in thickness
Pseudoglands	None to rare or very focal	Common
Vascular invasion	Absent	Present

[a]Modified from Table 2-4 from Ishak KG, Goodman ZD, Stocker JT. Tumors of the liver and intrahepatic bile ducts. Third series, Fascicle 31, 2001, American Registry of Pathology, Armed Forces Institute of Pathology.

Table 2-4

SUBTYPES OF HEPATOCELLULAR ADENOMA

Subtype	Clinical and Genetic Features	Pathologic Features
HNF-1α inactivated HCA[a]	Somatic inactivation of *HNF-1α* gene 30% of HCA Associated with MODY-3 Malignant transformation: very rare	Single or multiple Steatosis within tumor common
β-catenin activated HCA	Activated mutation of *β-catenin* gene 10-15% of HCA Can occur in male individuals May be associated with anabolic steroid Glycogen storage disease Malignant transformation occurs (50%)	Cytoarchitectural atypia may be seen
Inflammatory HCA	Mutation of *IL6ST*, *STAT3*, or *GNAS* 35-50% of HCA (most common) Obesity and excessive alcohol use Elevated CRP in serum Activated mutation of *β-catenin* in 10% Malignant transformation occurs	Telangiectatic changes in tumor Pseudo-portal tracts in tumor Ductular reaction within tumor Inflammation within tumor
Unclassified HCA	Up to 10% of HCA No known mutations	No distinctive features

[a]HNF = hepatocyte nuclear factor; HCA = hepatocellular adenoma; CRP = C-reactive protein.

Table 2-5

IMMUNOHISTOCHEMICAL FINDINGS IN HEPATOCELLULAR ADENOMA SUBTYPES

HCA[a] subtype	LFABP	GS	β-Catenin (nuclear stain)	CRP/SAA
HNF-1α inactivated	Loss	Negative	Negative	Negative
β-catenin mutated	No loss	Diffusely positive	Positive	Negative
Inflammatory	No loss	Negative (except if *β-catenin* mutated)	Negative (except if *β-catenin* mutated)	Positive
Unclassified	No loss	Negative	Negative	Negative

[a]HCA = hepatocellular adenoma; HNF = hepatocyte nuclear factor; LFABP = liver fatty acid binding protein; GS = glutamine synthetase; CRP/SAA = C-reactive protein/serum amyloid A.

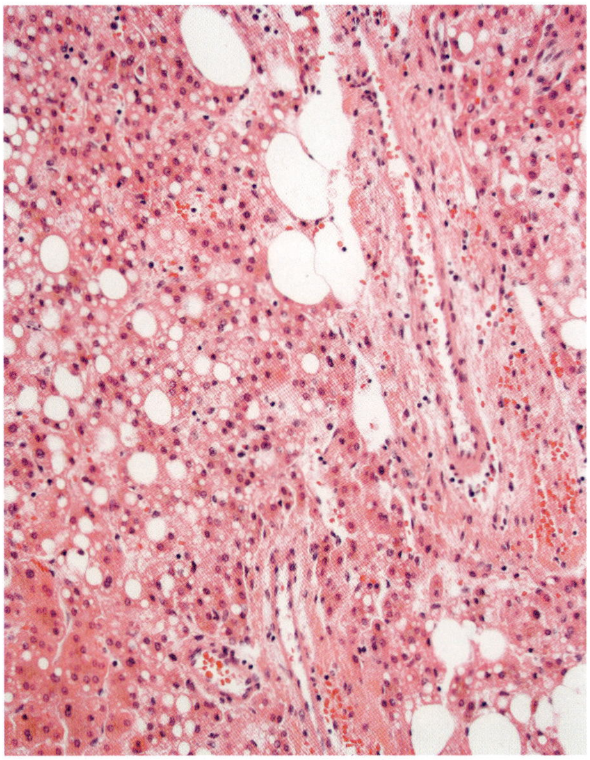

Figure 2-26

HEPATOCELLULAR ADENOMA, *HNF-1α*–MUTATED SUBTYPE

Steatosis within the tumor is very common in this subtype.

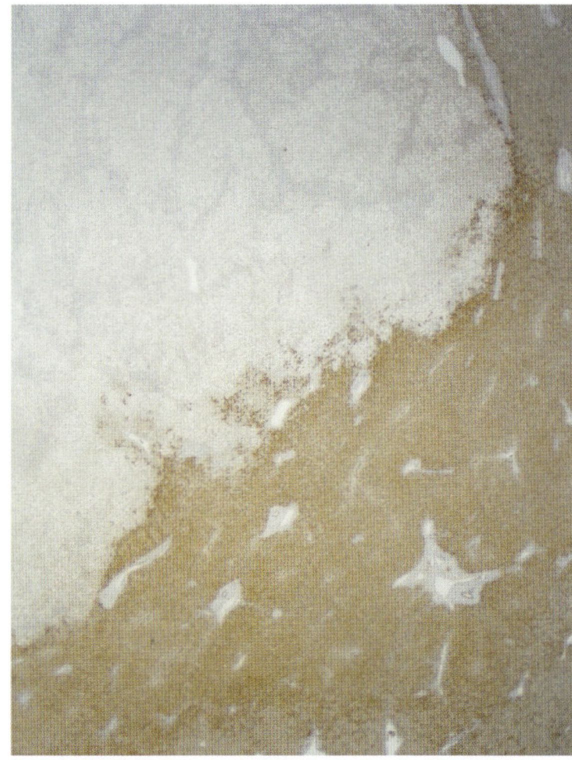

Figure 2-27

HEPATOCELLULAR ADENOMA, *HNF-1α*–MUTATED SUBTYPE

Immunohistochemistry for liver fatty acid binding protein (LFABP) shows there is loss of staining in the tumor cells (top left), while there is no loss of staining in the nontumoral hepatocytes. There is marked steatosis within the tumor.

Liver fatty acid binding protein (LFABP) is a lipid trafficking protein normally expressed in hepatocytes. It is positively regulated by HNF-1α. Downregulation of LFABP expression is a characteristic feature of H-HCA (54). As a result of the *HNF-1α* gene mutation, absent immunohistochemical staining confirms the diagnosis of H-HCA (fig. 2-27).

β-Catenin Mutated HCA (β-HCA). This subtype accounts for 10 to 15 percent of hepatocellular adenomas (26,49,50,55,56). It occurs in females as well as males, and may be associated with anabolic steroid use or hereditary glycogen storage disease. One of the β-catenin downstream target genes, glutamine synthetase (*GS*), is greatly overexpressed when compared to nontumor tissues, and is now typically used for subtyping hepatocellular adenomas.

Half of β-HCAs display both inflammatory and β-catenin-activated phenotypes (βI-HCA) (57). The βI-HCA subtype typically shows cytologic abnormalities with only very focal pseudoacinar or pseudoglandular formations that fall short of a diagnosis of hepatocellular carcinoma. Steatosis within the tumor is not common. Malignant transformation to hepatocellular carcinoma often occurs.

The diagnosis of β-HCA depends on immunohistochemical stains for β-catenin and glutamine synthetase, which show strong, diffuse, homogeneous, and cytoplasmic expression of GS and nuclear and cytoplasmic immunohistochemical staining for β-catenin (fig. 2-28). Lesions with hot spot mutations other than the common exon 3 at *CTNNB1* encoding β-catenin, such as exons 7-8, show weak and patchy GS staining without nuclear β-catenin staining (56), which may cause challenges in diagnosis; molecular testing may be necessary.

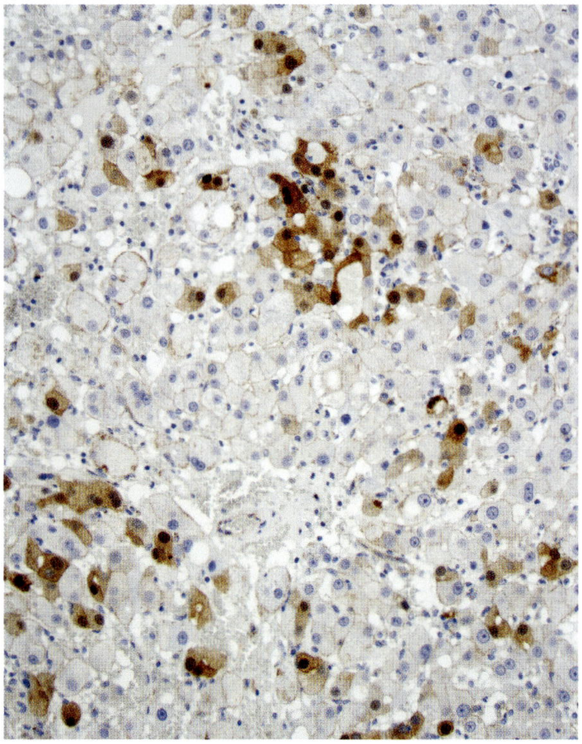

Figure 2-28

HEPATOCELLULAR ADENOMA, *β-CATENIN*–MUTATED SUBTYPE

Immunohistochemical staining for β-catenin shows nuclear and cytoplasmic positivity.

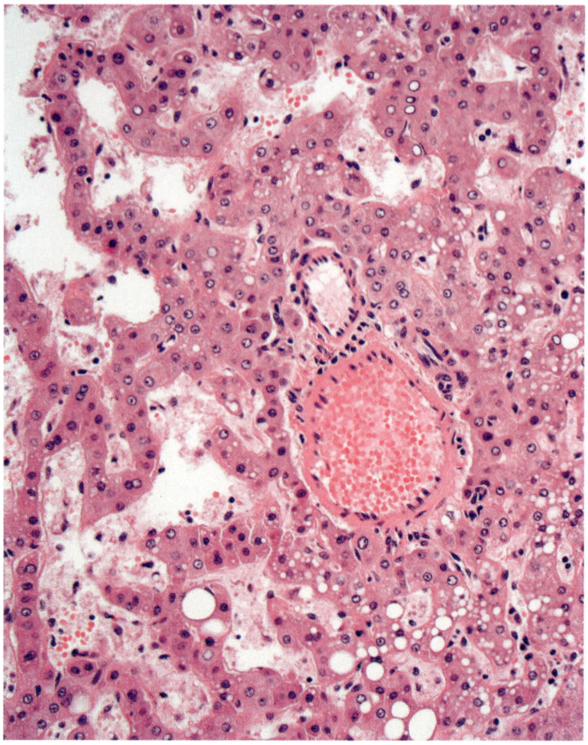

Figure 2-29

HEPATOCELLULAR ADENOMA, INFLAMMATORY SUBTYPE

Telangiectatic changes with sinusoidal dilatation are seen within the tumor. Unpaired arteries are present.

Inflammatory Hepatocellular Adenoma (I-HCA). I-HCA is the most common subtype of hepatocellular adenomas, accounting for 35 to 50 percent of cases (45,50). Up to 60 percent of I-HCA cases are caused by somatic mutation of *IL6ST,* which activates gp130 (58,59). The remaining I-HCAs are mutated for *STAT3* (60) or *GNAS* (61). This subtype is associated with obesity and excessive alcohol use. C-reactive protein (CRP) is typically elevated in serum, a manifestation of an inflammatory syndrome.

Within the tumor, real portal tracts are absent but fibrous structures containing dystrophic and thick muscular-walled arteries, and inflammatory infiltrate with ductular reaction at the periphery, are prominent, also known as pseudo-portal tracts, as they do not contain real bile ducts (see fig. 2-14). There are also telangiectatic changes, i.e., sinusoidal dilatation and hemorrhage within the tumor (fig. 2-29), termed the *telangiectatic subtype* of hepatocellular adenoma (21).

Unlike H-HCAs, steatosis is not common within the tumor, but the background liver is usually fatty (fig. 2-30) or even shows steatohepatitis. As the JAK-STAT pathway is activated, acute phase inflammatory proteins, such as serum amyloid A (SAA) and CRP, are induced and overexpressed within the tumor and are used as diagnostic markers for I-HCA (fig. 2-31). Unlike the H-HCA, there is no loss of LFABP within the tumor (fig. 2-32).

A subset of I-HCA (approximately 10 percent) shows activating mutations of the β-catenin pathway (49,50), and also has a higher risk of malignant potential, similar to the β-HCA subtype. This subset shows diffuse GS staining. The tumoral cells also show nuclear β-catenin staining (fig. 2-33) as well as atypical morphology including nuclear atypia and focal pseudoacinar formation.

Unclassified Hepatocellular Adenoma (U-HCA). Hepatocellular adenomas that do not show the typical immunohistochemical or histologic profiles described in the above three subtypes are currently categorized as unclassified HCA, hence a diagnosis of exclusion. They do not possess mutations in *HNF-1*α or β-*catenin* genes, nor do they have mutations in the inflammatory pathways. U-HCAs account for 5 to 10 percent of all HCA cases (45). Further stratification of exact underlying molecular mechanisms in this group await further investigation.

Ultrastructural Findings. Electron microscopy generally is not useful for the routine diagnosis of hepatocellular adenoma. On ultrastructural examination, the neoplastic cells typically show findings seen in normal hepatocytes, including the presence of bile canaliculi with tight junctions and desmosomes, but there may be excessive accumulation of glycogen as well as enlarged and distorted mitochondria containing dense bodies (62).

The perisinusoidal cells are replaced by myofibroblasts (63). The thickness of the endothelial cells is not regular. While there is capillarization of the sinusoids with loss of fenestrae, its degree is less prominent than in hepatocellular carcinoma (64–66).

Cytologic Findings. Hepatocellular adenomas typically exhibit tumor cells that are

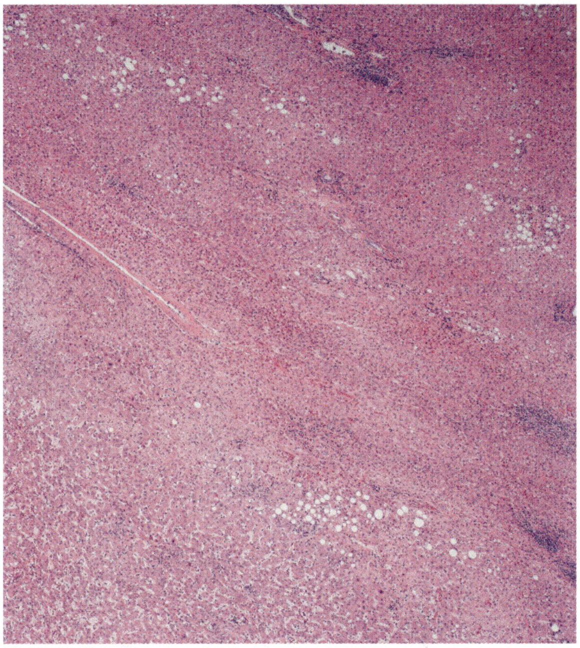

Figure 2-30

HEPATOCELLULAR ADENOMA, INFLAMMATORY SUBTYPE

The background liver at the top shows fatty changes due to underlying obesity in this patient, whereas the tumor at the bottom shows telangiectatic changes.

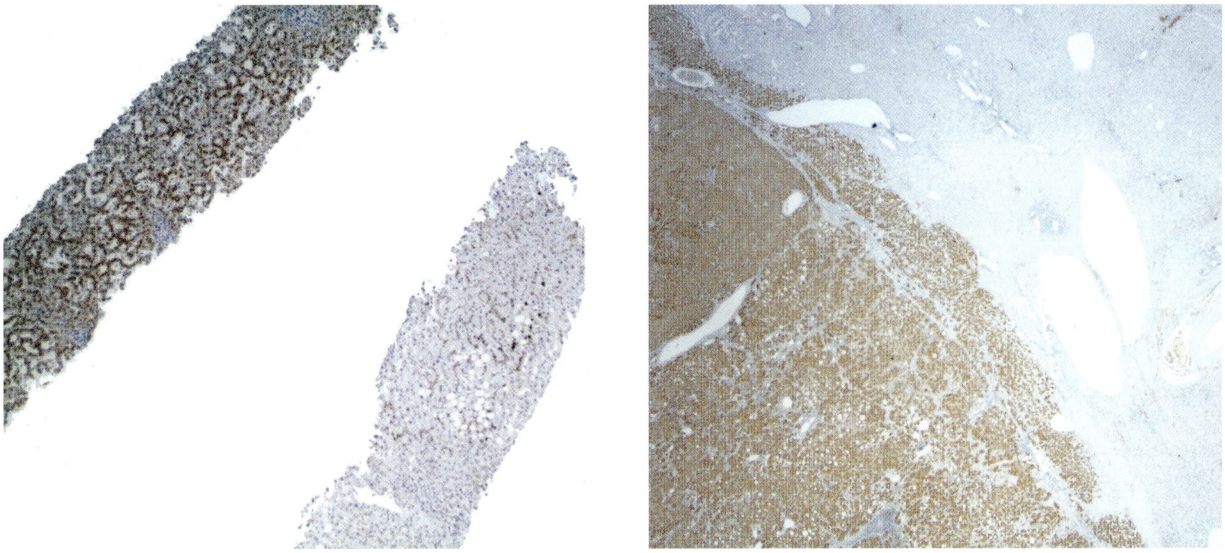

Figure 2-31

HEPATOCELLULAR ADENOMA, INFLAMMATORY SUBTYPE

Left: Immunohistochemical stain for serum amyloid A (SAA) is positive in the tumor (left core biopsy), but negative in the nontumoral liver (right core biopsy).

Right: C-reactive protein (CRP) is positive in the tumor (left side of image), but negative in the nontumoral liver (right side of image).

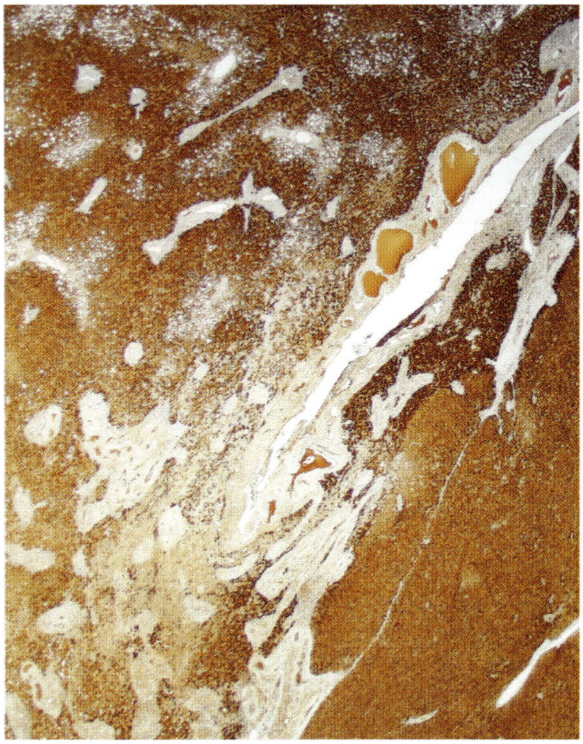

Figure 2-32

HEPATOCELLULAR ADENOMA, INFLAMMATORY SUBTYPE

Immunohistochemical stain for LFABP shows no loss of staining in the tumor (lower right).

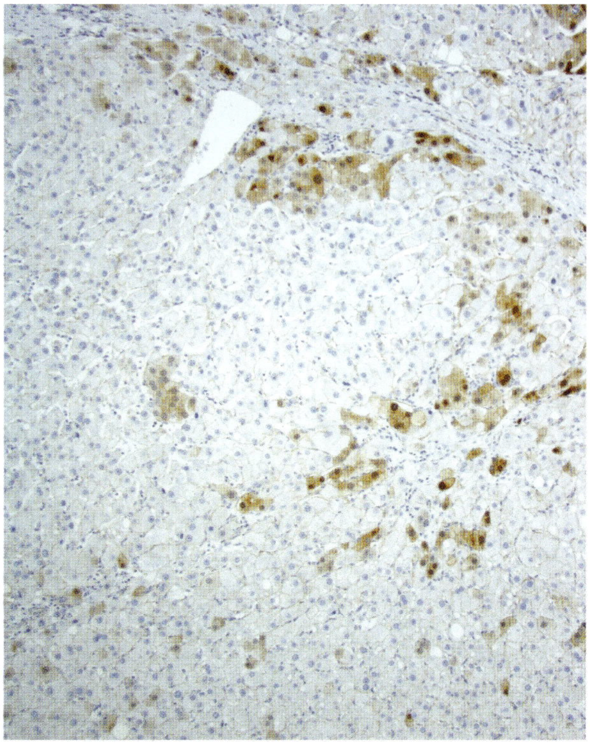

Figure 2-33

HEPATOCELLULAR ADENOMA, INFLAMMATORY SUBTYPE WITH *β-CATENIN* MUTATION

Immunohistochemical stain for β-catenin shows nuclear and cytoplasmic staining.

bland appearing, with a normal nuclear to cytoplasmic ratio, abundant cytoplasm, and minimal atypia (67). Cytology specimens usually contain hepatocytes only. Aspirates are hypercellular and composed of a monotonous population of well-differentiated hepatocytes, but features of hemorrhage or necrosis may be present. The hepatocytes exist singly or in two-cell–thick cords (fig. 2-34). Bile duct epithelium is absent. The hepatocytes may show clear cell change due to glycogen, fatty change, or bile (68,69).

Molecular Genetic Findings. While molecular testing currently is not routinely performed for the diagnosis and subtyping of hepatocellular adenoma, it may offer an option for cases with equivocal immunohistochemical results, including next-generation sequencing (70).

Differential Diagnosis. *Well-Differentiated Hepatocellular Carcinoma.* Although hepatocellular carcinoma (HCC) is distinguished by the thickened trabecula, loss of reticulin framework, pseudoglandular structures, and cytologic atypia (high nuclear to cytoplasmic ratio, pleomorphic nuclei, and mitotic figures) well-differentiated HCC often shows features that overlap with hepatocellular adenoma, especially the β-catenin-activated subtype that poses a major diagnostic challenge. These adenomas often harbor HCC at the time of initial diagnosis or give rise to HCC during follow-up, adding further difficulties in diagnosis, especially in biopsy specimens (49,50,71). The loss of the reticulin framework in HCC, as highlighted by a reticulin stain, may be a distinguishing feature, but focal loss of reticulin in adenoma, especially fatty adenomas (see fig. 2-23, right), has also been recognized as a diagnostic pitfall (72,73).

Combined use of immunohistochemical stains such as glypican-3 and heat shock protein 70 (HSP70) may help to distinguish between hepatocellular adenoma and well-differentiated HCC given their high specificities. Positive results of these malignant markers argue against

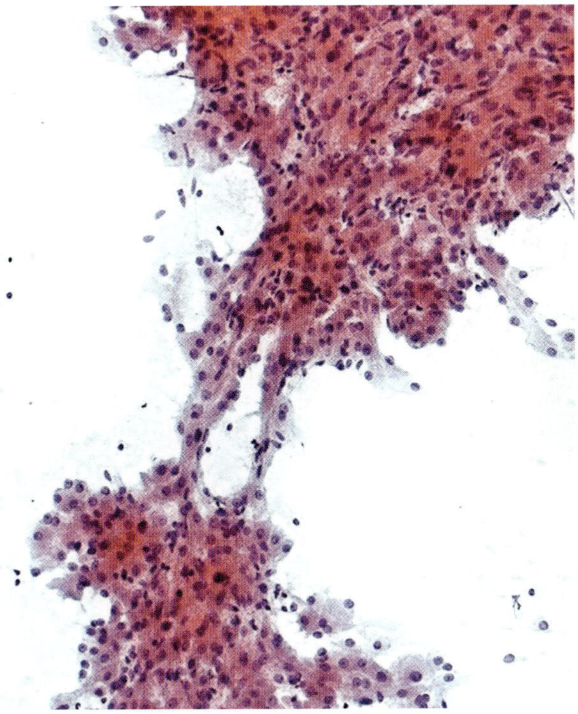

Figure 2-34

HEPATOCELLULAR ADENOMA

The hypercellular fine-needle aspirate is composed predominantly of hepatocytes with round central nuclei, distinct nucleoli, ample cytoplasm, and a normal nuclear-cytoplasmic ratio. There is no nuclear atypia. Obvious admixed spindled nuclei, representing either endothelial cells or Kupffer cells, are present, indicating that the trabeculae are not unduly broadened. There is a lack of bile ductal elements in the background (Papanicolaou stain). (Courtesy of Dr. Aileen Wee, Singapore.)

typical hepatocellular adenoma but negative results are not as useful due to their low sensitivities (73–75).

In cases of hepatocellular adenomas with atypical morphologic features, such as focal cytologic or architectural atypia (thickened trabeculae or pseudoglandular formation), focal loss of reticulin stain, or *β-catenin*-activated mutation that fall short of reaching a definitive diagnosis of HCC, the term *well-differentiated hepatocellular neoplasm of uncertain malignant potential* (HUMP) has been proposed. This entity also applies to hepatocellular adenomas with atypical clinical presentations including female patients older than 50 or younger than 15 years of age, or male patients (76,77).

Focal Nodular Hyperplasia. Focal nodular hyperplasia is an important entity that needs to be distinguished from hepatocellular adenoma, as it does not pose a risk for malignant transformation, and does not require surgical intervention unless it causes symptoms. While both hepatocellular adenoma and focal nodular hyperplasia have benign-appearing hepatocytes, there are distinguishing features. Typically seen in hyperplasia, but uncommon in adenoma, are thick fibrous septa containing thick-walled blood vessels, ductular reaction, mixed inflammatory cell infiltrates, and periseptal cholate stasis (36). These features, however, are not always apparent in focal nodular hyperplasia. On the other hand, the pseudo-portal tract seen in inflammatory hepatocellular adenoma is a diagnostic pitfall that may mimic hyperplasia. Immunohistochemical stains for glutamine synthetase showing the characteristic map-like pattern is the ultimate biological marker for diagnosing focal nodular hyperplasia (27).

Nodular Regenerative Hyperplasia. Although nodular regenerative hyperplasia, which typically presents as diffuse nodules ranging from 1 to 3 mm in diameter throughout the liver, is easily distinguished from hepatocellular adenoma and does not pose a diagnostic challenge, occasionally the nodules may coalesce into a large tumor nodule and the portal tracts and terminal hepatic venules are not easily recognizable as the interlobular bile ducts become atrophic and vanish. When sampled by biopsy, it may mimic hepatocellular adenoma, especially I-HCA with features such as sinusoidal dilatation, telangiectasia, and atrophy of hepatocytic cords (4,78–80). In addition, both lesions may have clear-appearing cytoplasm within the hepatocytes due to accumulated fat or glycogen. The presence of underlying vascular pathology in nodular regenerative hyperplasia, including portal venopathy or arteriopathy that shows thrombi or occlusions within the blood vessels, may help to distinguish it from hepatocellular adenoma (6,7,81,82).

Angiomyolipoma. There are three components in variable amounts in angiomyolipoma; smooth muscle cells, fat, and blood vessels (83), which may resemble hepatocellular adenoma on imaging (84) as well as on histopathology, especially due to the latter two elements. HMB-45 and melan-A are immunoreactive in angiomyolipoma (fig. 2-35), but not in hepatocellular adenoma and are useful markers for diagnosing

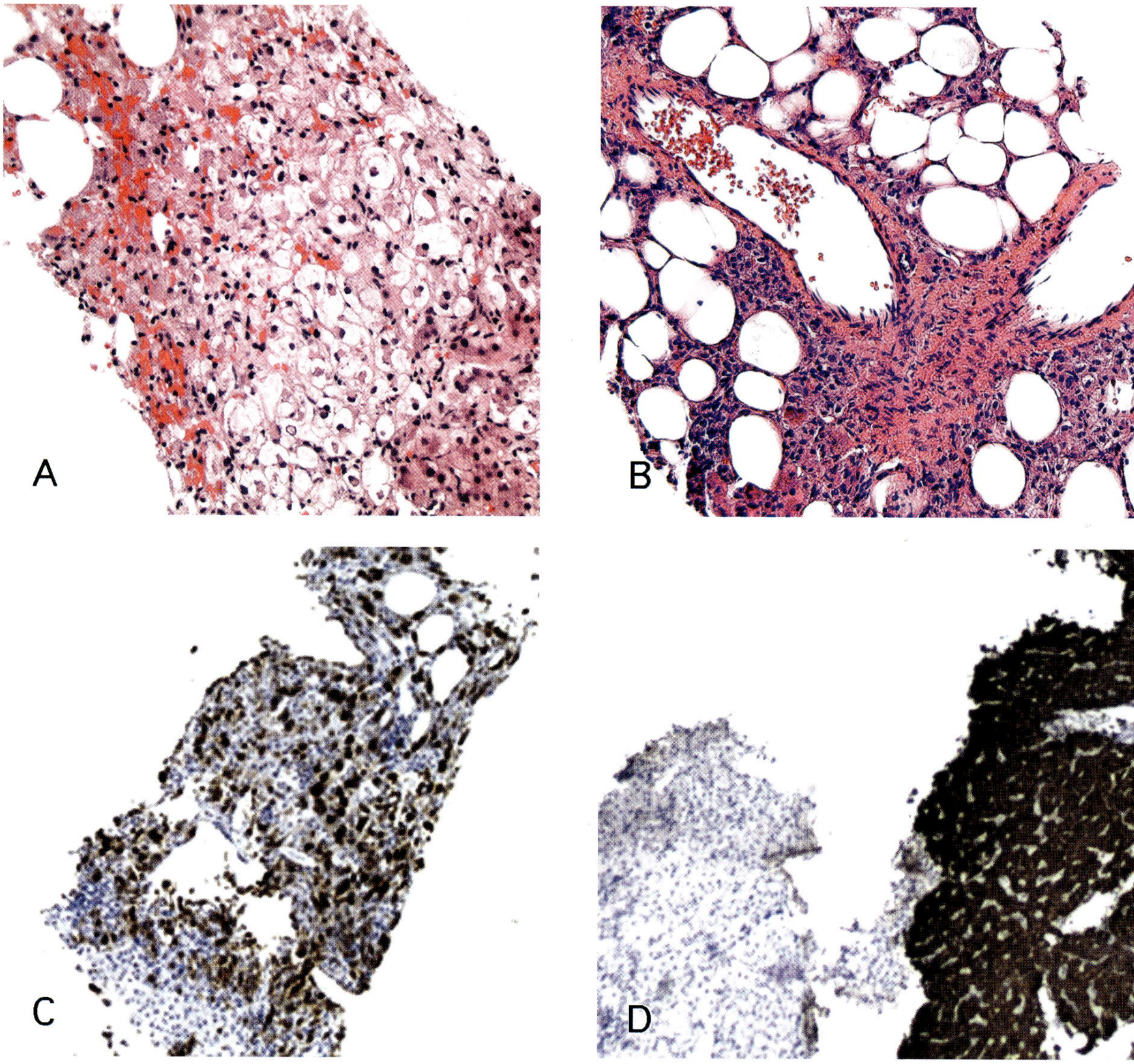

Figure 2-35

ANGIOMYOLIPOMA

A: Fat and epithelioid neoplastic cells are present, which may resemble hepatocytes.

B: The vascular component in angiomyolipoma may be mistaken as unpaired arteries and thus misdiagnosed as hepatocellular adenoma.

C: Immunohistochemical stains are positive for HMB-45 in angiomyolipoma, but not in adjacent uninvolved hepatocytes.

D: Unlike hepatocellular adenoma, the neoplastic cells in angiomyolipoma on the left are negative for HepPar1, whereas the adjacent hepatocytes on the right are positive.

angiomyolipoma (83,85,86). Unlike hepatocellular adenoma, the neoplastic cells in angiomyolipoma are negative for hepatocellular markers such as HepPar1 and arginase-1 (fig. 2-35).

Treatment and Prognosis. There is no consensus on the management of hepatocellular adenoma, but considering the risk of hemorrhage and potential malignant transformation, resection of lesions larger than 5 cm that persist after cessation of hormonal therapy is generally recommended (39,84,87). It has also been suggested hepatocellular adenomas in male patients should be resected irrespective of size, due to the high likelihood of malignant transformation (84,87). Hepatocellular adenomas harboring HCC or dysplastic foci, or containing β-catenin-activated mutations should also be resected (88).

The cessation of hormonal therapy in hepatocellular adenomas smaller than 5 cm in female patients is generally recommended, with regular imaging follow-up (84). The interval of imaging follow-up may differ depending on the subtype: experts recommend twice a year follow-up for patients with I-HCA and annual follow-up for those with noninflammatory hepatocellular adenomas for at least 5 consecutive years. The use of other less invasive modalities than surgical resection, such as locoregional therapies including transarterial embolization and radiofrequency ablation, has gained popularity. Liver transplantation for hepatocellular adenoma is currently not a standard treatment except for multiple unresectable adenomas in male patients and in patients with glycogen storage disease who do not respond to medical therapies (84).

Bleeding and malignant transformation are the two major complications of hepatocellular adenoma. The size of the tumor is correlated with the risk of bleeding: tumors larger than 5 cm carry a higher risk of bleeding (89,90). While the overall malignant transformation rate for hepatocellular adenoma is estimated to range from 4 to 5 percent (73,84,91,92), the data were mostly gathered from studies of resection specimens, so it may have been overestimated, especially in women (84). Recent reports have suggested hepatocellular adenomas with lipofuscin pigment have an increased risk of atypia and malignancy, particularly in men (93,94).

The outcome of liver resection for hepatocellular adenoma in well-selected patients is generally good. Recurrence rates after long-term follow-up are low (0 to less than 10 percent) (89,95,96,97).

REFERENCES

1. Steiner PE. Nodular regenerative hyperplasia of the liver. Am J Pathol 1959;35:943-953.
2. Hartleb M, Gutkowski K, Milkiewicz P. Nodular regenerative hyperplasia: evolving concepts on underdiagnosed cause of portal hypertension. World J Gastroenterol 2011;17:1400-1409.
3. Morris JM, Oien KA, McMahon M, et al. Nodular regenerative hyperplasia of the liver: survival and associated features in a UK case series. Eur J Gastroenterol Hepatol 2010;22:1001-1005.
4. Reshamwala PA, Kleiner DE, Heller T. Nodular regenerative hyperplasia: not all nodules are created equal. Hepatology 2006;44:7-14.
5. Schouten JN, Garcia-Pagan JC, Valla DC, Janssen HL. Idiopathic noncirrhotic portal hypertension. Hepatology 2011;54:1071-1081.
6. Wanless IR, Godwin TA, Allen F, Feder A. Nodular regenerative hyperplasia of the liver in hematologic disorders: a possible response to obliterative portal venopathy. A morphometric study of nine cases with an hypothesis on the pathogenesis. Medicine (Baltimore) 1980;59:367-379.
7. Wanless IR. Micronodular transformation (nodular regenerative hyperplasia) of the liver: a report of 64 cases among 2,500 autopsies and a new classification of benign hepatocellular nodules. Hepatology 1990;11:787-797.
8. Nakanuma Y. Nodular regenerative hyperplasia of the liver: retrospective survey in autopsy series. J Clin Gastroenterol 1990;12:460-465.
9. Cotte L, Benet T, Billioud C, et al. The role of nucleoside and nucleotide analogues in nodular regenerative hyperplasia in HIV-infected patients: a case control study. J Hepatol 2011;54:489-496.
10. Hussain N, Feld JJ, Kleiner DE, et al. Hepatic abnormalities in patients with chronic granulomatous disease. Hepatology 2007;45:675-683.
11. Klein R, Goller S, Bianchi L. Nodular regenerative hyperplasia (NRH) of the liver—a manifestation of 'organ-specific antiphospholipid syndrome'? Immunobiology 2003;207:51-57.
12. Malamut G, Ziol M, Suarez F, et al. Nodular regenerative hyperplasia: the main liver disease in patients with primary hypogammaglobulinemia and hepatic abnormalities. J Hepatol 2008;48:74-82.
13. Mallet VO, Varthaman A, Lasne D, et al. Acquired protein S deficiency leads to obliterative portal venopathy and to compensatory nodular regenerative hyperplasia in HIV-infected patients. AIDS 2009;23:1511-1518.
14. O'Brien K, Hussain N, Warady BA, et al. Nodular regenerative hyperplasia and severe portal hypertension in cystinosis. Clin Gastroenterol Hepatol 2006;4:387-394.

15. Vigano L, Rubbia-Brandt L, De Rosa G, et al. Nodular regenerative hyperplasia in patients undergoing liver resection for colorectal metastases after chemotherapy: risk factors, preoperative assessment and clinical impact. Ann Surg Oncol 2015;22:4149-4157.
16. Rubbia-Brandt L, Lauwers GY, Wang H, et al. Sinusoidal obstruction syndrome and nodular regenerative hyperplasia are frequent oxaliplatin-associated liver lesions and partially prevented by bevacizumab in patients with hepatic colorectal metastasis. Histopathology 2010;56:430-439.
17. Dumortier J, Boillot O, Chevallier M, et al. Familial occurrence of nodular regenerative hyperplasia of the liver: a report on three families. Gut 1999;45:289-294.
18. Rothweiler S, Terracciano L, Tornillo L, Dill MT, Heim MH, Semela D. Downregulation of the endothelial genes Notch1 and ephrinB2 in patients with nodular regenerative hyperplasia. Liver Int 2014;34:594-603.
19. International Working Party. Terminology of nodular hepatocellular lesions. Hepatology 1995; 22:983-993.
20. Sato Y, Harada K, Sasaki M, Nakanuma Y. Altered intrahepatic microcirculation of idiopathic portal hypertension in relation to glutamine synthetase expression. Hepatol Res 2015;45:1323-1330.
21. Bioulac-Sage P, Blanc JF, Rebouissou S, Balabaud C, Zucman-Rossi J. Genotype phenotype classification of hepatocellular adenoma. World J Gastroenterol 2007;13:2649-2654.
22. Mahamid J, Miselevich I, Attias D, Laor R, Zuckerman E, Shaoul R. Nodular regenerative hyperplasia associated with idiopathic thrombocytopenic purpura in a young girl: a case report and review of the literature. J Pediatr Gastroenterol Nutr 2005;41:251-255.
23. Sood A, Cox GA 2nd, McWilliams JP, Wang HL, Saab S. Patients with nodular regenerative hyperplasia should be considered for hepatocellular carcinoma screening. Hepatol Res 2014;44:689-693.
24. Bioulac-Sage P, Laumonier H, Rullier A, et al. Over-expression of glutamine synthetase in focal nodular hyperplasia: a novel easy diagnostic tool in surgical pathology. Liver Int 2009;29:459-465.
25. Bioulac-Sage P, Cubel G, Balabaud C, Zucman-Rossi J. Revisiting the pathology of resected benign hepatocellular nodules using new immunohistochemical markers. Semin Liver Dis 2011;31:91-103.
26. Bioulac-Sage P, Balabaud C, Wanless I. Focal nodular hyperplasia and hepatocellular adenoma. In: Bosman FT, Carneiro F, Hruban RH, Theise ND, eds. World Health Organization classification of tumours of the digestive system, 4th ed. Lyon: IARC Press; 2010:198-204.
27. Bioulac-Sage P, Cubel G, Taouji S, et al. Immunohistochemical markers on needle biopsies are helpful for the diagnosis of focal nodular hyperplasia and hepatocellular adenoma subtypes. Am J Surg Pathol 2012;36:1691-1699.
28. Nguyen BN, Flejou JF, Terris B, Belghiti J, Degott C. Focal nodular hyperplasia of the liver: a comprehensive pathologic study of 305 lesions and recognition of new histologic forms. Am J Surg Pathol 1999;23:1441-1454.
29. Wanless IR, Albrecht S, Bilbao J, et al. Multiple focal nodular hyperplasia of the liver associated with vascular malformations of various organs and neoplasia of the brain: a new syndrome. Mod Pathol 1989;2:456-462.
30. Rebouissou S, Bioulac-Sage P, Zucman-Rossi J. Molecular pathogenesis of focal nodular hyperplasia and hepatocellular adenoma. J Hepatol 2008;48:163-170.
31. Wanless IR, Mawdsley C, Adams R. On the pathogenesis of focal nodular hyperplasia of the liver. Hepatology 1985;5:1194-1200.
32. Wanless IR, Sapp H, Guindy M, Olshansky D, Takayam A. The pathogenesis of focal nodular hyperplasia/an hypothesis based on histological review of 20 lesions including 3 occurring in early biliary cirrhosis. Hepatology 2006;(Suppl 1):491A.
33. Paradis V, Laurent A, Flejou JF, Vidaud M, Bedossa P. Evidence for the polyclonal nature of focal nodular hyperplasia of the liver by the study of X-chromosome inactivation. Hepatology 1997;26:891-895.
34. Paradis V, Bieche I, Dargere D, et al. A quantitative gene expression study suggests a role for angiopoietins in focal nodular hyperplasia. Gastroenterology 2003;124:651-659.
35. Rebouissou S, Couchy G, Libbrecht L, et al. The beta-catenin pathway is activated in focal nodular hyperplasia but not in cirrhotic FNH-like nodules. J Hepatol 2008;49:61-71.
36. Makhlouf HR, Abdul-Al HM, Goodman ZD. Diagnosis of focal nodular hyperplasia of the liver by needle biopsy. Hum Pathol 2005;36:1210-1216.
37. Deniz K, Moreira RK, Yeh MM, Ferrell LD. Steatohepatitis-like changes in focal nodular hyperplasia, a finding to distinguish from steatohepatitic variant of hepatocellular carcinoma. Am J Surg Pathol 2017;41:277-281.
38. Ruschenburg I, Droese M. Fine needle aspiration cytology of focal nodular hyperplasia of the liver. Acta Cytol 1989;33:857-860.
39. Balabaud C, Al-Rabih WR, Chen PJ, et al. Focal nodular hyperplasia and hepatocellular adenoma around the world viewed through the scope of the immunopathological classification. Int J Hepatol 2013;2013:268625.
40. Salomao M, Remotti H, Vaughan R, Siegel AB, Lefkowitch JH, Moreira RK. The steatohepatitic variant of hepatocellular carcinoma and its association with underlying steatohepatitis. Hum Pathol 2012;43:737-746.

41. Halankar JA, Kim TK, Jang HJ, Khalili K, Masoom HA. Understanding the natural history of focal nodular hyperplasia in the liver with MRI. Indian J Radiol Imaging 2012;22:116-120.
42. Rifai K, Mix H, Krusche S, Potthoff A, Manns MP, Gebel MJ. No evidence of substantial growth progression or complications of large focal nodular hyperplasia during pregnancy. Scand J Gastroenterol 2013;48:88-92.
43. Venkatesh SK, Chandan V, Roberts LR. Liver masses: a clinical, radiologic, and pathologic perspective. Clin Gastroenterol Hepatol 2014;12:1414-1429.
44. Koehne de Gonzalez AK, Salomao MA, Lagana SM. Current concepts in the immunohistochemical evaluation of liver tumors. World J Hepatol 2015;7:1403-1411.
45. Bioulac-Sage P, Laumonier H, Couchy G, et al. Hepatocellular adenoma management and phenotypic classification: the Bordeaux experience. Hepatology 2009;50:481-489.
46. Rooks JB, Ory HW, Ishak KG, et al. Epidemiology of hepatocellular adenoma. The role of oral contraceptive use. JAMA 1979;242:644-648.
47. Cassiman D, Libbrecht L, Verslype C, et al. An adult male patient with multiple adenomas and a hepatocellular carcinoma: mild glycogen storage disease type Ia. J Hepatol 2010;53:213-217.
48. Bioulac-Sage P, Taouji S, Possenti L, Balabaud C. Hepatocellular adenoma subtypes: the impact of overweight and obesity. Liver Int 2012;32:1217-1221.
49. Bioulac-Sage P, Rebouissou S, Thomas C, et al. Hepatocellular adenoma subtype classification using molecular markers and immunohistochemistry. Hepatology 2007;46:740-748.
50. Zucman-Rossi J, Jeannot E, Nhieu JT, et al. Genotype-phenotype correlation in hepatocellular adenoma: new classification and relationship with HCC. Hepatology 2006;43:515-524.
51. Stueck AE, Qu Z, Huang MA, Camprecios G, Ferrell LD, Thung SN. Hepatocellular carcinoma arising in an HNF-1alpha-mutated adenoma in a 23-year-old woman with maturity-onset diabetes of the young: a case report. Semin Liver Dis 2015;35:444-449.
52. Bluteau O, Jeannot E, Bioulac-Sage P, et al. Bi-allelic inactivation of TCF1 in hepatic adenomas. Nat Genet 2002;32:312-315.
53. Nault JC, Bioulac-Sage P, Zucman-Rossi J. Hepatocellular benign tumors—from molecular classification to personalized clinical care. Gastroenterology 2013;144:888-902.
54. Inoue M, Takahashi Y, Fujii T, Kitagawa M, Fukusato T. Significance of downregulation of liver fatty acid-binding protein in hepatocellular carcinoma. World J Gastroenterol 2014;20:17541-17551.
55. Chen YJ, Chen PJ, Lee MC, Yeh SH, Hsu MT, Lin CH. Chromosomal analysis of hepatic adenoma and focal nodular hyperplasia by comparative genomic hybridization. Genes Chromosomes Cancer 2002;35:138-143.
56. Roncalli M, Sciarra A, Tommaso LD. Benign hepatocellular nodules of healthy liver: focal nodular hyperplasia and hepatocellular adenoma. Clin Mol Hepatol 2016;22:199-211.
57. Pilati C, Letouze E, Nault JC, et al. Genomic profiling of hepatocellular adenomas reveals recurrent FRK-activating mutations and the mechanisms of malignant transformation. Cancer Cell 2014;25:428-441.
58. Poussin K, Pilati C, Couchy G, et al. Biochemical and functional analyses of gp130 mutants unveil JAK1 as a novel therapeutic target in human inflammatory hepatocellular adenoma. Oncoimmunology 2013;2:e27090.
59. Rebouissou S, Amessou M, Couchy G, et al. Frequent in-frame somatic deletions activate gp130 in inflammatory hepatocellular tumours. Nature 2009;457:200-204.
60. Pilati C, Amessou M, Bihl MP, et al. Somatic mutations activating STAT3 in human inflammatory hepatocellular adenomas. J Exp Med 2011;208:1359-1366.
61. Nault JC, Fabre M, Couchy G, et al. GNAS-activating mutations define a rare subgroup of inflammatory liver tumors characterized by STAT3 activation. J Hepatol 2012;56:184-191.
62. Kay S, Schatzki PF. Ultrastructure of a benign liver cell adenoma. Cancer 1971;28:755-762.
63. Bioulac-Sage P, Lamouliatte H, Saric J, Merlio JP, Balabaud C. Ultrastructure of sinusoidal cells in a benign liver cell adenoma. Ultrastruct Pathol. 1986;10:49-54.
64. Balazs M. Primary hepatocellular tumours during long-term androgenic steroid therapy. A light and electron microscopic study of 11 cases with emphasis on microvasculature of the tumours. Acta Morphol Hung 1991;39:201-216.
65. Balazs M. Comparative electron-microscopic studies of benign hepatoma and icterus in patients on oral contraceptives. Virchows Arch A Pathol Anat Histol 1978;381:97-109.
66. Haratake J, Hisaoka M, Yamamoto O, Horie A. An ultrastructural comparison of sinusoids in hepatocellular carcinoma, adenomatous hyperplasia, and fetal liver. Arch Pathol Lab Med 1992;116:67-70.
67. Suen KC. Diagnosis of primary hepatic neoplasms by fine-needle aspiration cytology. Diagn Cytopathol 1986;2:99-109.
68. Chhieng DC. Fine needle aspiration biopsy of liver - an update. World J Surg Oncol 2004;2:5.
69. Wee A. Fine needle aspiration biopsy of hepatocellular carcinoma and hepatocellular nodular lesions: role, controversies and approach to diagnosis. Cytopathology 2011;22:287-305.
70. Margolskee E, Bao F, de Gonzalez AK, et al. Hepatocellular adenoma classification: a comparative evaluation of immunohistochemistry and targeted mutational analysis. Diagn Pathol 2016;11:27.

71. Micchelli ST, Vivekanandan P, Boitnott JK, Pawlik TM, Choti MA, Torbenson M. Malignant transformation of hepatic adenomas. Mod Pathol 2008;21:491-497.
72. Singhi AD, Jain D, Kakar S, Wu TT, Yeh MM, Torbenson M. Reticulin loss in benign fatty liver: an important diagnostic pitfall when considering a diagnosis of hepatocellular carcinoma. Am J Surg Pathol 2012;36:710-715.
73. Dhingra S, Fiel MI. Update on the new classification of hepatic adenomas: clinical, molecular, and pathologic characteristics. Arch Pathol Lab Med 2014;138:1090-1097.
74. Nguyen TB, Roncalli M, Di Tommaso L, Kakar S. Combined use of heat-shock protein 70 and glutamine synthetase is useful in the distinction of typical hepatocellular adenoma from atypical hepatocellular neoplasms and well-differentiated hepatocellular carcinoma. Mod Pathol 2016; 29:283-292.
75. Lagana SM, Salomao M, Bao F, Moreira RK, Lefkowitch JH, Remotti HE. Utility of an immunohistochemical panel consisting of glypican-3, heat-shock protein-70, and glutamine synthetase in the distinction of low-grade hepatocellular carcinoma from hepatocellular adenoma. Appl Immunohistochem Mol Morphol 2013;21:170-176.
76. Bedossa P, Burt AD, Brunt EM, et al. Well-differentiated hepatocellular neoplasm of uncertain malignant potential: proposal for a new diagnostic category. Hum Pathol 2014;45:658-660.
77. Evason KJ, Grenert JP, Ferrell LD, Kakar S. Atypical hepatocellular adenoma-like neoplasms with beta-catenin activation show cytogenetic alterations similar to well-differentiated hepatocellular carcinomas. Hum Pathol 2013;44:750-758.
78. Ames JT, Federle MP, Chopra K. Distinguishing clinical and imaging features of nodular regenerative hyperplasia and large regenerative nodules of the liver. Clin Radiol 2009;64:1190-1195.
79. Dachman AH, Ros PR, Goodman ZD, Olmsted WW, Ishak KG. Nodular regenerative hyperplasia of the liver: clinical and radiologic observations. AJR Am J Roentgenol 1987;148:717-722.
80. Wang HM, Lo GH, Hsu PI, et al. Nodular regenerative hyperplasia of the liver. J Chin Med Assoc 2008;71:523-527.
81. Wanless IR, Lentz JS, Roberts EA. Partial nodular transformation of liver in an adult with persistent ductus venosus. Review with hypothesis on pathogenesis. Arch Pathol Lab Med 1985;109:427-432.
82. Wanless IR, Gryfe A. Nodular transformation of the liver in hereditary hemorrhagic telangiectasia. Arch Pathol Lab Med 1986;110:331-335.
83. Nonomura A, Enomoto Y, Takeda M, Takano M, Morita K, Kasai T. Angiomyolipoma of the liver: a reappraisal of morphological features and delineation of new characteristic histological features from the clinicopathological findings of 55 tumours in 47 patients. Histopathology 2012;61:863-880.
84. Belghiti J, Cauchy F, Paradis V, Vilgrain V. Diagnosis and management of solid benign liver lesions. Nat Rev Gastroenterol Hepatol 2014;11:737-749.
85. Tsui WM, Colombari R, Portmann BC, et al. Hepatic angiomyolipoma: a clinicopathologic study of 30 cases and delineation of unusual morphologic variants. Am J Surg Pathol 1999;23:34-48.
86. Tsui WM, Yuen AK, Ma KF, Tse CC. Hepatic angiomyolipomas with a deceptive trabecular pattern and HMB-45 reactivity. Histopathology 1992;21:569-573.
87. Blanc JF, Frulio N, Chiche L, et al. Hepatocellular adenoma management: call for shared guidelines and multidisciplinary approach. Clin Res Hepatol Gastroenterol 2015;39:180-187.
88. Vijay A, Elaffandi A, Khalaf H. Hepatocellular adenoma: an update. World J Hepatol 2015;7:2603-2609.
89. Dokmak S, Paradis V, Vilgrain V, et al. A single-center surgical experience of 122 patients with single and multiple hepatocellular adenomas. Gastroenterology 2009;137:1698-1705.
90. Deneve JL, Pawlik TM, Cunningham S, et al. Liver cell adenoma: a multicenter analysis of risk factors for rupture and malignancy. Ann Surg Oncol 2009;16:640-648.
91. Farges O, Dokmak S. Malignant transformation of liver adenoma: an analysis of the literature. Dig Surg 2010;27:32-38.
92. Stoot JH, Coelen RJ, De Jong MC, Dejong CH. Malignant transformation of hepatocellular adenomas into hepatocellular carcinomas: a systematic review including more than 1600 adenoma cases. HPB (Oxford) 2010;12:509-522.
93. Hechtman JF, Raoufi M, Fiel MI, et al. Hepatocellular carcinoma arising in a pigmented telangiectatic adenoma with nuclear beta-catenin and glutamine synthetase positivity: case report and review of the literature. Am J Surg Pathol 2011;35:927-932.
94. Mounajjed T, Yasir S, Aleff PA, Torbenson MS. Pigmented hepatocellular adenomas have a high risk of atypia and malignancy. Mod Pathol 2015;28:1265-1274.
95. Karkar AM, Tang LH, Kashikar ND, et al. Management of hepatocellular adenoma: comparison of resection, embolization and observation. HPB (Oxford) 2013;15:235-243.
96. Hoffmann K, Unsinn M, Hinz U, et al. Outcome after a liver resection of benign lesions. HPB (Oxford) 2015;17:994-1000.
97. de'Angelis N, Memeo R, Calderaro J, et al. Open and laparoscopic resection of hepatocellular adenoma: trends over 23 years at a specialist hepatobiliary unit. HPB (Oxford) 2014;16:783-788.

3 HEPATOCELLULAR CARCINOMA

PRECURSOR HEPATOCELLULAR CARCINOMA LESIONS

Several hepatocytic lesions have been studied as possible precursors of hepatocellular carcinoma. Some are microscopic findings only, while others are macroscopic nodular lesions. Essentially all of the lesions with the most compelling evidence of being a hepatocellular carcinoma precursor are found in cirrhotic livers. While about 20 percent of hepatocellular carcinomas occur in noncirrhotic livers, no convincing precursor lesion has emerged.

Small Cell Change

Small cell change, also referred to as *small cell dysplasia*, histologically consists of small discrete aggregates of hepatocytes with a reduced volume of cytoplasm and mild nuclear hyperchromasia, but otherwise normal nuclear and cytoplasmic cytology (fig. 3-1). These foci often stand out best at low-power magnification. Foci of small cell change may be clonal (1) and show chromosomal damage, telomere shortening, and other DNA changes that support a role as a precursor of hepatocellular carcinoma (2–4).

Large Cell Change

Hepatocytes with *large cell change* have larger and more hyperchromatic nuclei than those seen in the background liver. They are easily spotted at low-power magnification (fig. 3-2). However, the increased nuclear size is accompanied by increased volume of cytoplasm, leading to preservation of a normal, or near normal, nuclear to cytoplasmic ratio.

Large cell change is associated with DNA damage, but it remains controversial whether large cell change is a direct precursor of malignancy itself. Data suggest that large cell change is a genetically heterogeneous finding and is directly premalignant in only a minority of cases, with most cases representing degenerative or senescent changes (2,3,5,6).

Glycogen Storing Foci

Glycogen storing foci have been proposed as potential premalignant lesions (7,8). At this point, however, the data do not strongly support a major role for these lesions in carcinoma risk. They are polyclonal (1) and can be found in the background liver of 10 percent of hepatocellular carcinomas arising in cirrhotic livers and 20 percent arising in noncirrhotic livers (9). In some cases, glycogen storing foci have intermediate hepatocyte-like cells that stain for CK7 (10).

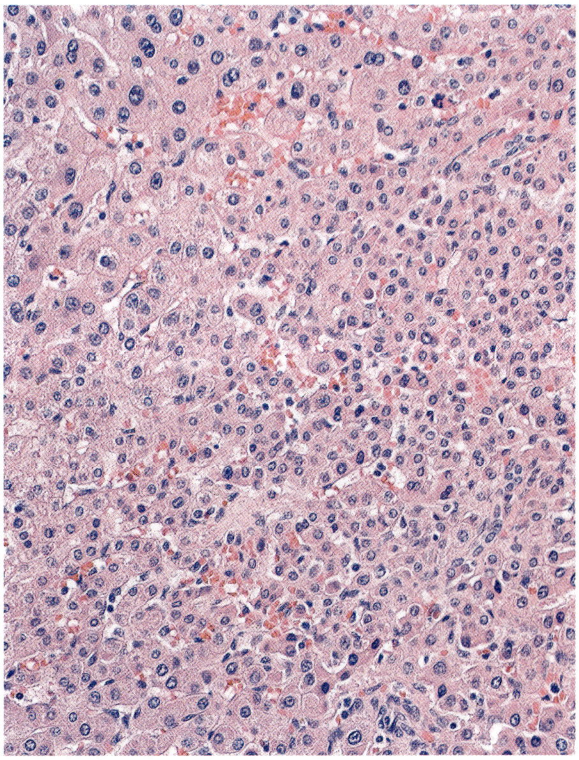

Figure 3-1

SMALL CELL CHANGE

Small cell change is seen in the hepatocytes on the right side of the image, with an increased nuclear/cytoplasmic ratio and mild nuclear hyperchromasia.

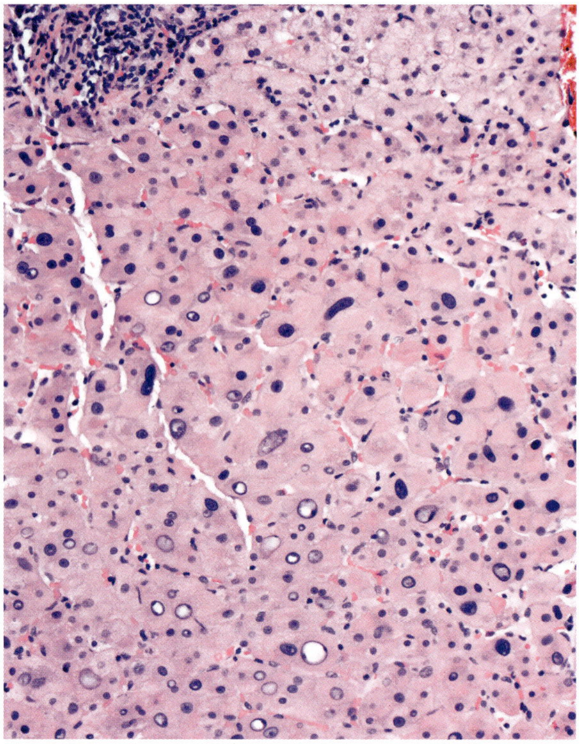

Figure 3-2

LARGE CELL CHANGE

This cirrhotic liver had chronic hepatitis C infection and hepatocellular carcinoma was present elsewhere on the biopsy. In this field, large cell change is evident, with scattered hepatocytes showing large atypical nuclei, but with a preserved nuclear/cytoplasmic ratio.

Macroregenerative Nodule

Macroregenerative nodules are defined as nodular lesions that are at least 10 mm in diameter and stand out from the background liver because they have differences in color and texture (usually softer), or because they bulge out more than other cirrhotic nodules from the cut surface. Most macroregenerative nodules are between 10 and 20 mm: two large studies both found an average size of 12 mm (11,12). Multiple macroregenerative nodules are found in about two thirds of cases with cirrhosis (11). Rarely, there is a large number of macroregenerative nodules, too many to count at a practical level (11).

Almost all macroregenerative nodules are found in cirrhotic livers, with 15 to 30 percent of cirrhotic livers having macroregenerative nodules (11,12). Noncirrhotic livers rarely can develop macroregenerative nodules, primarily when the liver has extensive parenchymal loss, leading to large areas of panacinar collapse, such as seen after fulminant autoimmune hepatitis. In the latter setting, the surviving hepatocytes can grow as large nodules that suggest carcinoma on imaging studies and on gross examination, but on histology show the features of benign regenerative nodules. Sometimes this pattern is also called *post-necrotic macroregenerative nodules*.

The distinction between a macroregenerative nodule and a low-grade dysplastic nodule is subjective, without well-accepted criteria. However, the basic notion of a macroregenerative nodule is simple: a cirrhotic nodule that stands out on gross examination because it is significantly larger than its peers (usually the nodule is larger than 10 mm) or has a different color or texture, yet shows no or minimal cytologic atypia. One useful approach to the diagnosis of a macroregenerative nodule is that the hepatocytes in the nodule should look cytologically identical to the hepatocytes in the rest of the liver. The hepatocytes within macroregenerative nodules may show patchy large cell change when the background liver shows similar changes, but there should be no other cytologic atypia. There should be no small cell change. Scattered portal tracts are typically present in macroregenerative nodules (fig. 3-3). Their malignant potential is probably not much greater than that of the background liver, but some studies suggest an increased risk of malignant transformation (13).

Focal Nodular Hyperplasia-Like Lesions

Vascular shunts in the cirrhotic liver can lead to nodules that look and stain like focal nodular hyperplasia (14). They are called *focal nodular hyperplasia-like lesions* and do not have neoplastic potential (15). In keeping with vascular shunting as their etiology, these lesions are more common after chemoembolization and in individuals with esophageal varices (15). However, these lesions do not appear to be identical to typical focal nodular hyperplasia based on transcriptome profiling (16).

Dysplastic Nodules

The most widely accepted precursor lesions of hepatocellular carcinoma are *dysplastic nodules*. Dysplastic nodules are found only in cirrhotic livers and are further divided into those with low-grade versus high-grade dysplasia. Portal

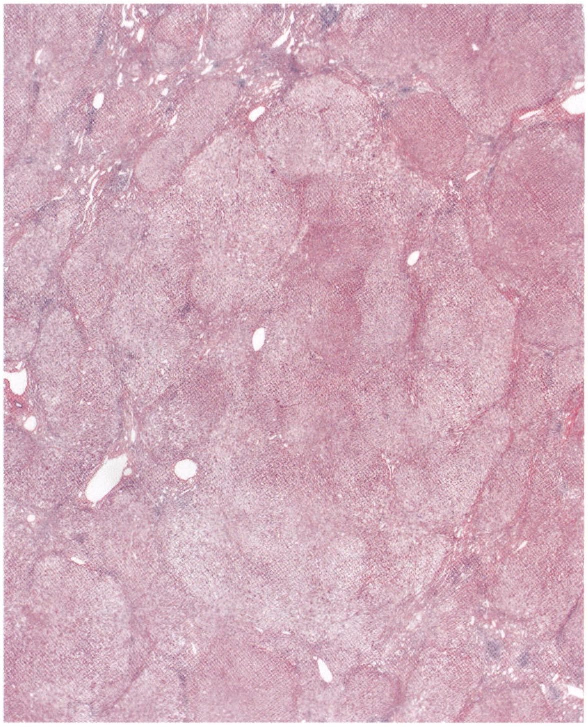

Figure 3-3

MACROREGENERATIVE NODULE

This macroregenerative nodule stands out from the background liver because of its size and slightly different color. Histologically, the nodule shows more fatty change than the rest of the cirrhotic nodules. Portal tracts are present throughout the nodule.

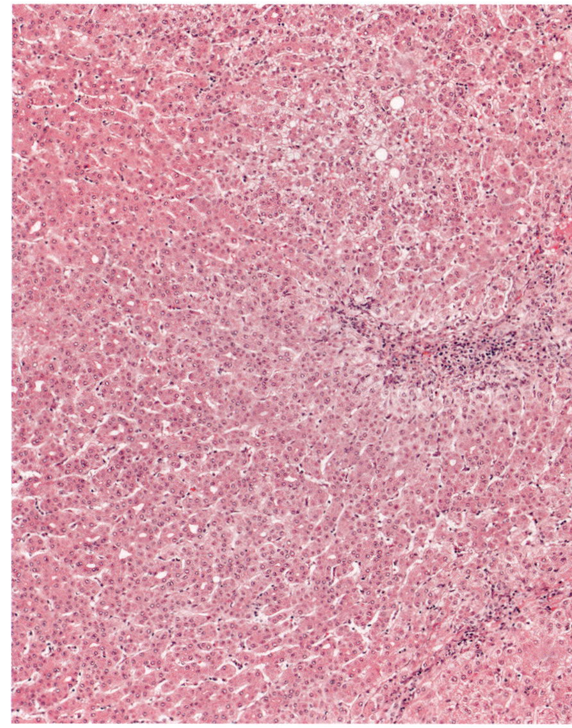

Figure 3-4

DYSPLASTIC NODULE: LOW GRADE

The nodule shows residual portal tracts but histologically stands out from the background liver, with a higher nuclear/cytoplasmic ratio, focal fatty change, and focal areas with a pseudoglandular architecture.

tracts are typically present within the dysplastic nodules. Dysplastic nodules show cytologic and architectural atypia that make them distinct from background cirrhotic liver nodules, but do not have the full histologic features of malignancy. The cytologic atypia, although greater than in the background liver, is usually mild. Either large cell or small cell change may be present in high-grade dysplastic nodules. The architectural atypia includes pseudogland formation (less helpful in cholestatic livers), vague nodule within nodule growth, or lobular arterioles (unpaired arteries). Lobular arterialization is often accompanied by strong and diffuse staining with CD34, but this pattern of staining is not specific and is found in some ordinary cirrhotic nodules.

In contrast to hepatocellular carcinoma, dysplastic nodules show no loss of reticulin and have no or rare mitotic figures. Immunostains are negative for alpha-fetoprotein (AFP) and beta-catenin nuclear accumulation. Glypican 3 results alone do not always separate high-grade dysplastic nodules from hepatocellular carcinoma because some high-grade nodules are focally positive and many well-differentiated hepatocellular carcinomas are negative. Nonetheless, when a nodule is strongly and diffusely positive for glypican 3, hepatocellular carcinoma should be carefully excluded. Strong and diffuse staining for glutamine synthetase also favors hepatocellular carcinoma. When available, staining for heat-shock protein (HSP)-70 may also suggest hepatocellular carcinoma (17).

Once a diagnosis of a dysplastic nodule is made, it is further categorized as high-grade or low-grade dysplasia. This approach can be difficult to implement on needle biopsy specimens, but works reasonably well in resection specimens. Low-grade dysplastic nodules (fig. 3-4) continue to show portal tracts but have more

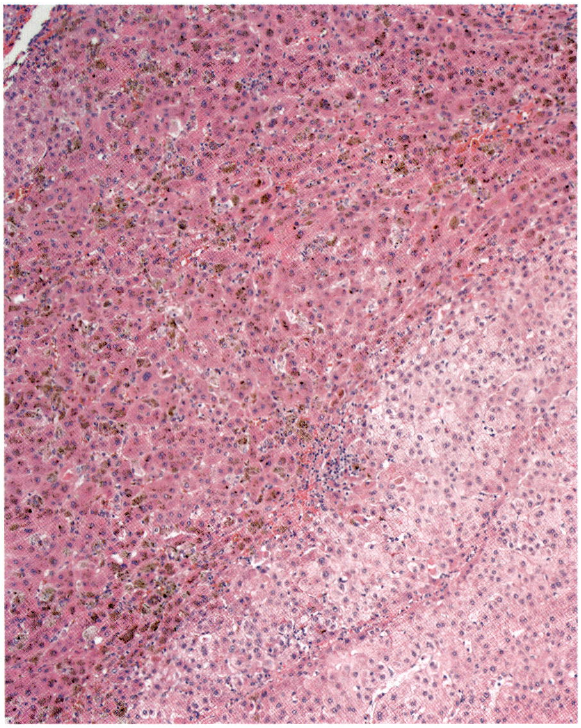

Figure 3-5

DYSPLASTIC NODULE: HIGH GRADE

Compared to the background liver (lower right), this nodule (upper left) shows an increased nuclear/cytoplasmic ratio, focal nuclear pleomorphism, and marked cholestasis.

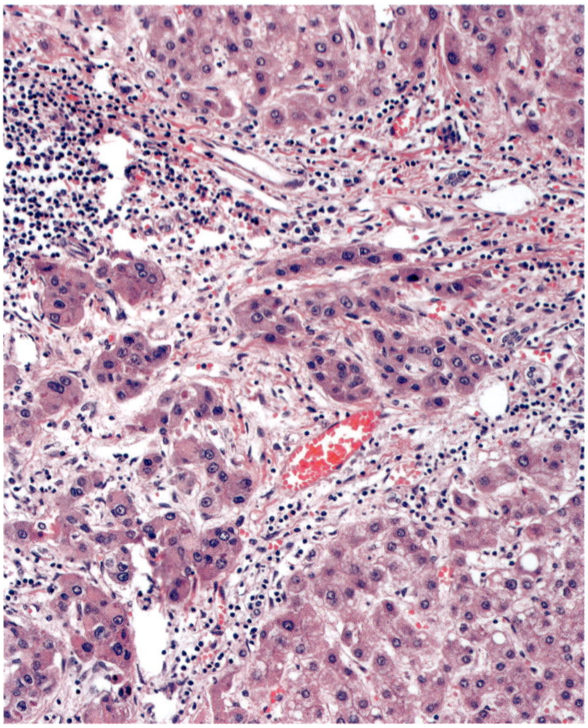

Figure 3-6

HEPATOCELLULAR CARCINOMA: STROMAL INVASION

Non-neoplastic cirrhotic liver is seen on both the lower and upper portion of this image. The hepatocellular carcinoma has invaded along the fibrous septum, extending from the main tumor mass, which is below and not seen in this image.

cytologic atypia than the background liver. They have small numbers of unpaired arteries, but no other architectural abnormalities (such as nodule within nodule growth). In contrast, high-grade dysplastic nodules (fig. 3-5) have more striking architectural abnormalities. They show loss of many or nearly all portal tracts, have increased numbers of unpaired arteries, and are more likely to have small cell change, an overall increase in cell density, and increased nuclear hyperchromasia. Pseudoglands and vague nodule within nodule growth can be seen in some cases. Similar to low-grade dysplastic nodules, there should be no reticulin loss.

The main entity in the differential diagnosis of dysplastic nodule is well-differentiated hepatocellular carcinoma. The degree of cytologic atypia can overlap with that of hepatocellular carcinomas, but hepatocellular carcinomas have mitotic figures, frequently an increased Ki-67 proliferative rate compared to the background liver, and definite loss of reticulin stain. In addition, almost all hepatocellular carcinomas no longer have the retained portal structures found in most dysplastic nodules. As discussed above, immunostains for HSP-70, glypican 3, and glutamine synthetase are helpful, as strong diffuse positivity favors hepatocellular carcinoma. Dysplastic nodules also do not show nuclear accumulation of beta-catenin and are AFP negative, but neither marker is very sensitive for the diagnosis of hepatocellular carcinoma.

Stromal invasion has been suggested as a histologic finding that can be used to identify well-differentiated hepatocellular carcinomas and separate them from high-grade dysplastic nodules (18–20). Stromal invasion is defined as malignant cells that invade the stroma of portal tracts or fibrous bands surrounding a nodule (fig. 3-6). Stromal invasion is challenging to reproducibly identify, even on full resections, and its use has not been clearly demonstrated in biopsy material.

In addition, stromal invasion is best seen in cases that are obviously hepatocellular carcinomas and much more challenging to confidently identify in well-differentiated lesions, for which more help is needed. Because of these challenges, the use of CK7 and CK19 immunostains has been advocated, as a ductular reaction (highlighted by the keratin stains) is typically absent at the edges of hepatocellular carcinomas with stromal invasion, but present at the edges of high-grade dysplastic nodules and cirrhotic nodules (21).

These stains may be helpful, but the criterion of stromal invasion remains difficult to implement with needle biopsy specimens. Unfortunately, some clinical management guidelines for hepatocellular carcinoma have prematurely considered stromal invasion to be a key criterion for diagnosing hepatocellular carcinoma. Many tumor biopsies are confidently diagnosed as well-differentiated hepatocellular carcinoma, yet the biopsies are all tumor and do not contain the tumor and nontumor interface. In other cases, also confidently diagnosed as well-differentiated hepatocellular carcinoma, the interface is present yet fails to show stromal invasion.

Livers with dysplastic nodules are at increased risk for the development of hepatocellular carcinoma. One study followed dysplastic nodules for a median of about 2 years by imaging studies and found that 46 percent disappeared on imaging, but 12 percent progressed to hepatocellular carcinoma (22). Interestingly, an additional 24 percent of individuals developed hepatocellular carcinoma outside of the dysplastic nodule that was being followed. Another study found that 9 percent of low-grade dysplastic nodules and 32 percent of high-grade dysplastic nodules transformed to hepatocellular carcinoma, with a median of 36 months of follow-up (23). The high risk for malignant transformation in dysplastic nodules was confirmed in another large study that found 42 percent of dysplastic nodules underwent malignant transformation during a median of 39 months (13).

Formal guidelines for the clinical management of small lesions are based more on lesion size and imaging findings, but in general, low-grade dysplastic nodules are followed radiographically every 6 months until they either disappear or enlarge. If they enlarge, biopsies are often performed to determine whether hepatocellular carcinoma has developed. As noted above, high-grade dysplastic nodules have a much greater risk of progression to hepatocellular carcinoma than low-grade dysplastic nodules. The optimal treatment guidelines for these nodules remain uncertain, but current management in most centers is similar to that of low-grade dysplastic nodules, with careful follow-up every 6 months by imaging studies until the lesion disappears or progresses. The data are mixed on early ablation or other treatments for high-grade dysplastic nodules, but some centers use ablation therapies (24,25). Classically, macroregenerative nodules and dysplastic nodules have been described as hypovascular or isovascular on imaging studies. Other studies, however, have reported high numbers of hypervascular lesions on imaging studies (26).

DEFINITION OF HEPATOCELLULAR CARCINOMA

Primary liver tumors are hepatocellular carcinomas when they are composed of malignant epithelial cells with hepatocytic differentiation as their main line of differentiation.

There are several terms used to subdivide hepatocellular carcinomas for research purposes. *Small hepatocellular carcinoma* refers to any hepatocellular carcinoma that is less than 2 cm. Some but not all small hepatocellular carcinomas can be further classified as either *early hepatocellular carcinomas* versus *progressed hepatocellular carcinomas*, as detailed below. One example of a small hepatocellular carcinoma that would not fit into either an early or progressed hepatocellular carcinoma category is a small but poorly differentiated hepatocellular carcinoma. Another example is malignant transformation of a hepatocellular adenoma.

For hepatocellular carcinomas that are less than 2 cm, the terms *vaguely nodular hepatocellular carcinoma, small hepatocellular carcinoma with indistinct margins*, and *early hepatocellular carcinoma* are used when the tumor is grossly ill-defined and on histology shows a well-differentiated hepatocellular carcinoma that has focal areas with residual portal tracts, suggesting it arose out of a high-grade dysplastic nodule.

The term *progressed hepatocellular carcinoma* is used for hepatocellular carcinomas that are less than 2 cm but with more distinct gross margins and moderately differentiated histology.

Angiolymphatic invasion is more common than in early hepatocellular carcinomas.

CLINICAL FEATURES

Patients with hepatocellular carcinomas typically present with nonspecific signs and symptoms. Vague abdominal pain, fatigue, and anorexia are the most commonly reported symptoms, while weight loss is the most common sign (27). Many carcinomas are identified in asymptomatic individuals through screening programs focusing on those at high risk for hepatocellular carcinoma. Outside the setting of screening programs, most individuals have advanced disease at the time of clinical presentation.

DEMOGRAPHICS

Hepatocellular carcinomas have been reported at almost all ages and in both genders. However, most hepatocellular carcinomas present clinically after the age of 5 years. Pediatric hepatocellular carcinomas arise primarily in the setting of chronic hepatitis B, especially in hepatitis B endemic areas, or in children with metabolic disease, such as glycogen storage disease or tyrosinemia.

In adults, 80 percent of hepatocellular carcinomas are associated with underlying chronic liver disease. In this setting, the incidence of hepatocellular carcinoma begins to rise around age 40 years and peaks at approximately age 65. Men are at greater risk than women. There is a less striking male predominance for hepatocellular carcinomas in noncirrhotic livers, which are more likely to develop in older individuals (40 percent of patients are age 70 or older) (27–29). The hepatocellular carcinomas in noncirrhotic livers also tend to be larger than those in cirrhotic livers (29).

SERUM FINDINGS

Hepatocellular carcinomas secrete proteins that are detectable in blood and serve as tumor markers. AFP is the best known, but others include lens culinaris agglutinin-reactive AFP (AFP-L3) and des-gamma carboxyprothrombin (DCP). In addition to their historic use in screening and their current use in diagnosis, all of these markers have prognostic value, with positive testing indicating a worse prognosis (30).

Normal serum levels of AFP are less than 20 ng/mL in healthy adults. These levels are elevated in approximately one third of patients with hepatocellular carcinomas, although the frequency varies and is lower in smaller tumors. Serum AFP may also be mildly elevated in inflamed livers that do not have tumors. Because of specificity concerns, serum AFP levels have been dropped as part of the screening strategies proposed by a number of medical groups (31). Significant increases above baseline, however, are strong indicators of hepatocellular carcinoma risk in cirrhotic livers when there is no evidence for a hepatitis flare. As a result, serum AFP is still commonly used as part of the workup of a mass lesion in the liver. Using a cut-off of 20 ng/mL, the sensitivity and specificity for hepatocellular carcinoma in one large multicenter study was 69 and 90 percent, respectively (32). For diagnostic purposes, cut-off values vary in different studies and treatment guidelines, but 400 ng/mL is commonly used as diagnostic of hepatocellular carcinoma in the setting of a radiologically consistent mass lesion.

AFP-L3 is the fraction of AFP that is glycosylated, a form of AFP that is more specific for hepatocellular carcinoma. A cut-off of 10 percent is commonly used, with a sensitivity and specificity for hepatocellular carcinoma of 42 and 97 percent, respectively (32). When levels reach 35 percent, the specificity increases to nearly 100 percent (33).

DCP is an abnormal form of prothrombin that is also known as prothrombin induced by vitamin K absence II (PIVKA II). The sensitivity and specificity for hepatocellular carcinoma are approximately 74 and 70 percent, respectively (32). DCP performs better when viral hepatitis is the cause of the liver disease (32).

ETIOLOGY

Most hepatocellular carcinomas occur because of chronic injury to the liver, with 80 percent developing in cirrhotic livers. The most frequent underlying liver diseases associated with hepatocellular carcinoma are chronic hepatitis B, chronic hepatitis C, and alcohol abuse, with the frequency for each cause varying in different parts of the world (34). Chronic hepatitis B is the most common risk for hepatocellular carcinoma worldwide, with the highest frequency found in Asia. Chronic hepatitis C is currently the most common etiology in the United States, much

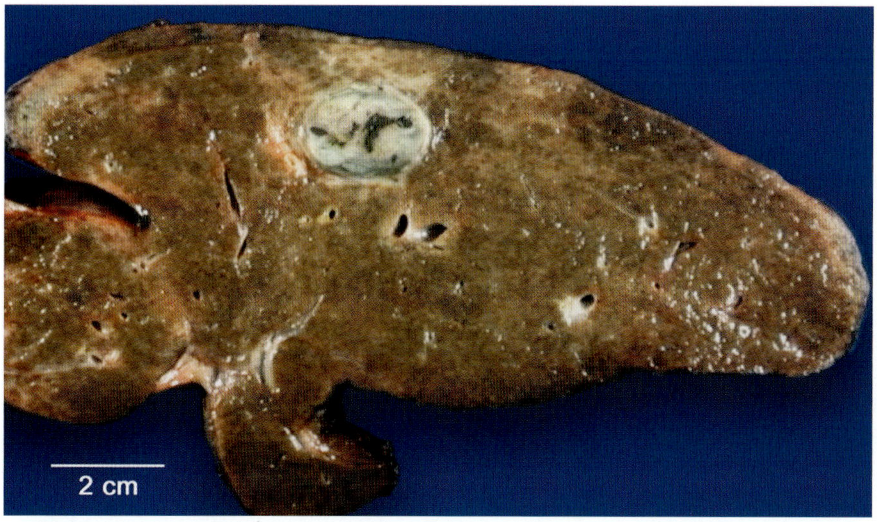

Figure 3-7

HEPATOCELLULAR CARCINOMA

The hepatocellular carcinoma stands out from the background liver.

of Europe, and Japan, but will likely diminish with the new antiviral agents available to treat chronic hepatitis C. Nevertheless, successful treatment of chronic hepatitis C does not completely eliminate the risk of hepatocellular carcinoma (35,36), probably because mutations have already been "locked into" the DNA of hepatocytes and/or stem cells.

The metabolic syndrome and fatty liver disease-associated cirrhosis are growing risk factors throughout the world (37). In parts of Africa, chronic aflatoxin B1 exposure is an important risk factor for hepatocellular carcinoma. Aflatoxin is produced by Aspergillus, a fungus that grows on food stored in warm, damp conditions (38).

Not all forms of cirrhosis carry the same risk of hepatocellular carcinoma. One study found the following 5-year cumulative risk incidences for different causes of cirrhosis: hereditary hemochromatosis (21 percent), chronic hepatitis C (17 percent), chronic hepatitis B virus (10 percent), and biliary cirrhosis (5 percent) (39).

In cirrhotic livers from all causes, other cofactors contribute to hepatocellular carcinoma risk. For example, the metabolic syndrome increases the risk of hepatocellular carcinoma in individuals with chronic viral hepatitis C cirrhosis (40). Alcohol use considerably increases cancer risk for those with chronic viral hepatitis (39). Likewise, hepatic siderosis contributes to cancer development in cirrhotic livers from many causes, even when the underlying liver disease is not genetic hemochromatosis. This risk was demonstrated in a study of over 5,000 explanted livers, where histologic iron deposits were shown to increase the risk of hepatocellular carcinoma, even after adjusting for the major cause of liver disease (41).

For the approximately 20 percent of hepatocellular carcinomas that develop in noncirrhotic livers, about half have a recognized a risk factor and many have mild fibrosis. Most of these risk factors fall into one of these categories: chronic hepatitis B (42), chronic hepatitis C (43), genetic-related iron overload (44), fatty liver disease (45,46), malignant transformation of hepatocellular adenomas (47), or chronic vascular disease (48–50).

GROSS FINDINGS

Hepatocellular carcinomas vary in color from yellow to green to light tan (fig. 3-7), but most are some shade of brown/tan. Tumors with fat tend to be more yellow and those with bile more green. Necrosis and hemorrhage are common and can lead to a variegated appearance. In other cases, different areas of tumor have different colors and should be individually targeted for sectioning. Most hepatocellular carcinomas are soft and bulge out from the cut surface of the liver. In contrast, carcinomas with abundant intratumoral fibrosis can be firm. Some hepatocellular carcinomas, in particular those in cirrhotic livers, have a pseudocapsule of inflamed, fibrotic tissue that clearly separates the tumor from the background liver.

Hepatocellular carcinomas have one of four main growth patterns on gross examination.

In the first pattern, the carcinoma forms a single distinct tumor nodule. In the second pattern, the carcinoma grows as multiple distinct tumor nodules, with a large dominant nodule and multiple smaller "satellite" nodules, usually within 2 cm of the dominant nodule. This pattern results from local spread of the large dominant nodule. The third pattern consists of multiple distinct nodules of hepatocellular carcinoma that are sufficiently separate that they would not be satellite tumors, for example, multiple small carcinomas in both the right and left lobes of the liver. This pattern generally represents foci of independent hepatocellular carcinomas. For tumor staging, separate nodules of carcinoma are considered multifocal disease, whether they are satellite tumors or not. The fourth pattern is the least common, seen in less than 1 percent of cases, and is called "diffuse" or "cirrhotomimetic." The carcinoma grows as many small tumor nodules (dozens to hundreds) that are approximately the same size and shape as cirrhotic nodules. With this growth pattern, the tumor burden is almost always greater than recognized on imaging studies.

Some unifocal hepatocellular carcinomas are pedunculated, protruding from the surface of the liver. In one study, 4 percent of all hepatocellular carcinomas had a pedunculated growth pattern (51). These tumors may have a better prognosis, but data are limited and mixed (51,52). This distinctive gross pattern does not have any unique histologic correlates (53). On imaging studies, pedunculated hepatocellular carcinomas and metastases to the adrenal gland may have a similar appearance (54).

A careful gross examination report comments on the margin, tumor size, percent of tumor necrosis (estimated to the nearest 10 percent), and presence or absence of gross vascular invasion. The margin should be carefully examined for tumor because a positive margin, either grossly or microscopically, carries a greater risk of recurrence (55). For negative margins, the clinical relevance of the distance from tumor to the closest resection margin is not completely resolved (56,57), but it seems prudent to include this measurement in the pathology evaluation. One prospective study found that patients with resections with a 2-cm margin had better disease-free and overall survival rates compared to those with a 1-cm margin (58). Microscopic vascular invasion is a well-recognized risk factor for disease recurrence. The tumor-nontumor interface is the best place to identify vascular invasion. The optimal number of sections to submit on a hepatocellular carcinoma specimen has not been well defined, but the general rule of one section per centimeter of tumor is reasonable as a baseline. Additional sections should be taken as needed depending on gross findings.

MICROSCOPIC FINDINGS

Diagnosis

The hematoxylin and eosin (H&E) findings are the foundation for making a diagnosis of hepatocellular carcinoma. In most cases, these findings are supplemented with immunohistochemistry. Immunohistochemical stains are essentially never interpreted in isolation and should be used with the H&E results: there is great synergy in using them together; synergy that is lost when used separately. Currently, molecular methods have no significant role in the diagnosis of conventional hepatocellular carcinoma for clinical care.

Hepatocellular carcinomas are characterized by architectural and cytologic abnormalities. Identifying these abnormalities is often best approached by examining H&E-stained slides at low-power magnification for populations of cells that look different from the background liver. There are three key architectural changes used to differentiate tumor from nontumor, but do not separate benign from malignant lesions. First, hepatocellular neoplasms do not have normal portal tracts (fig. 3-8). There can be fibrous septa with vascular structures within the tumor, but true portal tracts are absent. Occasionally, hepatocellular carcinomas have entrapped normal portal tracts, usually at the edge of the tumor. However, even in these cases, the lack of normal numbers and spacing of the portal tracts provide important clues that the tissue is neoplastic. The second finding is abnormal arterialization of the hepatic lobules (fig. 3-9). Normally, arterioles are present only in the portal tracts. Hepatocellular neoplasms, however, frequently show small arterioles or unpaired (naked) arteries in the hepatic lobules. This finding, though helpful, should not be used in isolation, as nontumorous hepatic parenchyma can show

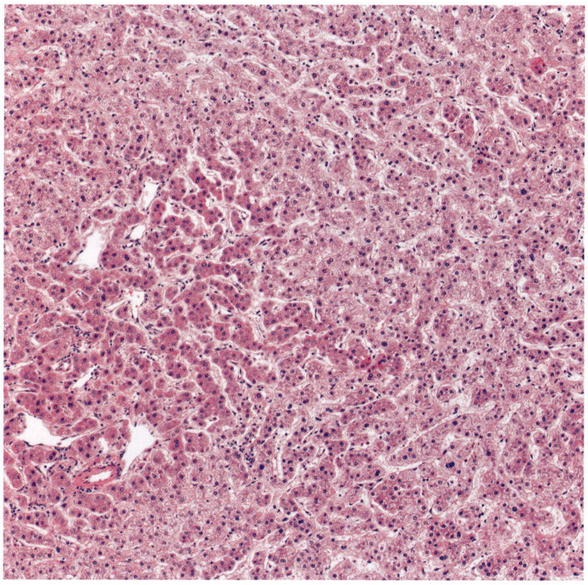

Figure 3-8

HEPATOCELLULAR CARCINOMA: NO PORTAL TRACTS

No portal tracts are seen in this well-differentiated hepatocellular carcinoma.

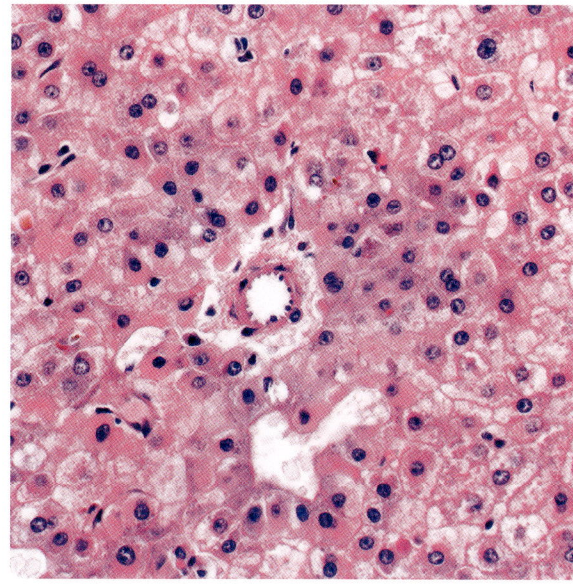

Figure 3-9

HEPATOCELLULAR CARCINOMA: ABNORMAL LOBULAR ARTERY

A naked artery is seen within this well-differentiated hepatocellular carcinoma.

arterialization as well. This occurs when there are vascular flow abnormalities in nonfibrotic livers (fig. 3-10) or with advanced fibrosis. The third architectural feature is abnormal hepatocellular cord organization. In the normal liver, the hepatocellular cords are one to two cells in thickness and are regularly organized. In neoplasms, the cords of hepatocytes often show abnormal growth patterns, including plate thickening and pseudoacinar structures.

Cytologic abnormalities are related to either nuclear or cytoplasmic changes. These changes vary from tumor to tumor, but most hepatocellular carcinomas have at least some of these changes. Nuclear changes include hyperchromasia, nuclear membrane irregularities (fig. 3-11), variation in size, multinucleation (fig. 3-12), and prominent nucleoli. Cytoplasmic changes include reduced cytoplasmic volume, leading to an increased nuclear to cytoplasmic ratio. The cytoplasm often becomes more basophilic when the volume is reduced. Some hepatocellular carcinomas retain abundant pink cytoplasm, but often show increased lipofuscin deposits (fig. 3-13). Other hepatocellular carcinomas have abundant cytoplasm that can be filled with glycogen or show fatty

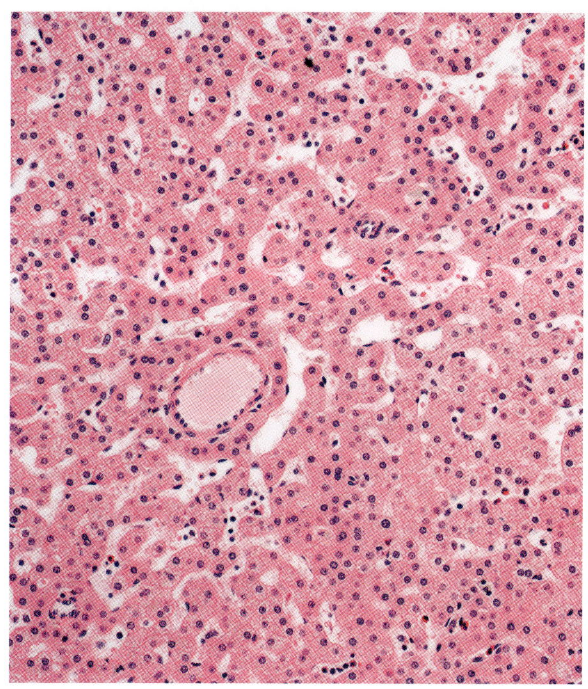

Figure 3-10

ABERRANT ARTERIOLE IN NONTUMOR

Several small arterioles are present in the lobules, even though this is not a biopsy of a tumor. This case had vascular flow abnormalities.

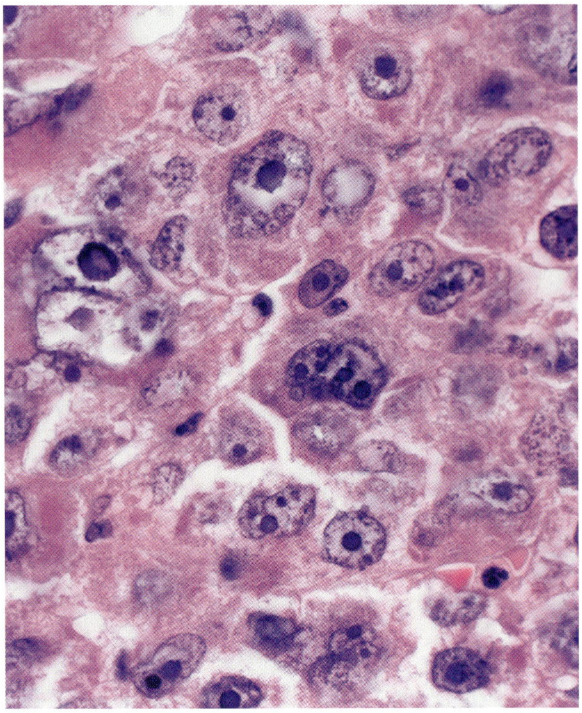

Figure 3-11

HEPATOCELLULAR CARCINOMA: NUCLEAR ABNORMALITIES

This hepatocellular carcinoma shows marked nuclear pleomorphism with variably prominent nucleoli.

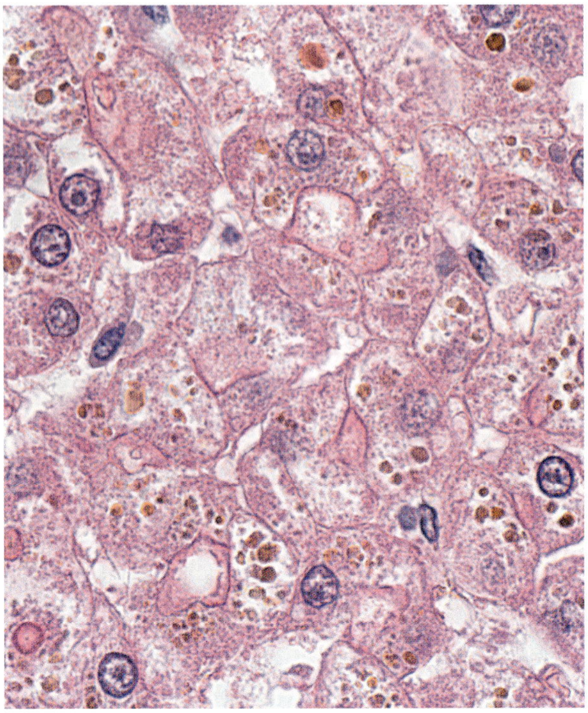

Figure 3-13

HEPATOCELLULAR CARCINOMA: LIPOFUSCIN

The tumor cells have abundant eosinophilic cytoplasm with no significant increase in their nuclear/cytoplasmic ratios. Abundant lipofuscin is also present.

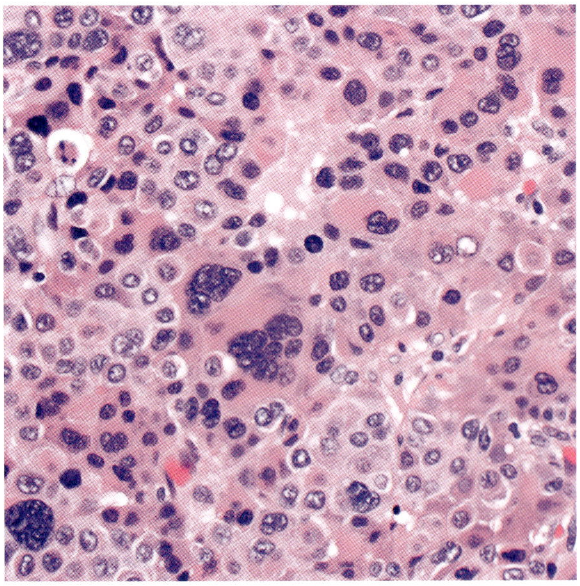

Figure 3-12

HEPATOCELLULAR CARCINOMA: MULTINUCLEATION

Scattered tumor cells are multinucleated.

change. Some hepatocellular carcinomas have distinctive inclusions in their cytoplasm, including hyaline bodies, Mallory-Denk bodies, or pale bodies (figs. 3-14–3-16). Hepatocellular carcinomas with hyaline bodies have a worse prognosis, but there is no known clinical impact for Mallory-Denk bodies or pale bodies.

Growth Patterns

Hepatocellular carcinomas have four major growth patterns (figs. 3-17–3-20) (59): trabecular (70 percent), solid (also known as compact, 20 percent), pseudoglandular (also known as pseudoacinar, 10 percent), and macrotrabecular (1 percent). By custom, each of these patterns is defined solely by the H&E findings. The trabecular growth pattern shows tumor cells growing in trabeculae separated by sinusoidal spaces, while the solid growth pattern shows a sheet-like pattern without well-defined trabeculae. In the pseudoglandular pattern, pseudoglands form when tumor cells cluster around a central

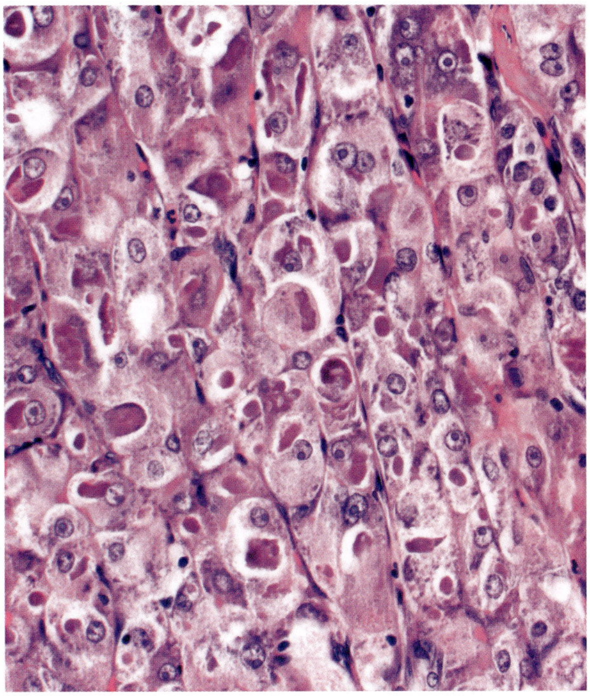

Figure 3-14

HEPATOCELLULAR CARCINOMA: HYALINE BODIES

The hyaline bodies are round to oval and deeply eosinophilic.

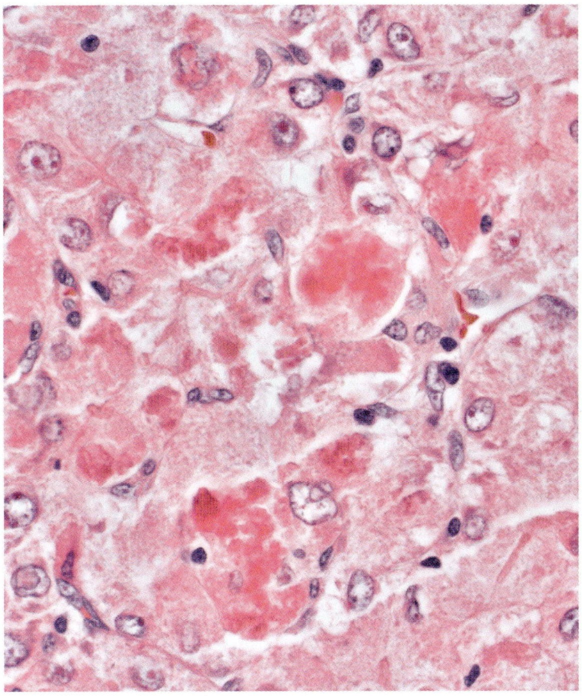

Figure 3-15

HEPATOCELLULAR CARCINOMA: MALLORY-DENK BODIES

The Mallory-Denk bodies are striking.

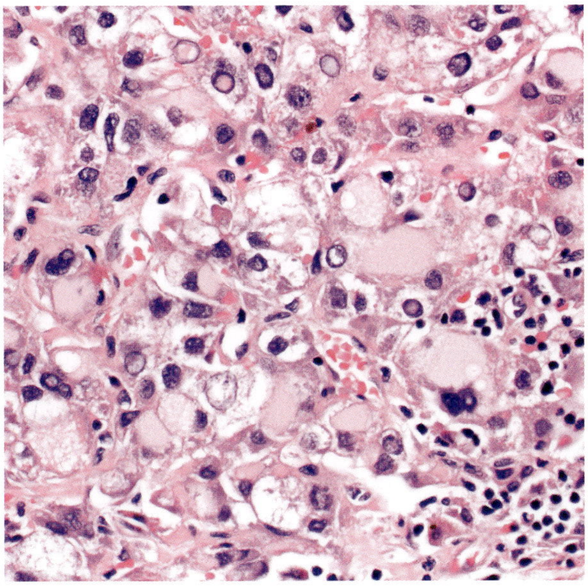

Figure 3-16

HEPATOCELLULAR CARCINOMA: PALE BODIES

Cytoplasmic pale bodies are seen in this conventional hepatocellular carcinoma. The pale bodies are round and amphophilic.

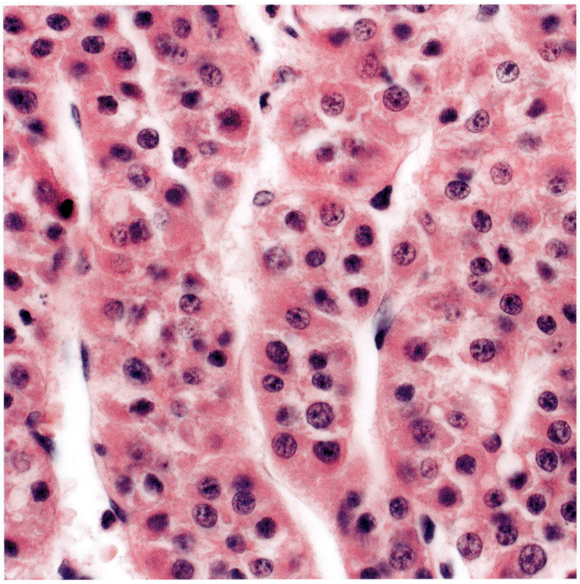

Figure 3-17

HEPATOCELLULAR CARCINOMA: TRABECULAR GROWTH PATTERN

The tumor cells grow as thickened trabeculae.

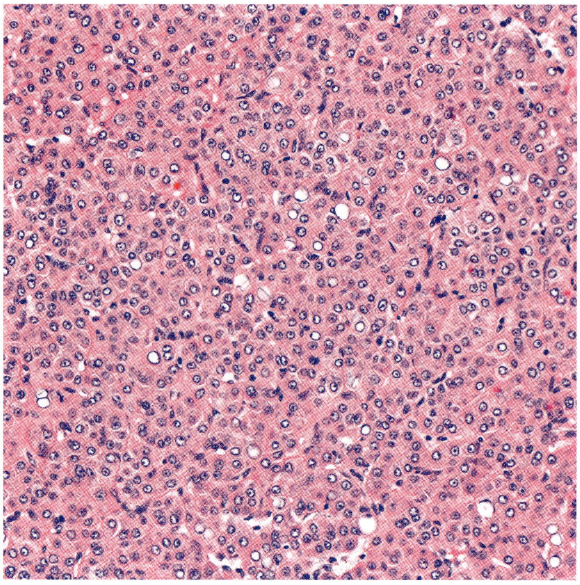

Figure 3-18

HEPATOCELLULAR CARCINOMA: SOLID GROWTH PATTERN

The tumor cells grow as solid sheets.

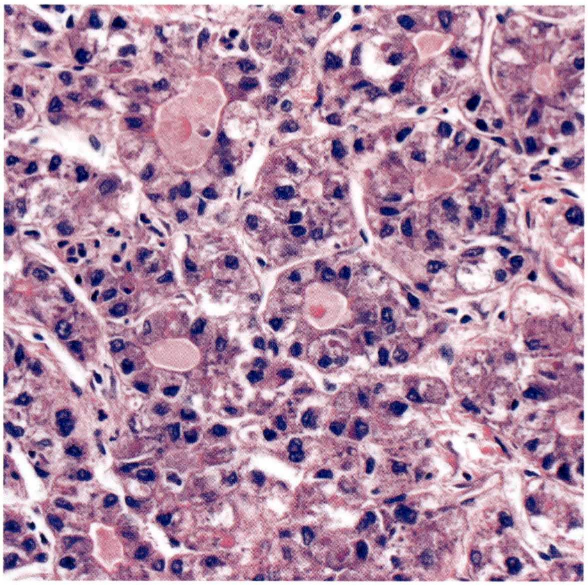

Figure 3-19

HEPATOCELLULAR CARCINOMA: PSEUDOGLANDULAR GROWTH PATTERN

This hepatocellular carcinoma has small pseudoglands formed by rings of hepatocytes around dilated canalicular-type structures.

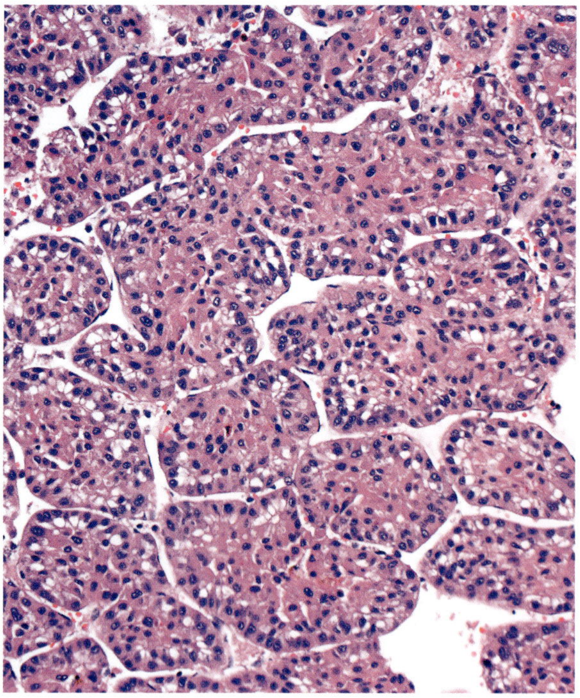

Figure 3-20

HEPATOCELLULAR CARCINOMA: MACROTRABECULAR GROWTH PATTERN

The trabeculae are greatly thickened in this hepatocellular carcinoma.

dilated space, which often contains bile or other inspissated secretions. When pseudoglands are large, they can be filled with thin, granular material, a pattern of growth sometimes called acinar or pseudocyst (fig. 3-21). The macrotrabecular pattern is defined as a tumor showing trabeculae of at least 10 cells in thickness. These growth patterns are different from hepatocellular carcinoma variants, discussed later in this chapter, which can be composed of tumor cells showing any of the four growth patterns.

There are challenges in determining the frequencies of these growth patterns. First, the trabecular and solid growth patterns can be difficult to reliably distinguish. Second, about 50 percent of resection specimens have mixed patterns, usually trabecular plus one or two others. For this reason, the minimum percent needed to score a growth pattern as present can significantly alter results. Third, the macrotrabecular growth pattern is defined differently in various studies, leading to different frequencies. Despite the variable reported frequencies, all studies show that the macrotrabecular growth pattern is the least common. One study found

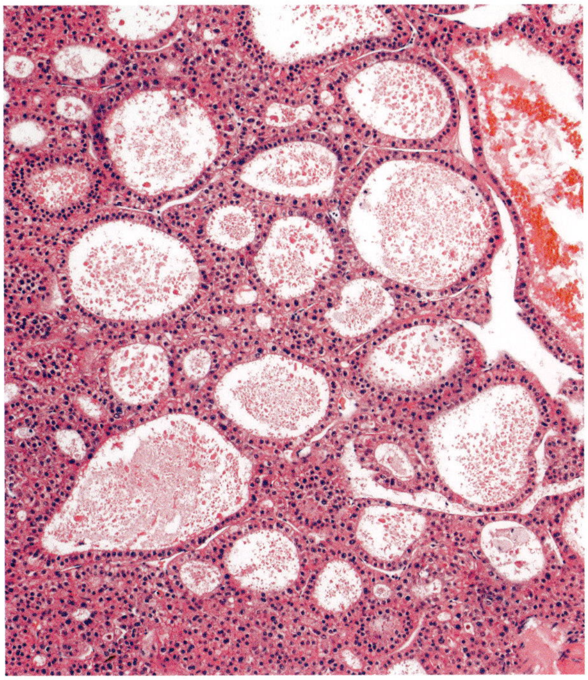

Figure 3-21

HEPATOCELLULAR CARCINOMA: LARGE PSEUDOCYST

The pseudocysts are large and dilated, filled with thin flocculent material.

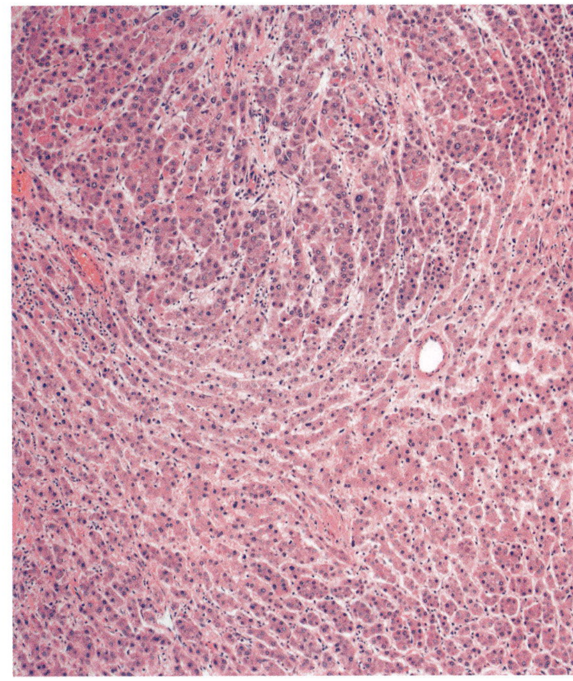

Figure 3-22

HEPATOCELLULAR CARCINOMA: NODULE WITHIN NODULE

A distinct nodule with an increased nuclear/cytoplasmic ratio has developed within the setting of a well-differentiated hepatocellular carcinoma.

that patients with the macrotrabecular pattern have a worse prognosis when compared to those with the solid growth pattern (60). In those cases in which the macrotrabecular pattern is associated with small basophilic tumor cells, serum AFP levels are typically elevated and extensive angiolymphatic invasion is seen.

Other changes can be superimposed on the above growth patterns. A subset of hepatocellular carcinomas has smaller tumor nodules within the main tumor mass, nodules that show distinctly different morphologies from the main tumor, a finding called "nodule within a nodule" (fig. 3-22). In most cases, this appears to represent the emergence of a more aggressive tumor clone, as evidenced by the smaller nodules showing higher-grade cytology. In addition to the nodule within a nodule pattern, other hepatocellular carcinomas have multiple adjacent nodules that have distinctly different morphologies (fig. 3-23). Other findings include peliosis-like areas, with large pools of blood dissecting the tumor trabeculae (fig. 3-24), or large numbers of benign macrophages filling the tumor sinusoids (fig. 3-25). The significance of these latter two changes is unclear. Some hepatocellular carcinomas show bile accumulation within tumor canalicular structures (fig. 3-26).

Changes after Chemoembolization Therapy

With current management algorithms, a large proportion of hepatocellular carcinomas are treated with chemoembolization or ablation prior to resection. This therapy often shrinks the tumor, making a previously unresectable tumor amenable to surgery, and can affect the gross appearance and the microscopic findings. Irrespective of preoperative therapy, hepatocellular carcinomas are staged in the same fashion, but the pathology report should also comment on tumor necrosis. The percent of necrosis should be estimated using the gross and histologic findings; estimations to the nearest 10 percent are a reasonable approach. At a minimum, the pathology report should indicate whether the tumor is 100 percent viable, totally necrotic,

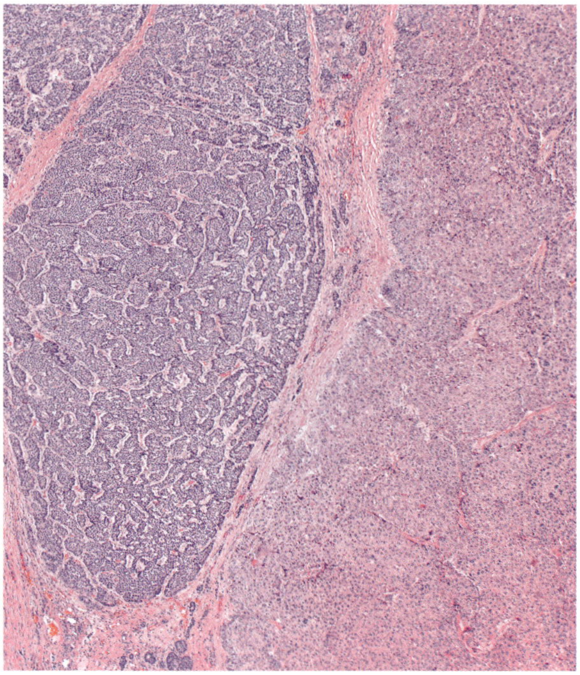

Figure 3-23

HEPATOCELLULAR CARCINOMA:
NODULES WITH DIFFERENT PATTERNS

This hepatocellular carcinoma has multiple nodules with distinct morphologic patterns.

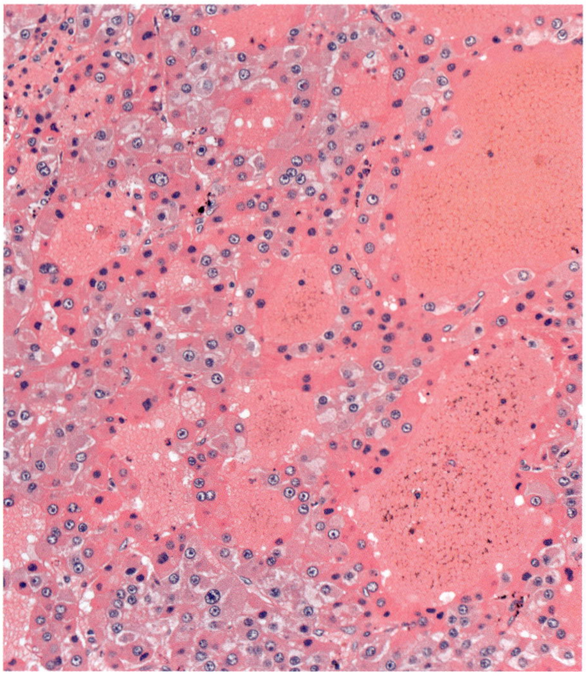

Figure 3-24

HEPATOCELLULAR CARCINOMA:
PELIOSIS-LIKE CHANGES

The tumor sinusoids are markedly dilated and congested.

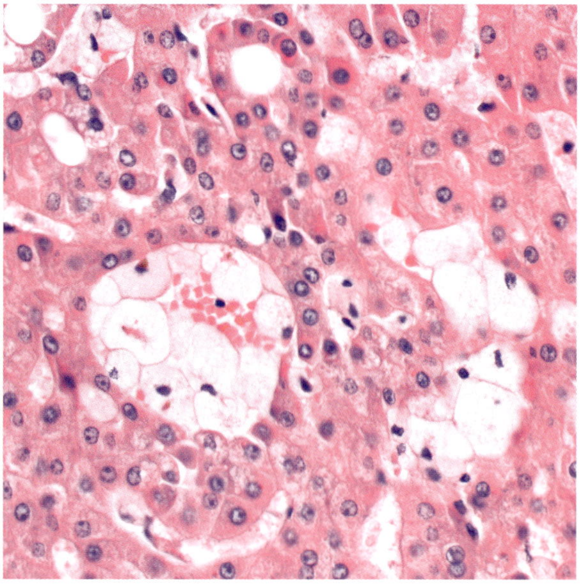

Figure 3-25

HEPATOCELLULAR CARCINOMA:
MACROPHAGES IN SINUSOIDS

Distinct clusters of benign macrophages are seen within the tumor sinusoids.

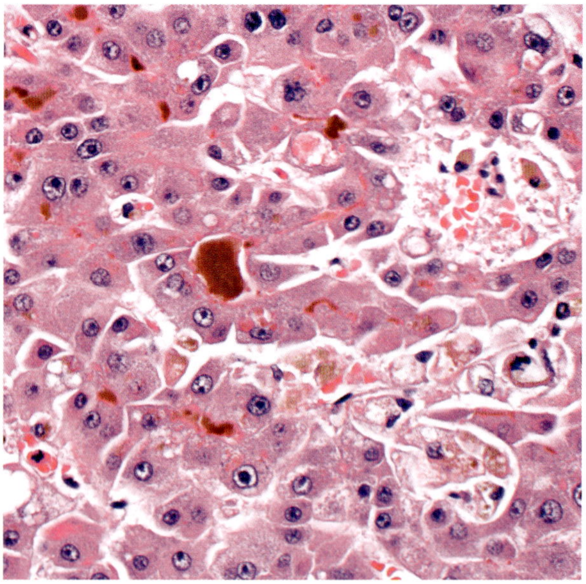

Figure 3-26

HEPATOCELLULAR CARCINOMA: BILE PRODUCING

This hepatocellular carcinoma produces bile that is retained in the tumor canalicular structures.

Table 3-1

MODIFIED EDMONDSON-STEINER GRADING SYSTEM FOR HEPATOCELLULAR CARCINOMA

Grade	Criteria
1	Abundant cytoplasm; minimal nuclear atypia
2	Mild nuclear atypia with prominent nucleoli, hyperchromasia, and nuclear irregularity
3	Moderate nuclear atypia with greater hyperchromasia and nuclear irregularity
4	Marked nuclear pleomorphism, marked hyperchromasia, and anaplastic giant cells

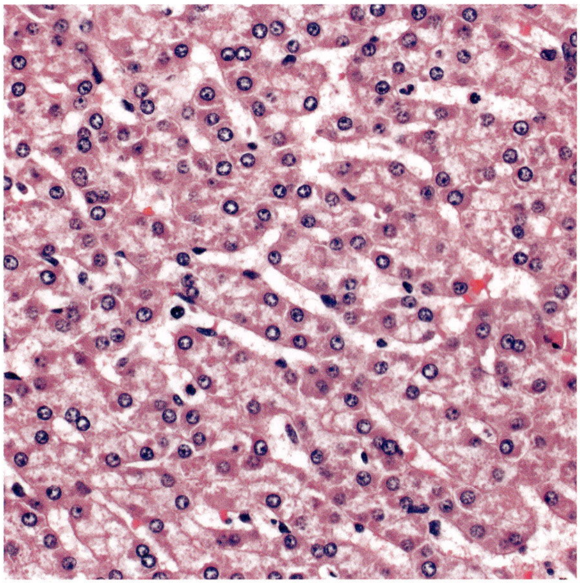

Figure 3-27

HEPATOCELLULAR CARCINOMA: VERY WELL DIFFERENTIATED

This hepatocellular carcinoma closely resembles an adenoma, with no significant nuclear pleomorphism. A slight increase in the nuclear/cytoplasmic ratio is evident.

or has some necrosis present with viable tumor. When estimating the percent of tumor necrosis, there is no reliable way to distinguish treatment-related necrosis from spontaneous tumor necrosis and all necrosis is included in the estimate. Embolic beads can also be seen in the tumor and often in the adjacent nontumor liver.

Treatment can lead to other histologic changes beyond necrosis, including increased intratumoral inflammation and intratumoral fibrosis. Treatment can increase the expression of CK19 and lead to areas of growth with a biliary and/or spindled cell morphology (61,62). The potential effect of treatment on tumor grade has not been well studied.

Evaluating the Background Liver

When evaluating resection specimens, sections from the background liver are needed to assess for ongoing liver disease and fibrosis. Of note, sections for this purpose should avoid the non-tumor boundary with the hepatocellular carcinoma, which can be secondarily inflamed and fibrotic because of proximity to the tumor. Sections of the background liver should be taken as far away from the tumor as possible, ideally at least 1 cm. Sections taken to evaluate the background liver should also avoid areas with cautery effect.

HISTOLOGIC GRADING

Hepatocellular carcinomas are graded for prognosis, as tumor grade predicts overall patient survival and disease-free survival in all major clinical settings when the tumor is resected with curative intent, including after resections in cirrhotic (63,64) and noncirrhotic livers (65), and after liver transplantation (63,66). Tumor grade has several important correlates, including tumor size and angiolymphatic invasion, but has independent prognostic value.

In research studies, the Edmondson-Steiner grading system and the modified Edmonson-Steiner grading system are the most frequently used grading schemes (Table 3-1) (59). When a tumor has two or more nuclear grades, the predominant tumor grade and the worst tumor grade should be reported. The worst grade tends to drive prognosis (67).

While the Edmondson-Steiner grading system works reasonably well for research, grading in clinical practice is more commonly based on a three-tier system: well-differentiated, moderately differentiated, and poorly differentiated tumors. Some pathologists use additional categories on either or both ends of the spectrum: very well differentiated and undifferentiated. By common practice, tumors that are very well differentiated should appear "adenoma-like" (fig. 3-27), with only focal reticulin loss and mild cytologic atypia. Well-differentiated hepatocellular carcinomas show definite and convincing hepatocellular differentiation on H&E-stained

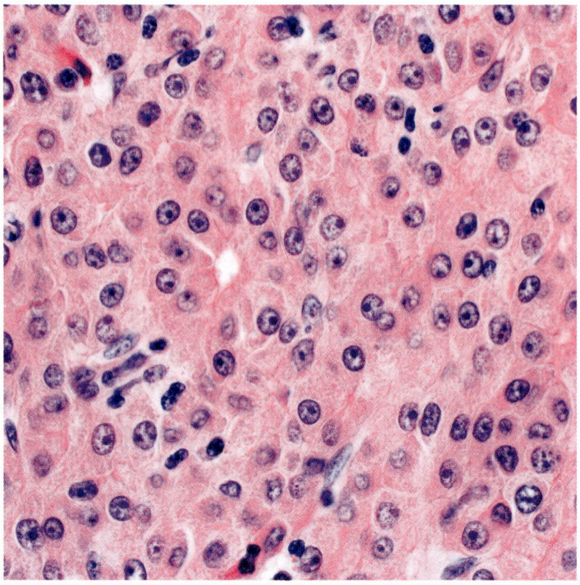

Figure 3-28

HEPATOCELLULAR CARCINOMA: WELL DIFFERENTIATED

Nuclear atypia is minimal and the cells have abundant eosinophilic cytoplasm. The tumor nuclei lack the regular, orderly spacing of benign proliferations.

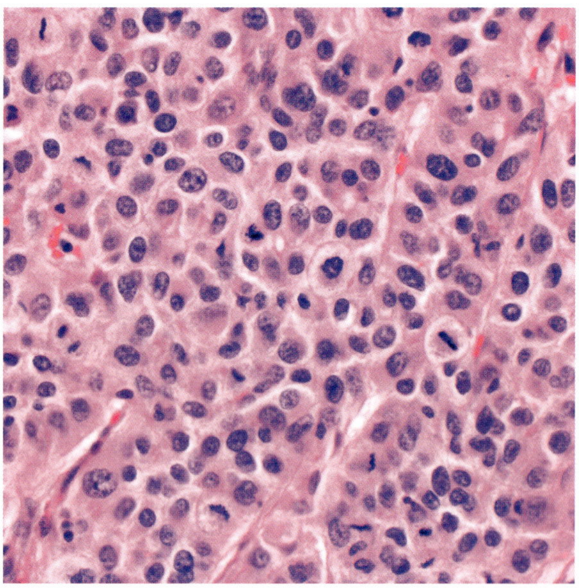

Figure 3-29

HEPATOCELLULAR CARCINOMA: MODERATELY DIFFERENTIATED

Nuclear atypia is striking, but the tumor shows morphologic evidence of hepatocellular differentiation with a trabecular growth pattern and abundant, granular, eosinophilic cytoplasm.

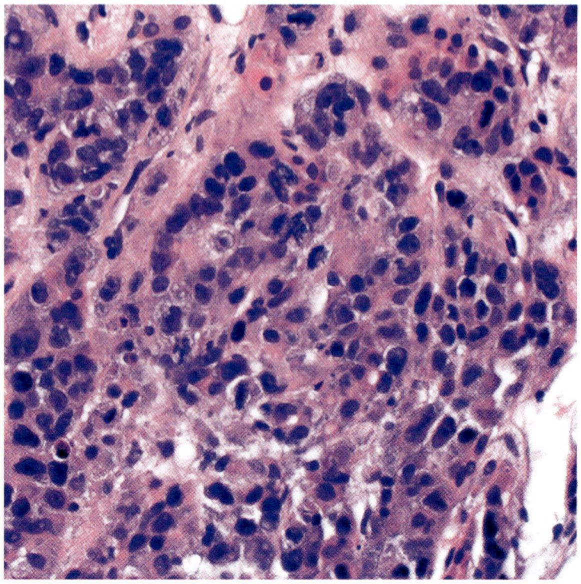

Figure 3-30

HEPATOCELLULAR CARCINOMA: POORLY DIFFERENTIATED

This poorly differentiated hepatocellular carcinoma can be confidently classified only with special stains.

slides, and additional stains are necessary to make sure the tumors are malignant (fig. 3-28).

Clearly, there is significant potential overlap between very well and well-differentiated hepatocellular carcinomas, with the extent of cytologic atypia the main differentiating feature. Moderately differentiated hepatocellular carcinomas are clearly malignant on H&E-stained slides and the overall morphology strongly suggests a hepatocellular origin, but stains are helpful to confirm hepatocellular differentiation (fig. 3-29). Poorly differentiated hepatocellular carcinomas are also clearly malignant with H&E, but the morphology is consistent with a range of poorly differentiated carcinomas, and immunostains are needed to confirm hepatocellular differentiation (fig. 3-30). Undifferentiated carcinomas of the liver have no morphologic features of hepatocellular differentiation or glandular differentiation with H&E, and stains are needed to prove that the neoplasm is epithelial, as the H&E differential diagnosis includes lymphoma, melanoma, and mesenchymal tumors. Undifferentiated carcinomas are keratin positive but lack expression of hepatocellular markers such as HepPar1, arginase, and glypican 3. Such tumors

Table 3-2

STAINS THAT HELP DISTINGUISH BENIGN FROM MALIGNANT HEPATOCYTIC LESIONS

Stains	Comment
Reticulin	Rarely, well-differentiated hepatocellular carcinomas have no obvious reticulin loss
Ki-67	Most helpful if significantly higher than background liver; not all hepatocellular carcinomas have a high proliferative rate
CD34	Strong diffuse staining is more common in hepatocellular carcinoma than in an adenoma, but there is considerable overlap
Glypican 3	Positive in about 50 percent of well-differentiated hepatocellular carcinomas; also stains lipofuscin, benign hepatocytes with significant inflammation (focal), some inflammatory adenomas (focal), and some dysplastic nodules
Alpha-fetoprotein	Positive in about one third of all hepatocellular carcinomas

Table 3-3

STAINS THAT HELP DEMONSTRATE HEPATOCELLULAR DIFFERENTIATION IN AN OBVIOUS MALIGNANCY[a]

Stains	Comment
Arginase 1	Positive in 90% of all hepatocellular carcinomas; poorly differentiated hepatocellular carcinomas are most likely to be negative; negative in 10% of well-differentiated hepatocellular carcinomas
HepPar1	Positive in 90% of all hepatocellular carcinomas
Glypican 3	Positive in 80-90% of hepatocellular carcinomas
In situ hybridization for albumin	Positive in >95% of hepatocellular carcinomas and about 80-95% of cholangiocarcinomas
Polyclonal CEA[b] (canalicular pattern)	Positive in 60-80% of hepatocellular carcinomas; the stain tends to be more confusing than helpful in poorly differentiated carcinomas
CD10 (canalicular pattern)	Performance is similar to that of polyclonal CEA
Alpha-fetoprotein	Positive in about one third of hepatocellular carcinomas

[a]None of these stains are 100% specific and all are best used in combination with clinical findings and H&E morphology.
[b]CEA = carcinoembryonic antigen.

are rare, but the differential for undifferentiated carcinomas includes cholangiocarcinoma and metastatic neoplasm. Once metastatic neoplasm is excluded by imaging studies and immunohistochemistry, these tumors can be classified as primary to the liver.

IMMUNOHISTOCHEMICAL FINDINGS

Special stains are used in two distinctly different situations when evaluating liver tumors. The first is to decide whether a tumor that is clearly hepatic on the H&E stain is benign or malignant. The second situation is to decide whether a clearly malignant tumor is hepatocellular carcinoma, cholangiocarcinoma, or another malignant neoplasm.

Stains that are useful in the first setting are shown in Table 3-2. The differential for a tumor in a noncirrhotic liver is focal nodular hyperplasia, hepatocellular adenoma, and hepatocellular carcinoma. In a cirrhotic liver, the differential diagnosis changes to focal nodular hyperplasia-like lesion, macroregenerative nodule, dysplastic nodule, and hepatocellular carcinoma. Some nodules in cirrhotic livers express C-reactive protein (CRP) or serum amyloid A (SAA) (68,69), but the term hepatocellular adenoma for these lesions is best avoided, both because it leads to unnecessary confusion for the clinical team and because there is no evidence that such lesions behave clinically like a hepatocellular adenoma.

In the second setting, the H&E findings clearly show a malignant neoplasm, but the question is what type of malignancy. A diagnosis of hepatocellular carcinoma depends on detecting proteins or RNA transcripts that indicate hepatocellular differentiation. The most commonly used stains are shown in Table 3-3.

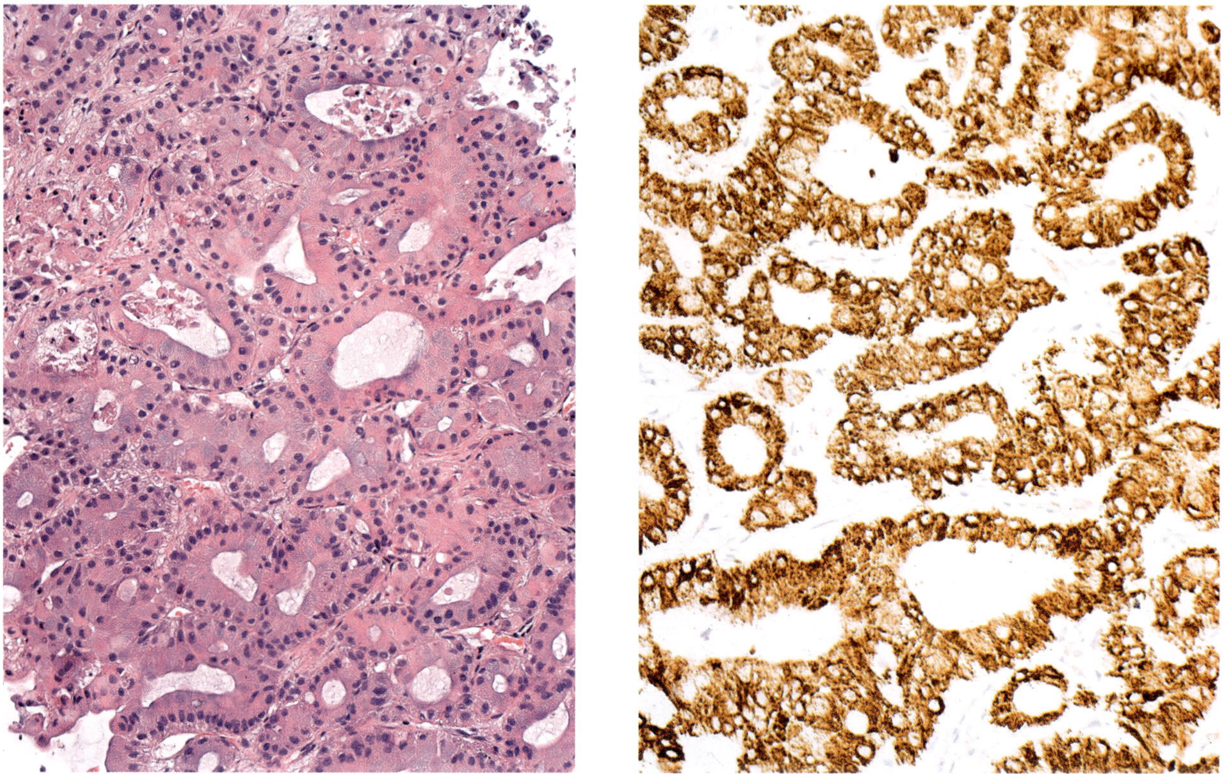

Figure 3-31

ADENOCARCINOMA METASTATIC TO THE LIVER

Left: The morphologic findings are clearly that of an adenocarcinoma.

Right: An immunostain for HepPar1 is positive, but there is no diagnostic dilemma when the morphology (see left) is incorporated into the stain's interpretation.

Laws of Immunohistochemistry

When applying immunohistochemical stains in diagnostic pathology, there are four fundamental, immutable laws governing their use.

Law 1. *All special stains should be used in conjunction with the H&E findings.* Immunostains are very powerful, an exciting part of the current and future practice of modern surgical pathology. But even with this bright future, we should not forget the past, anchoring our interpretation of immunostains to the morphology evident with the use of H&E. The powers of immunostains are greatly amplified when they are used with the H&E findings. The medical literature is rich with reports showing that a subset of neoplasms from all over the body can be positive for the key markers of hepatocellular differentiation, including albumin in situ hybridization, glypican 3, HepPar1, and arginase 1. This of course is a problem for those pathologists who don't use the H&E morphology and rely on a single immunostain to make their diagnosis. However, these observations do not strongly reduce the value of these stains, as most of the tumors from other organs that stain for these hepatic markers do not look like hepatocellular carcinoma on the H&E slide (fig. 3-31). Likewise, the wise pathologist evaluates cases that show more challenging morphology with multiple markers to rule in hepatocytic differentiation and multiple markers to rule out other tumors. Correlation of the H&E results with positive immunostains is also important because sometimes entrapped hepatocytes within a metastatic tumor can stain strongly with hepatocytic markers, which can be misinterpreted as evidence for hepatocytic differentiation within the tumor (fig. 3-32). The incorporation of clinical and radiologic findings is also critical for proper tumor evaluation.

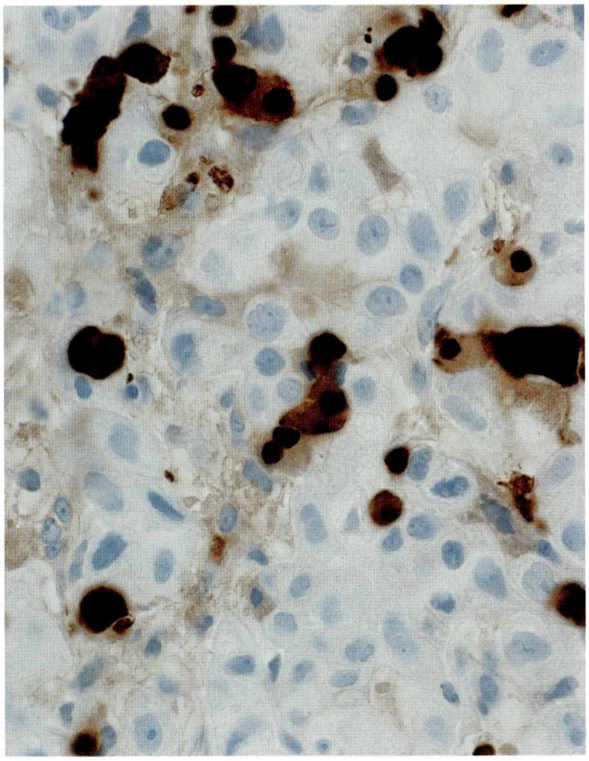

Figure 3-32

METASTATIC CARCINOMA TO THE LIVER: ARGINASE 1

The positive staining in this section is only within entrapped hepatocytes.

Law 2. *The sensitivity and specificity of immunostains invariably get worse as more studies are done.* The first study is the best. As additional studies look at a wider range of tumors, the performance of stains diminishes, and the sensitivity and the specificity fall. A given stain's performance can also be influenced by differences in staining platforms and other laboratory practices, so internal validation of a stain's performance is very important.

Several tumor-specific factors can strongly affect the results of studies of immunostains used to demonstrate hepatocytic differentiation, including the most commonly used markers glypican 3, HepPar1 and arginase. These factors include tumor grade, the type of underlying liver disease, and the presence or absence of cirrhosis. As one example, glypican 3 is more likely to be positive in hepatocellular carcinomas arising in cirrhotic livers than in noncirrhotic livers (70). Specific subtypes of hepatocellular carcinoma also have different staining characteristics. This can be seen, for example, with scirrhous hepatocellular carcinomas, which have the lowest frequency of positivity for HepPar1 (71).

Many papers report a statistical superiority of one stain over another, but such data should be interpreted cautiously as results can be influenced by the degree of differentiation, underlying liver disease, and other tumor-specific factors. Thus, laboratory decisions on adding a new stain or dropping an old stain should be made cautiously in the first several years after a new stain is reported. Currently, most expert liver pathologists rely on a panel of the top performing stains to document hepatocytic differentiation in their daily practice, as wisely chosen stains will complement each other, helping to mitigate individual weaknesses.

Law 3. *In cases for which there is a discrepancy between the morphology and immunohistochemical findings, additional studies must be performed.* The diagnostic path is easily lost when one discrepant result is arbitrarily chosen over another. In this situation, review of the H&E results is critical. Resection specimens often benefit from submitting more sections. The discrepant immunostain can also be repeated to make sure the result is reproducible. Additional immunostains are often needed to clarify the diagnosis.

Law 4. *A difficult case is simply the wrong time to first use a stain you're not familiar with.* There are many shipwrecks in uncharted waters. Before using a stain, it is important to understand how the stain performs in typical cases, in variants, and in tumors that commonly enter the differential diagnosis. Once you have charted these familiar waters, then you will be ready to use the test in more challenging cases. Also, once you start using an immunostain, you should use it often enough to maintain skill in its interpretation.

Cytokeratin and Other Stains

Essentially all hepatocellular carcinomas are positive for CK8 and CK18. CAM5.2, which targets CK8 and to a lesser degree CK7, is also positive in essentially all hepatocellular carcinomas (72). CK7 staining is found in 20 to 40 percent of hepatocellular carcinomas (73,74) while CK20 positivity is seen in 5 percent (fig. 3-33). Interestingly, CK20 staining almost always occurs with CK7 positivity. CK19 expression is an

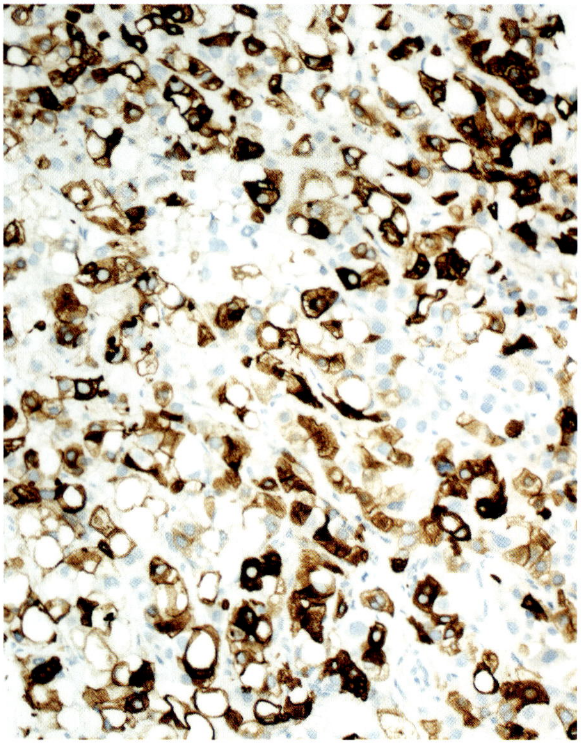

Figure 3-33

HEPATOCELLULAR CARCINOMA: CK20

CK20 staining is patchy but strong.

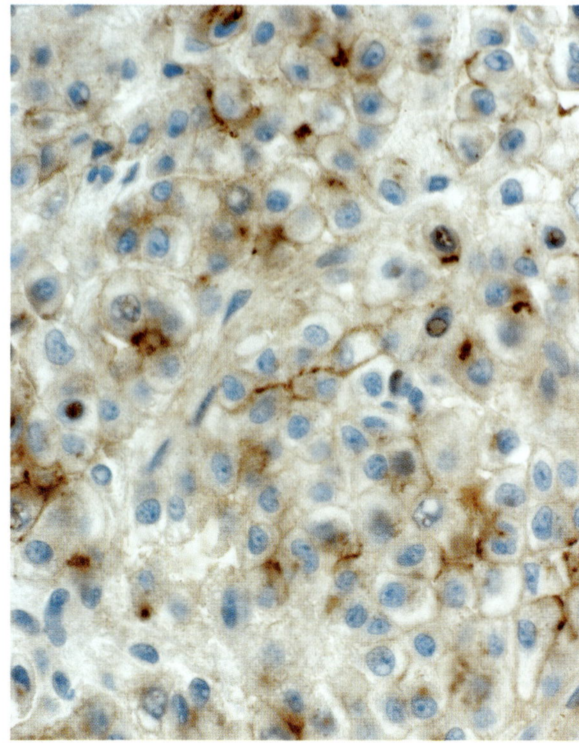

Figure 3-34

HEPATOCELLULAR CARCINOMA: POLYCLONAL CARCINOEMBRYONIC ANTIGEN

This moderately differentiated hepatocellular carcinoma shows focal canalicular staining.

indicator of a worse prognosis and is found in 10 to 15 percent of hepatocellular carcinomas (73–75). Similar to CK20 expression, hepatocellular carcinomas that express CK19 are usually CK7 positive (73,74). CK5/6 is negative in most hepatocellular carcinomas (76), while AE1/AE3 is positive in about 15 percent of cases (77).

A wide variety of immunostains is frequently used to work up poorly differentiated tumors, including various markers of epithelial differentiation and markers of cell lineage. Table 3-4 shows the frequency of positive staining in hepatocellular carcinomas for some of the more commonly used stains.

Stains to Identify Hepatocytic Differentiation

AFP, CD10, and polyclonal CEA (pCEA) have largely been replaced by more sensitive markers of hepatocytic differentiation: HepPar1, glypican 3, arginase 1, and albumin in situ hybridization. None of these stains is perfect and difficult cases are often best approached using multiple stains.

CD10 and pCEA. CD10 and pCEA have sensitivities for hepatocellular carcinoma of about 55 percent and 75 percent, respectively. A canalicular staining pattern is needed to specifically indicate hepatocytic differentiation (fig. 3-34). About one third of the hepatocellular carcinomas with canalicular staining also show cytoplasmic or membranous staining. As long as some convincing canalicular staining is seen, the results support a diagnosis of hepatocellular carcinoma. An additional 10 to 15 percent of hepatocellular carcinomas lack the canalicular staining pattern and instead show only membranous or cytoplasmic staining (fig. 3-35), a pattern acceptable for a diagnosis of hepatocellular carcinoma, but not specific for hepatocytic differentiation.

Both CD10 and pCEA canalicular staining is most likely to be seen in well-differentiated and moderately differentiated hepatocellular carcinomas, but they perform badly in poorly differentiated hepatocellular carcinomas. Even when

Table 3-4

FREQUENCY OF POSITIVITY FOR NONHEPATOCELLULAR MARKERS IN HEPATOCELLULAR CARCINOMA

Immunostain	Approximate Frequency	Comments
Epithelial markers		
CAM5.2[a]	>99%	
Cytokeratin AE1/AE3	15%	
CK19	15%	Positive tumors have a worse prognosis; positive cases typically coexpress CK7
CK7	30%	Hepatocellular carcinomas that are cholestatic or occur in younger individuals (<40 years) are positive in the majority of cases
CK20	5%	Positive cases typically coexpress CK7
CK5/6	1%	
EMA	5%	
Stains for site of origin		
CDX2	5%	Staining is focal in hepatocellular carcinoma; 20-30% of cholangiocarcinomas are CDX2 positive
TTF1	0%	TTF1 can show cytoplasmic staining with some antibodies, but not nuclear staining
PAX8	0%	Limited data
SALL4	45%	May be a marker of "stemness"
Villin	30%	Staining is typically strong and cytoplasmic and can have a membranous accentuation
Stains commonly used to evaluate for mesothelioma		
MOC31	35%	Usually focal; strong diffuse staining is seen in many cholangiocarcinomas
WT1	>80%	
Calretinin	0%	Limited data
D240	0%	Limited data
Stains used to subtype hepatocellular adenomas		
LFABP	20%	
CRP	50%	
SAA	15%	
Beta-catenin (nuclear)	30%	
Glutamine synthetase	50%	
Nonepithelial markers		
CD117 (C-KIT)	70%	
CD138	65%	Non-neoplastic hepatocytes are also positive; membranous staining is seen in both tumor and nontumor
Vimentin	10%	About 10% of typical hepatocellular carcinomas are positive. Vimentin expression is associated with more aggressive behavior and with epithelial to mesenchymal transition; sarcomatoid hepatocellular carcinomas are positive in most cases

[a]CAM = cell adhesion molecule; EMA = epithelial membrane antigen; TTF = thyroid transcription factor; LFABP = liver fatty acid binding protein; CRP = C reactive protein; SAA = serum amyloid A.

positive in poorly differentiated hepatocellular carcinomas, a canalicular staining pattern is often focal and equivocal, making it difficult to identify with much confidence, and leading to significant inter- and intraobserver variability. For these reasons, these two stains have largely been replaced by better markers.

HepPar1. HepPar1 is directed against carbamoyl phosphate synthetase 1, a mitochondrial protein in the urea cycle (78). Positivity is seen in 85 to 95 percent of hepatocellular carcinomas, with a granular cytoplasmic staining pattern (fig. 3-36) (79,80). Benign liver tissue is strongly and diffusely positive, while staining can be focal within hepatocellular carcinomas. HepPar1 performs best in well- and moderately differentiated hepatocellular carcinomas, with reduced sensitivity in poorly differentiated tumors.

A number of carcinomas from other sites can be HepPar1 positive (81): gastric adenocarcinomas (up to 40 percent), ovarian clear cell and ovarian mucinous carcinoma (up to 35 percent each), adrenal cortical carcinoma (up to 15 percent), lung adenocarcinoma (up to 15 percent),

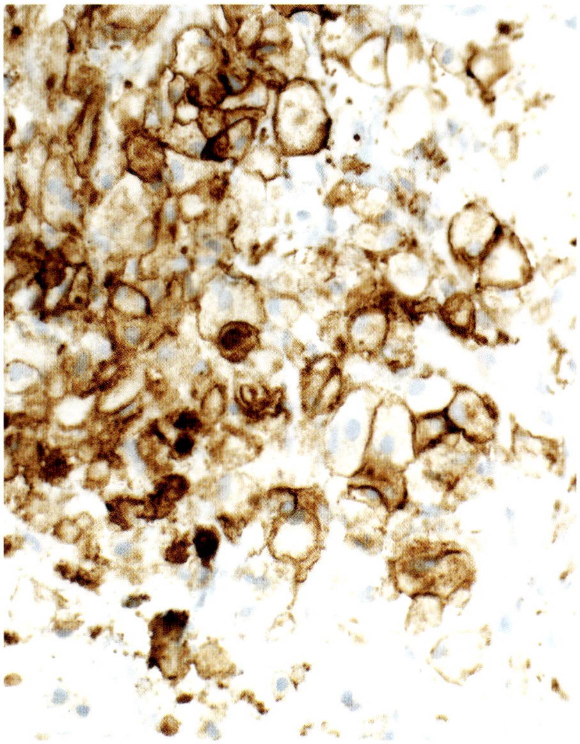

Figure 3-35

HEPATOCELLULAR CARCINOMA: CD10 WITH NONCANALICULAR STAINING

Membranous and cytoplasmic staining are seen, but there is no compelling evidence for canalicular staining.

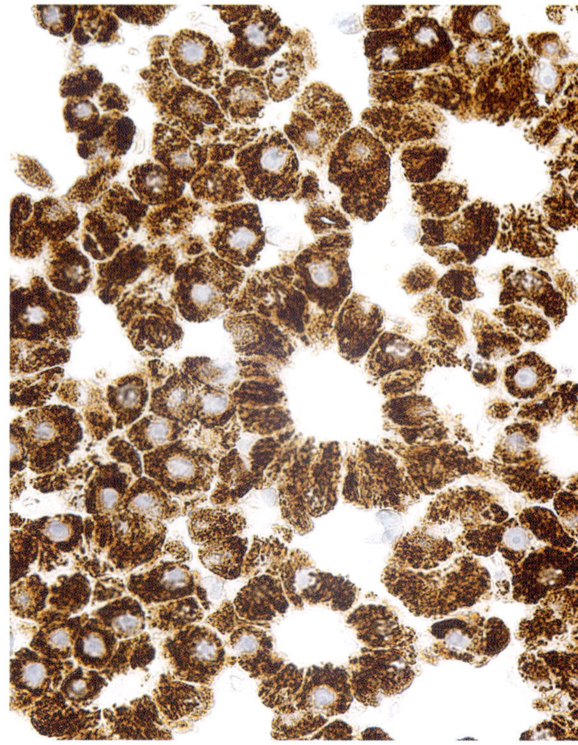

Figure 3-36

HEPATOCELLULAR CARCINOMA: HEPPAR1

A HepPar1 stain shows strong cytoplasmic granular staining.

cholangiocarcinoma (up to 10 percent), and neuroendocrine carcinoma (up to 10 percent). In most cases, these carcinomas do not look like hepatocellular carcinoma on the H&E-stained slide, so there is little risk of confusion. However, there can be challenges with ovarian clear cell carcinomas, neuroendocrine carcinomas, and adrenal cortical carcinomas, all of which can resemble hepatocellular carcinoma on the H&E. This problem is mitigated by incorporating the clinical and imaging findings and by the wise use of a panel of immunostains to both rule in hepatocellular carcinoma and rule out potential mimics, as suggested by the clinical, radiologic, or morphologic findings.

Glypican 3. Cytoplasmic staining supports hepatocellular differentiation when used in association with H&E morphology (fig. 3-37). Compatible morphology is critical to interpreting the glypican 3 stain, as many carcinomas from other organs can be positive, including yolk sac tumors (95 to 100 percent), squamous cell carcinoma of the lung (50 percent), chromophobe renal carcinoma (40 percent), and cholangiocarcinoma (10 percent) (82).

Overall, 80 to 90 percent of hepatocellular carcinomas are positive for glypican 3, but staining is often focal, and some studies show that only 50 percent of biopsies and fine-needle aspirates are positive (83). Tumor grade also strongly influences the stain's performance, as only 50 percent of well-differentiated hepatocellular carcinomas are positive. The frequency of glypican 3 staining is also lower in hepatocellular carcinomas arising in noncirrhotic livers (84) and in the scirrhous variant of hepatocellular carcinoma (71). On the other hand, glypican 3 performs very well in poorly differentiated carcinomas and in hepatitis B-related hepatocellular carcinomas (85).

Glypican 3 is negative in normal hepatocytes, so positive staining is concerning for hepatocellular carcinoma. There are several caveats, however. First, the non-neoplastic liver tissue can be focally positive when there is significant

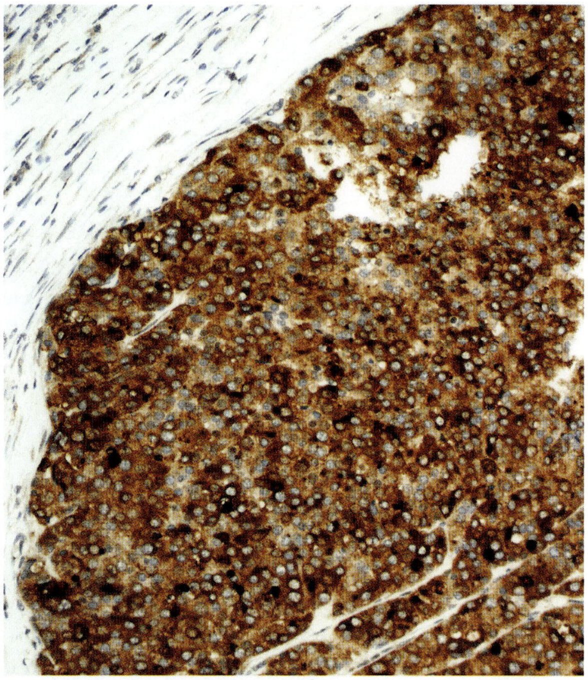

Figure 3-37

HEPATOCELLULAR CARCINOMA: GLYPICAN 3

An immunostain for glypican 3 shows strong cytoplasmic staining.

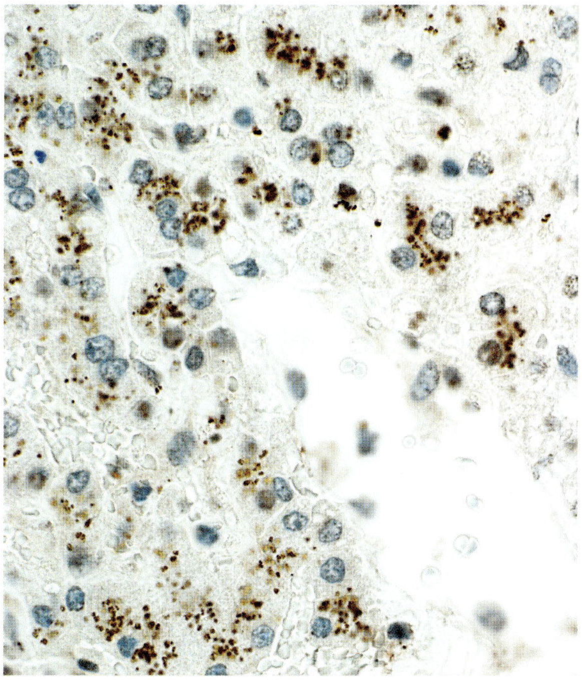

Figure 3-38

BENIGN HEPATOCYTES WITH LIPOFUSCIN: GLYPICAN 3

Mild lipofuscin deposits in this HNF1 alpha-inactivated hepatocellular adenoma are highlighted by a glypican 3 stain, which may result an overdiagnosis of hepatocellular carcinoma.

inflammation (86). Second, focal nodular hyperplasias and hepatocellular adenomas are negative for strong and diffuse staining (84,87,88). However, otherwise typical inflammatory adenomas rarely show weak focal staining. Third, glypican 3 stains lipofuscin (fig. 3-38) and the H&E results should be double checked to make sure that positive glypican 3 staining in a tumor is not due to lipofuscin deposition. Finally, macroregenerative nodules and dysplastic nodules in cirrhotic livers can be focally glypican 3 positive (84), so a diagnosis of carcinoma should not rely solely on glypican 3 staining in this situation.

Arginase 1. Arginase 1 is positive in benign and malignant hepatocytes (89). Positive staining can be cytoplasmic or nuclear (fig. 3-39). Arginase 1 tends to perform better than HepPar1 in poorly differentiated hepatocellular carcinomas, but performs worse in well-differentiated tumors, which are almost all HepPar1 positive, but about 10 percent are arginase 1 negative (fig. 3-40). Both arginase 1 and HepPar1 are positive in hepatoid adenocarcinomas from many sites (90). Other tumors that can be arginase 1

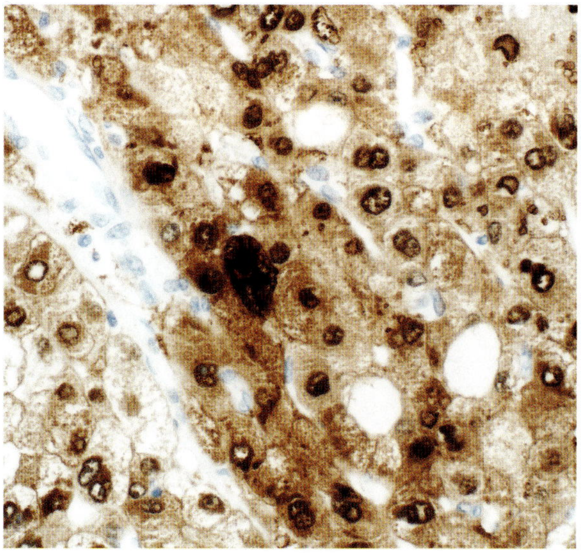

Figure 3-39

HEPATOCELLULAR CARCINOMA: ARGINASE 1

Nuclear and cytoplasmic staining are evident in a hepatocellular carcinoma.

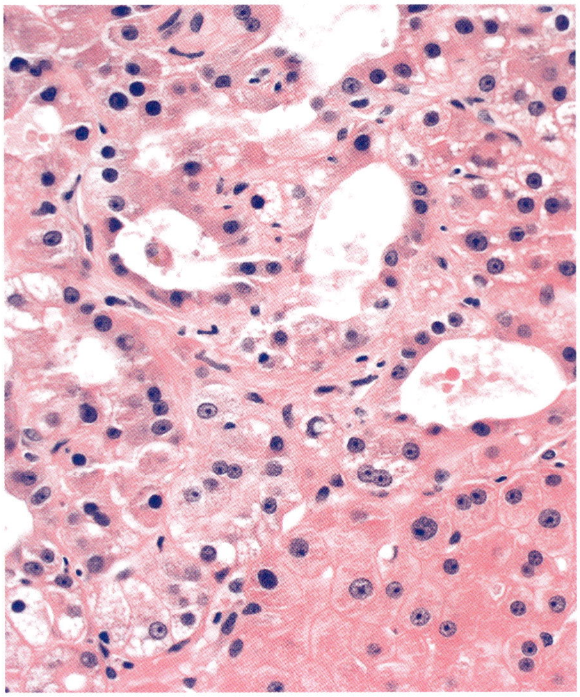

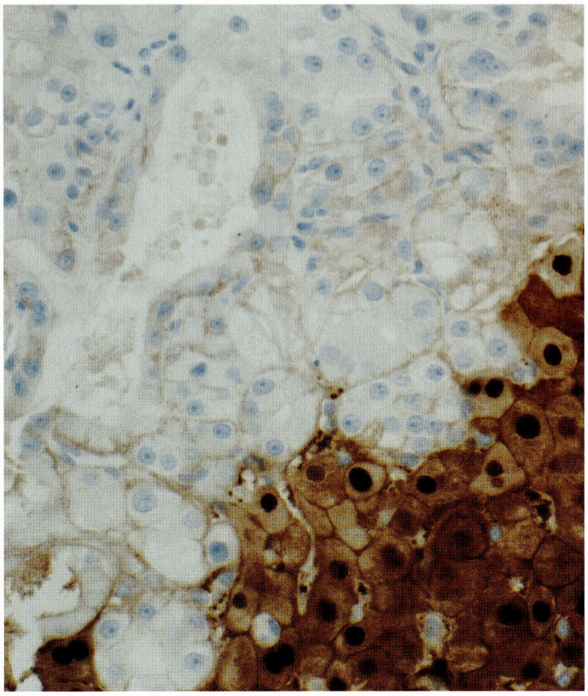

Figure 3-40

HEPATOCELLULAR CARCINOMA

Left: The hepatocellular carcinoma is well differentiated, but an arginase 1 stain is negative (hematoxylin and eosin [H&E] stain).

Right: The arginase 1 stain is positive in the adjacent nontumor liver, seen in the lower right, but is negative in the tumor itself.

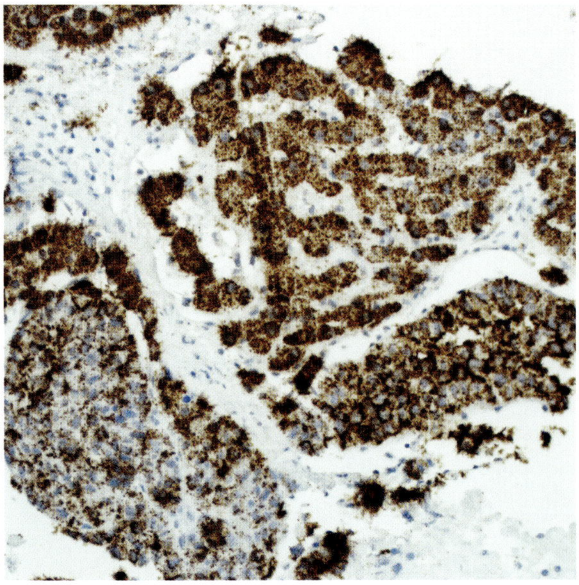

Figure 3-41

HEPATOCELLULAR CARCINOMA: ALBUMIN IN SITU HYBRIDIZATION

Staining is cytoplasmic, strong, and granular.

positive include rare cholangiocarcinomas and metastatic carcinomas from the breast, pancreas, and colon (83,91,92).

Albumin In Situ Hybridization. In situ hybridization for albumin is less widely available but is another useful technique for identifying hepatocytic differentiation. Staining is cytoplasmic (fig. 3-41). As always, correlation with morphology is important as hepatoid adenocarcinomas can be positive for albumin in situ hybridization (90), as are about 50 percent of acinar cell carcinomas of the pancreas (93). Cholangiocarcinomas are also frequently positive (reported range, 77 to 95 percent) (93,94). Also positive are occasional neuroendocrine carcinomas and adenocarcinomas of the lung (fig. 3-42), breast, and gallbladder.

As with any stain, morphology and clinical-radiologic findings matter. Positive in situ hybridization for albumin in a carcinoma should not be the sole basis for classifying the tumor as hepatocellular carcinoma, or for classifying an adenocarcinoma as a cholangiocarcinoma.

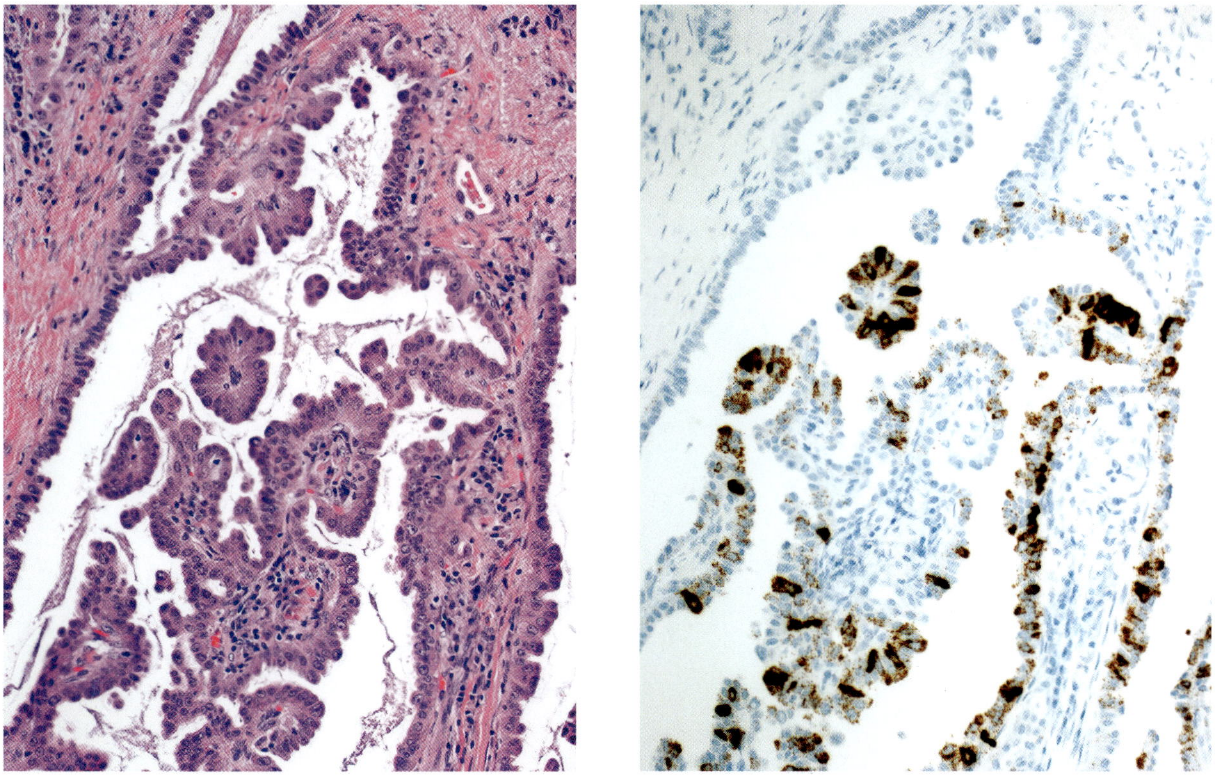

Figure 3-42

PAPILLARY CARCINOMA OF THE LUNG

Left: Papillary carcinoma of the lung.
Right: Albumin in situ hybridization.

Alpha-Fetoprotein. Alpha-fetoprotein shows cytoplasmic staining in approximately one third of hepatocellular carcinomas (fig. 3-43), but the low sensitivity and the high background staining that is commonly present with this immunostain limits its usefulness as a routine marker of hepatocellular carcinoma. The stain is occasionally helpful in very poorly differentiated hepatocellular carcinomas that are negative or equivocal for other markers of hepatocytic differentiation. Because of the high background staining, a tumor should show strong and bright staining to be called positive, with staining that is clearly more intense than the background.

Stains to Separate Benign from Malignant Hepatocytes

Reticulin. For over 40 years, the reticulin stain has been used to diagnose hepatocellular carcinoma (95–97). The field of diagnostic pathology has made great progress in identifying markers of

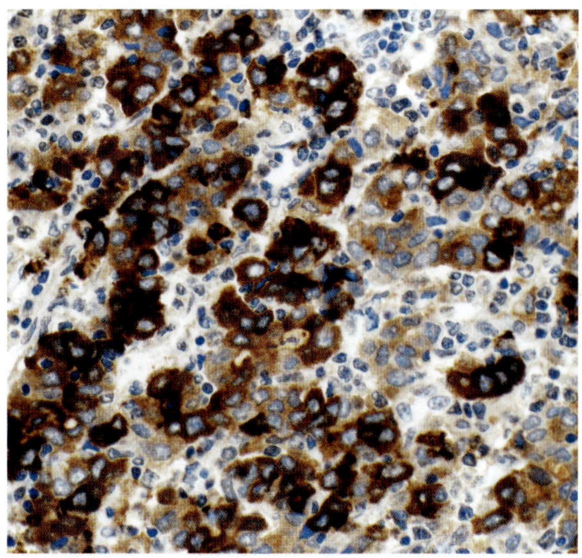

Figure 3-43

HEPATOCELLULAR CARCINOMA: ALPHA-FETOPROTEIN

Strong cytoplasmic staining is seen.

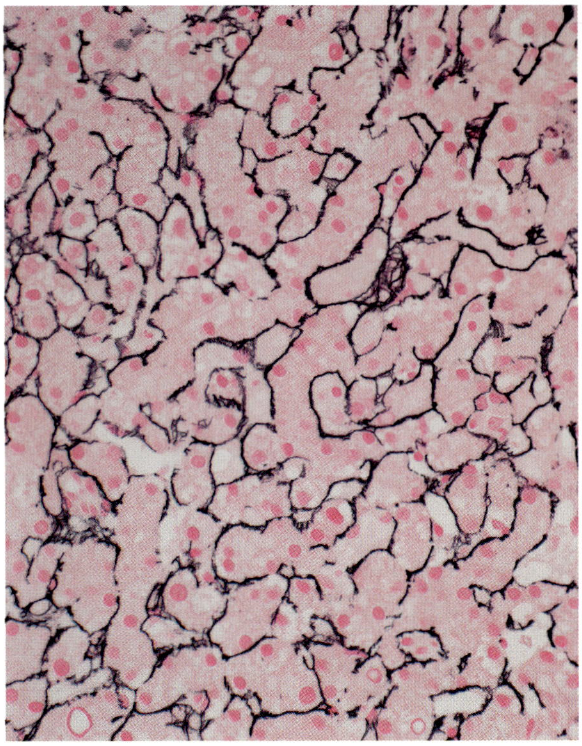

Figure 3-44

HEPATOCELLULAR ADENOMA: RETICULIN STAIN

There is no loss of reticulin; every hepatocyte touches reticulin on at least one of its cytoplasmic membranes.

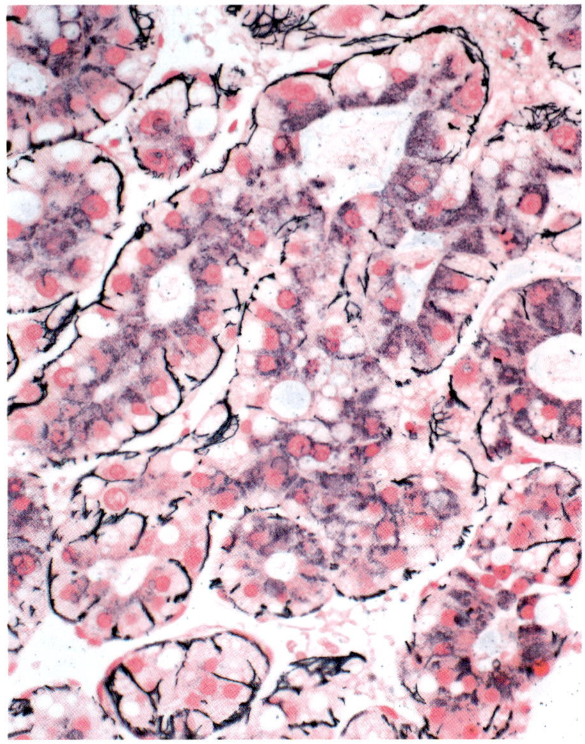

Figure 3-45

HEPATOCELLULAR CARCINOMA: RETICULIN LOSS

Focal mild reticulin loss is seen.

hepatocytic differentiation, but distinguishing a benign hepatocytic proliferation from well-differentiated hepatocellular carcinoma continues to be an important diagnostic challenge. The reticulin stain continues to be widely used in this setting because it demonstrates thin hepatic trabeculae that are composed of a single or double layer of cells in benign proliferations (fig. 3-44), with reticulin touching essentially all cells on at least one of their borders. There is focal reticulin loss in well-differentiated hepatocellular carcinomas, with thickened trabeculae and/or areas of hepatocytes that are not touching reticulin on any of their borders (fig. 3-45).

Hepatocellular carcinomas show a range of reticulin loss: some show near total absence of reticulin (fig. 3-46), but most show more focal loss. Reticulin loss as a diagnostic tool is very useful but needs to be used in conjunction with the morphology and with common sense. For example, focal equivocal reticulin loss is insufficient for a diagnosis of hepatocellular carcinoma in isolation.

There are four main caveats with using the reticulin stain to support a diagnosis of hepatocellular carcinoma. First, non-neoplastic liver trabeculae can be three to four cells thick in rapidly regenerating livers, but this is rarely a true diagnostic dilemma because the clinical situations are different, with a mass in one setting versus acute liver injury in the other. Second, the reticulin stain has to be performed properly to be informative. A poor quality reticulin stain can show artifactual loss of reticulin that mimics hepatocellular carcinoma. The non-neoplastic liver, when present, serves as an excellent internal control. If the reticulin staining in the background liver is not strong and crisp, the stain should be repeated. Third, benign liver with fatty change often shows focal loss of reticulin that can mimic hepatocellular carcinoma (fig. 3-47) (97,98). The least fatty areas of the tumor should be evaluated with the reticulin stain when possible. When only fatty areas are seen in the specimen, the reticulin

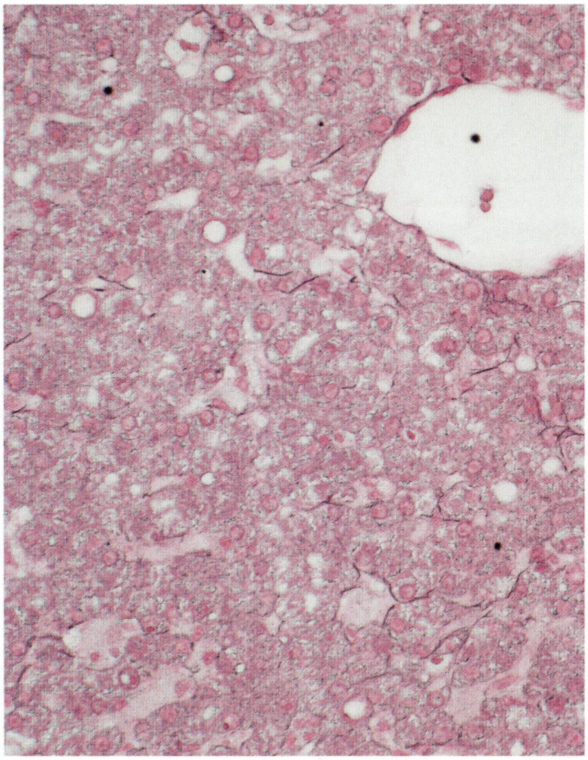

Figure 3-46

HEPATOCELLULAR CARCINOMA: EXTENSIVE RETICULIN LOSS

Extensive reticulin loss is evident. Reticulin loss does not always correlate with the tumor's differentiation, as can be seen in this well-differentiated hepatocellular carcinoma.

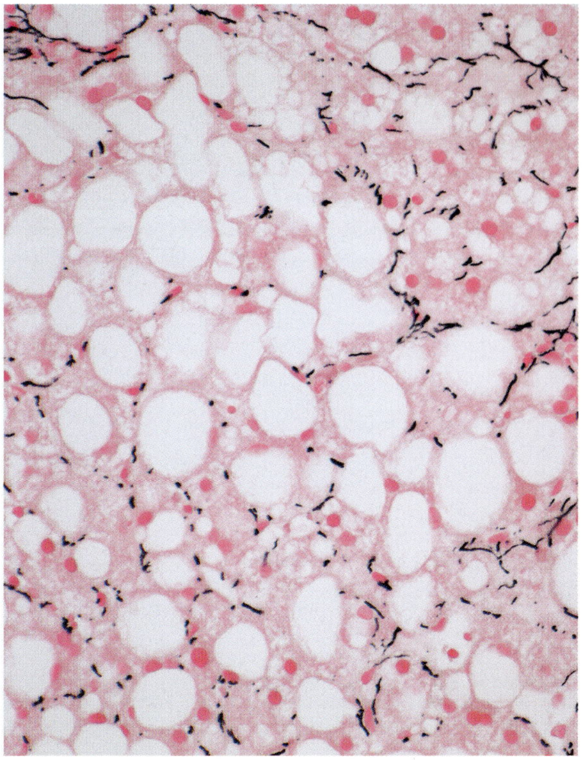

Figure 3-47

NONTUMOR LIVER WITH FATTY CHANGE: RETICULIN STAIN

Reticulin loss is seen in the non-neoplastic liver when there is fatty change.

loss should be substantial and widespread to be informative. Finally, a small number of well-differentiated hepatocellular carcinomas (less than 1 percent) show no loss of reticulin staining on biopsy specimens (99,100) and even more rarely on resection specimens. Almost all of these cases have dense intratumoral fibrosis, such as with the scirrhous variant of hepatocellular carcinoma. When there is no convincing reticulin loss (fig. 3-48), the final diagnosis of hepatocellular carcinoma rests on other findings, principally cytologic atypia, increased proliferative rates, and strong aberrant expression of proteins such as AFP or glypican 3.

CD34. In the normal liver, CD34 staining is limited to the endothelial cells lining the sinusoids in zone 1. In contrast, in hepatocellular carcinomas, CD34 frequently shows a strong and diffuse sinusoidal staining pattern (fig. 3-49) (101). However, there are a number of caveats that limit the routine use of this stain. First, some well-differentiated and some poorly differentiated hepatocellular carcinomas do not show this staining pattern (88). Second, a subset of both hepatocellular adenoma and focal nodular hyperplasia have a diffuse pattern that is essentially indistinguishable from that of hepatocellular carcinoma (88,102–104). In addition to a role in tumor diagnosis, strong and diffuse CD34 staining in hepatocellular carcinoma can predict resistance to transarterial chemoembolization (105).

Ki-67. Increased Ki-67 staining can help distinguish benign hepatocellular tumors from well-differentiated hepatocellular carcinoma, as a high proliferate rate favors malignancy. The stain is most useful when the background non-neoplastic liver is present on the same stained section as the tumor. There is no well-established cut-off that indicates malignancy,

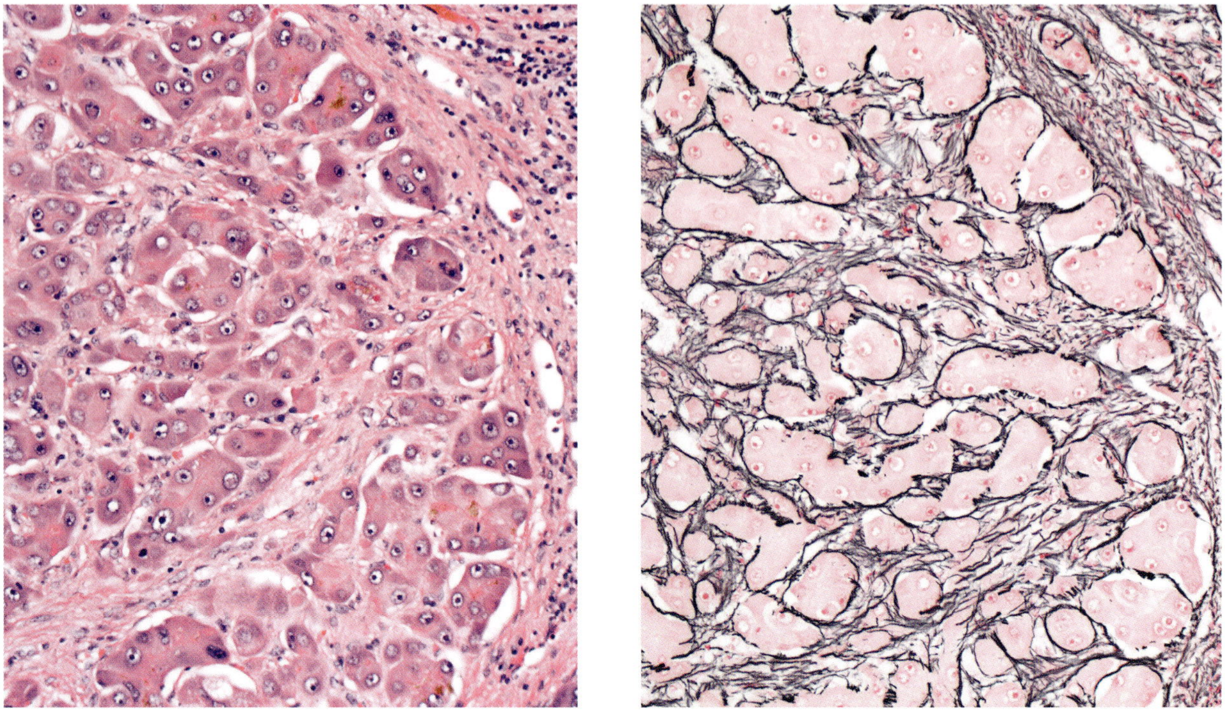

Figure 3-48

HEPATOCELLULAR CARCINOMA

Left: This hepatocellular carcinoma has significant intratumoral fibrosis.
Right: No reticulin loss is seen.

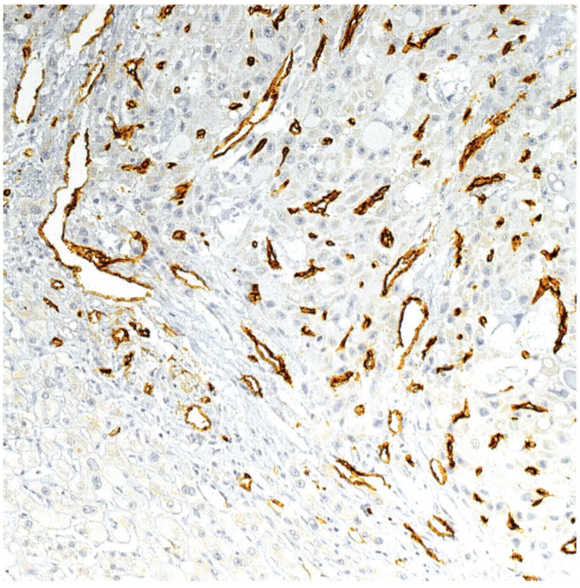

Figure 3-49

HEPATOCELLULAR CARCINOMA: CD34

The tumor sinusoids are strongly and diffusely positive. Compare to the nontumor liver in the lower left.

but benign hepatocellular lesions have a proliferative rate of less than 2 percent in general. In contrast, hepatocellular carcinomas tend to have a bimodal distribution of proliferative rates, with about half of tumors showing a rate of 20 to 60 percent and the other half less than 10 percent (106,107). Some well-differentiated hepatocellular carcinomas have proliferative rates similar to those of benign lesions, so only significantly elevated rates are informative. Pathologists need to be certain they are examining tumor nuclei and not inflammatory cells when evaluating the Ki-67 stain.

Glypican 3. The glypican 3 stain is only informative when positive. Approximately 50 percent of well-differentiated hepatocellular carcinomas are negative for glypican 3 (84,108), so negative staining does not favor benign over malignant. Positive glypican 3 stains are used in two diagnostic settings: in poorly differentiated carcinomas, glypican 3 staining can support a diagnosis of hepatocellular differentiation; in well-differentiated tumors, especially those arising in noncirrhotic livers, glypican 3 staining suggests malignancy. In either setting, the stain should be used in correlation with the H&E morphology.

When evaluating well-differentiated lesions, there are four settings where positive glypican 3 staining should be interpreted with great caution. First, glypican 3 can focally stain benign hepatocytes in markedly inflamed livers (86). Second, lipofuscin in benign hepatocytes is frequently strongly glypican 3 positive. Third, a subset of inflammatory adenomas has weak and focal glypican 3 staining, without any other features to suggest malignancy. Finally, the stain is less helpful in distinguishing dysplastic nodules from hepatocellular carcinoma, as focal glypican 3 is positive in about 50 percent of high-grade and 5 percent of macroregenerative/low-grade dysplastic nodules (70). Nonetheless, strong and diffuse staining favors hepatocellular carcinoma.

HISTOLOGIC SUBTYPES

A number of hepatocellular carcinoma subtypes (or variants) have been described. Subtypes are different from growth patterns (growth patterns are trabecular, solid, pseudoglandular, and macrotrabecular) and different growth patterns can be seen within each of the hepatocellular carcinoma variants. A subtype of hepatocellular carcinoma is defined by the following four features (109): 1) unique H&E findings that are consistently and reproducibly present; 2) unique results from immunostains or other special studies that can confirm the H&E morphology; 3) unique clinical correlates; and 4) unique molecular findings.

These four features are not equally well developed when a subtype is first defined, but true subtypes develop each of these characteristics over time. An estimated 35 percent of all hepatocellular carcinomas can be classified as unique subtypes (Table 3-5). Except for fibrolamellar carcinoma, all of the subtypes occur in both cirrhotic and noncirrhotic livers.

Carcinosarcoma

Fewer that 1 percent of hepatocellular carcinomas are primary *carcinosarcomas*. They have an epithelial component that is either cholangiocarcinoma or hepatocellular carcinoma, as well as a spindle cell component that is clearly malignant and shows morphologic and immunohistochemical evidence of sarcomatous differentiation (fig. 3-50). If the epithelial component is hepatocytic and the spindle cell component shows no differentiation toward a specific mesenchymal lineage, then the term *sarcomatoid hepatocellular carcinoma* is used.

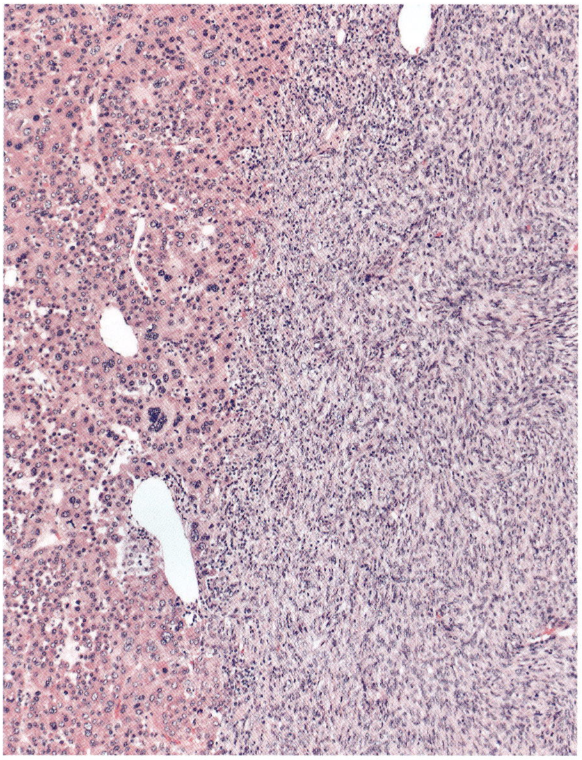

Figure 3-50

CARCINOSARCOMA

A fibrosarcoma (right) and a hepatocellular carcinoma (left).

These strict definitions are not always followed and sometimes these two terms are used interchangeably by authors, with still other authors using terms such as spindle cell hepatocellular carcinoma, sarcomatous carcinoma, and, most unfortunately, adult hepatoblastoma. The inconsistent use of these terms makes it challenging to understand these rare tumors and it is safe to say that carcinosarcomas are one of the least understood tumors of the liver.

The sarcoma component of carcinosarcomas can show differentiation toward leiomyosarcoma, rhabdomyosarcoma, chondrosarcoma, fibrosarcoma, or osteosarcoma (110–112). Some cases also secrete granulocyte colony stimulating factor and

Table 3-5

HEPATOCELLULAR CARCINOMA SUBTYPES

Subtype	Frequency	Prognosis[a]
Steatohepatitic	20%	similar
Clear cell	7%	better
Scirrhous	4%	similar to better
Cirrhotomimetic	1%	worse
Combined hepato-cellular-cholangio-carcinoma	1%	worse
Combined hepatocel-lular-neuroendocrine	<1%	worse
Granulocyte colony-stimulating factor producing	<1%	worse
Sarcomatoid	<1%	worse
Carcinosarcoma	<1%	worse
Lymphocyte rich	<1%	better

[a]Compared to conventional hepatocellular carcinoma.

have numerous intratumoral neutrophils (111). The prognosis is worse than for patients with conventional hepatocellular carcinoma (113).

Carcinosarcoma with Osteoclast-like Giant Cells. In some cases, the sarcoma component of the carcinosarcoma is histologically similar to a giant cell tumor of the bone. In these cases, the hepatocellular carcinoma component varies from well differentiated to poorly differentiated. The two components are found as adjacent nodules or can be admixed, but the transition between the two components is abrupt. The sarcomatous component typically shows the following findings (114–118): 1) extensive hemorrhage, cystic change, and necrosis. The hemorrhage is of varying ages and numerous pigment-laden macrophages are also present in many tumors; 2) the tumor is composed of sheets of mononuclear, plump to spindled tumor cells (fig. 3-51) that are negative or very focally positive for keratins, negative for markers of hepatocytic differentiation, and negative for markers of specific mesenchymal linage differentiation; and 3) admixed within the mononuclear spindled cells are scattered osteoclast-like giant cells. These giant cells have numerous nuclei, often up to 30, but are benign, staining strongly for CD68 (fig. 3-52) and other markers that indicate osteoclast-like differentiation (114,115,119).

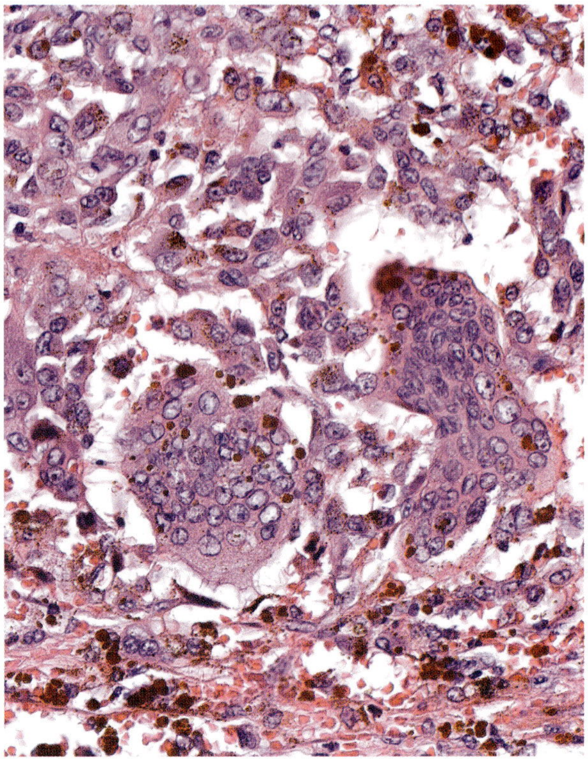

Figure 3-51

CARCINOSARCOMA WITH OSTEOCLAST-LIKE GIANT CELLS

The sarcomatous component in this case shows spindled mononuclear tumor cells admixed with benign osteoclast-like giant cells. Hemosiderin deposits are also evident.

This variant of carcinosarcoma is clinically aggressive (119). Metastases from these tumors can contain the osteoclast-like giant cell morphology (120,121). A hepatocellular carcinoma component is required to classify these cases as a carcinosarcoma subtype of hepatocellular carcinoma, as cholangiocarcinomas and metastatic carcinomas rarely have areas of sarcomatous differentiation with this same osteoclast-like giant cell morphology.

Cirrhotomimetic Hepatocellular Carcinoma

The *cirrhotomimetic variant of hepatocellular carcinoma* (also termed *diffuse hepatocellular carcinoma* and *cirrhosis-like hepatocellular carcinoma*) is the only subtype defined by gross findings. Because the histologic findings are variable, it remains unclear whether this truly represents a subtype with unique molecular findings or a rare growth pattern that can be seen in both

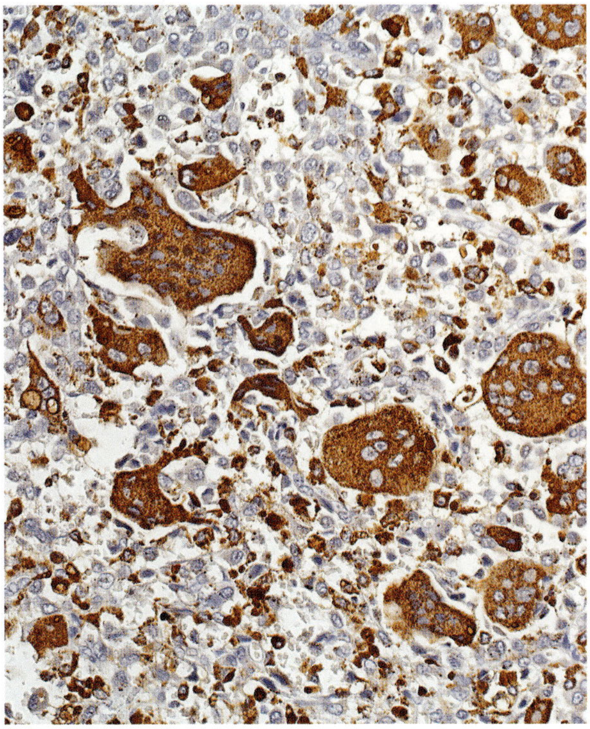

Figure 3-52

CARCINOSARCOMA WITH OSTEOCLAST-LIKE GIANT CELLS

A CD68 immunostain highlights the osteoclast-like giant cells.

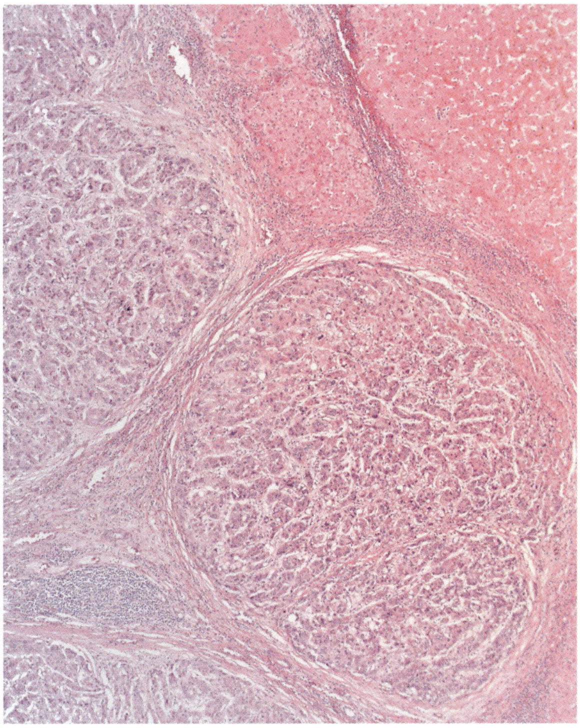

Figure 3-53

CIRRHOTOMIMETIC HEPATOCELLULAR CARCINOMA

This subtype of hepatocellular carcinoma is defined by its growth pattern. The tumor grows as numerous small nodules that are the same size as cirrhotic nodules.

conventional and other variants of hepatocellular carcinoma. Nonetheless, this subtype is currently defined by numerous small tumor nodules that closely resemble the nodules in the background cirrhotic liver (fig. 3-53), being similar in size and shape and often in color to benign cirrhotic nodules. In fact, the hepatocellular carcinoma can so closely mimic ordinary cirrhosis that both imaging studies and gross examination can either miss or significantly underestimate the tumor burden (122).

Almost all cases are found in cirrhotic livers, but rarely noncirrhotic livers have a similar pattern of carcinoma spread, with innumerable small nodules of tumor throughout the liver. The frequency is estimated to be 1 percent.

In many specimens, the tumor nodules focally coalesce to form a larger mass, a finding that is still consistent with the cirrhotomimetic variant of hepatocellular carcinoma. However, the term cirrhotomimetic carcinoma should not be used for cases with a dominant nodule of hepatocellular carcinoma and scattered satellite nodules, even if the satellite nodules were not seen well on imaging or gross examination. In these cases, the satellite nodules are typically found in a narrow strip of liver surrounding the dominant nodule, typically within a few centimeters. If there are enough satellite nodules, a subtle gradient can sometimes be appreciated, with larger and more numerous satellite nodules closer to the main tumor. In contrast, the nodules in cirrhotomimetic hepatocellular carcinoma are more widely dispersed and more evenly distributed. There is no data-driven cut-off for the number of small cirrhosis-like nodules needed for the diagnosis of cirrhotomimetic hepatocellular carcinoma, but most have more than 30. The explanation for the distinctive growth pattern has not been fully resolved. To date, the best explanation appears to be that there is early tumor spread to the large hilar portal vein branches, leading to subsequent seeding of the rest of the liver with tumor (123,124).

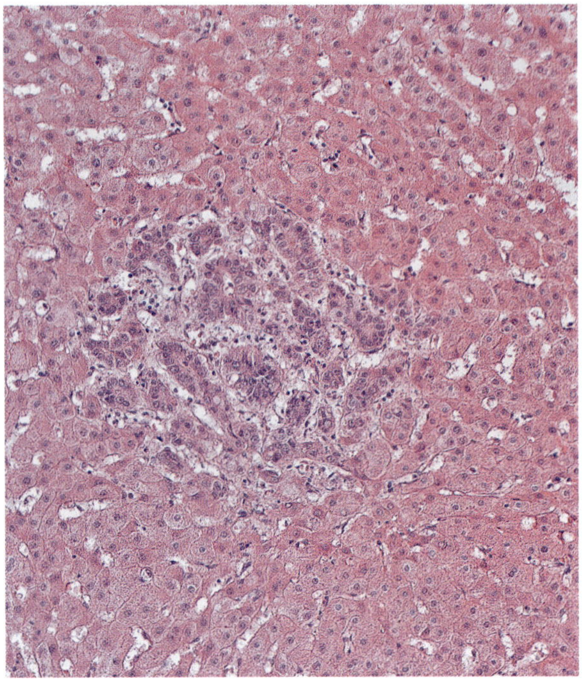

Figure 3-54

CIRRHOTOMIMETIC HEPATOCELLULAR CARCINOMA TUMORLET

A small cluster of tumor cells is present in the center of a benign cirrhotic nodule.

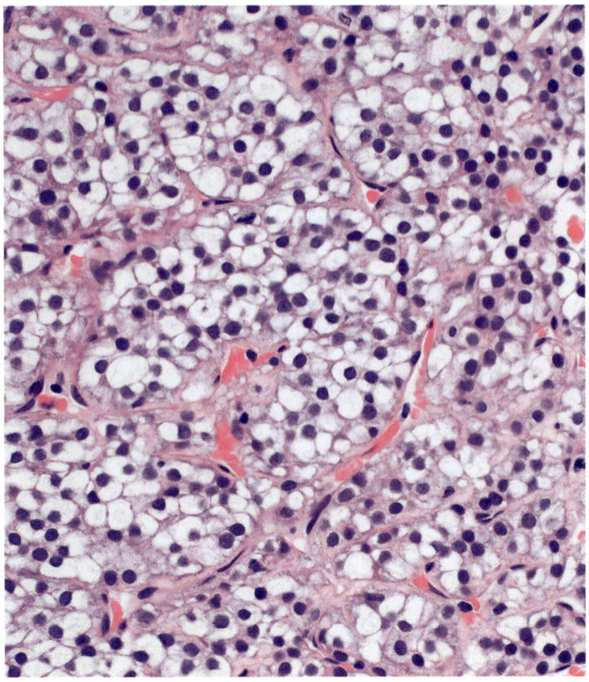

Figure 3-55

CLEAR CELL HEPATOCELLULAR CARCINOMA

The tumor cells are well differentiated and show abundant clear cytoplasm.

The tumor is typically moderately to poorly differentiated. Any of the three major growth patterns can be found including solid, trabecular, and pseudoglandular. Even though the tumor nodules are small, some show central necrosis because they are not arterialized like conventional hepatocellular carcinoma. Some may have clear cell or fatty change. While data are limited, one study found that a clear cell pattern was associated with a better prognosis (125). Most of the small nodules that form the tumor are entirely composed of hepatocellular carcinoma, however, sections can also show scattered tumorlets of a few dozen cells growing in the center of non-neoplastic cirrhotic nodules (fig. 3-54). While published information is limited, this variant appears to stain like conventional hepatocellular carcinomas.

Both the rarity of this variant and the use of various definitions make it difficult to determine the prognosis with certainty, but in many cases the prognosis is poor (123). While successful liver transplants have been reported (125,126), the tumor tends to recur and behave aggressively after transplantation or resection. Those patients with lower total tumor burden tend to do better clinically (125).

Clear Cell Hepatocellular Carcinoma

Clear cell hepatocellular carcinoma has abundant clear cytoplasm (fig. 3-55). The clear cell change is easy to identify in most cases, but a single uniform definition on the percent of clear cells needed for the diagnosis has not found widespread usage. Thus, the literature may be confusing. A reasonable minimum definition is that at least 50 percent of the neoplastic cells should have clear cell change. A purer group of tumors would be achieved using a higher threshold, such as 90 percent of cells with clear cell change. Focal or patchy clear cell change involving less than 50 percent of neoplastic cells is of unclear significance and these tumors are best classified as ordinary hepatocellular carcinomas. With the caveat of problematic definitions, the frequency of clear cell hepatocellular carcinoma is approximately 7 percent, based on the

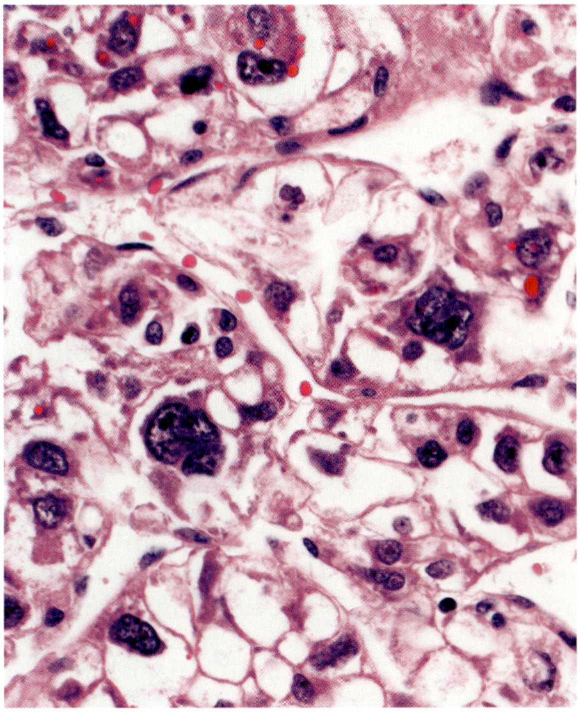

Figure 3-56

CLEAR CELL HEPATOCELLULAR CARCINOMA: HIGH-GRADE CYTOLOGY

The tumor cells show high-grade nuclear cytology but retain abundant clear cytoplasm.

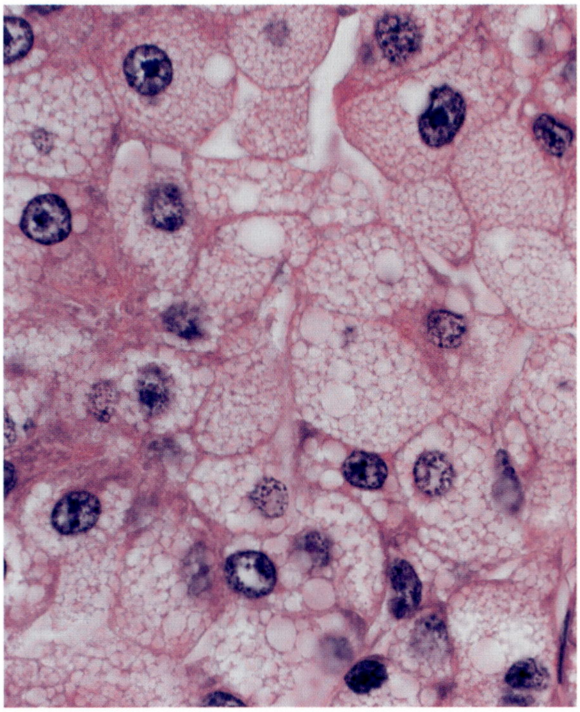

Figure 3-57

LIPID-RICH HEPATOCELLULAR CARCINOMA

This moderately differentiated hepatocellular carcinoma has abundant pale cytoplasm and can mimic clear cell hepatocellular carcinoma, but instead of glycogen, the cytoplasm is filled with small lipid droplets.

combined results from several published series, with a total of over 1,400 cases (127).

Some hepatocellular carcinomas grow as adjacent but separate nodules that show distinctly different morphologies, occasionally with one of the nodules having clear cell change. This pattern is sufficiently different from conventional clear cell carcinoma that it probably should be studied separately.

The reported clinical correlates of clear cell hepatocellular carcinoma are not entirely consistent, but the general trend is that patients with clear cell carcinoma have a better outcome (128–130). The tumors tend to be smaller than nonclear cell hepatocellular carcinomas (129,130) and tend to be better differentiated (129), with lower rates of vascular invasion (128–130).

The tumor cells in clear cell hepatocellular carcinoma are large and polygonal, with abundant clear cytoplasm (fig. 3-55). Most cases are well or moderately differentiated. A smaller subset is poorly differentiated, with high-grade nuclear cytology despite the abundant clear cytoplasm (fig. 3-56). The tumors have any of the four major growth patterns (trabecular, solid, pseudoacinar, macrotrabecular) and rare cases have a cirrhotomimetic or diffuse growth pattern (125,131). One third of clear cell hepatocellular carcinomas also have fatty change (132), which can be focal or involve a significant percentage of the tumor cells.

The clear cell morphology can mimic clear cell carcinomas from other organs, but clear cell hepatocellular carcinomas stain like conventional hepatocellular carcinomas and are positive for HepPar1 or arginase 1. Clear cell carcinomas of the kidney are HepPar1 negative (133), but about 35 percent of clear cell carcinomas of the ovary are HepPar1 positive (81), a potential diagnostic pitfall.

Rarely, hepatocellular carcinomas have clear cell change that is not secondary to glycogen but to diffuse lipid accumulation (fig. 3-57) (134,135). Periodic acid–Schiff (PAS) stains are

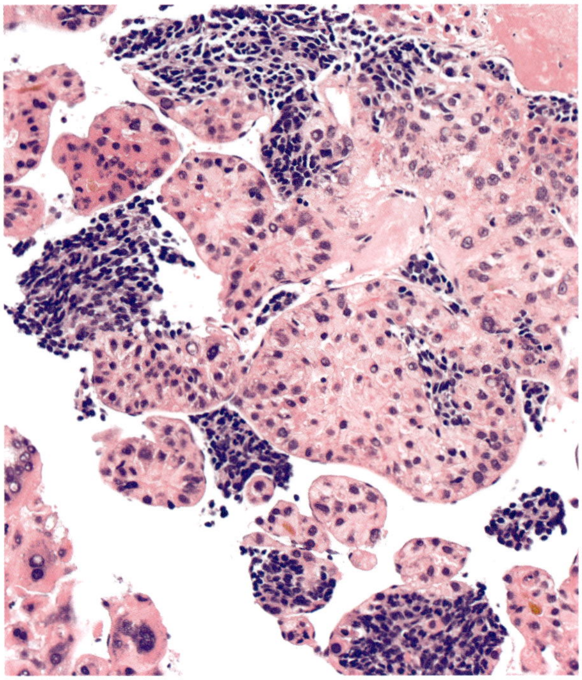

Figure 3-58

COMBINED HEPATOCELLULAR-NEUROENDOCRINE CARCINOMA

Nests of small cell neuroendocrine carcinoma are growing within the tumor sinusoids of well-differentiated hepatocellular carcinoma.

negative. These uncommon cases should not be classified as clear cell hepatocellular carcinoma and most likely represent a unique but very rare hepatocellular carcinoma subtype called lipid rich hepatocellular carcinoma.

Double Primary Carcinomas

Double primary carcinomas are different from combined hepatocellular carcinoma-cholangiocarcinoma (discussed in chapter 8), but unfortunately they are often lumped together in studies. In double primary carcinomas, the liver has widely separate and clearly distinct nodules of hepatocellular carcinoma and cholangiocarcinoma. A large study of over 14,000 primary liver tumors reported the frequency of double primary carcinomas to be 0.2 percent (136). Individual tumors should be graded and staged separately, but the prognosis in most cases is driven by the cholangiocarcinomas, since recurrent and metastatic disease mostly occurs with the cholangiocarcinoma component (136).

Combined Hepatocellular and Neuroendocrine Carcinoma

Combined hepatocellular and neuroendocrine carcinoma consists of two distinctly different components in a single tumor: hepatocellular carcinoma and neuroendocrine carcinoma. The two components are typically intermingled but also may be adjacent to each other. The frequency is less than 1 percent.

Specimens are not called combined hepatocellular and neuroendocrine carcinoma if the two components are clearly separate tumors, with no admixing of the tumors and the nodules are not adjacent. Instead, such tumors are best classified as separate primaries.

Combined hepatocellular and neuroendocrine carcinoma have been reported in cirrhotic and noncirrhotic livers (137,138). There is no clear association with any specific underlying liver disease, as most occur in the setting of chronic hepatitis C and B, which are the major drivers of hepatocellular carcinoma in general.

The hepatocellular component of combined hepatocellular and neurocarcinoma shows a conventional hepatocellular carcinoma morphology, while the neuroendocrine component typically has a small cell morphology (fig. 3-58), but rarely can have a large cell morphology. The neuroendocrine component commonly grows as nests, distending the sinusoids in the hepatocellular carcinoma. In these cases, the bulk of the tumor is typically composed of the hepatocellular component, although rarely, the hepatocellular carcinoma is a minor component of the neuroendocrine carcinoma (137). Less commonly, there may be two distinct but adjacent nodules, one with hepatocellular carcinoma and one with a neuroendocrine component. In this setting, focal transitional areas are often found with sufficient sectioning (137). One reported case also had sarcomatoid change in the neuroendocrine component (139). Metastatic disease can be purely neuroendocrine.

Regardless of growth pattern, the hepatocellular component should have a typical immunohistochemical profile, with evidence of hepatocytic differentiation by hepatocytic markers such as HepPar1 or arginase. The neuroendocrine component should likewise show positive staining for neuroendocrine markers such as synaptophysin or chromogranin and be negative for markers

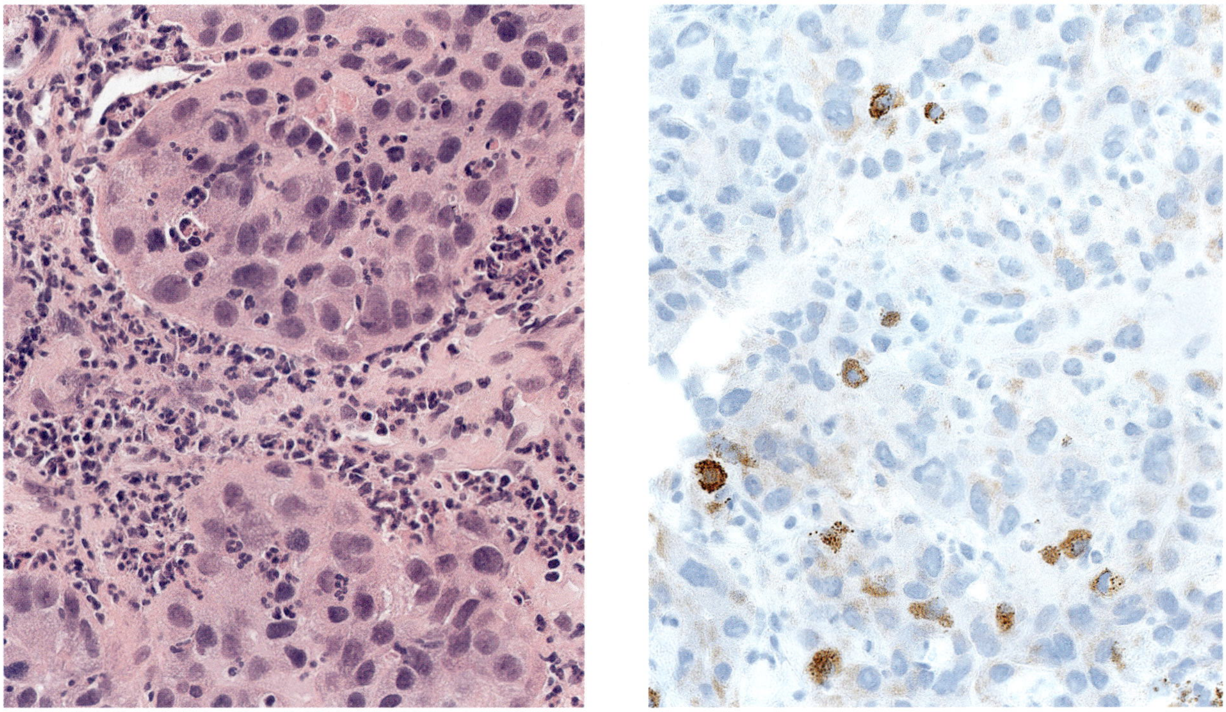

Figure 3-59

GRANULOCYTE COLONY-STIMULATING FACTOR–PRODUCING (GCSFP) HEPATOCELLULAR CARCINOMA

Left: The hepatocellular carcinoma is poorly differentiated and shows numerous tumor-infiltrating neutrophils. Right: Focal HepPar1 staining.

of hepatocytic differentiation. Of note, and this is important, there must be two independent morphologies, as a positive immunostain for both hepatocellular differentiation and neuroendocrine differentiation in a monomorphic tumor is insufficient for the diagnosis of a combined hepatocellular and neuroendocrine carcinoma. As one example, a small proportion of conventional neuroendocrine carcinomas stain focally for HepPar1 or glypican 3 (82,140). On the other hand, a subset of conventional hepatocellular carcinomas, especially when cholestatic, are focally positive for chromogranin, synaptophysin, or CD56 (141,142), but these findings do not qualify for a combined hepatocellular and neuroendocrine carcinoma.

Granulocyte Colony-Stimulating Factor–Producing Hepatocellular Carcinoma

Individuals with the *granulocyte colony-stimulating factor–producing* (GCSFP) subtype of hepatocellular carcinoma present with markedly elevated peripheral white blood cell counts, elevated serum IL-6 levels (111,143–145), and often with elevated serum CRP levels (111,143–146). Histologically, this variant is defined by striking neutrophilic infiltrates within the tumor sinusoids. The frequency is much less than 1 percent (111,143–148). Some cases of conventional hepatocellular carcinoma show foci of necrosis and intense neutrophilia following chemoembolization, but this finding should not be mistaken for the GCSFP variant of hepatocellular carcinoma. Most GCSFP hepatocellular carcinomas occur in older individuals. The prognosis is poor (111,143–145).

Most tumors are poorly differentiated and areas of sarcomatoid dedifferentiation are common (111,143–145). The epithelial component has large numbers of neutrophils within the tumor sinusoids (fig. 3-59, left). The neutrophilia can be less striking or absent in the sarcomatoid areas. Since other poorly differentiated carcinomas rarely produce GCSF, including cholangiocarcinomas (149) and metastatic carcinomas (150), hepatocytic differentiation

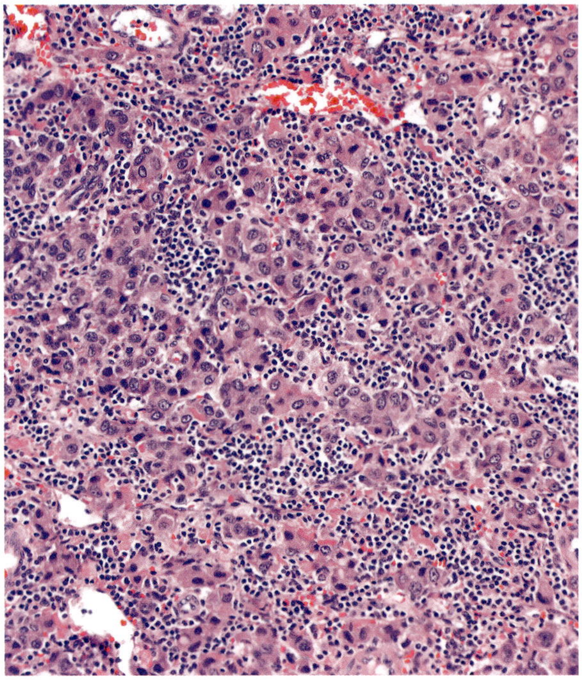

Figure 3-60

LYMPHOCYTE-RICH HEPATOCELLULAR CARCINOMA

The tumor-infiltrating lymphocytes outnumber the tumor cells.

in the epithelial component should be proven with immunostains (fig. 3-59, right). The sarcomatoid areas, if present, are typically negative for markers of hepatocytic differentiation.

GCSF may be produced by the hepatocellular carcinoma component (111,146,147), the sarcomatoid component (143,144), or both components (145). The role played by GCSF in the tumor's biology is not clear. Some studies that examined GCSFP tumors from non-liver sites have suggested these tumors also produce the GCSF receptor, leading to an autocrine loop that stimulates growth, possibly explaining their aggressive behavior (151). This remains unproven, however, and the GCSF receptor in GCSFP hepatocellular carcinomas has not been well studied and in some cases is negative (146).

Lymphocyte-Rich Hepatocellular Carcinoma and Lymphoepithelioma-Like Hepatocellular Carcinoma

Lymphocyte-rich hepatocellular carcinomas are defined by marked lymphocytic inflammation (fig. 3-60). This variant is rare, with a frequency of less than 1 percent. Authors have used variable definitions, but the lymphocytic inflammation should be diffuse and striking. The best definition is as follows: a carcinoma with definite evidence of hepatocellular differentiation and diffuse lymphocytosis, where the number of lymphocytes is greater than the number of tumor cells in most fields. Many conventional hepatocellular carcinomas have focal areas of dense inflammation or have a mild and more generalized lymphocytosis; these do not meet the minimum definition for lymphocyte-rich hepatocellular carcinoma. Other names have been used in the literature for this subtype, including *hepatocellular carcinoma with lymphoid-rich stroma* and *inflammatory hepatocellular carcinoma*, but the preferred term is lymphocyte-rich hepatocellular carcinoma.

There are no strong etiologic associations. While the data to date are very limited, several studies have suggested that patients with lymphocyte-rich hepatocellular carcinomas have a better prognosis than conventional hepatocellular carcinomas (152–154). These carcinomas are typically well to moderately differentiated (152,154) and are found in both cirrhotic and noncirrhotic livers (152,153). The inflammation is composed mostly of lymphocytes, with occasional plasma cells. The tumor sinusoids are diffusely infiltrated, but the background liver is not involved, although other chronic inflammatory diseases may be present such as chronic hepatitis B or C. Germinal centers are usually present within the tumor (fig. 3-61). The lymphocytes are reactive T cells, with B cells located in the germinal centers (152). Rarely, plasma cells are prominent (fig. 3-62). Many lymphocyte-rich hepatocellular carcinomas focally show pale bodies within the tumor cells.

Sometimes the term *lymphoepithelioma-like hepatocellular carcinoma* is used as a synonym for lymphocyte-rich hepatocellular carcinoma. However, lymphoepithelioma-like hepatocellular carcinomas are by definition poorly differentiated (fig. 3-63). They have islands or sheets of epithelial cells, often with indistinct cell borders, giving a syncytial appearance. Hepatocytic differentiation must be proven by immunostains, as cholangiocarcinomas and metastatic disease can have similar findings. The relationship between lymphoepithelioma-like hepatocellular carcinoma and lymphocyte-rich hepatocellular carcinoma is unclear, but it is prudent to keep them as

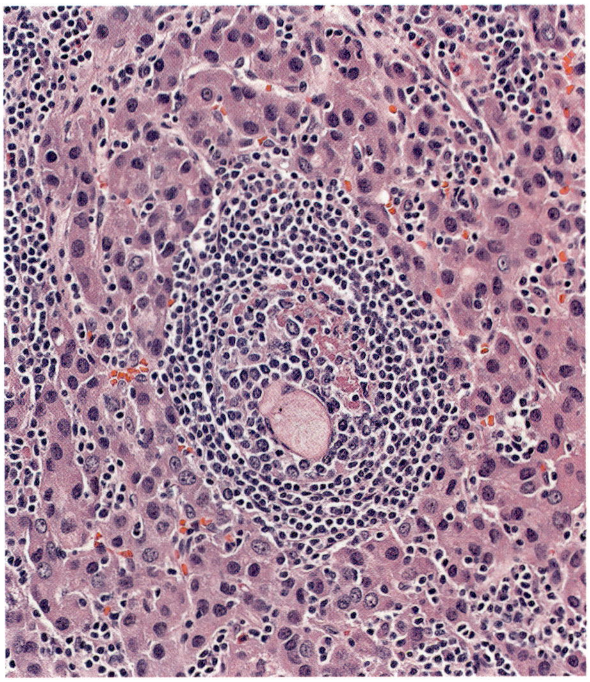

Figure 3-61

LYMPHOCYTE-RICH HEPATOCELLULAR CARCINOMA

A reactive lymphoid follicle is seen.

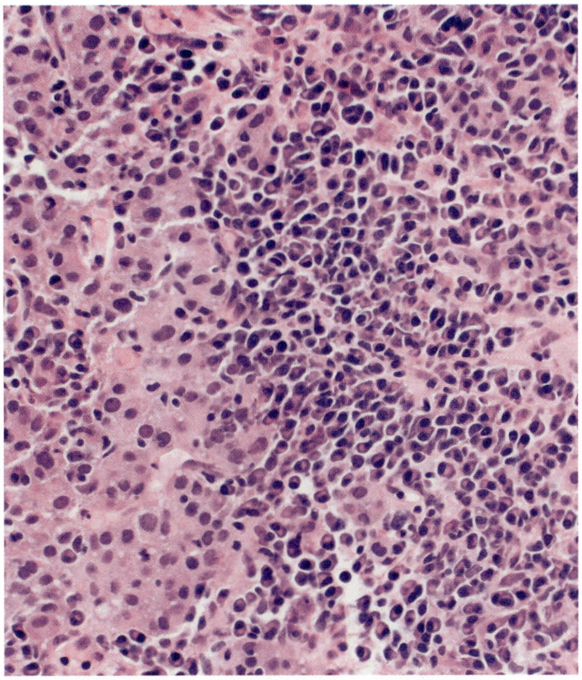

Figure 3-62

LYMPHOCYTE-RICH HEPATOCELLULAR CARCINOMA

Scattered areas are plasma cell rich.

separate entities until this is resolved. It is often assumed that lymphocyte-rich hepatocellular carcinoma can dedifferentiate into lymphoepithelioma-like hepatocellular carcinoma, but this has not been convincingly shown to date.

Because lymphoepithelioma-like hepatocellular carcinomas are poorly differentiated (155, 156), multiple sections and immunostains are often needed to identify areas of hepatocellular differentiation. Also, the epithelial component in both lymphoepithelioma-like hepatocellular carcinoma and in lymphocyte-rich hepatocellular carcinoma is Epstein-Barr virus (EBV) negative (153,155,156), in contrast to the EBV-positive lymphoepithelioma-like cholangiocarcinoma (157).

Sarcomatoid Hepatocellular Carcinomas

Sarcomatoid hepatocellular carcinomas have both an epithelial component of hepatocellular carcinoma and a major spindle cell component (fig. 3-64). There is no well-defined minimum amount of spindle cell change, but in most cases, the spindle cell component is prominent. The spindle cell component should not show specific mesenchymal differentiation by

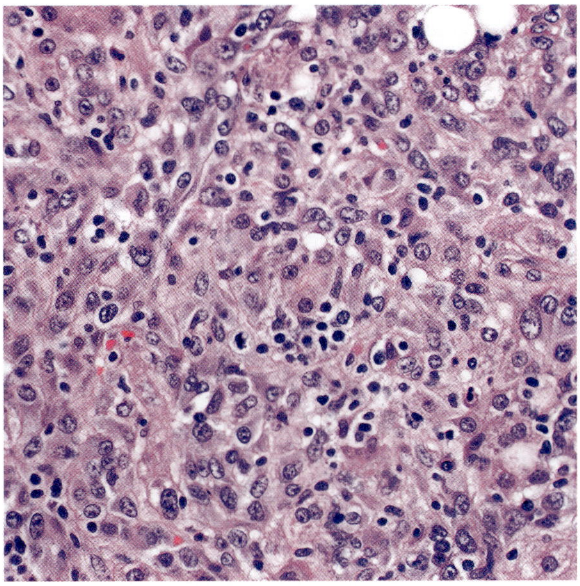

Figure 3-63

LYMPHOEPITHELIOMA-LIKE HEPATOCELLULAR CARCINOMA

The carcinoma is poorly differentiated and the epithelial nature is less evident on H&E stain. Numerous tumor infiltrating lymphocytes are seen.

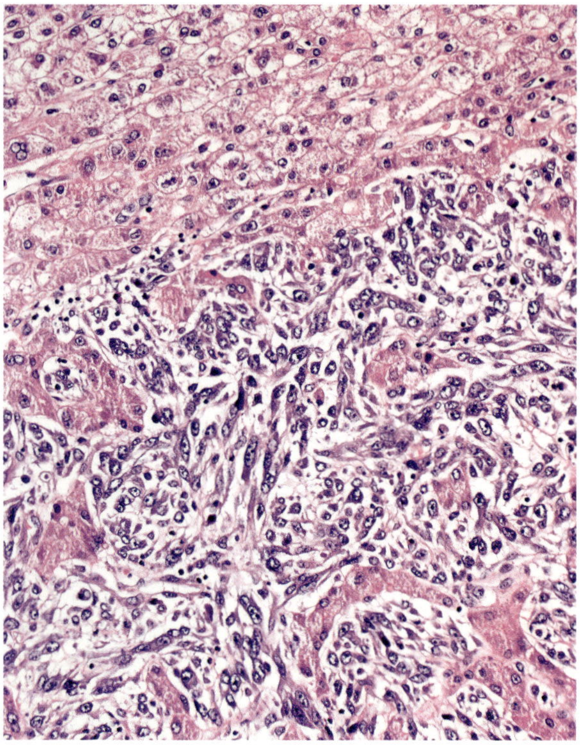

Figure 3-64

SARCOMATOID HEPATOCELLULAR CARCINOMA

An area of spindle cell growth is seen in the center of this hepatocellular carcinoma.

morphology or by immunostains; if it does, then the tumor is classified as a carcinosarcoma. Sarcomatoid hepatocellular carcinomas are rare, with a frequency of less than 1 percent.

The hepatocellular carcinoma component is most commonly high grade, but can be moderately differentiated. There are no other morphologic findings that strongly correlate with the development of a spindle cell component and the hepatocellular component stains in an ordinary fashion with keratins and other markers of hepatocytic differentiation.

The sarcomatoid component is most commonly found as a distinct nodule of tumor growth and can be at the periphery of the tumor or within the center. The spindled tumor cells are vimentin positive, usually at least focally keratin positive, but are negative or only focally and equivocally positive for markers of hepatocytic differentiation. If a biopsy specimen only shows a spindle cell neoplasm, then metastatic disease should be carefully excluded, even in a cirrhotic liver.

Scirrhous Hepatocellular Carcinoma

Scirrhous hepatocellular carcinoma is defined by striking intratumoral fibrosis involving over 50 percent of the tumor. In areas of intratumoral fibrosis, the fibrosis should make up at least 50 percent of the surface area. In larger tumors, the central areas are often densely sclerotic with few or no tumor cells. The frequency ranges from 2 to 6 percent (158–160). The prognosis is similar to (158,159) or better than (160,161) that of conventional hepatocellular carcinoma.

Scirrhous hepatocellular carcinomas occur in both cirrhotic and noncirrhotic livers, but they are more common in noncirrhotic livers (159,162). They are most commonly found beneath the liver capsule, but can be located elsewhere. They tend to grow as a cluster of closely approximated tumor nodules. Scirrhous hepatocellular carcinomas are not encapsulated, and entrapped intratumoral portal tracts are common at the growing front of the tumor (158–160,162,163).

Histologically, the tumor most commonly has a trabecular growth pattern. Usually the trabeculae are thin (fig. 3-65, left), but they can be thick and bulbous (fig. 3-65, right). In other areas, the tumor can have a solid growth pattern. Most scirrhous hepatocellular carcinomas are well to moderately differentiated. Some have either fatty change or clear cell change. Cytoplasmic inclusions are also common and include hyaline bodies or pale bodies.

The intratumoral fibrosis is often haphazard but can be lamellar in areas, closely mimicking fibrolamellar carcinoma. The tumor cells can also have prominent nucleoli, further raising the possibility of fibrolamellar carcinoma. In other cases, the striking intratumoral fibrosis can suggest cholangiocarcinoma. Radiologists can make the same mistake and scirrhous hepatocellular carcinomas are commonly misdiagnosed by imaging studies as cholangiocarcinomas (159,160).

Reticulin stains may show no loss of reticulin in some cases, but the tumors are clearly malignant based on the cytology, and the question of benign versus malignant is rarely an issue. In fact, the most common diagnostic issue is separating scirrhous hepatocellular carcinomas from other malignancies, including fibrolamellar carcinoma (fig. 3-66), cholangiocarcinoma, and metastatic carcinoma. Markers of hepatocytic differentiation help separate scirrhous hepatocellular carcinoma

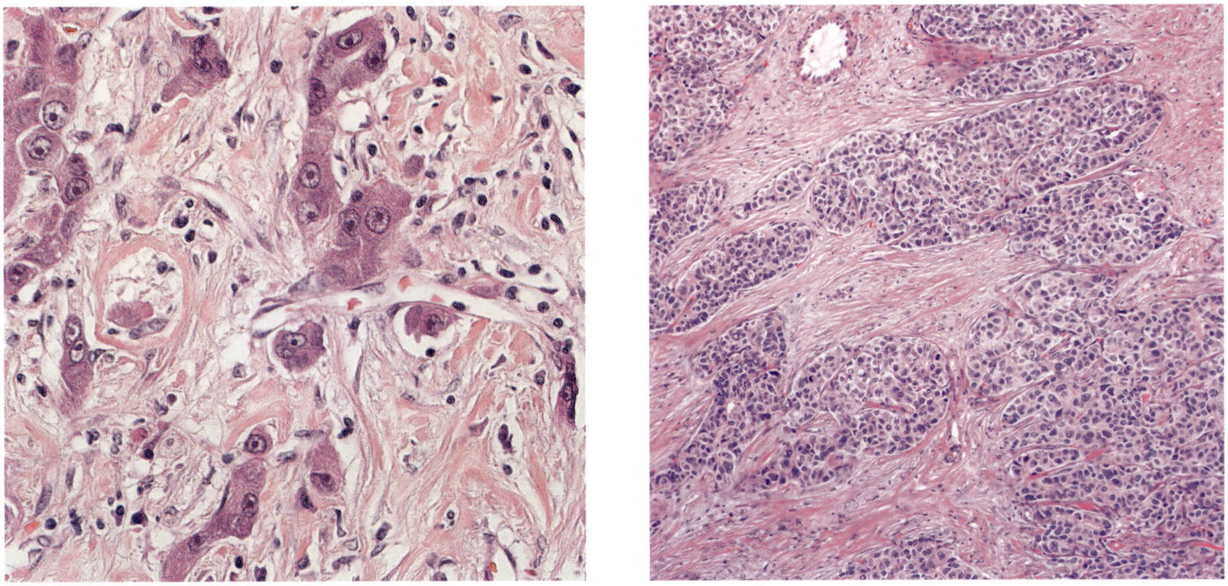

Figure 3-65

SCIRRHOUS HEPATOCELLULAR CARCINOMA

Left: The tumor cells are growing as thin trabeculae in a dense desmoplastic background.
Right: The tumor cells are growing in thick and somewhat more chunky trabeculae, with a dense desmoplastic background.

from metastatic disease and from cholangiocarcinoma. In this regard, arginase is a more sensitive marker of hepatocytic differentiation than HepPar1, as HepPar1 is positive in only about 40 percent of cases (71,158,161). Co-expression of CK7 and CD68 or molecular studies can be used to evaluate for fibrolamellar carcinoma (164).

Steatohepatitic Hepatocellular Carcinoma

The *steatohepatitic variant of hepatocellular carcinoma* has histologic findings of steatohepatitis that are similar to those in non-neoplastic liver, including macrovesicular steatosis, balloon cells, Mallory-Denk bodies, inflammation, and pericellular fibrosis (165,166). There is some variation in the literature on both the precise requirements needed for each of these components and on what percent of the tumor needs to show a steatohepatitic pattern to qualify for the diagnosis. At least 5 percent of the tumor should consist of macrovesicular steatosis (166) but a cut-off of 33 percent fatty change has also been used (165). As a best approach, the steatohepatitic changes should be a dominant part of the histology and not a focal finding; a cut-off of 50 percent of the tumor having a steatohepatitic morphology is reasonable (165,166). The frequency of the steatohepatitic

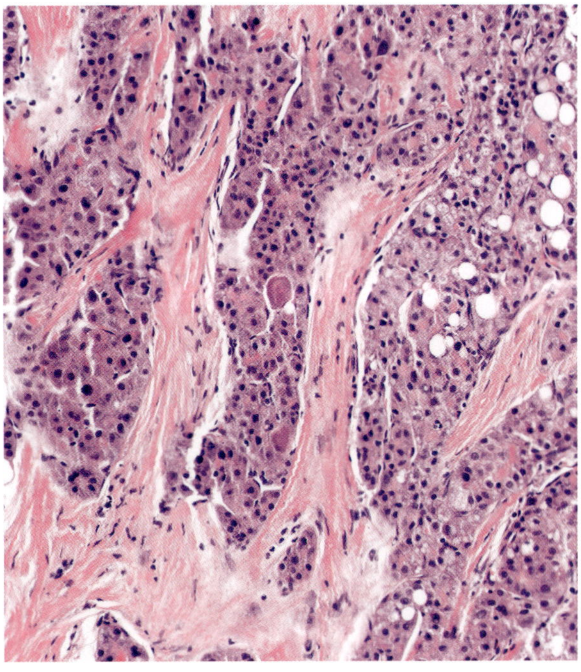

Figure 3-66

SCIRRHOUS HEPATOCELLULAR CARCINOMA

This case was originally diagnosed as fibrolamellar carcinoma. The histologic findings in these two entities may be similar. Molecular studies and immunostains confirmed this was not fibrolamellar carcinoma.

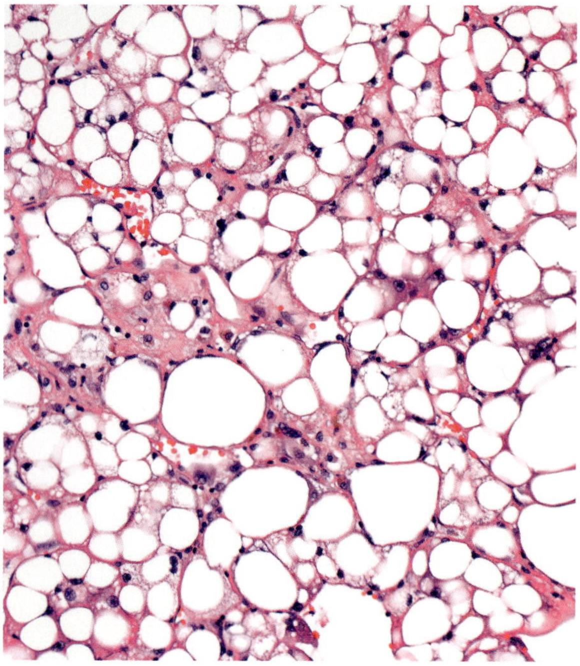

Figure 3-67

STEATOHEPATITIC HEPATOCELLULAR CARCINOMA

Marked diffuse macrovesicular steatosis is present.

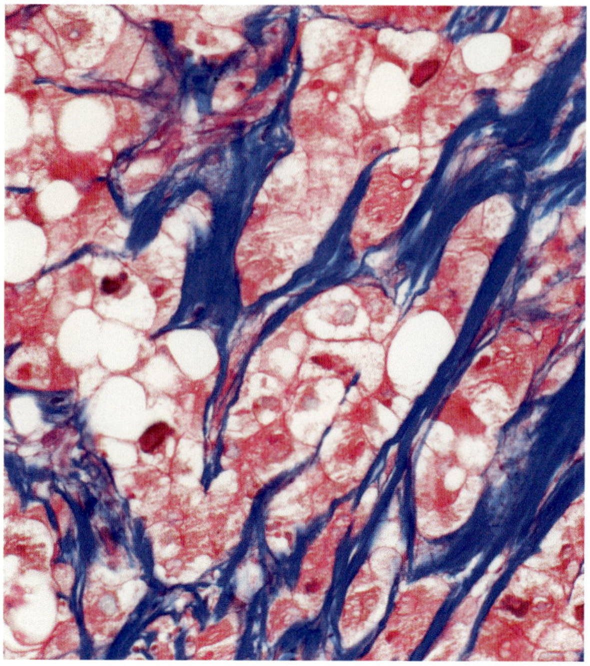

Figure 3-69

STEATOHEPATITIC HEPATOCELLULAR CARCINOMA

A trichrome stain highlights the intratumoral fibrosis.

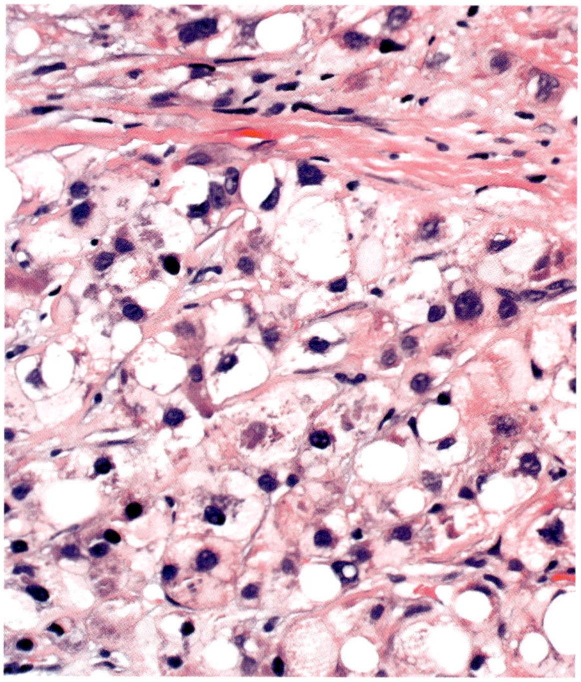

Figure 3-68

STEATOHEPATITIC HEPATOCELLULAR CARCINOMA

Ballooned hepatocytes and Mallory-Denk bodies are easily seen.

variant of hepatocellular carcinoma ranges from 13 to 31 percent in different studies, in part because of differences in how this variant is defined (165,167,168). Survival is similar to that of conventional hepatocellular carcinomas without the steatohepatitic morphology (165).

In addition to fat (fig. 3-67), steatohepatitic hepatocellular carcinomas show at least mild intratumoral inflammation, principally lymphocytic. Balloon cells should also be present and some may have Mallory-Denk bodies (fig. 3-68). This subtype also shows intratumoral fibrosis deposited in a pericellular pattern, similar to that seen in steatohepatitis in non-neoplastic liver. The pericellular fibrosis is often best seen with a trichrome stain (fig. 3-69). In most cases, the steatohepatitic morphology is diffuse, although it may be limited to a distinct nodule in tumors that have multiple morphologies. Most steatohepatitic hepatocellular carcinomas are well to moderately differentiated and show a solid or trabecular growth pattern.

This subtype is strongly associated with the metabolic syndrome and the background non-neoplastic liver in most cases shows nonalcoholic fatty liver disease (165,167,168).

Steatohepatitic hepatocellular carcinoma can also develop in the setting of alcoholic liver disease (165). Interestingly, the steatohepatitic changes are often more striking in the tumor than in the background non-neoplastic liver (167). The explanation for this distinctive histologic finding is presumably that the tumor cells are sufficiently well differentiated that they can respond to the same factors (metabolic syndrome or ethanol) inducing steatohepatitis in the background liver. In rare cases, however, the steatohepatitic variant of hepatocellular carcinoma is found in livers where there is no clinical evidence of the metabolic syndrome or ethanol use and the background liver has no fatty change (169). In these cases, the steatohepatitic changes in the tumor are typically diffuse and striking, and presumably represent tumor-specific mutations or epigenetic changes.

The most important diagnostic pitfall is that some cases are diagnosed as steatohepatitis and the hepatocellular carcinoma is missed. The same mistake can occur with focal nodular hyperplasia, which also occasionally shows steatohepatitic changes (170). The diagnosis of hepatocellular carcinoma is made by recognizing the usual histologic findings of cytologic atypia, increased proliferation, and loss of reticulin. The reticulin stain should be interpreted carefully in these cases, focusing on those areas of the tumor that have no or minimal fatty change, as fatty change can lead to reticulin loss even in non-neoplastic liver tissue (98). The same general approach applies to focal nodular hyperplasia with a steatohepatitis morphology, which is diagnosed in the usual fashion.

Molecular studies have found that the steatohepatitic variant of hepatocellular carcinoma is less likely than conventional hepatocellular carcinoma to show beta-catenin mutations or diffuse glutamine synthesis staining (171). They also are more likely to express the sonic hedgehog ligand (171).

PROVISIONAL SUBTYPES OF HEPATOCELLULAR CARCINOMA

These subtypes are categorized as provisional because of limited published data.

Chromophobe Hepatocellular Carcinoma

The neoplastic cells in *chromophobe hepatocellular carcinoma* show amphophilic to eosinophilic cytoplasm with scattered cystic spaces.

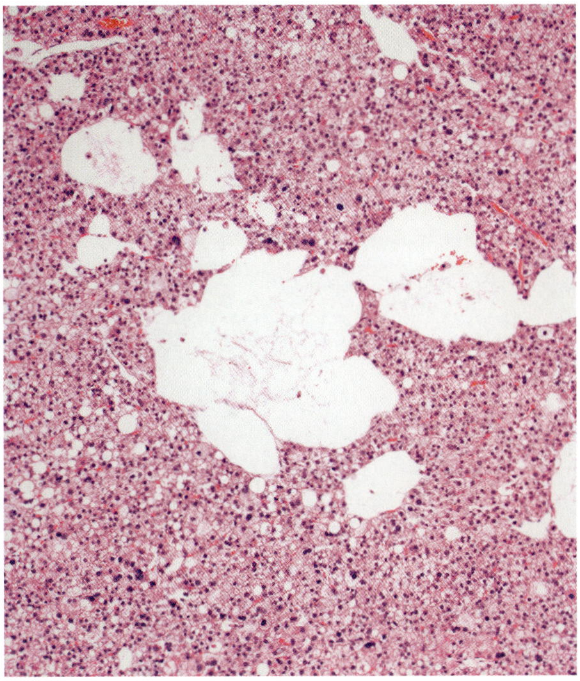

Figure 3-70

CHROMOPHOBE HEPATOCELLULAR CARCINOMA

Irregular cyst-like spaces are found in many of these tumors, especially as they get larger.

The cystic spaces are not lined by tumor cells and are filled with a thin serum-like substance (fig. 3-70). Bland nuclei are seen throughout most of the tumor, but there are also scattered discrete foci of tumor cells with more striking nuclear anaplasia (fig. 3-71).

Chromophobe hepatocellular carcinoma is strongly associated with a molecular finding of alternative lengthening of telomeres (109). Such tumors maintain their telomeres not by activating telomerase, but instead by a telomere-independent mechanism involving homologous recombination of the telomeres (172).

Lipid-Rich Hepatocellular Carcinoma

Lipid-rich hepatocellular carcinomas may be confused with clear cell hepatocellular carcinoma at low power because they have abundant clear cytoplasm and tend to be well to moderately differentiated. On higher-power examination, however, the cytoplasm does not have clear cell change, but instead is filled with numerous tiny droplets of fat, similar to that seen in microvesicular steatosis (fig. 3-72). Lipid-rich

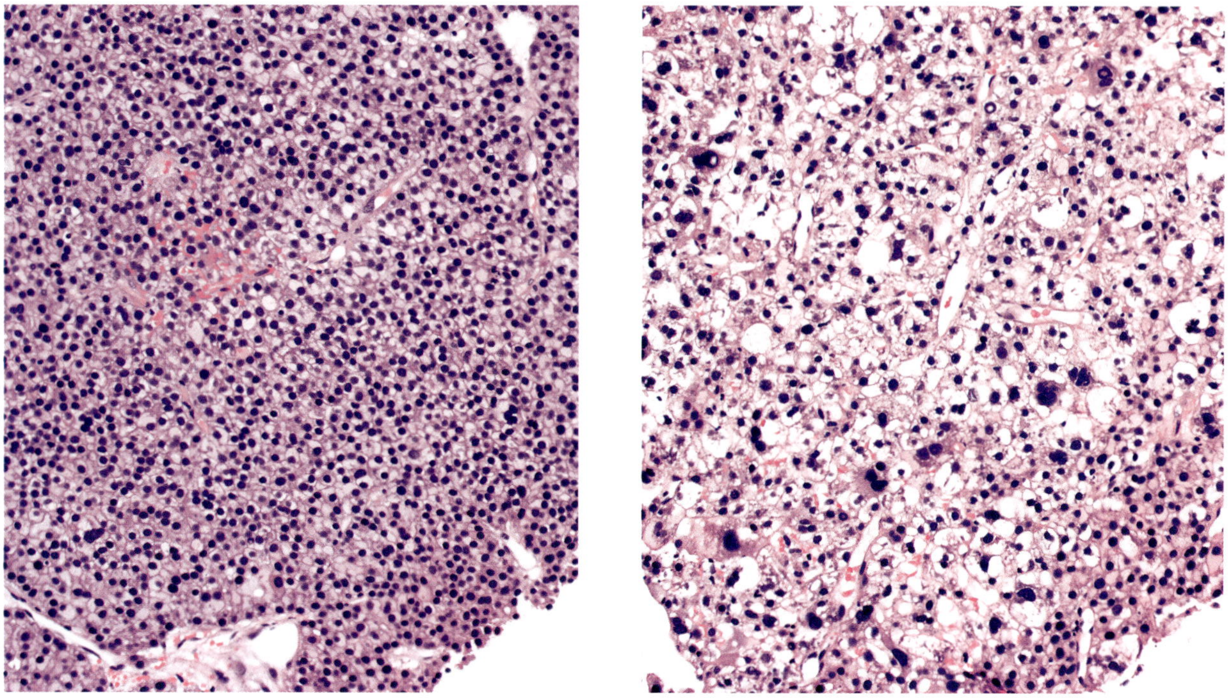

Figure 3-71

CHROMOPHOBE HEPATOCELLULAR CARCINOMA

Left: The tumor nuclei are generally bland and the tumor cells have moderately abundant amphophilic cytoplasm. Right: Scattered loosely aggregated tumor foci have striking nuclear anaplasia.

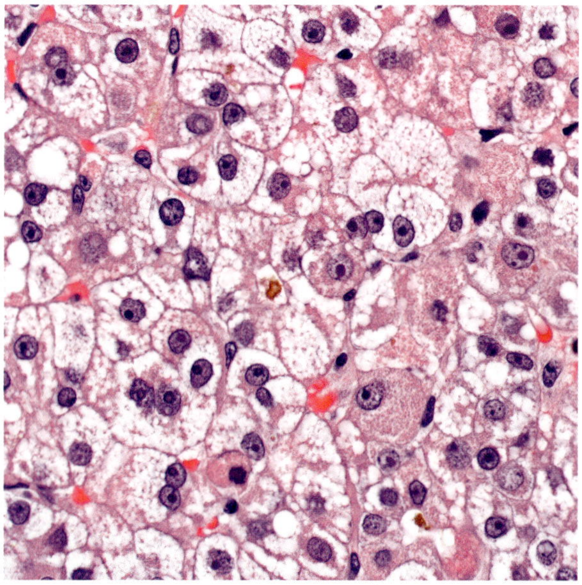

Figure 3-72

LIPID-RICH HEPATOCELLULAR CARCINOMA

The cytoplasm is filled with numerous small droplets of fat. Bile is within the canalicular structure at the center of the image, supporting its hepatocellular origin.

hepatocellular carcinoma should have diffuse microvesicular steatosis as the predominant pattern, although rare larger droplets of fat are acceptable. Too few cases have been reported to understand the clinical and morphologic findings in these cases. However, in one case report, the background liver showed nonalcoholic fatty liver disease and advanced fibrosis (135). Focal microvesicular steatosis can also be seen in the steatohepatitic subtype of hepatocellular carcinoma, but such cases should be classified as steatohepatitic hepatocellular carcinoma.

Myxoid Hepatocellular Carcinoma

As indicated by the name, *myxoid hepatocellular carcinoma* shows myxoid material dissecting the sinusoids of the tumor (fig. 3-73A). The myxoid material is alcian blue positive and can be weakly mucicarmine positive (fig. 3-73B,C). Some hepatocellular adenomas show similar changes, so the tumor needs to be fully evaluated to prove hepatocellular carcinoma. The cause of the myxoid deposits is not clear but these tumors should not be classified as cholangiocarcinoma. The tumor

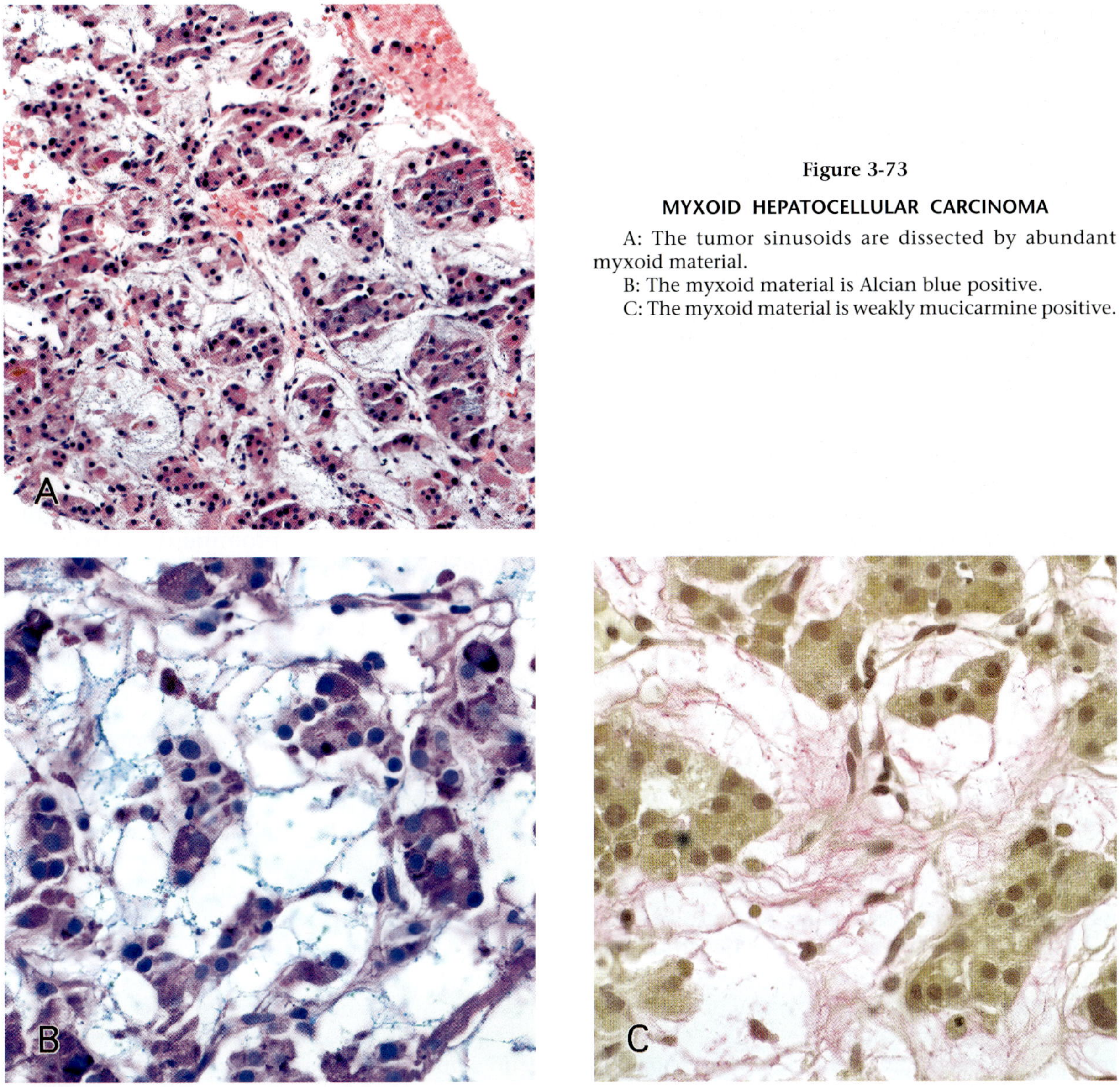

Figure 3-73

MYXOID HEPATOCELLULAR CARCINOMA

A: The tumor sinusoids are dissected by abundant myxoid material.

B: The myxoid material is Alcian blue positive.

C: The myxoid material is weakly mucicarmine positive.

does not show any true glandular differentiation. They stain strongly with HepPar1 and arginase and are CDX2 and CK19 negative. They often have loss of liver fatty acid binding protein (LFABP) staining and diffuse staining of glutamine synthetase (173). Unique radiologic findings have also been reported (174).

Hepatocellular Carcinoma with Syncytial Giant Cells

This variant was proposed in a case report that showed a well-differentiated hepatocellular carcinoma with numerous syncytial-type multinuclear giant cells, similar to those seen in infantile giant cell hepatitis (175). Other areas of the tumor showed smaller, less-differentiated nests of tumor cells in a desmoplastic background. The tumor stained with HepPar1 and was CK7 and CK19 negative. Aberrant nuclear beta-catenin expression was seen in the less-differentiated areas.

Transitional Liver Cell Tumor

Transitional liver cell tumor (fig. 3-74) is a term used for tumors in older children and adolescents that look like hepatocellular carcinomas on H&E but also have focal areas that suggest

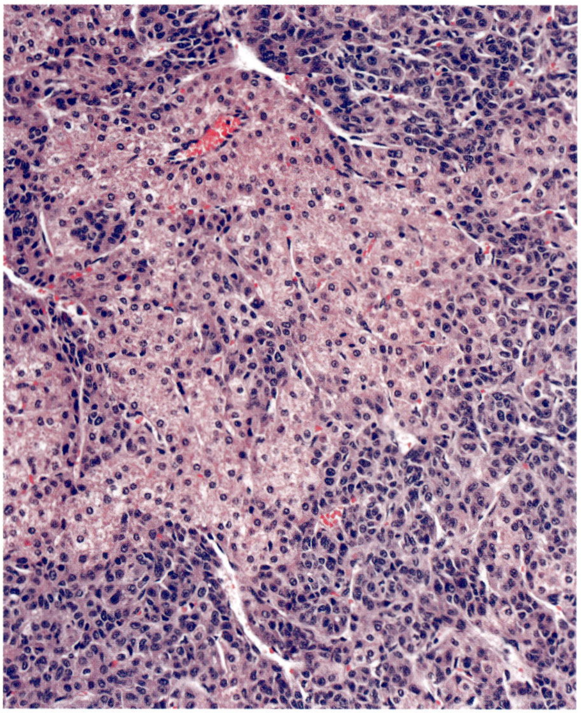

Figure 3-74

TRANSITIONAL CELL CARCINOMA

Most of the tumor shows changes of conventional hepatocellular carcinoma (middle of image), but there are rare scattered foci of more primitive appearing tumor cells (edges of image).

hepatoblastoma (176). These areas have small basophilic tumor cells similar to those seen in the embryonal growth pattern of hepatoblastoma. Nevertheless, the overall histologic findings are in most cases in keeping with conventional hepatocellular carcinoma. They behave clinically more like hepatocellular carcinoma than hepatoblastoma. This tumor is associated with elevated serum AFP levels.

It is not clear why these tumors have focal areas that suggest hepatoblastoma. Proposed explanations include "maturation" of a pure fetal hepatoblastoma, changes secondary to preoperative chemotherapy, or intrinsic genetic changes enriched in hepatocellular carcinomas arising in this young age group.

ULTRASTRUCTURAL FINDINGS

Ultrastructure studies are not currently used in the evaluation of hepatocellular carcinoma for clinical care. Research studies have shown that hepatocellular carcinomas have no distinct features. Well-differentiated hepatocellular carcinomas resemble mature hepatocytes, but as the tumors become less well differentiated, they show a reduction in the number of internal organelles, with varying amounts of glycogen, endoplasmic reticulum, lysosomes, and mitochondria (177). Secondary lysosomes are often prominent, and hyaline inclusions and Mallory-Denk bodies are frequently found. Capillarization of the tumor sinusoids is also evident (177).

CYTOLOGIC FINDINGS

On smears, findings that suggest hepatocytic differentiation include abundant eosinophilic and granular cytoplasm, fatty change, and bile production. Hepatocyte nuclei tend to be round and centrally placed, and have distinctive nuclear membranes with prominent nucleoli. Differentiating benign from malignant hepatocytes can be challenging on smears and may require correlation with the cell block or accompanying biopsy and the use of immunohistochemical stains (178).

Tumor cells can be smaller, the same size, or larger than benign hepatocytes (179). Evidence for malignancy includes tumor cells showing a high nuclear to cytoplasmic ratio and nuclear pleomorphism (178). Multinucleated cells and hyaline bodies also suggest malignancy (180). Other findings that favor malignancy include mitotic figures, pseudoacinar structures, or cells growing in thick trabeculae. The thick trabeculae are found as cohesive clusters and arborizing cords of tumor cells (fig. 3-75). These thick cords of cells are often "wrapped" by endothelial cells, which are seen as thin spindle-shaped cells surrounding thickened cords of neoplastic hepatocytes (179). Blood vessels may be seen running across or "transgressing" the thickened hepatocytic cords (fig. 3-76) (179). Naked tumor nuclei (fig. 3-77) or a dirty background with necrotic debris also supports a diagnosis of malignancy. In hepatocellular carcinoma smears, ductal cells are few or absent.

MOLECULAR GENETIC FINDINGS

Molecular methods do not currently play a role in diagnosis, other than with fibrolamellar carcinoma (181), which is discussed in its own chapter. Nor do molecular methods currently play a role in prognosis. Numerous papers have

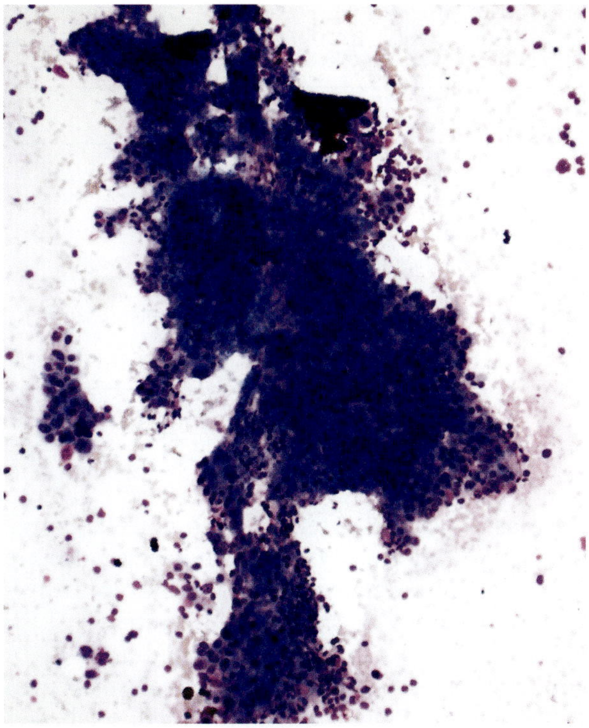

Figure 3-75

HEPATOCELLULAR CARCINOMA

The tumor cells are seen as three-dimensional cohesive clusters of arborizing cords of cells (Diff quick stain).

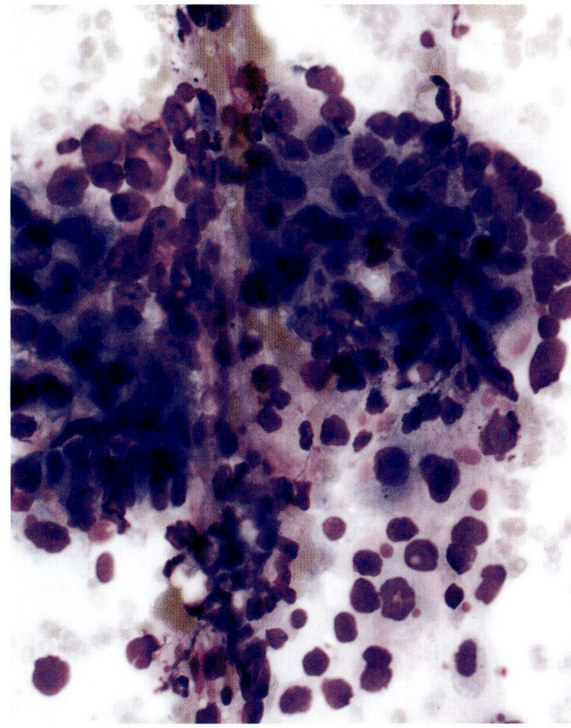

Figure 3-76

HEPATOCELLULAR CARCINOMA

A small vessel is seen running across a cluster of tumor cells (Diff quick stain).

proposed molecular subtypes of hepatocellular carcinoma based on gene expression, but to date, most reported findings are not reproducible and none have become widely accepted. However, this area of oncology research is still in its infancy and may change in time. There is considerable active research looking for molecular methods to help direct therapy, but currently these methods are used in specific clinical trials and are not used in routine clinical care.

DIFFERENTIAL DIAGNOSIS

The differential diagnosis for hepatocellular carcinoma depends on the degree of differentiation and on the presence or absence of cirrhosis in the background liver (Table 3-6). Focal nodular hyperplasia and hepatocellular adenoma arise in noncirrhotic livers and should have no or minimal cytologic atypia and no pseudoglands. Hepatocellular adenomas almost never show cholestasis with an H&E stain. One exception to the lack of cholestatic change and

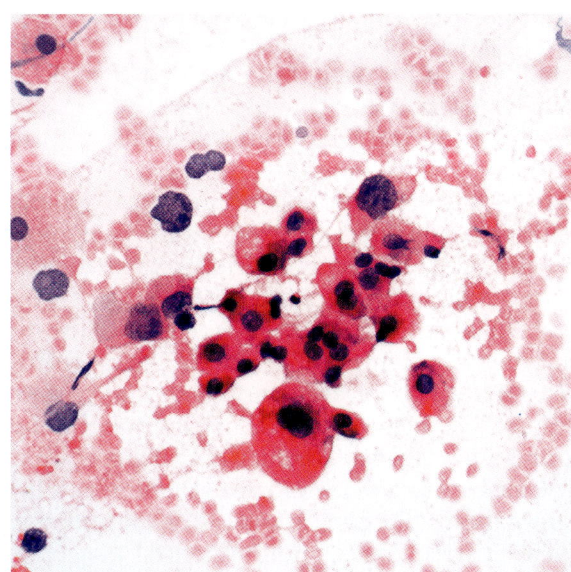

Figure 3-77

HEPATOCELLULAR CARCINOMA

A cluster of benign hepatocytes is juxtaposed to scattered single tumor nuclei with marked nuclear atypia (H&E stain).

Table 3-6

DIFFERENTIAL DIAGNOSIS FOR HEPATOCELLULAR CARCINOMA

	Well-Differentiated Hepatocytic Tumor	Moderately or Poorly Differentiated Hepatocytic Tumor
Noncirrhotic background liver	Focal nodular hyperplasia Hepatocellular adenoma Hepatocellular carcinoma	Hepatocellular carcinoma Cholangiocarcinoma Metastatic disease
Cirrhotic background liver	Focal nodular hyperplasia-like lesions[a] Macroregenerative nodule Low-grade dysplastic nodule High-grade dysplastic nodule Hepatocellular carcinoma	Hepatocellular carcinoma Cholangiocarcinoma Metastatic disease

[a]These lesions result from vascular shunting in the cirrhotic liver and look and stain similar to focal nodular hyperplasia in the noncirrhotic liver (14).

pseudoglands is the androgen-related adenoma. Hyaline inclusions are not present in the tumor cells of hepatocellular adenomas or focal nodular hyperplasia. There should be no evidence of a nodule within nodule growth pattern and no loss of reticulin staining, outside of areas of fatty change. Mitotic figures should be rare or absent and should never be atypical. The Ki-67 proliferative rate is low, typically less than 2 percent.

Rarely, biopsies show well-differentiated tumors that suggest an adenoma but have enough atypical findings that the tumor straddles the histologic dividing line between benign and malignant. In this setting, a reasonable approach is to use the term "well-differentiated hepatocellular neoplasm" and then provide a prioritized differential in the note/comment section of the pathology report, indicating the atypical features that do not fit well for adenoma. These tumors are often designated in the literature as atypical hepatocellular adenomas or hepatocellular tumors of uncertain malignant potential (HUMP) (182). All of these tumors benefit from careful follow-up and many benefit from resection. The diagnosis of HUMP or atypical adenoma should not be overused, as most hepatocellular tumors can be confidently classified as benign or malignant, even on biopsy, after full histologic evaluation and incorporation of the clinical and histologic findings.

In cirrhotic livers, the differential diagnosis for well-differentiated lesions includes macroregenerative and dysplastic nodules. Both typically contain portal tracts. Cytologic atypia is absent or mild and focal in macroregenerative and low-grade dysplastic nodules, while high-grade dysplastic nodules often show small cell change and more evident atypia. Proliferative rates are low (183) and there should be no atypical mitotic figures. There should be no reticulin loss. Some nodules in cirrhotic livers stain for CRP or SAA and have some morphologic features of an inflammatory adenoma (68,69). These should not be called hepatocellular adenoma in clinical practice because activation of a shared pathway does not make them the same tumor, and the natural history and other molecular changes in these cirrhotic nodules are unclear.

When epithelial tumors are clearly malignant, the differential diagnosis includes hepatocellular carcinoma, cholangiocarcinoma, and metastatic neoplasm. In a cirrhotic liver, hepatocellular carcinoma and cholangiocarcinoma are more common than metastatic neoplasms.

SPREAD AND METASTASES

Approximately 40 percent of individuals with hepatocellular carcinoma have metastatic disease at the time of first presentation (184). The most common sites of metastases are the lungs (50 percent), bones (30 percent), abdominal lymph nodes (30 percent), and adrenal glands (10 percent) (184,185). Because of the frequent involvement of lungs, chest imaging is performed as part of the initial staging of hepatocellular carcinoma. Bone scans are not currently part of most guidelines but instead are performed as indicated by clinical findings. Peritoneal spread (carcinomatosis) is uncommon but can be seen: one autopsy study found hepatocellular carcinoma had spread to the peritoneum focally (6 percent) or diffusely (3 percent), with risk factors that included tumor rupture, direct invasion of the diaphragm, or lymph node disease (186).

Needle Tract Seeding. The biopsy needle track can be seeded by hepatocellular carcinoma during biopsy or ablation therapies. There are a few outlier studies with higher frequencies, but overall this is considered a rare event, with a frequency of approximately 2.5 percent in older literature (187) and 0.25 percent in more recent and larger studies (188). More recent biopsy methods, such as the coaxial technique, can bring the risk of seeding down to essentially 0 percent (189). When needle track seeding occurs, the carcinoma is usually detected within the first 6 months (188). Seeding is most common with subcapsular tumors and with high-grade hepatocellular carcinomas. In most cases, tumor seeding can be treated locally and does not reduce life expectancy (190). There is no evidence that pretransplant biopsy of a hepatocellular carcinoma reduces post-transplant survival (191).

STAGING AND TREATMENT

Hepatocellular carcinomas are staged for clinical purposes using a variety of approaches, which tend to be based largely on tumor variables (imaging or pathology findings), underlying liver function (e.g., Child-Pugh score), or physiologic reserve (e.g., performance status). The American Joint Committee on Cancer (AJCC) system is the most commonly used staging approach for pathology information (Table 3-7). The Barcelona Clinic Liver Cancer (BCLC) staging system categorizes individuals into different stages, each with recommended therapies, by incorporating some tumor variables, underlying liver function, and overall health status. Patients with stage 0 and stage A tumors are candidates for surgery with curative intent; stage B tumors are not resectable and are instead treated with transarterial chemoembolization (TACE); stage C tumors are treated with sorafenib; and patients with stage D tumors are treated by supportive care.

Currently, pathologists' main roles are to provide a diagnosis and properly grade and stage the tumor. In the future, these responsibilities seem likely to expand. As targeted therapies mature, pathologists will look for the expression of specific proteins to guide the choice of therapy.

Table 3-7

AMERICAN JOINT COMMITTEE ON CANCER (AJCC) STAGING SYSTEM

T Category	T Criteria
TX	Primary tumor cannot be assessed
T0	No evidence of primary tumor
T1	Solitary tumor ≤2 cm, or >2 cm without vascular invasion
T1a	Solitary tumor ≤2 cm
T1b	Solitary tumor >2 cm without vascular invasion
T2	Solitary tumor >2 cm with vascular invasion, or multiple tumors, none >5 cm
T3	Multiple tumors, at least one of which is >5 cm
T4	Single tumor or multiple tumors of any size involving a major branch of the portal vein or hepatic vein, or tumor(s) with direct invasion of adjacent organs other than the gallbladder or with perforation of visceral peritoneum
N Category	**N Criteria**
NX	Regional lymph nodes cannot be assessed
N0	No regional lymph node metastasis
N1	Regional lymph node metastasis
M Category	**M Criteria**
M0	No distant metastasis
M1	Distant metastasis

[a]AJCC Cancer Staging Manual, 8th edition, 2017.

Currently, prognosis is sufficiently poor for all patients with hepatocellular carcinomas that sufficient prognostic information is obtained by classic staging information: tumor size, numbers of tumors, tumor grade, and angiolymphatic invasion. As therapies improve, immunohistochemistry and molecular-based studies will likely become increasingly important to provide more refined prognostic information.

Surgical resection with curative intent is the preferred treatment for solitary tumors in individuals with well-preserved liver function (192). Adequate liver function for surgery is defined as normal bilirubin levels and a hepatic venous pressure gradient ≤10 mmHg and/or platelet count ≥100,000. Anatomic resections are preferred and employed whenever possible. Ablation therapy is used for small tumors (less than 3 cm) that cannot be surgically resected because of location or comorbid conditions. The two most common ablation methods are radiofrequency ablation (RFA) and ethyl alcohol

(ETOH) injection. RFA kills tumor cells by producing high levels of heat through a high frequency electric current. RFA results in a lower local recurrence rate and better overall survival rate compared to ETOH injection and most treatment guidelines recommend RFA as the locoregional ablation therapy of choice, unless the tumor's anatomic location precludes RFA therapy. The use of RFA as primary therapy in tumors larger than 3 cm remains controversial (193), although it is often used to downstage larger tumors, as a bridge to transplantation or surgery (194). In some cases, RFA is combined with transarterial chemoembolization (TACE) for locoregional therapy (195,196).

TACE and radioembolization are used for unresectable tumors in patients who are not candidates for ablative therapy and do not have metastatic disease. Tumor invasion of the portal vein or Child-Pugh C cirrhosis are contraindications to TACE, while portal vein thrombosis or bilirubin levels greater than 3 mg/dL are relative contraindications (193). With TACE, microsphere beads are infused with chemotherapy agents and injected into the hepatic artery branches feeding the hepatocellular carcinoma. Radioembolization is similar to TACE, but the microspheres are loaded with Yttrium-90, which can deliver localized but high levels of radiation. Patients with hepatocellular carcinomas treated with TACE show better survival rates than non-treatment groups (197), but it is not curative. TACE has a high frequency of complications, largely resulting from beads extending outside the tumor, killing non-neoplastic liver. This can lead to acute hepatic decompensation in up to 20 percent of individuals, which is irreversible in about 3 percent (193).

Systemic chemotherapy is used when tumors invade the portal vein or when there is metastatic disease. Currently, sorafenib is the only therapy widely used (outside the setting of specific clinical trials). The sorafenib therapy in advanced hepatocellular carcinoma (SHARP) trial (198), considered a landmark study in hepatocellular carcinoma therapy, showed sorafenib is superior to placebo in a multicenter study, leading to better median overall survival (11 versus 8 months) in patients with Child-Pugh A cirrhosis. The usefulness of sorafenib in Child-Pugh B and C cirrhosis is under investigation.

PROGNOSIS

In most studies, the median survival time for patients with hepatocellular carcinoma is between 10 and 18 months (199–201). The most important prognostic factor is whether the tumor can be safely and completely resected, which depends on tumor size, tumor location, portal vein invasion, metastatic disease, and physiologic status. Successful resection dramatically improves survival, with a 5-year overall survival rate that ranges from 25 to 80 percent, with best results in those whose tumors are less than 2 cm (202). Liver transplantation is also an important therapy, providing a 5-year survival rate of approximately 75 percent, which is similar to transplantation without hepatocellular carcinoma (202). Liver transplantation has the added benefit of curing the underlying cirrhosis. However, this option is limited by organ shortages and comorbid medical conditions that may precluded transplantation, such as severe cardiovascular disease.

Following surgery with curative intent, hepatocellular carcinomas recur in approximately 60 percent of individuals, most commonly in the liver (203,204). Tumor recurrence is clonally related to the original tumor in about two thirds of cases; the remaining cases result from the development of a second primary in individuals with a background of cirrhosis (205,206).

Several good prognostic factors have been identified. Of these, resectability is by far the most important. Clinical parameters leading to a better prognosis include young age, female gender, and good overall health status. There are three powerful tumor-specific prognostic factors: tumor size, tumor grade, and angiolymphatic invasion. Not surprisingly, these factors are all correlated to some degree, as larger tumors are more likely to be poorly differentiated and are more likely to have angiolymphatic invasion. However, each of these factors also has independent prognostic value. The tumor subtype also has prognostic relevance, with a better prognosis for those with clear cell hepatocellular carcinoma and perhaps for lymphocyte-rich hepatocellular carcinoma, and a worse prognosis for those with combined hepatocellular carcinoma-cholangiocarcinoma, combined hepatocellular carcinoma-neuroendocrine carcinoma, cirrhotomimetic hepatocellular carcinoma, sarcomatoid hepatocellular carcinoma, GCSFP hepatocellular carcinoma, and carcinosarcoma. Pathology findings in the background liver that impart a better prognosis include lack of underlying liver disease and lack of advanced fibrosis (207).

Because tumor size is a major driver of prognosis, size is incorporated into all staging systems. Tumor size is defined as the maximum diameter measured in centimeters. There often are small discrepancies between gross measurements and radiologic measurements, in most cases a centimeter or less, but in some cases the disagreement is more substantial. Pathology staging is based on the gross measurements and not imaging findings.

Patients with larger tumors have a worse prognosis, as do those with multifocal tumors. Based on published data, there appears to be a threshold effect of about 4 cm for predicting prognosis based on tumor size. Tumors between 1 to 4 cm in size have no incremental impact on survival for each additional centimeter of tumor, while those larger than 5 cm have an incremental decrease in survival for each centimeter of increased size.

Angiolymphatic Invasion. Vascular invasion predicts tumor recurrence after both resection (63,65) and liver transplantation (66). One possible exception is tumors less than 2 cm in diameter, where one study found that microvascular invasion did not affect prognosis (208); other studies, however, have come to the opposite conclusion (209,210).

Macrovascular invasion is defined as tumor invading blood vessels that can be recognized by gross examination or by imaging. The frequency of macrovascular invasion is between 5 and 30 percent in most studies. The portal venous system and the central veins/vena cava are most commonly involved (211), while macroscopic invasion of the hepatic arteries is almost never seen.

Microvascular invasion is defined as vascular involvement that is evident only on histologic examination. An endothelial lining should be present to make the diagnosis of vascular invasion (fig. 3-78), as retraction artifact can sometimes mimic lymphatic or venous invasion. In addition, hepatocellular carcinomas are often friable and finding rare individual or small clusters of tumor cells floating freely in an otherwise empty vascular lumen in a resection specimen is generally interpreted as sectioning artifact and not true vascular invasion.

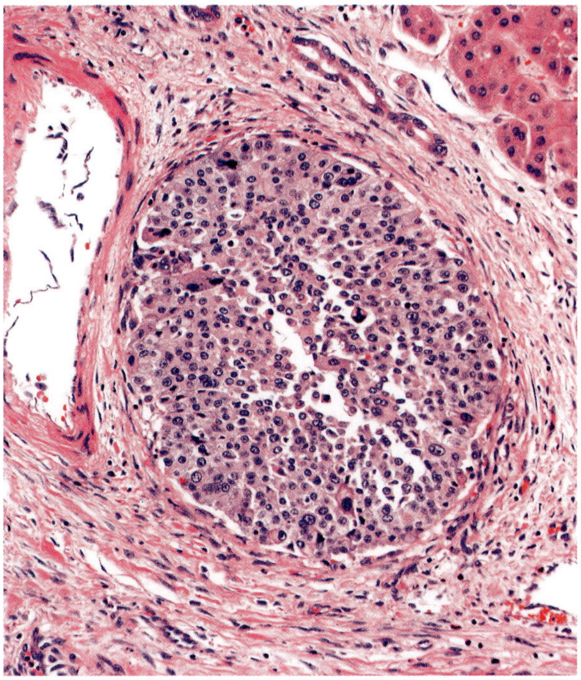

Figure 3-78

ANGIOLYMPHATIC INVASION

The portal vein shows a large plug of hepatocellular carcinoma.

Microvascular invasion is seen in approximately 30 percent of resected specimens, although the frequency ranges in studies from 15 to 57 percent (212). It is most commonly seen in sections taken at the tumor-nontumor interface. The portal veins are much more likely to be involved by cancer than the central veins, with a ratio of about 10 to 1 (213). Invasion of the hepatic arteries is even less common but is generally considered to confer a worse prognosis than venous invasion. Several studies have identified additional potential prognostic information by subclassification of vascular invasion, although these findings are not routinely found in surgical pathology reports. These factors include the number of foci of vascular invasion, the size of tumor deposits, whether or not the affected vessel has a muscular wall, and a distance of greater than 1 cm between the vascular invasion and the main tumor deposit (214,215).

REFERENCES

1. Gong L, Li YH, Su Q, Chu X, Zhang W. Clonality of nodular lesions in liver cirrhosis and chromosomal abnormalities in monoclonal nodules of altered hepatocytes. Histopathology 2010;56: 589-599.
2. Park YN. Update on precursor and early lesions of hepatocellular carcinomas. Arch Pathol Lab Med 2011;135:704-715.
3. Marchio A, Terris B, Meddeb M, et al. Chromosomal abnormalities in liver cell dysplasia detected by comparative genomic hybridisation. Mol Pathol 2001;54:270-274.
4. Plentz RR, Park YN, Lechel A, et al. Telomere shortening and inactivation of cell cycle checkpoints characterize human hepatocarcinogenesis. Hepatology 2007;45:968-976.
5. Lee RG, Tsamandas AC, Demetris AJ. Large cell change (liver cell dysplasia) and hepatocellular carcinoma in cirrhosis: matched case-control study, pathological analysis, and pathogenetic hypothesis. Hepatology 1997;26:1415-1422.
6. Niu ZS, Niu XJ, Wang WH, Zhao J. Latest developments in precancerous lesions of hepatocellular carcinoma. World J Gastroenterol 2016;22:3305-3314.
7. Su Q, Zerban H, Otto G, Bannasch P. Cytokeratin expression is reduced in glycogenotic clear hepatocytes but increased in ground-glass cells in chronic human and woodchuck hepadnaviral infection. Hepatology 1998;28(2):347-359.
8. Su Q, Benner A, Hofmann WJ, Otto G, Pichlmayr R, Bannasch P. Human hepatic preneoplasia: phenotypes and proliferation kinetics of foci and nodules of altered hepatocytes and their relationship to liver cell dysplasia. Virchows Arch 1997;431:391-406.
9. Klein WM, Molmenti EP, Colombani PM, et al. Primary liver carcinoma arising in people younger than 30 years. Am J Clin Pathol 2005;124:512-518.
10. Libbrecht L, Desmet V, Van Damme B, Roskams T. The immunohistochemical phenotype of dysplastic foci in human liver: correlation with putative progenitor cells. J Hepatol 2000;33:76-84.
11. Hytiroglou P, Theise ND, Schwartz M, Mor E, Miller C, Thung SN. Macroregenerative nodules in a series of adult cirrhotic liver explants: issues of classification and nomenclature. Hepatology 1995;21:703-708.
12. Furuya K, Nakamura M, Yamamoto Y, Togei K, Otsuka H. Macroregenerative nodule of the liver. A clinicopathologic study of 345 autopsy cases of chronic liver disease. Cancer 1988;61:99-105.
13. Sato T, Kondo F, Ebara M, et al. Natural history of large regenerative nodules and dysplastic nodules in liver cirrhosis: 28-year follow-up study. Hepatol Int 2015;9:330-336.
14. Quaglia A, Tibballs J, Grasso A, et al. Focal nodular hyperplasia-like areas in cirrhosis. Histopathology 2003;42:14-21.
15. Libbrecht L, Cassiman D, Verslype C, et al. Clinicopathological features of focal nodular hyperplasia-like nodules in 130 cirrhotic explant livers. Am J Gastroenterol 2006;101:2341-2346.
16. Rebouissou S, Couchy G, Libbrecht L, et al. The beta-catenin pathway is activated in focal nodular hyperplasia but not in cirrhotic FNH-like nodules. J Hepatol 2008;49:61-71.
17. Nguyen TB, Roncalli M, Di Tommaso L, Kakar S. Combined use of heat-shock protein 70 and glutamine synthetase is useful in the distinction of typical hepatocellular adenoma from atypical hepatocellular neoplasms and well-differentiated hepatocellular carcinoma. Mod Pathol 2016;29:283-292.
18. Nakano M, Saito A, Yamamoto M, Doi M, Takasaki K. Stromal and blood vessel wall invasion in well-differentiated hepatocellular carcinoma. Liver 1997;17:41-46.
19. Kojiro M, Roskams T. Early hepatocellular carcinoma and dysplastic nodules. Semin Liver Dis 2005;25:133-142.
20. Kondo F. Assessment of stromal invasion for correct histological diagnosis of early hepatocellular carcinoma. Int J Hepatol 2011;2011:241652.
21. Park YN, Kojiro M, Di Tommaso L, et al. Ductular reaction is helpful in defining early stromal invasion, small hepatocellular carcinomas, and dysplastic nodules. Cancer 2007;109:915-923.
22. Seki S, Sakaguchi H, Kitada T, et al. Outcomes of dysplastic nodules in human cirrhotic liver: a clinicopathological study. Clin Cancer Res 2000;6:3469-3473.
23. Iavarone M, Manini MA, Sangiovanni A, et al. Contrast-enhanced computed tomography and ultrasound-guided liver biopsy to diagnose dysplastic liver nodules in cirrhosis. Dig Liver Dis 2013;45:43-49.
24. Kim SH, Lim HK, Kim MJ, Choi D, Rhim H, Park CK. Radiofrequency ablation of high-grade dysplastic nodules in chronic liver disease: comparison with well-differentiated hepatocellular carcinoma based on long-term results. Eur Radiol 2008;18:814-821.
25. Cho YK, Wook Chung J, Kim Y, Je Cho H, Hyun Yang S. Radiofrequency ablation of high-grade dysplastic nodules. Hepatology 2011;54:2005-2011.

26. Ouedraogo NA, Danjoux-de-Volontat M, Auriol J, Peron JM, Rousseau H, Otal P. Dysplastic hepatic nodules: radiological abnormalities and histopathological correlations. Eur J Radiol 2011;79:232-236.
27. Dorfman JD, Schulick R, Choti MA, et al. Differences in characteristics of patients with and without known risk factors for hepatocellular carcinoma in the United States. World J Gastroenterol 2007;13:781-784.
28. Martin RC 2nd, Loehle J, Scoggins CR, McMasters KM. Kentucky hepatoma: epidemiologic variant or same problem in a different region? Arch Surg 2007;142:431-436; discussion 436-437.
29. van Meer S, van Erpecum KJ, Sprengers D, et al. Hepatocellular carcinoma in cirrhotic versus noncirrhotic livers: results from a large cohort in the Netherlands. Eur J Gastroenterol Hepatol 2016;28:352-359.
30. Toyoda H, Kumada T, Tada T, Sone Y, Kaneoka Y, Maeda A. Tumor markers for hepatocellular carcinoma: simple and significant predictors of outcome in patients with HCC. Liver Cancer 2015;4:126-136.
31. Song PP, Xia JF, Inagaki Y, et al. Controversies regarding and perspectives on clinical utility of biomarkers in hepatocellular carcinoma. World J Gastroenterol 2016;22:262-274.
32. Marrero JA, Feng Z, Wang Y, et al. Alpha-fetoprotein, des-gamma carboxyprothrombin, and lectin-bound alpha-fetoprotein in early hepatocellular carcinoma. Gastroenterology 2009;137:110-118.
33. Leerapun A, Suravarapu SV, Bida JP, et al. The utility of Lens culinaris agglutinin-reactive alpha-fetoprotein in the diagnosis of hepatocellular carcinoma: evaluation in a United States referral population. Clin Gastroenterol Hepatol 2007;5:394-402; quiz 267.
34. Sanyal AJ, Yoon SK, Lencioni R. The etiology of hepatocellular carcinoma and consequences for treatment. Oncologist 2010;15(Suppl 4):14-22.
35. Hirakawa M, Ikeda K, Arase Y, et al. Hepatocarcinogenesis following HCV RNA eradication by interferon in chronic hepatitis patients. Intern Med 2008;47:1637-1643.
36. Tokita H, Fukui H, Tanaka A, et al. Risk factors for the development of hepatocellular carcinoma among patients with chronic hepatitis C who achieved a sustained virological response to interferon therapy. J Gastroenterol Hepatol 2005;20:752-758.
37. Paradis V, Zalinski S, Chelbi E, et al. Hepatocellular carcinomas in patients with metabolic syndrome often develop without significant liver fibrosis: a pathological analysis. Hepatology 2009;49:851-859.
38. Kew MC. Aflatoxins as a cause of hepatocellular carcinoma. J Gastrointestin Liver Dis 2013;22: 305-310.
39. Fattovich G, Stroffolini T, Zagni I, Donato F. Hepatocellular carcinoma in cirrhosis: incidence and risk factors. Gastroenterology 2004;127 (Suppl 1):S35-50.
40. Wang CS, Yao WJ, Chang TT, Wang ST, Chou P. The impact of type 2 diabetes on the development of hepatocellular carcinoma in different viral hepatitis statuses. Cancer Epidemiol Biomarkers Prev 2009;18:2054-2060.
41. Ko C, Siddaiah N, Berger J, et al. Prevalence of hepatic iron overload and association with hepatocellular cancer in end-stage liver disease: results from the National Hemochromatosis Transplant Registry. Liver Int 2007;27:1394-1401.
42. Wang Q, Luan W, Villanueva GA, et al. Clinical prognostic variables in young patients (under 40 years) with hepatitis B virus-associated hepatocellular carcinoma. J Dig Dis 2012;13:214-218.
43. Yeh MM, Daniel HD, Torbenson M. Hepatitis C-associated hepatocellular carcinomas in non-cirrhotic livers. Mod Pathol 2010;23:276-283.
44. von Delius S, Lersch C, Schulte-Frohlinde E, et al. Hepatocellular carcinoma associated with hereditary hemochromatosis occurring in non-cirrhotic liver. Z Gastroenterol 2006;44:39-42.
45. Baffy G, Brunt EM, Caldwell SH. Hepatocellular carcinoma in non-alcoholic fatty liver disease: an emerging menace. J Hepatol 2012;56:1384-1391.
46. Alexander J, Torbenson M, Wu TT, Yeh MM. Non-alcoholic fatty liver disease contributes to hepatocellular carcinoma in non-cirrhotic liver: a clinical and pathological study. J Gastroenterol Hepatol 2013;28:848-54.
47. Micchelli ST, Vivekanandan P, Boitnott JK, Pawlik TM, Choti MA, Torbenson M. Malignant transformation of hepatic adenomas. Mod Pathol 2008;21:491-497.
48. Benedict M, Rodriguez-Davalos M, Emre S, Walther Z, Morotti RA. Congenital extrahepatic portosystemic shunt (Abernethy malformation type Ib) with associated hepatocellular carcinoma: case report and literature review. Pediatr Dev Pathol 2017;20:354-362.
49. Sharma VK, Ranade PR, Marar S, Nabi F, Nagral A. Long-term clinical outcome of Budd-Chiari syndrome in children after radiological intervention. Eur J Gastroenterol Hepatol 2016;28:567-575.
50. Dang X, Li L, Li S, et al. Studies on Budd-chiari syndrome complicated with hepatocellular carcinoma: most patients without inferior vena cava obstruction. Int J Clin Exp Med 2015;8:9071-9078.

51. Yeh CN, Lee WC, Jeng LB, Chen MF. Pedunculated hepatocellular carcinoma: clinicopathologic study of 18 surgically resected cases. World J Surg 2002;26:1133-1138.
52. Horie Y, Shigoku A, Tanaka H, et al. Prognosis for pedunculated hepatocellular carcinoma. Oncology 1999;57:23-28.
53. Anthony PP, James K. Pedunculated hepatocellular carcinoma. Is it an entity? Histopathology 1987;11:403-414.
54. M Mashfigul AS, Tan YM, Thng CH, et al. Pedunculated HCC or adrenal metastasis: a diagnostic conundrum. Singapore Med J 2007;48:e50-52.
55. Hirokawa F, Hayashi M, Asakuma M, Shimizu T, Inoue Y, Uchiyama K. Risk factors and patterns of early recurrence after curative hepatectomy for hepatocellular carcinoma. Surg Oncol 2016;25:24-29.
56. Lee JW, Lee YJ, Park KM, Hwang DW, Lee JH, Song KB. Anatomical Resection but not surgical margin width influence survival following resection for HCC, a propensity score analysis. World J Surg 2016;40:1429-1439.
57. Lafaro K, Grandhi MS, Herman JM, Pawlik TM. The importance of surgical margins in primary malignancies of the liver. J Surg Oncol 2016;113:296-303.
58. Shi M, Guo RP, Lin XJ, et al. Partial hepatectomy with wide versus narrow resection margin for solitary hepatocellular carcinoma: a prospective randomized trial. Ann Surg 2007;245:36-43.
59. Nzeako UC, Goodman ZD, Ishak KG. Comparison of tumor pathology with duration of survival of North American patients with hepatocellular carcinoma. Cancer 1995;76:579-588.
60. Lauwers GY, Terris B, Balis UJ, et al. Prognostic histologic indicators of curatively resected hepatocellular carcinomas: a multi-institutional analysis of 425 patients with definition of a histologic prognostic index. Am J Surg Pathol 2002;26:25-34.
61. Lai JP, Conley A, Knudsen BS, Guindi M. Hypoxia after transarterial chemoembolization may trigger a progenitor cell phenotype in hepatocellular carcinoma. Histopathology 2015;67:442-450.
62. Zen C, Zen Y, Mitry RR, et al. Mixed phenotype hepatocellular carcinoma after transarterial chemoembolization and liver transplantation. Liver Transpl 2011;17:943-954.
63. Benckert C, Jonas S, Thelen A, et al. Liver transplantation for hepatocellular carcinoma in cirrhosis: prognostic parameters. Transplant Proc 2005;37:1693-1694.
64. Zhou L, Rui JA, Wang SB, et al. Outcomes and prognostic factors of cirrhotic patients with hepatocellular carcinoma after radical major hepatectomy. World J Surg 2007;31:1782-1787.
65. Lang H, Sotiropoulos GC, Brokalaki EI, et al. Survival and recurrence rates after resection for hepatocellular carcinoma in noncirrhotic livers. J Am Coll Surg 2007;205:27-36.
66. Jonas S, Bechstein WO, Steinmuller T, et al. Vascular invasion and histopathologic grading determine outcome after liver transplantation for hepatocellular carcinoma in cirrhosis. Hepatology 2001;33:1080-1086.
67. Han DH, Choi GH, Kim KS, et al. Prognostic significance of the worst grade in hepatocellular carcinoma with heterogeneous histologic grades of differentiation. J Gastroenterol Hepatol 2013;28:1384-1390.
68. Sasaki M, Yoneda N, Kitamura S, Sato Y, Nakanuma Y. A serum amyloid A-positive hepatocellular neoplasm arising in alcoholic cirrhosis: a previously unrecognized type of inflammatory hepatocellular tumor. Mod Pathol 2012;25:1584-1593.
69. Calderaro J, Nault JC, Balabaud C, et al. Inflammatory hepatocellular adenomas developed in the setting of chronic liver disease and cirrhosis. Mod Pathol 2016;29:43-50.
70. Wang XY, Degos F, Dubois S, et al. Glypican-3 expression in hepatocellular tumors: diagnostic value for preneoplastic lesions and hepatocellular carcinomas. Hum Pathol 2006;37:1435-1441.
71. Krings G, Ramachandran R, Jain D, et al. Immunohistochemical pitfalls and the importance of glypican 3 and arginase in the diagnosis of scirrhous hepatocellular carcinoma. Mod Pathol 2013;26:782-791.
72. Han CP, Hsu JD, Koo CL, Yang SF. Antibody to cytokeratin (CK8/CK18) is not derived from CAM5.2 clone, and anticytokeratin CAM5.2 (Becton Dickinson) is not synonymous with the antibody (CK8/CK18). Hum Pathol 2010;41:616-617; author reply 617.
73. Durnez A, Verslype C, Nevens F, et al. The clinicopathological and prognostic relevance of cytokeratin 7 and 19 expression in hepatocellular carcinoma. A possible progenitor cell origin. Histopathology 2006;49:138-151.
74. Uenishi T, Kubo S, Yamamoto T, et al. Cytokeratin 19 expression in hepatocellular carcinoma predicts early postoperative recurrence. Cancer Sci 2003;94:851-857.
75. Kim H, Choi GH, Na DC, et al. Human hepatocellular carcinomas with "stemness"-related marker expression: keratin 19 expression and a poor prognosis. Hepatology 2011;54:1707-1717.
76. Vlasoff DM, Baschinsky DY, Frankel WL. Cytokeratin 5/6 immunostaining in hepatobiliary and pancreatic neoplasms. Appl Immunohistochem Mol Morphol 2002;10:147-151.

77. Christensen WN, Boitnott JK, Kuhajda FP. Immunoperoxidase staining as a diagnostic aid for hepatocellular carcinoma. Mod Pathol 1989;2:8-12.
78. Butler SL, Dong H, Cardona D, et al. The antigen for Hep Par 1 antibody is the urea cycle enzyme carbamoyl phosphate synthetase 1. Lab Invest 2008;88:78-88.
79. Wennerberg AE, Nalesnik MA, Coleman WB. Hepatocyte paraffin 1: a monoclonal antibody that reacts with hepatocytes and can be used for differential diagnosis of hepatic tumors. Am J Pathol 1993;143:1050-1054.
80. Chan ES, Yeh MM. The use of immunohistochemistry in liver tumors. Clin Liver Dis 2010;14:687-703.
81. Fan Z, van de Rijn M, Montgomery K, Rouse RV. Hep par 1 antibody stain for the differential diagnosis of hepatocellular carcinoma: 676 tumors tested using tissue microarrays and conventional tissue sections. Mod Pathol 2003;16:137-144.
82. Mounajjed T, Zhang L, Wu TT. Glypican-3 expression in gastrointestinal and pancreatic epithelial neoplasms. Hum Pathol 2013;44:542-550.
83. Fujiwara M, Kwok S, Yano H, Pai RK. Arginase-1 is a more sensitive marker of hepatic differentiation than HepPar-1 and glypican-3 in fine-needle aspiration biopsies. Cancer Cytopathol 2012;120:230-237.
84. Shafizadeh N, Ferrell LD, Kakar S. Utility and limitations of glypican-3 expression for the diagnosis of hepatocellular carcinoma at both ends of the differentiation spectrum. Mod Pathol 2008;21:1011-1018.
85. Yan B, Wei JJ, Qian YM, et al. Expression and clinicopathologic significance of glypican 3 in hepatocellular carcinoma. Ann Diagn Pathol 2011;15:162-169.
86. Abdul-Al HM, Makhlouf HR, Wang G, Goodman ZD. Glypican-3 expression in benign liver tissue with active hepatitis C: implications for the diagnosis of hepatocellular carcinoma. Hum Pathol 2008;39:209-212.
87. Libbrecht L, Severi T, Cassiman D, et al. Glypican-3 expression distinguishes small hepatocellular carcinomas from cirrhosis, dysplastic nodules, and focal nodular hyperplasia-like nodules. Am J Surg Pathol 2006;30:1405-1411.
88. Coston WM, Loera S, Lau SK, et al. Distinction of hepatocellular carcinoma from benign hepatic mimickers using Glypican-3 and CD34 immunohistochemistry. Am J Surg Pathol 2008;32:433-444.
89. Yan BC, Gong C, Song J, et al. Arginase-1: a new immunohistochemical marker of hepatocytes and hepatocellular neoplasms. Am J Surg Pathol 2010;34:1147-1154.
90. Chandan VS, Shah SS, Torbenson MS, Wu TT. Arginase-1 is frequently positive in hepatoid adenocarcinomas. Hum Pathol 2016;55:11-16.
91. Radwan NA, Ahmed NS. The diagnostic value of arginase-1 immunostaining in differentiating hepatocellular carcinoma from metastatic carcinoma and cholangiocarcinoma as compared to HepPar-1. Diagn Pathol 2012;7:149.
92. Geramizadeh B, Seirfar N. Diagnostic Value of Arginase-1 and Glypican-3 in differential diagnosis of hepatocellular carcinoma, cholangiocarcinoma and metastatic carcinoma of liver. Hepat Mon 2015;15:e30336.
93. Terris B, Hergli I, Lin-Marq N, Rubbia-Brandt L. Letter to the editor with regard to the article entitled: "Branched chain in situ hybridization for albumin as a marker of hepatocellular differentiation." Am J Surg Pathol 2015;39:1156-1157.
94. Ferrone CR, Ting DT, Shahid M, et al. The ability to diagnose intrahepatic cholangiocarcinoma definitively using novel branched DNA-enhanced albumin RNA in situ hybridization technology. Ann Surg Oncol 2016;23:290-296.
95. Noorredam K. Primary carcinoma of the liver. A histological study of 27 cases of primary carcinoma of the liver from Malawi. Acta Pathol Microbiol Scand A 1977;85:461-469.
96. Koelma IA, Nap M, Huitema S, Krom RA, Houthoff HJ. Hepatocellular carcinoma, adenoma, and focal nodular hyperplasia. Comparative histopathologic study with immunohistochemical parameters. Arch Pathol Lab Med 1986;110:1035-1040.
97. Bergman S, Graeme-Cook F, Pitman MB. The usefulness of the reticulin stain in the differential diagnosis of liver nodules on fine-needle aspiration biopsy cell block preparations. Mod Pathol 1997;10:1258-1264.
98. Singhi AD, Jain D, Kakar S, Wu TT, Yeh MM, Torbenson M. Reticulin loss in benign fatty liver: an important diagnostic pitfall when considering a diagnosis of hepatocellular carcinoma. Am J Surg Pathol 2012;36:710-715.
99. Hong H, Patonay B, Finley J. Unusual reticulin staining pattern in well-differentiated hepatocellular carcinoma. Diagn Pathol 2011;6:15.
100. Wilkens L, Becker T, Schlegelberger B, Kreipe HH, Flemming P. Preserved reticulin network in a case of hepatocellular carcinoma. Histopathology 2006;48:876-878.
101. Ruck P, Xiao JC, Kaiserling E. Immunoreactivity of sinusoids in hepatocellular carcinoma. An immunohistochemical study using lectin UEA-1 and antibodies against endothelial markers, including CD34. Arch Pathol Lab Med 1995;119:173-178.

102. Ahmad I, Iyer A, Marginean CE, et al. Diagnostic use of cytokeratins, CD34, and neuronal cell adhesion molecule staining in focal nodular hyperplasia and hepatic adenoma. Hum Pathol 2009;40:726-734.
103. Kong CS, Appenzeller M, Ferrell LD. Utility of CD34 reactivity in evaluating focal nodular hepatocellular lesions sampled by fine needle aspiration biopsy. Acta Cytol 2000;44:218-222.
104. Bellamy CO, Maxwell RS, Prost S, Azodo IA, Powell JJ, Manning JR. The value of immunophenotyping hepatocellular adenomas: consecutive resections at one UK centre. Histopathology 2013;62:431-445.
105. Sciarra A, Ronot M, Di Tommaso L, et al. TRIP: a pathological score for transarterial chemoembolization resistance individualized prediction in hepatocellular carcinoma. Liver Int 2015;35:2466-2473.
106. Nolte M, Werner M, Nasarek A, et al. Expression of proliferation associated antigens and detection of numerical chromosome aberrations in primary human liver tumours: relevance to tumour characteristics and prognosis. J Clin Pathol 1998;51:47-51.
107. van Dekken H, Verhoef C, Wink J, et al. Cell biological evaluation of liver cell carcinoma, dysplasia and adenoma by tissue micro-array analysis. Acta Histochem 2005;107:161-171.
108. Shirakawa H, Suzuki H, Shimomura M, et al. Glypican-3 expression is correlated with poor prognosis in hepatocellular carcinoma. Cancer Sci 2009;100:1403-1407.
109. Wood LD, Heaphy CM, Daniel HD, et al. Chromophobe hepatocellular carcinoma with abrupt anaplasia: a proposal for a new subtype of hepatocellular carcinoma with unique morphological and molecular features. Mod Pathol 2013;26:1586-1593.
110. Lao XM, Chen DY, Zhang YQ, et al. Primary carcinosarcoma of the liver: clinicopathologic features of 5 cases and a review of the literature. Am J Surg Pathol 2007;31:817-826.
111. Aita K, Seki K. Carcinosarcoma of the liver producing granulocyte-colony stimulating factor. Pathol Int 2006;56:413-419.
112. Xiang S, Chen YF, Guan Y, Chen XP. Primary combined hepatocellular-cholangiocellular sarcoma: An unusual case. World J Gastroenterol 2015;21:7335-7342.
113. Lu J, Zhang J, Xiong XZ, et al. Primary hepatic sarcomatoid carcinoma: clinical features and prognosis of 28 resected cases. J Cancer Res Clin Oncol 2014;140:1027-1035.
114. Lee KB. Sarcomatoid hepatocellular carcinoma with mixed osteoclast-like giant cells and chondroid differentiation. Clin Mol Hepatol 2014;20:313-316.
115. Kuwano H, Sonoda T, Hashimoto H, Enjoji M. Hepatocellular carcinoma with osteoclast-like giant cells. Cancer 1984;54:837-842.
116. Hood DL, Bauer TW, Leibel SA, McMahon JT. Hepatic giant cell carcinoma. An ultrastructural and immunohistochemical study. Am J Clin Pathol. 1990;93(1):111-116.
117. Sasaki A, Yokoyama S, Nakayama I, Nakashima K, Kim YI, Kitano S. Sarcomatoid hepatocellular carcinoma with osteoclast-like giant cells: case report and immunohistochemical observations. Pathol Int 1997;47:318-324.
118. Tanahashi C, Nagae H, Nukaya T, Hasegawa M, Yatabe Y. Combined hepatocellular carcinoma and osteoclast-like giant cell tumor of the liver: possible clue to histogenesis. Pathol Int 2009;59:813-816.
119. Dioscoridi L, Bisogni D, Freschi G. Hepatocellular carcinoma with osteoclast-like giant cells: report of the seventh case in the literature. Case Rep Surg 2015;2015:836105.
120. Dahm HH. Immunohistochemical evaluation of a sarcomatoid hepatocellular carcinoma with osteoclastlike giant cells. Diagn Pathol 2015;10:40.
121. Ikeda T, Seki S, Maki M, et al. Hepatocellular carcinoma with osteoclast-like giant cells: possibility of osteoclastogenesis by hepatocyte-derived cells. Pathol Int 2003;53:450-456.
122. Jakate S, Yabes A, Giusto D, et al. Diffuse cirrhosis-like hepatocellular carcinoma: a clinically and radiographically undetected variant mimicking cirrhosis. Am J Surg Pathol 2010;34:935-941.
123. Okuda K, Noguchi T, Kubo Y, Shimokawa Y, Kojiro M, Nakashima T. A clinical and pathological study of diffuse type hepatocellular carcinoma. Liver 1981;1:280-289.
124. Kanematsu M, Semelka RC, Leonardou P, Mastropasqua M, Lee JK. Hepatocellular carcinoma of diffuse type: MR imaging findings and clinical manifestations. J Magn Reson Imaging 2003;18:189-195.
125. Clayton EF, Malik S, Bonnel A, et al. Liver transplantation and cirrhotomimetic hepatocellular carcinoma: classification and outcomes. Liver Transpl 2014;20:765-774.
126. Han YS, Choi DL, Park JB. Cirrhotomimetic type hepatocellular carcinoma diagnosed after liver transplantation—eighteen months of follow-up: a case report. Transplant Proc 2008;40:2835-2836.
127. Emile JF, Lemoine A, Azoulay D, Debuire B, Bismuth H, Reynes M. Histological, genomic and clinical heterogeneity of clear cell hepatocellular carcinoma. Histopathology 2001;38:225-231.

128. Liu Z, Ma W, Li H, Li Q. Clinicopathological and prognostic features of primary clear cell carcinoma of the liver. Hepatol Res 2008;38:291-299.
129. Li T, Fan J, Qin LX, et al. Risk factors, prognosis, and management of early and late intrahepatic recurrence after resection of primary clear cell carcinoma of the liver. Ann Surg Oncol 2011;18:1955-1963.
130. Xu W, Ge P, Liao W, et al. Edmondson grade predicts survival of patients with primary clear cell carcinoma of liver after curative resection: A retrospective study with long-term follow-up. Asia Pac J Clin Oncol 2016. [Epub ahead of print]
131. Buchanan TF, Jr., Huvos AG. Clear-cell carcinoma of the liver. A clinicopathologic study of 13 patients. Am J Clin Pathol 1974;61:529-539.
132. Yang SH, Watanabe J, Nakashima O, Kojiro M. Clinicopathologic study on clear cell hepatocellular carcinoma. Pathol Int 1996;46:503-509.
133. Murakata LA, Ishak KG, Nzeako UC. Clear cell carcinoma of the liver: a comparative immunohistochemical study with renal clear cell carcinoma. Mod Pathol 2000;13:874-881.
134. Noro T, Gotohda N, Kojima M, et al. Hepatocellular carcinoma with foamy histiocyte-like appearance: a deceptively clear cell carcinoma appearing variant. Case Rep Gastroenterol 2010;4:286-292.
135. Orikasa H, Ohyama R, Tsuka N, Eyden BP, Yamazaki K. Lipid-rich clear-cell hepatocellular carcinoma arising in non-alcoholic steatohepatitis in a patient with diabetes mellitus. J Submicrosc Cytol Pathol 2001;33:195-200.
136. Cao J, Huang L, Liu C, et al. Double primary hepatic cancer (hepatocellular carcinoma and intrahepatic cholangiocarcinoma) in a single patient: a clinicopathologic study of 35 resected cases. J Gastroenterol Hepatol 2013;28:1025-1031.
137. Yang CS, Wen MC, Jan YJ, Wang J, Wu CC. Combined primary neuroendocrine carcinoma and hepatocellular carcinoma of the liver. J Chin Med Assoc 2009;72:430-433.
138. Yamaguchi R, Nakashima O, Ogata T, Hanada K, Kumabe T, Kojiro M. Hepatocellular carcinoma with an unusual neuroendocrine component. Pathol Int 2004;54:861-865.
139. Nakanishi C, Sato K, Ito Y, et al. Combined hepatocellular carcinoma and neuroendocrine carcinoma with sarcomatous change of the liver after transarterial chemoembolization. Hepatol Res 2012;42:1141-1145.
140. Chu PG, Ishizawa S, Wu E, Weiss LM. Hepatocyte antigen as a marker of hepatocellular carcinoma: an immunohistochemical comparison to carcinoembryonic antigen, CD10, and alpha-fetoprotein. Am J Surg Pathol 2002;26:978-988.
141. Jin M, Zhou X, Yearsley M, Frankel WL. Liver metastases of neuroendocrine tumors rarely show overlapping immunoprofile with hepatocellular carcinomas. Endocr Pathol 2016;27:253-258.
142. Huang XF, Wang CM, Dai XW, et al. Expressions of chromogranin A and cathepsin D in human primary hepatocellular carcinoma. World J Gastroenterol 2000;6:693-698.
143. Kohno M, Shirabe K, Mano Y, et al. Granulocyte colony-stimulating-factor-producing hepatocellular carcinoma with extensive sarcomatous changes: report of a case. Surg Today 2012;43:439-445.
144. Amano H, Itamoto T, Emoto K, Hino H, Asahara T, Shimamoto F. Granulocyte colony-stimulating factor-producing combined hepatocellular/cholangiocellular carcinoma with sarcomatous change. J Gastroenterol 2005;40:1158-1159.
145. Araki K, Kishihara F, Takahashi K, et al. Hepatocellular carcinoma producing a granulocyte colony-stimulating factor: report of a resected case with a literature review. Liver Int 2007;27:716-721.
146. Joshita S, Nakazawa K, Koike S, et al. A case of granulocyte-colony stimulating factor-producing hepatocellular carcinoma confirmed by immunohistochemistry. J Korean Med Sci 2010;25:476-480.
147. Yamamoto S, Takashima S, Ogawa H, et al. Granulocyte-colony-stimulating-factor-producing hepatocellular carcinoma. J Gastroenterol 1999;34:640-644.
148. Snyder RA, Liu E, Merchant NB. Granulocyte colony stimulating factor secreting hepatocellular carcinoma. Am Surg 2012;78:821-822.
149. Takenaka M, Akiba J, Kawaguchi T, et al. Intrahepatic cholangiocarcinoma with sarcomatous change producing granulocyte-colony stimulating factor. Pathol Int 2013;63:233-235.
150. Shimakawa T, Asaka S, Usuda A, et al. Granulocyte-colony stimulating factor (G-CSF)-producing esophageal squamous cell carcinoma: a case report. Int Surg 2014;99:280-285.
151. Tachibana M, Murai M. G-CSF production in human bladder cancer and its ability to promote autocrine growth: a review. Cytokines Cell Mol Ther 1998;4:113-120.
152. Wada Y, Nakashima O, Kutami R, Yamamoto O, Kojiro M. Clinicopathological study on hepatocellular carcinoma with lymphocytic infiltration. Hepatology 1998;27:407-414.
153. Emile JF, Adam R, Sebagh M, et al. Hepatocellular carcinoma with lymphoid stroma: a tumour with good prognosis after liver transplantation. Histopathology 2000;37:523-529.

154. Park HS, Jang KY, Kim YK, Cho BH, Moon WS. Hepatocellular carcinoma with massive lymphoid infiltration: a regressing phenomenon? Pathol Res Pract 2009;205:648-652.
155. Chen CJ, Jeng LB, Huang SF. Lymphoepithelioma-like hepatocellular carcinoma. Chang Gung Med J 2007;30:172-177.
156. Patel KR, Liu TC, Vaccharajani N, Chapman WC, Brunt EM. Characterization of Inflammatory (lymphoepithelioma-like) hepatocellular carcinoma: a study of 8 cases. Arch Pathol Lab Med 2014;138:1193-1202.
157. Si MW, Thorson JA, Lauwers GY, DalCin P, Furman J. Hepatocellular lymphoepithelioma-like carcinoma associated with epstein barr virus: a hitherto unrecognized entity. Diagn Mol Pathol 2004;13:183-189.
158. Matsuura S, Aishima S, Taguchi K, et al. 'Scirrhous' type hepatocellular carcinomas: a special reference to expression of cytokeratin 7 and hepatocyte paraffin 1. Histopathology 2005;47:382-390.
159. Lee JH, Choi MS, Gwak GY, et al. Clinicopathologic characteristics and long-term prognosis of scirrhous hepatocellular carcinoma. Dig Dis Sci 2012;57:1698-1707.
160. Kurogi M, Nakashima O, Miyaaki H, Fujimoto M, Kojiro M. Clinicopathological study of scirrhous hepatocellular carcinoma. J Gastroenterol Hepatol 2006;21:1470-1477.
161. Sugiki T, Yamamoto M, Taka K, Nakano M. Specific characteristics of scirrhous hepatocellular carcinoma. Hepatogastroenterology 2009;56:1086-1089.
162. Fujii T, Zen Y, Harada K, et al. Participation of liver cancer stem/progenitor cells in tumorigenesis of scirrhous hepatocellular carcinoma—human and cell culture study. Hum Pathol 2008;39:1185-1196.
163. Seok JY, Na DC, Woo HG, et al. A fibrous stromal component in hepatocellular carcinoma reveals a cholangiocarcinoma-like gene expression trait and epithelial-mesenchymal transition. Hepatology 2012;55:1776-1786.
164. Limaiem F, Bouraoui S, Sboui M, Bouslama S, Lahmar A, Mzabi S. Fibrolamellar carcinoma versus scirrhous hepatocellular carcinoma : diagnostic usefulness of CD68. Acta Gastroenterol Belg 2015;78:393-398.
165. Salomao M, Remotti H, Vaughan R, Siegel AB, Lefkowitch JH, Moreira RK. The steatohepatitic variant of hepatocellular carcinoma and its association with underlying steatohepatitis. Hum Pathol 2012;43:737-746.
166. Salomao M, Yu WM, Brown RS Jr, Emond JC, Lefkowitch JH. Steatohepatitic hepatocellular carcinoma (SH-HCC): a distinctive histological variant of HCC in hepatitis C virus-related cirrhosis with associated NAFLD/NASH. Am J Surg Pathol 2010;34:1630-1636.
167. Shibahara J, Ando S, Sakamoto Y, Kokudo N, Fukayama M. Hepatocellular carcinoma with steatohepatitic features: a clinicopathological study of Japanese patients. Histopathology 2014;64:951-962.
168. Jain D, Nayak NC, Kumaran V, Saigal S. Steatohepatitic hepatocellular carcinoma, a morphologic indicator of associated metabolic risk factors: a study from India. Arch Pathol Lab Med 2013;137:961-966.
169. Yeh MM, Liu Y, Torbenson M. Steatohepatitic variant of hepatocellular carcinoma in the absence of metabolic syndrome or background steatosis: a clinical, pathological, and genetic study. Hum Pathol 2015;46:1769-1775.
170. Deniz K, Moreira RK, Yeh MM, Ferrell LD. Steatohepatitis-like changes in focal nodular hyperplasia, a finding to distinguish from steatohepatitic variant of hepatocellular carcinoma. Am J Surg Pathol 2017;41:277-281.
171. Ando S, Shibahara J, Hayashi A, Fukayama M. β-catenin alteration is rare in hepatocellular carcinoma with steatohepatitic features: immunohistochemical and mutational study. Virchows Arch 2015;467:535-542.
172. Heaphy CM, Subhawong AP, Hong SM, et al. Prevalence of the alternative lengthening of telomeres telomere maintenance mechanism in human cancer subtypes. Am J Pathol 2011;179:1608-1615.
173. Salaria SN, Graham RP, Aishima S, Mounajjed T, Yeh MM, Torbenson MS. Primary hepatic tumors with myxoid change: morphologically unique hepatic adenomas and hepatocellular carcinomas. Am J Surg Pathol 2015;39:318-324.
174. Young JT, Kurup AN, Graham RP, Torbenson MS, Venkatesh SK. Myxoid hepatocellular neoplasms: imaging appearance of a unique mucinous tumor variant. Abdom Radiol (NY) 2016;41:2115-2122.
175. Atra A, Al-Asiri R, Wali S, Al-Husseini H, Al-Bassas A, Zimmermann A. Hepatocellular carcinoma, syncytial giant cell: a novel variant in children: a case report. Ann Diagn Pathol 2007;11:61-63.
176. Prokurat A, Kluge P, Kosciesza A, Perek D, Kappeler A, Zimmermann A. Transitional liver cell tumors (TLCT) in older children and adolescents: a novel group of aggressive hepatic tumors expressing beta-catenin. Med Pediatr Oncol 2002;39:510-518.
177. Dominguez-Malagon H, Gaytan-Graham S. Hepatocellular carcinoma: an update. Ultrastruct Pathol 2001;25:497-516.

178. Wee A, Nilsson B. Highly well differentiated hepatocellular carcinoma and benign hepatocellular lesions. Can they be distinguished on fine needle aspiration biopsy? Acta Cytol 2003;47:16-26.
179. Wee A. Fine-needle aspiration biopsy of hepatocellular carcinoma and related hepatocellular nodular lesions in cirrhosis: controversies, challenges, and expectations. Patholog Res Int 2011;2011:587936.
180. Soyuer I, Ekinci C, Kaya M, Genc Y, Bahar K. Diagnosis of hepatocellular carcinoma by fine needle aspiration cytology. Cellular features. Acta Cytol 2003;47:581-589.
181. Graham RP, Jin L, Knutson DL, et al. DNAJB1-PRKACA is specific for fibrolamellar carcinoma. Mod Pathol 2015;28:822-829.
182. Bedossa P, Burt AD, Brunt EM, et al. Well-differentiated hepatocellular neoplasm of uncertain malignant potential: proposal for a new diagnostic category. Hum Pathol 2014;45:658-660.
183. Yeh MM, Larson AM, Campbell JS, Fausto N, Rulyak SJ, Swanson PE. The expression of transforming growth factor-alpha in cirrhosis, dysplastic nodules, and hepatocellular carcinoma: an immunohistochemical study of 70 cases. Am J Surg Pathol 2007;31:681-689.
184. Katyal S, Oliver JH 3rd, Peterson MS, Ferris JV, Carr BS, Baron RL. Extrahepatic metastases of hepatocellular carcinoma. Radiology 2000;216:698-703.
185. Aino H, Sumie S, Niizeki T, et al. Clinical characteristics and prognostic factors for advanced hepatocellular carcinoma with extrahepatic metastasis. Mol Clin Oncol 2014;2:393-398.
186. Matsukuma S, Sato K. Peritoneal seeding of hepatocellular carcinoma: clinicopathological characteristics of 17 autopsy cases. Pathol Int 2011;61:356-362.
187. Silva MA, Hegab B, Hyde C, Guo B, Buckels JA, Mirza DF. Needle track seeding following biopsy of liver lesions in the diagnosis of hepatocellular cancer: a systematic review and meta-analysis. Gut 2008;57:1592-1596.
188. Chen QW, Cheng CS, Chen H, et al. Effectiveness and complications of ultrasound guided fine needle aspiration for primary liver cancer in a Chinese population with serum alpha-fetoprotein levels ≤/=200 ng/ml—a study based on 4,312 patients. PLoS One 2014;9:e101536.
189. Maturen KE, Nghiem HV, Marrero JA, et al. Lack of tumor seeding of hepatocellular carcinoma after percutaneous needle biopsy using coaxial cutting needle technique. AJR Am J Roentgenol 2006;187:1184-1187.
190. Mullhaupt B, Durand F, Roskams T, Dutkowski P, Heim M. Is tumor biopsy necessary? Liver Transpl 2011;17(Suppl 2):S14-25.
191. Jain D. Tissue diagnosis of hepatocellular carcinoma. J Clin Exp Hepatol 2014;4(Suppl 3):S67-73.
192. Guo W, He X, Li Z, Li Y. Combination of transarterial chemoembolization (TACE) and radiofrequency ablation (RFA) vs. Surgical resection (SR) on survival outcome of early hepatocellular carcinoma: a meta-analysis. Hepatogastroenterology 2015;62:710-714.
193. Fong ZV, Tanabe KK. The clinical management of hepatocellular carcinoma in the United States, Europe, and Asia: a comprehensive and evidence-based comparison and review. Cancer 2014;120:2824-2838.
194. Parikh ND, Waljee AK, Singal AG. Downstaging hepatocellular carcinoma: a systematic review and pooled analysis. Liver Transpl 2015; 21:1142-1152.
195. Iezzi R, Pompili M, Posa A, Coppola G, Gasbarrini A, Bonomo L. Combined locoregional treatment of patients with hepatocellular carcinoma: State of the art. World J Gastroenterol 2016;22:1935-1942.
196. Wang Y, Deng T, Zeng L, Chen W. Efficacy and safety of radiofrequency ablation and transcatheter arterial chemoembolization for treatment of hepatocellular carcinoma: a meta-analysis. Hepatol Res 2016;46:58-71.
197. Llovet JM, Real MI, Montana X, et al. Arterial embolisation or chemoembolisation versus symptomatic treatment in patients with unresectable hepatocellular carcinoma: a randomised controlled trial. Lancet 2002;359:1734-1739.
198. Llovet JM, Ricci S, Mazzaferro V, et al. Sorafenib in advanced hepatocellular carcinoma. N Engl J Med 2008;359:378-390.
199. Greten TF, Papendorf F, Bleck JS, et al. Survival rate in patients with hepatocellular carcinoma: a retrospective analysis of 389 patients. Br J Cancer 2005;92:1862-1868.
200. op den Winkel M, Nagel D, Sappl J, et al. Prognosis of patients with hepatocellular carcinoma. Validation and ranking of established staging-systems in a large western HCC-cohort. PLoS One 2012;7:e45066.
201. Tandon P, Garcia-Tsao G. Prognostic indicators in hepatocellular carcinoma: a systematic review of 72 studies. Liver Int 2009;29:502-510.
202. Earl TM, Chapman WC. Hepatocellular carcinoma: resection versus transplantation. Semin Liver Dis 2013;33:282-292.
203. Tabrizian P, Jibara G, Shrager B, Schwartz M, Roayaie S. Recurrence of hepatocellular cancer after resection: patterns, treatments, and prognosis. Ann Surg 2015;261:947-955.

204. Lee SY, Konstantinidis IT, Eaton AA, et al. Predicting recurrence patterns after resection of hepatocellular cancer. HPB (Oxford) 2014;16:943-953.
205. Li Q, Wang J, Juzi JT, et al. Clonality analysis for multicentric origin and intrahepatic metastasis in recurrent and primary hepatocellular carcinoma. J Gastrointest Surg 2008;12:1540-1547.
206. Ng IO, Guan XY, Poon RT, Fan ST, Lee JM. Determination of the molecular relationship between multiple tumour nodules in hepatocellular carcinoma differentiates multicentric origin from intrahepatic metastasis. J Pathol 2003;199:345-353.
207. Koike Y, Shiratori Y, Sato S, et al. Risk factors for recurring hepatocellular carcinoma differ according to infected hepatitis virus-an analysis of 236 consecutive patients with a single lesion. Hepatology 2000;32:1216-1223.
208. Shindoh J, Andreou A, Aloia TA, et al. Microvascular invasion does not predict long-term survival in hepatocellular carcinoma up to 2 cm: reappraisal of the staging system for solitary tumors. Ann Surg Oncol 2013;20:1223-1229.
209. Hsieh CH, Wei CK, Yin WY, et al. Vascular invasion affects survival in early hepatocellular carcinoma. Mol Clin Oncol 2015;3:252-256.
210. Nathan H, Schulick RD, Choti MA, Pawlik TM. Predictors of survival after resection of early hepatocellular carcinoma. Ann Surg 2009;249:799-805.
211. Pesi B, Ferrero A, Grazi GL, et al. Liver resection with thrombectomy as a treatment of hepatocellular carcinoma with major vascular invasion: results from a retrospective multicentric study. Am J Surg 2015;210:35-44.
212. Rodriguez-Peralvarez M, Luong TV, Andreana L, Meyer T, Dhillon AP, Burroughs AK. A systematic review of microvascular invasion in hepatocellular carcinoma: diagnostic and prognostic variability. Ann Surg Oncol 2013;20:325-339.
213. Ohashi M, Wakai T, Korita PV, Ajioka Y, Shirai Y, Hatakeyama K. Histological evaluation of intracapsular venous invasion for discrimination between portal and hepatic venous invasion in hepatocellular carcinoma. J Gastroenterol Hepatol 2010;25:143-149.
214. Roayaie S, Blume IN, Thung SN, et al. A system of classifying microvascular invasion to predict outcome after resection in patients with hepatocellular carcinoma. Gastroenterology 2009;137:850-855.
215. Fujita N, Aishima S, Iguchi T, et al. Histologic classification of microscopic portal venous invasion to predict prognosis in hepatocellular carcinoma. Hum Pathol 2011;42:1531-1538.

4 FIBROLAMELLAR CARCINOMA

Fibrolamellar carcinoma is a malignant tumor composed of neoplastic hepatocytes, with prominent intratumoral fibrosis but without underlying liver disease or fibrosis. It is diagnosed by the unique findings on hematoxylin and eosin (H&E)-stained slides with confirmation by immunostains or by molecular tests for either the deletion leading to the *DNAJB1-PRKACA* fusion transcript, or the fusion transcript itself.

CLINICAL FEATURES

Individuals with fibrolamellar carcinoma often present with vague, nonspecific signs and symptoms, such as abdominal pain, weight loss, and malaise (1,2). Another recurrent presentation is biliary obstruction, resulting from either direct tumor growth into the biliary tree or from compression of the extrahepatic bile duct by metastatic deposits in hilar lymph nodes (Table 4-1). A wide range of less common presentations has been reported (Table 4-1). Of these, gynecomastia in males is a rare but distinctive finding.

Fibrolamellar carcinomas make up less than 1 percent of all hepatocellular carcinomas. Prior studies suggested a frequency of around 5 percent, but more recent data from larger studies indicate a frequency closer to 0.5 to 1.0 percent (3–6). Fibrolamellar carcinomas occur throughout the world, but solid epidemiologic data are lacking for most parts of the world. In the United States, one study found no differences in the frequency of fibrolamellar carcinoma among white, black, Hispanic, and Asian populations (4). In terms of gender distribution, a slight male predominance has been reported in some studies (4), while other studies have found a slight female predominance (1,6). Regardless of how this point is sorted out in the end, it is clear that there is no striking male predominance, as is seen in typical hepatocellular carcinomas, and no striking female predominance, as is true for hepatocellular adenomas and focal nodular hyperplasia.

Fibrolamellar carcinomas are strongly enriched in younger individuals: 50 percent of cases occur between the ages of 17 and 30 years, while 80 percent occur between the ages of 10 to 35 years (7). Nonetheless, this key observation can also be a diagnostic pitfall, predisposing to a diagnosis of fibrolamellar carcinoma only because the patient is young and the background liver is noncirrhotic. In fact, typical hepatocellular carcinomas are still the most common form of liver cancer in children and young adults, accounting for 60 to 80 percent of cases, a finding that has been repeatedly observed in studies for many decades (3,8–11). Also of note, one recent data-base study found a second peak of fibrolamellar carcinomas in the 60- to 69-year-old age group, but this is currently an isolated observation and one that also lacks solid histologic data (12). This uncertain finding awaits potential confirmation.

Table 4-1

PRESENTING SIGNS AND SYMPTOMS IN FIBROLAMELLAR CARCINOMA

Category	Presentation (References)
Vascular flow abnormalities	Budd-Chiari syndrome (82,83) Caval compression/obstruction (84) Growth into and obstruction of inferior vena cava (85)
Systemic symptoms	Hyperammonemia (86–90) Hypoglycemia (91) Increased beta-hCG (92) Systemic AA amyloid deposition (41)
Biliary manifestations	Obstructive jaundice (62,93–96) Background disease of ulcerative colitis and primary sclerosing cholangitis (97)
Miscellaneous	Nonbacterial thrombotic endocarditis (98) Ascites from intraperitoneal metastases (99) Mimicking a liver abscess (100) Bone metastases (101) Gynecomastia (15,102–105) Cold agglutinin disease (106) Spontaneous rupture of tumor (13,107)

LABORATORY FINDINGS

Serum alpha-fetoprotein (AFP) levels are normal in individuals with fibrolamellar carcinoma. In about 5 percent of cases, serum AFP levels are mildly elevated (1,13,14), typically less than 100 ng/mL, but this is a nonspecific finding and immunohistochemistry consistently shows no AFP production by the tumor. A higher level of serum AFP (above 400 ng/mL), however, is an important clue that a diagnosis of fibrolamellar carcinoma is most likely wrong. In contrast, serum levels of PIVKA-II (protein induced by vitamin K absence/antagonist-II) are commonly elevated in many fibrolamellar carcinomas and many conventional hepatocellular carcinomas (15). PIVKA-II is an abnormally glycosylated form of prothrombin, which also goes by the name of des-gamma carboxyprothrombin (DCP).

A number of other serum proteins are elevated in individuals who have fibrolamellar carcinoma, including the vitamin B12-binding proteins, transcobalamin 1 (16,17), transcobalamin 2 (13), and transcobalamin 3 (13). Serum neurotensin levels can also be elevated. Neurotensin is expressed normally only in the fetal liver and in the adult small bowel (18), but is abnormally expressed by fibrolamellar carcinomas (19,20), leading to elevated serum levels (21). To date none of these serum markers are widely used clinically, as none are sufficiently sensitive or specific, although they are useful in individual cases for monitoring response to therapy and tumor recurrence.

ETIOLOGY

The etiology of fibrolamellar carcinoma is unknown. Rare cases have been reported in the setting of hepatocellular adenomas (7,22,23) as well as a few well-defined inherited syndromes: Carney complex (36), Fanconi anemia (37), and familial adenomatous polyposis (54). These observations may be by chance, however, and fibrolamellar carcinoma has not been convincingly shown to be part of any of these syndromes, except for the Carney complex.

By light microscopy, the background livers are essentially normal, with no consistent findings to indicate underlying chronic liver disease (9), and no histologic precursor lesion to fibrolamellar carcinoma has been identified. Hepatitis B viral proteins or DNA has been reported in rare cases of fibrolamellar carcinoma (24–26), but this observation is most likely by chance, given the high worldwide prevalence of chronic hepatitis B infection, and there are no compelling data that hepatitis B is an etiologic agent. Likewise, fibrolamellar carcinoma has been reported as a second malignancy following treatment for lymphoma (27), but this also appears to be a chance observation, and most individuals with fibrolamellar carcinoma have no such history.

GROSS FINDINGS

Fibrolamellar carcinomas are slightly more common in the left lobe of the liver than the right lobe, but not enough to be clinically or biologically informative. In 80 to 90 percent of cases, a single large tumor is present (28). Even when there is multifocal disease, there is no evidence for a "field effect" with multiple independent tumors. Instead, one nodule is typically dominant, with smaller adjacent satellite tumors.

Fibrolamellar carcinomas tend to be large at the time of resection, commonly measuring 10 cm or more in greatest dimension. They range in color from yellow to pale tan (fig. 4-1) and range in consistency from soft to firm. The tumors can feel gritty when microcalcifications are prominent. In cases with prominent pseudoglands, the tumors can be tacky and mucinous. A central scar is found in about two thirds of cases. Occasionally, the tumors may contain small foci of necrosis or areas of intratumoral hemorrhage. Gross vascular invasion is seen in up to 25 percent of cases (29). The background liver is noncirrhotic, but a rim of inflamed and fibrotic tissue is often present where the fibrolamellar carcinoma interfaces with the nontumor parenchyma. Sections from this area are helpful and important when seeking angiolymphatic invasion, but are not useful for examining the background liver for underlying liver disease.

MICROSCOPIC FINDINGS

Fibrolamellar carcinomas are composed of large tumor cells that are polygonal, have abundant eosinophilic cytoplasm that is rich in mitochondria and lysosomes, and have nuclei with vesicular chromatin and large nucleoli (fig. 4-2). Fortunately, most tumors adhere to this classic description. Intratumoral fibrosis

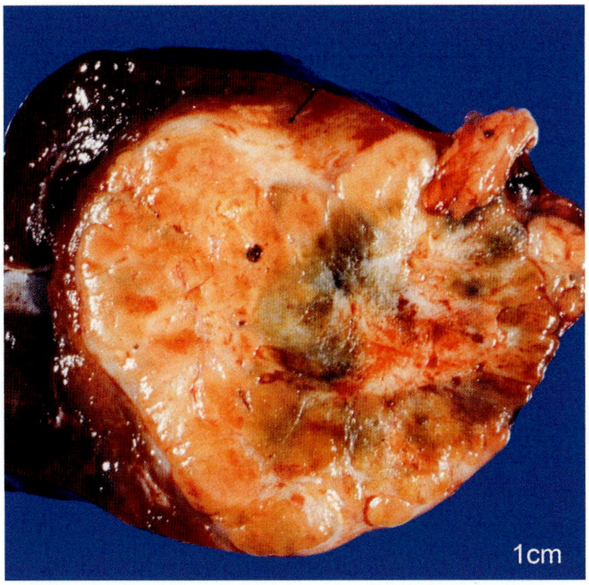

Figure 4-1

FIBROLAMELLAR CARCINOMA

The tumor is yellow and firm, with an ill-defined central area of hemorrhage and scarring.

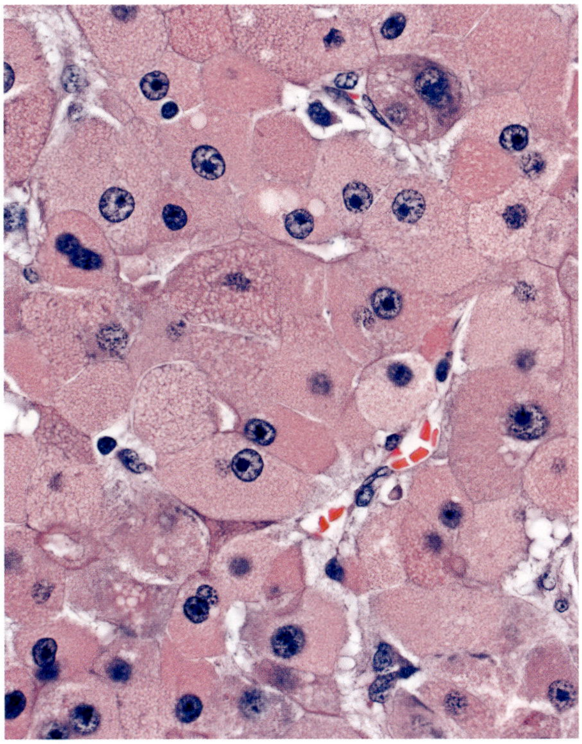

Figure 4-2

FIBROLAMELLAR CARCINOMA

The tumor is composed of large polygonal cells with abundant eosinophilic cytoplasm and prominent nucleoli.

is also a distinctive feature of fibrolamellar carcinoma. The collagen is often deposited in parallel bands, providing the impetus for the term "lamellar" in "fibrolamellar carcinoma" (fig. 4-3), but can also have a more haphazard arrangement (fig. 4-4).

The center of the tumor can become almost acellular, replaced by dense heavy scar tissue. However, some full resection specimens and some biopsies have areas of tumor where the fibrosis is inconspicuous. In these areas, the tumor retains the typical cytology of fibrolamellar carcinoma, but the tumor cells grow in solid sheets and trabeculae without significant intratumoral fibrosis (fig. 4-5). The frequency of this finding is not well defined, but one study found 3 of 28 (10 percent) fibrolamellar carcinomas had focal areas that resembled typical hepatocellular carcinoma (30). In adequately sampled specimens, there always are areas of more typical fibrolamellar carcinoma containing intratumoral fibrosis. The characteristic molecular deletion, leading to the *DNAJB1/PRACA* fusion transcript, is present in the areas lacking the typical intratumoral fibrosis (31), further affirming that these cases should not be called combined hepatocellular carcinoma-

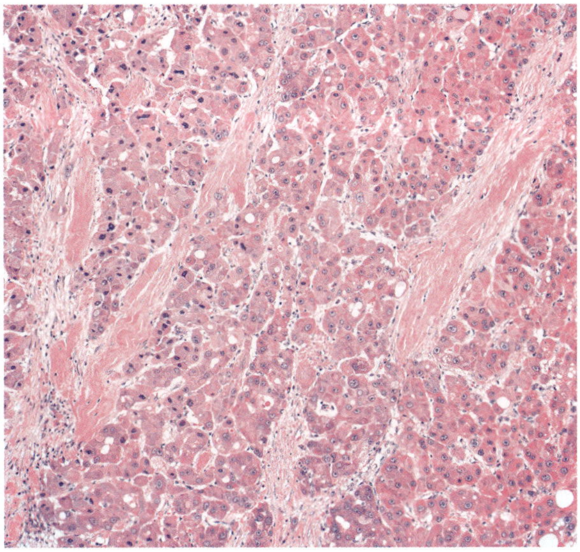

Figure 4-3

FIBROLAMELLAR CARCINOMA: LAMELLAR FIBROSIS

The intratumoral fibrosis is deposited in parallel bands.

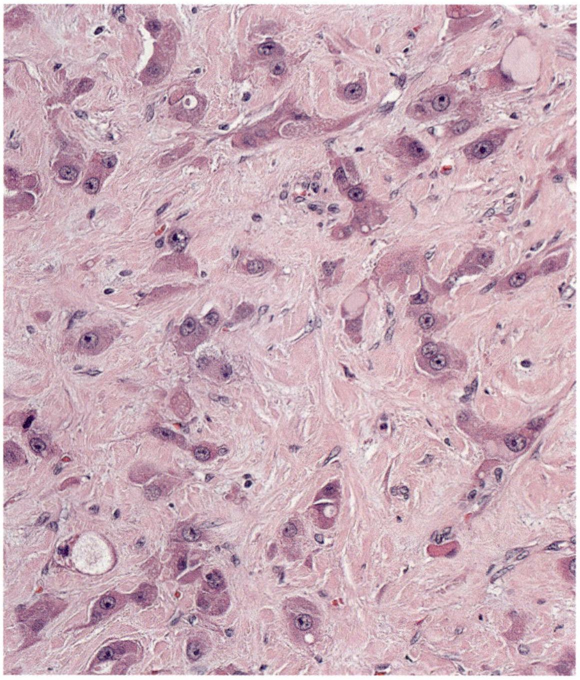

Figure 4-4

FIBROLAMELLAR CARCINOMA: IRREGULAR FIBROSIS

The intratumoral fibrosis is heavier and more haphazard than in figure 4-3, without a distinctive lamellar pattern.

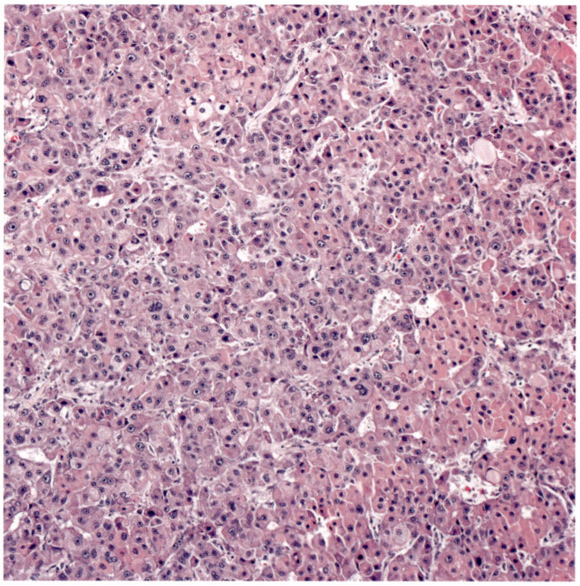

Figure 4-5

FIBROLAMELLAR CARCINOMA: SOLID GROWTH AREA

Areas of more solid growth, without much intratumoral fibrosis, can be seen in some fibrolamellar carcinomas and should not be diagnosed as combined hepatocellular carcinoma-fibrolamellar carcinoma.

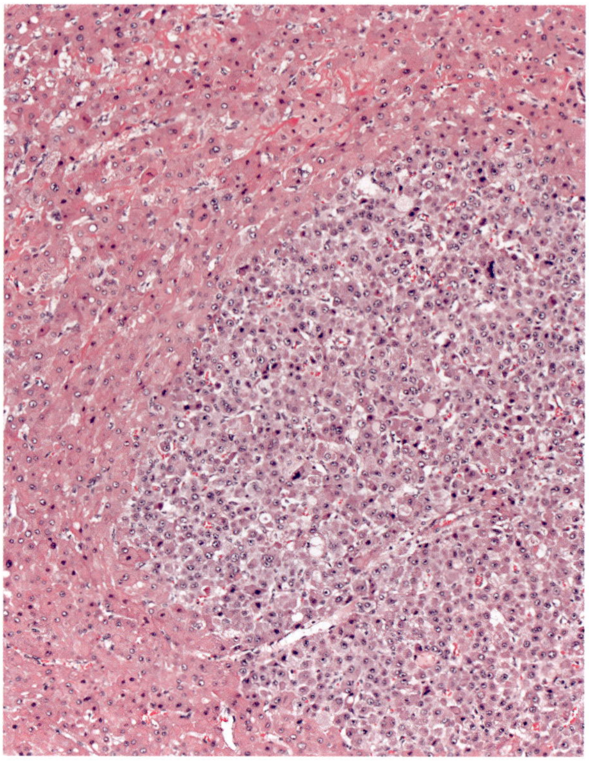

Figure 4-6

FIBROLAMELLAR CARCINOMA

Within the fibrolamellar carcinoma, a distinct nodule of dedifferentiated carcinoma shows reduced and more basophilic cytoplasm. Fluorescence in situ hybridization (FISH) demonstrated the same *DNAJB1-PRKACA* fusion in both components.

fibrolamellar carcinoma based solely on variable intratumoral fibrosis. In rare cases, a distinctive nodule of more poorly differentiated carcinoma can develop within the fibrolamellar carcinoma (fig. 4-6), a finding that represents tumor progression and not combined hepatocellular carcinoma-fibrolamellar carcinoma.

Fibrolamellar carcinomas commonly have some or all of an additional set of core findings: pale bodies, pink bodies, intratumoral cholestasis, and variably dilated pseudoglands. Some of the pseudoglands become sufficiently dilated to tempt the unwary into a diagnosis of adenocarcinoma. None of these four findings are specific for fibrolamellar carcinoma, however, and all can be found in ordinary hepatocellular carcinomas. Likewise, these four findings are not sensitive for a diagnosis of fibrolamellar carcinoma, so a pathologist can feel confident about diagnosing

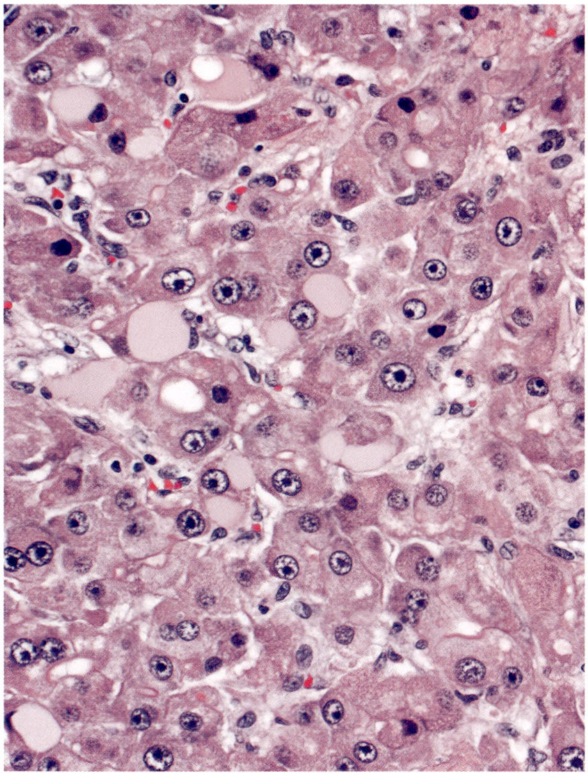

Figure 4-7

FIBROLAMELLAR CARCINOMA: PALE BODIES

Large, pale cytoplasmic inclusions are seen.

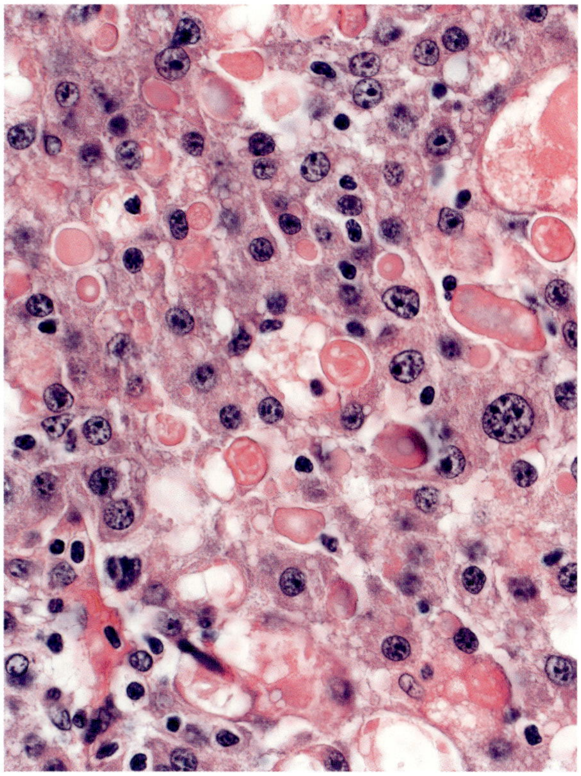

Figure 4-8

FIBROLAMELLAR CARCINOMA: PINK BODIES

Round, pink globules are clustered in a small area in this tumor.

fibrolamellar carcinoma even if pale bodies or pink bodies are not seen, for example.

Pale bodies are round cytoplasmic inclusions that appear pale gray on H&E-stained slides (fig. 4-7). There is typically a single pale body per cell. The composition of pale bodies is uncertain, but they probably contain a number of different proteins, including fibrinogen. By electron microscopy, pale bodies appear to arise from intracellular lumens (32) that are filled with unknown secretions composed of fine granular material. Electron microscopy also suggests that pale bodies may eventually condense to form the pink bodies seen on H&E-stained slides (32). Pink bodies are also called hyaline bodies or hyaline globules. They appear as distinctive, pink globules in the cytoplasm of tumor cells (fig. 4-8). The frequency of pale bodies and hyaline bodies has not been well studied, but overall, pale bodies are found in about half of cases and hyaline bodies in about one third. The frequency of both these inclusions is probably even higher if they are specifically searched for.

Intratumoral cholestasis is found in nearly all cases, when specimens are examined carefully. The bile pigment can be cytoplasmic or can be located within the small canalicular-type structures that lie between cells or within cells (fig. 4-9). The cholestatic features likely explain the finding of copper deposition within occasional tumor cells, as copper is normally excreted through the bile and bile retention leads to copper retention in all kinds of benign and malignant liver diseases.

Small dilated pseudoglands are very common in fibrolamellar carcinoma (fig. 4-10), and often appear to arise from dilated canalicular structures. In approximately 10 percent of cases, the pseudoglands reach much larger sizes (fig. 4-11) and produce mucinous material that is Alcian blue positive and often weakly to moderately

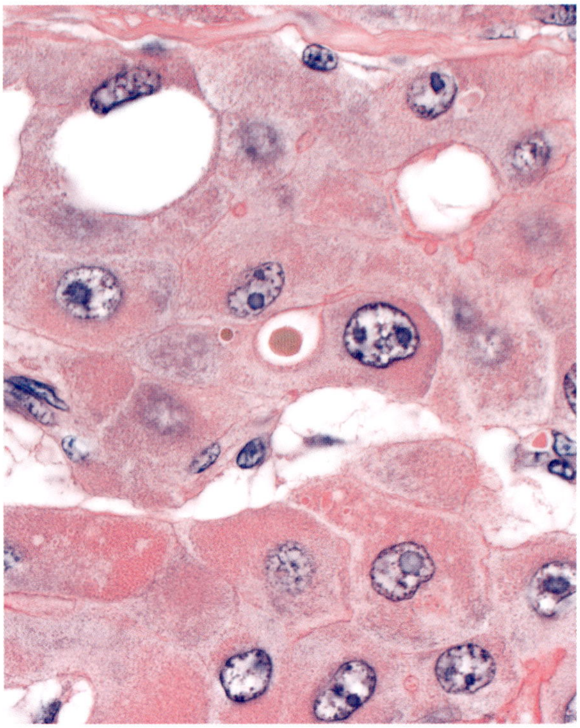

Figure 4-9

FIBROLAMELLAR CARCINOMA: CHOLESTASIS

Cholestasis is a common finding. In this case, the bile deposits are located in small vacuolar structures that suggest intracytoplasmic lumens.

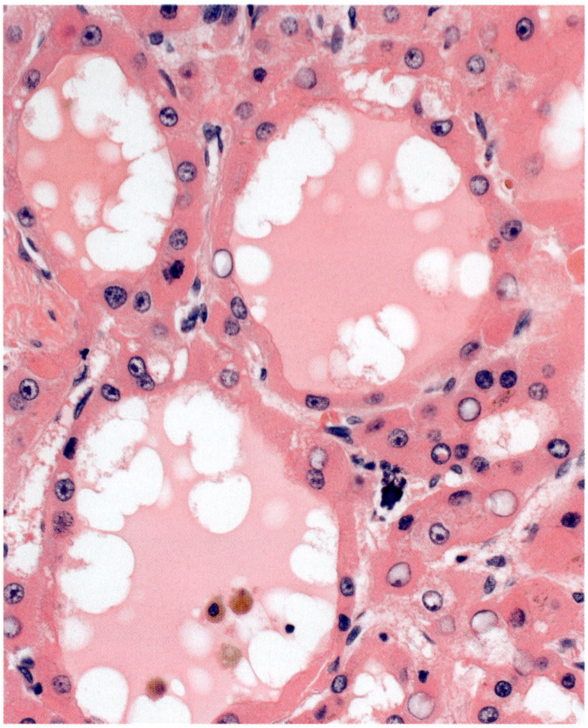

Figure 4-11

FIBROLAMELLAR CARCINOMA: LARGE PSEUDOGLANDS

Several large pseudoglands are seen.

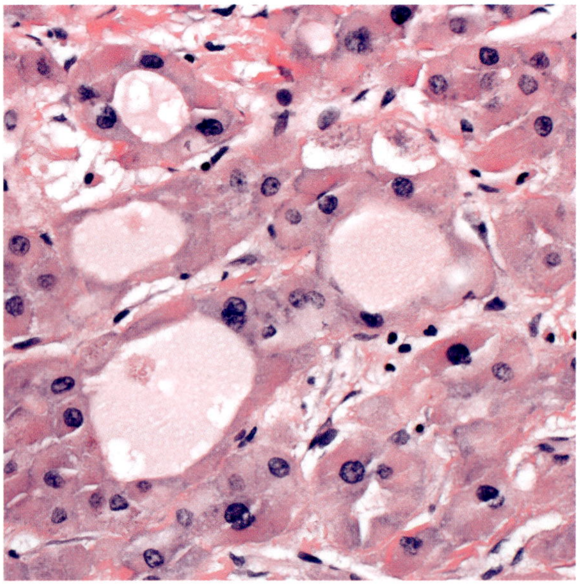

Figure 4-10

FIBROLAMELLAR CARCINOMA: SMALL PSEUDOGLANDS

Several small variably sized pseudoglands are seen.

positive on mucicarmine stains (33). Mucin can be detected within both individual neoplastic cells as well the pseudoglands (fig. 4-12). In one study, mucicarmine was positive in just over half the cases and Alcian blue in essentially all cases (33).

The pseudoglands are typically ovoid, cystic structures lined by neoplastic cells, which in some cases may be smaller than the cells in the more typical areas of the tumor, but are otherwise cytologically similar. There is almost always a continuum of pseudoglandular dilatation, from small to medium to large, and immunostains show that the tumor cells lining the pseudoglands retain their hepatocytic differentiation, even for the very large pseudoglands. One case report has shown the tumor cells lining the pseudoglands have increased expression of carcinoembryonic antigen, compared to the rest of the tumor (34). Despite the pseudoglandular structures and the mucin production, these changes are not evidence of adenocarcinoma

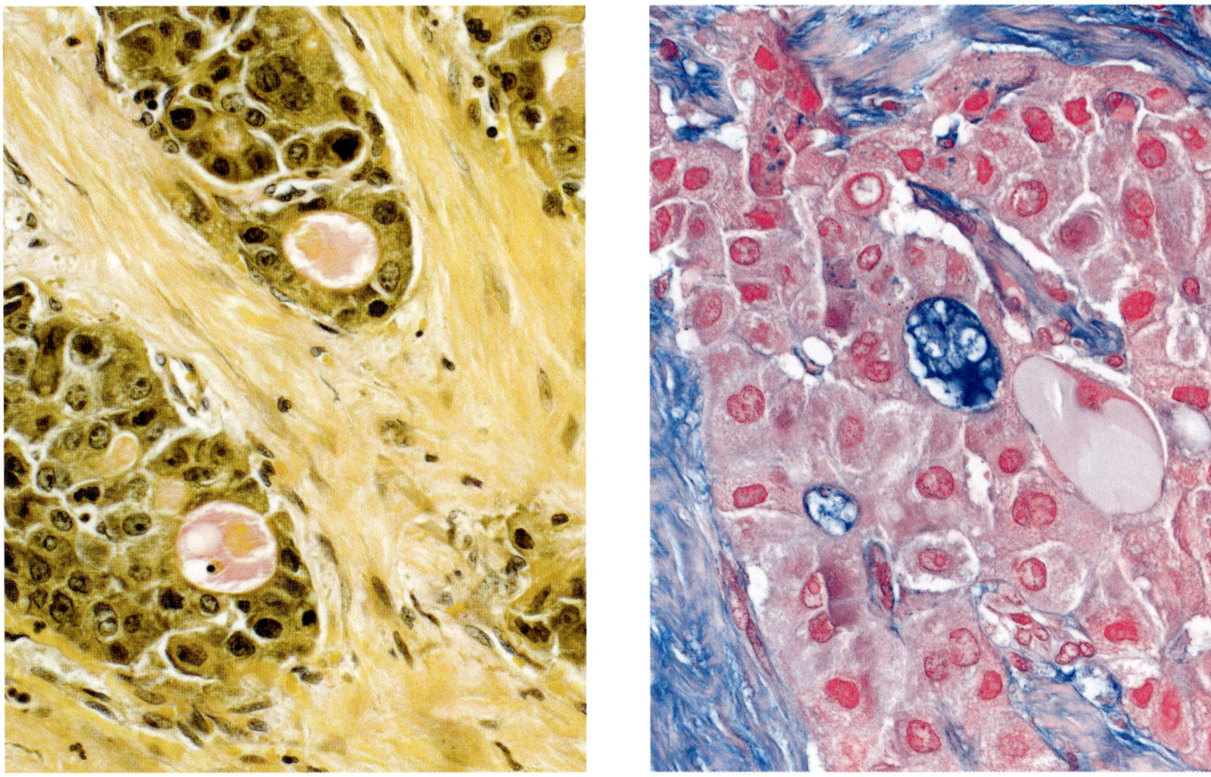

Figure 4-12

FIBROLAMELLAR CARCINOMA: MUCIN IN PSEUDOGLANDS

Left: Mucicarmine stain highlights the mucin.
Right: Mucin is highlighted by Alcian blue stain.

and tumors with this finding should not be called a combined cholangiocarcinoma-fibrolamellar carcinoma.

There are a number of other histologic findings that can be present in fibrolamellar carcinomas. Some tumors have microcalcifications, with either dystrophic calcifications or microcalcifications of single tumor cells (fig. 4-13). Calcifications are seen in up to two thirds of cases on computerized tomography (CT) scans (35). Histologically, dystrophic calcifications are found in areas of remote necrosis or fibrosis, or in the walls of larger vessels. Single tumor cells with microcalcifications tend to be scattered irregularly throughout the tumor. In addition, tumors frequently show scattered single tumor cells that have the distinctive "bubbly" cytoplasm of microvesicular steatosis (fig. 4-14). Mild macrovesicular fatty change can occasionally be seen within the tumor, even if there is no fat in the background liver (fig. 4-15). Benign isolated bile ducts are occasionally entrapped within the tumor. In other cases, the carcinoma directly invades into large bile ducts (fig. 4-16).

Association with Other Tumors

Rare reports have described hepatocellular adenomas in association with fibrolamellar carcinoma (7,22,23,36). Morphologically, the adenomas often show steatosis (fig. 4-17) and are subclassified as type 1 adenomas with liver fatty acid binding protein (LFABP) loss by immunohistochemistry (23). Because of the rarity of these reports, it is unclear whether these are coincidental findings.

Early studies of fibrolamellar carcinomas also noted a possible association with focal nodular hyperplasia (37–40). However, fibrolamellar carcinomas do not arise from focal nodular hyperplasia. Instead, some fibrolamellar carcinomas induce a secondary, reactive nodular hyperplasia at their periphery (fig. 4-18), perhaps

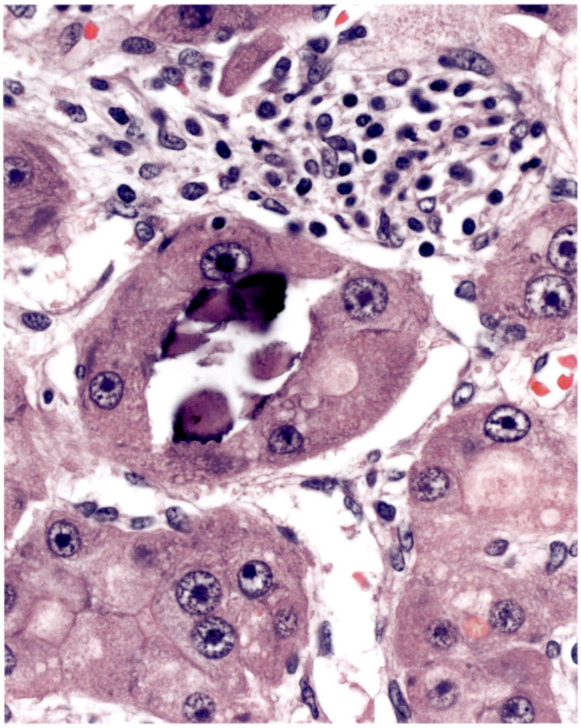

Figure 4-13

FIBROLAMELLAR CARCINOMA: MICROCALCIFICATIONS

This tumor had small calcifications. In this image, the microcalcifications appear to be in small pseudoglands.

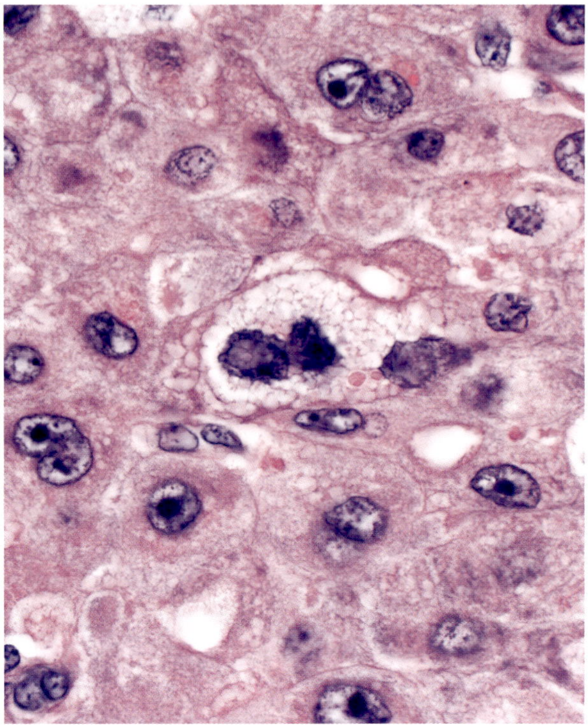

Figure 4-14

FIBROLAMELLAR CARCINOMA: VACUOLATED CYTOPLASM

The cytoplasm of several of the tumor cells has a distinctive bubbly appearance, caused by numerous tiny vacuoles.

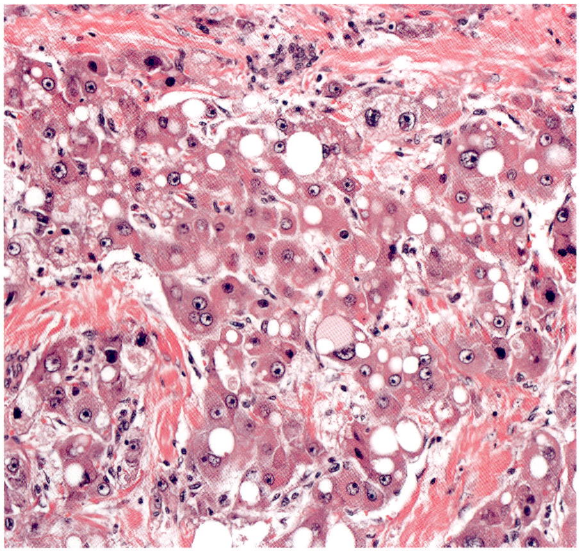

Figure 4-15

FIBROLAMELLAR CARCINOMA: STEATOSIS

Mild macrovesicular steatosis, without balloon cells.

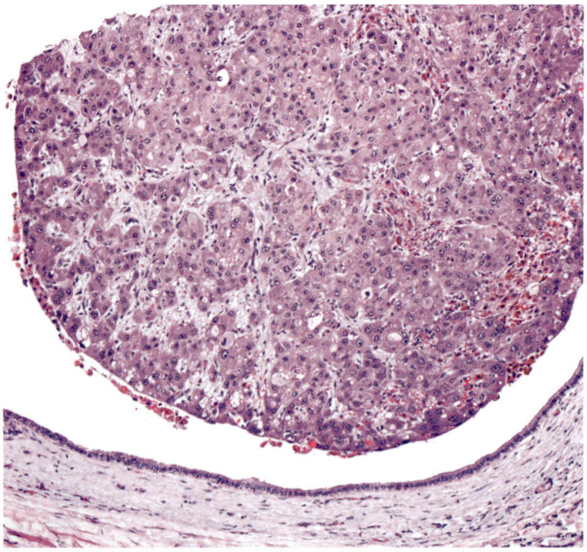

Figure 4-16

FIBROLAMELLAR CARCINOMA: BILE DUCT

The carcinoma is growing within the lumen of a large bile duct.

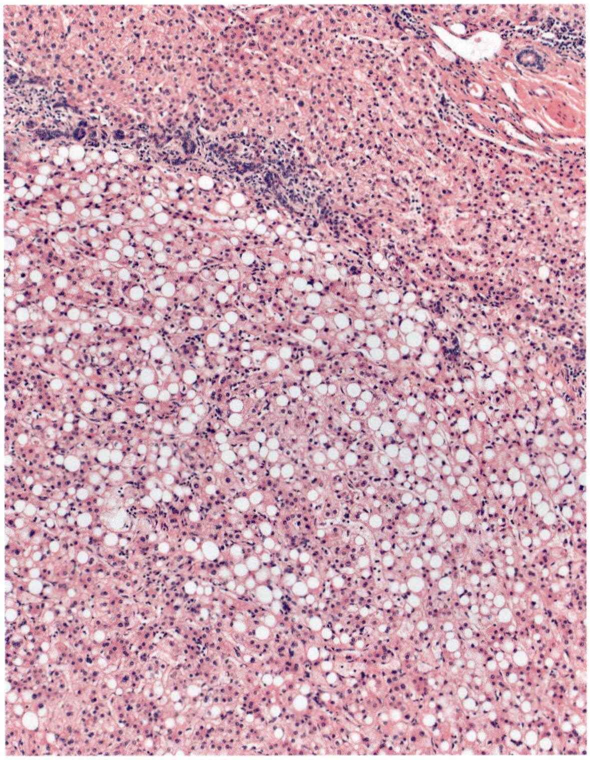

Figure 4-17

HEPATOCELLULAR ADENOMA

The background liver in this individual with fibrolamellar carcinoma had a hepatic adenoma, HNF1-alpha inactivated subtype.

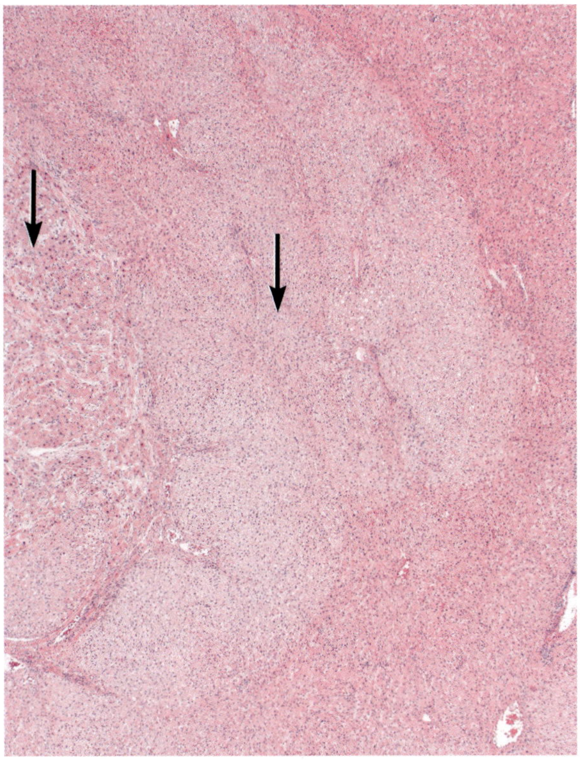

Figure 4-18

FIBROLAMELLAR CARCINOMA AND FOCAL NODULAR HYPERPLASIA

The fibrolamellar carcinoma (left arrow) is surrounded by a rim of reactive, nodular hepatocytes with the morphology and immunohistochemical findings of focal nodular hyperplasia (right arrow). This is a rare finding, but can be dramatic when present.

due to increased arterialization of the parenchyma surrounding the tumor (39). This reactive, nodular hyperplasia shows a "map-like" pattern with glutamine synthetase, similar to focal nodular hyperplasia (see chapter 2).

HISTOLOGIC GRADING

Most fibrolamellar carcinomas are cytologically homogeneous. Overall, they lack the range of differentiation seen in ordinary hepatocellular carcinomas, which range from well differentiated to undifferentiated. However, most tumor templates require a tumor grade and, for this purpose, essentially all primary fibrolamellar carcinomas are classified as moderately differentiated. Most recurrent and metastatic fibrolamellar carcinomas are also moderately differentiated. In fact, a diagnosis of poorly differentiated fibrolamellar carcinoma is sufficiently unusual that molecular confirmation may be needed. Rarely, fibrolamellar carcinomas have nodules of more poorly differentiated tumor, representing tumor progression (see fig. 4-6). These cases should not be called combined fibrolamellar carcinoma-hepatocellular carcinoma.

IMMUNOHISTOCHEMICAL FINDINGS

A wide variety of immunostains have been applied to fibrolamellar carcinoma for basic science and clinical studies, but this section will focus on those stains used in diagnostic surgical pathology (Table 4-2). Fibrolamellar carcinomas are positive for markers of hepatocellular differentiation, such as HepPar1 and arginase. Polyclonal carcinoembryonic antigen (pCEA) is better than CD10 immunostaining for highlighting a canalicular staining pattern, but in both cases, true canalicular staining can be

Table 4-2

IMMUNOSTAINS IN FIBROLAMELLAR CARCINOMA

Immunostain	Frequency of Positive Staining	Representative References and Comments
Markers of Hepatic Differentiation		
HepPar1	100%	(9,34,43)
Arginase 1	100%	
Glypican 3	20-60%	(43,108)
Albumin-ISH[a]	100%	(43)
Polyclonal CEA	80%	Canalicular pattern (43)
CD10	30%	Canalicular pattern (43)
AFP	0%	The occasional reported cases with AFP positivity may be misdiagnosed (43,44,109)
Markers for Diagnosis		
CD68	100%	Fibrolamellar carcinomas co-express CD68 (KP-1) and CK7 (46)
CK7	100%	(9,43,47,108,110,111)
Keratin Expression		
CK8 and 18	100%	(111,112)
CAM5.2	100%	(113)
CK19	0-25%	(9,43,108,111,112)
Neuroendocrine Markers		
CD56	90%	Most cases with focal staining (43)
Chromogranin	0%	Rare case reports of positive tumors (44)
Synaptophysin	0%	(44)
Other Stains		
EMA	100%	(43)
CD34	100%	Sinusoidal staining (108)
EGFR	80-100%	(112,114,115)
Ep-CAM (MOC-31)	20-80%	(43,116)
Ki-67	0-30%	(44,110,117)
Monoclonal CEA	10 %	(43)
CA19-9	0%	(43)
LFABP	100% (lost or reduced)	(23)

[a]ISH = in situ hybridization; CEA = carcinoembryonic antigen; AFP = alpha-fetoprotein; EMA = epithelial membrane antigen; CAM = cell adhesion molecule; LFABP = liver fatty acid binding protein.

sparse. Fibrolamellar carcinomas are negative for alpha-fetoprotein (AFP) and one third to two thirds of cases are glypican 3 positive.

Neuroendocrine features have been noted in fibrolamellar carcinomas using electron microscopy (41,42) and molecular studies (20). Rare cases are chromogranin positive (41), but most fibrolamellar carcinomas are negative for chromogranin and synaptophysin by immunohistochemistry (43,44). Some neuroendocrine carcinomas have a morphology that closely mimics that of fibrolamellar carcinoma. Furthermore, a subset of neuroendocrine tumors can be HepPar1 positive (45), so arginase 1 or polyclonal CEA have advantages in this setting. CD68 (KP-1 clone) highlights the lysosomes of fibrolamellar carcinoma, and together with CK7 coexpression, helps establish the correct diagnosis.

The H&E impression of fibrolamellar carcinoma is sometimes wrong. Time has shown that the H&E findings are very sensitive, as essentially all fibrolamellar carcinomas look alike, but they are not entirely specific, as typical hepatocellular carcinomas occasionally have cytologic features that closely mimic fibrolamellar carcinoma (fig. 4-19). Thus, additional studies to confirm a diagnosis of fibrolamellar carcinoma are important. One useful approach is to confirm the H&E findings with CK7 and CD68 (KP-1 clone) (fig. 4-20). Cases that are negative for either CK7 or CD68 most likely are not fibrolamellar carcinoma. Both CK7 and CD68 can show patchy staining, but the stains still perform well on biopsy material. The benign bile ducts should be strongly CK7 positive and the Kupffer cells within the tumor and nontumor should be strongly and brightly CD68 positive. If the internal control cells are not strongly positive, the stains should be repeated. Immunostains for CK7 and CD68 should be used together, as a small proportion of typical hepatocellular carcinomas can be CD68 positive (46), and a significant minority of typical hepatocellular carcinomas is CK7 positive. Molecular tests are also important tools for confirming the diagnosis and are discussed below. A proper diagnosis requires both the typical morphology plus confirmatory tests. Either alone is insufficient, but when combined with morphology, the genetic tests or CK7/CD68 coexpression are essentially 100 percent specific.

HISTOLOGIC TYPES

Several potential variants of fibrolamellar carcinoma have been proposed, but at this point essentially all of these appear to reflect regional morphologic variation in an otherwise typical fibrolamellar carcinoma and no well-accepted

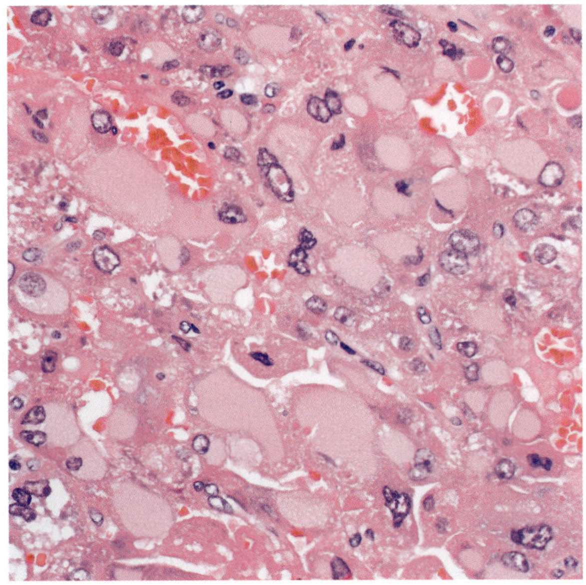

Figure 4-19

HEPATOCELLULAR CARCINOMA

This hepatocellular carcinoma had focal areas that closely mimic fibrolamellar carcinoma, including eosinophilic cells, pale bodies, and hyaline bodies. A subtle clue that this tumor is not fibrolamellar carcinoma is the absence of prominent nucleoli. Immunostains for CK7/CD68 and molecular testing were negative.

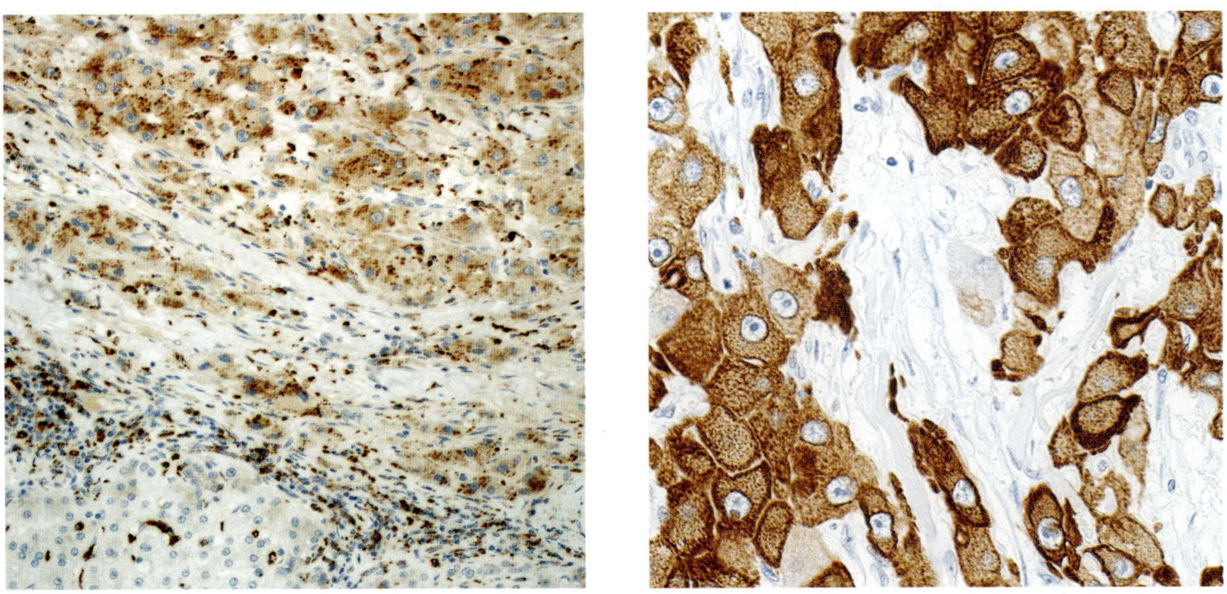

Figure 4-20

FIBROLAMELLAR CARCINOMA

Left: The CD68 (KP1 clone) shows granular staining in the tumor cytoplasm. The background liver (lower left) shows staining in the Kupffer cells.

Right: The tumor is strongly CK7 positive

variants have been defined. Pseudoglands, complete with mucin production (33), can be prominent, but do not appear to represent a unique variant. Mucicarmine staining in rare individual cells is also acceptable for a diagnosis of fibrolamellar carcinoma. The mucin production reflects the observation that fibrolamellar carcinomas have an unusual morphology that appears to combine both biliary and hepatocellular features.

About 10 percent of resected fibrolamellar carcinomas have focal, solid areas within the tumor that look cytologically like fibrolamellar carcinoma, but lack prominent intratumoral fibrosis. These cases are best classified as fibrolamellar carcinoma and not combined hepatocellular carcinoma-fibrolamellar carcinoma (31,47). In addition, rare fibrolamellar carcinomas can have an internal nodule of dedifferentiated tumor (see fig. 4-6). For example, one case report illustrated a large typical fibrolamellar carcinoma with a distinct central portion of the tumor showing de-differentiation, leading to a cytologically and immunohistochemically distinct nodule (48). These represent tumor progression and not mixed fibrolamellar carcinoma-hepatocellular carcinoma. Molecular studies have also attempted to define a mixed fibrolamellar-hepatocellular carcinoma subtype (49), but concern remains that such mixed tumors could have better original diagnoses, and may represent, for example, conventional hepatocellular carcinoma misclassified as fibrolamellar carcinoma because of focal areas of tumor growth that resemble fibrolamellar carcinoma.

Rare cases of fibrolamellar carcinoma with clear cell features have been reported (50,51). Except for the clear cytoplasm, the cases are reported to be histologically typical of fibrolamellar carcinoma. Both reported cases were in somewhat older individuals (59 and 66 years), and the significance of the clear cell change is unclear.

ULTRASTRUCTURAL FINDINGS

Electron microscopy is not useful for routine diagnosis or prognosis. On ultrastructural examination, the neoplastic cells show abundant mitochondria and lysosomes (32,52,53). The abundant lysosomes are the reason for the CD68 immunopositivity (KP1 clone) in fibrolamellar carcinomas. Neurosecretory granules or other features of neuroendocrine differentiation have been found in fibrolamellar carcinomas (41,42,53). The tumor cells can also show intracellular lumens that may contain microvilli, and sometimes bile (54–56). As noted above, pale bodies appear to begin as intracellular lumens, then eventually develop deposits that lead to the H&E findings of pale bodies (32).

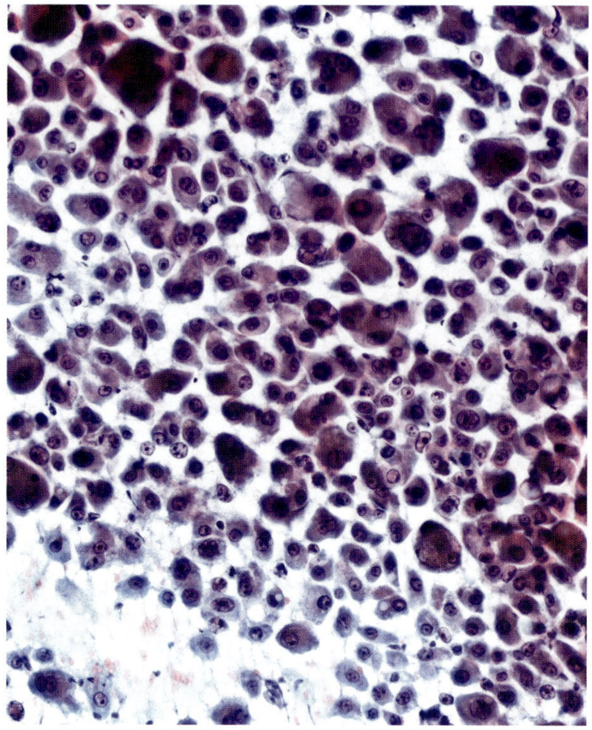

Figure 4-21

FIBROLAMELLAR CARCINOMA

The touch preparation is cellular, with sheets of discohesive cells (touch prep).

CYTOLOGIC FINDINGS

On smears and touch preparations, fibrolamellar carcinomas show monotonous sheets and large discohesive clusters of atypical hepatocytes (fig. 4-21). Aspirates can range from high cellularity (57) to low cellularity (58). Overall, cytopathologists are able to routinely make a diagnosis of fibrolamellar carcinoma on fine-needle aspirate specimens, with a low misclassification rate (59).

The tumor cells are typically large with abundant granular cytoplasm (fig. 4-22), being significantly larger than benign hepatocytes as well

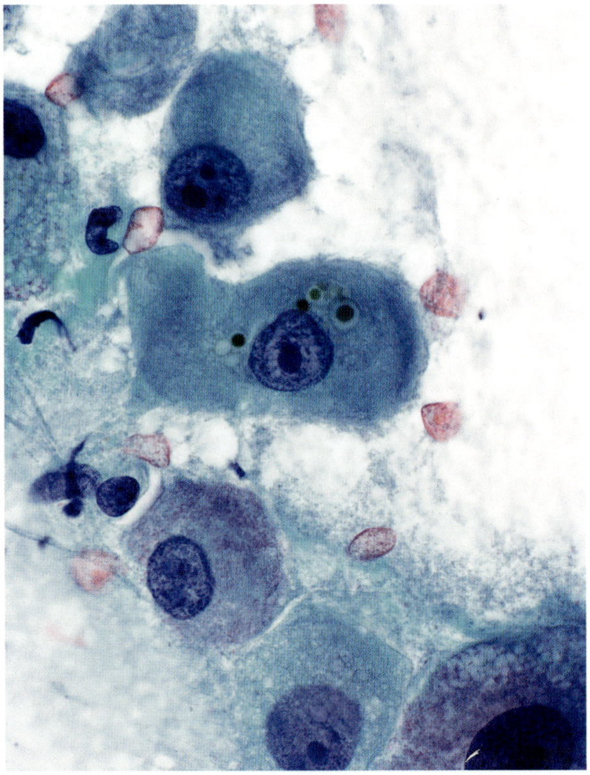

Figure 4-22

FIBROLAMELLAR CARCINOMA

The tumor cells have prominent nucleoli and abundant granular cytoplasm, occasionally with small intracytoplasmic vacuoles containing bile (touch prep; Papanicolaou stain).

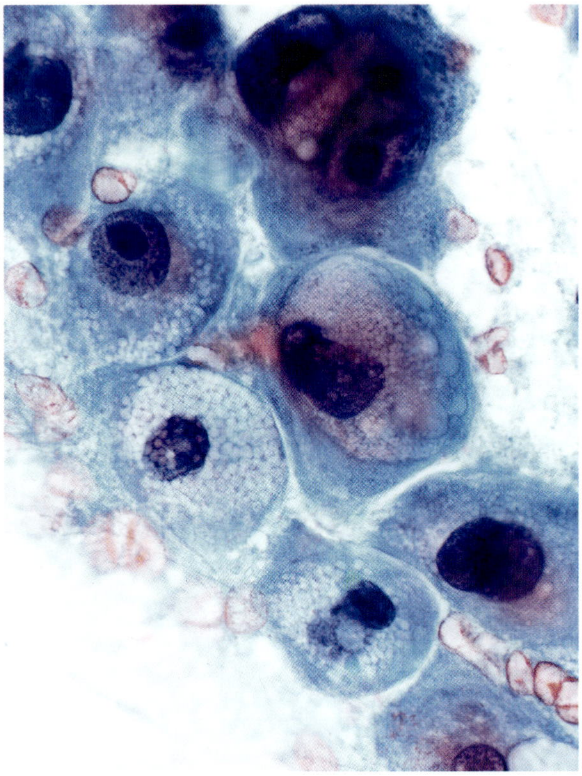

Figure 4-23

FIBROLAMELLAR CARCINOMA

Some tumor cells also have cytoplasm filled with numerous small, clear vacuoles (touch prep; Papanicolaou stain).

as the tumor cells of ordinary hepatocellular carcinoma (57,60,61). The fibrolamellar carcinoma cells also have classic findings of large central nuclei with prominent nucleoli (fig. 4-23). Binucleated tumor cells are often present. Nuclear pseudoinclusions can be prominent (62). Naked nuclei are seen in a subset of cases. Irregular fragments of collagen are sometimes present (61–63). Pale bodies and hyaline bodies are useful histologic clues and were present in all five fine-needle aspirates in one series (57). Other findings include bile production, cytoplasmic microvacules, and phagocytosis of neutrophils (57,63,64).

The cytologic features of typical hepatocellular carcinoma are usually absent, such as the narrow arborescent vascular channels intertwined with neoplastic trabeculae (57). The cytology of metastatic disease is similar to that of primary tumors (58,63).

MOLECULAR GENETIC FINDINGS

Molecular methods are excellent tools to confirm a diagnosis of fibrolamellar carcinoma. Essentially all fibrolamellar carcinomas with careful histologic confirmation have a fusion transcript between the *DNAJB1* gene and the *PRKACA* gene. *PRKACA* encodes the catalytic subunit of protein kinase A. As a rare exception, fibrolamellar carcinomas arising in the Carney complex can be negative for the translocation, instead having germline mutations in *PRKAR1A*, the regulatory subunit of protein kinase A.

The *DNAJB1-PRKACA* gene fusion is caused by a microdeletion on chromosome 19 (65). Protein kinase A is an important serine/threonine kinase that can phosphorylate a large number of cytoplasmic and nuclear proteins. The downstream target of the kinase in fibrolamellar carcinoma is not known. Reverse transcriptase-polymerase chain reaction (RT-PCR) can detect the

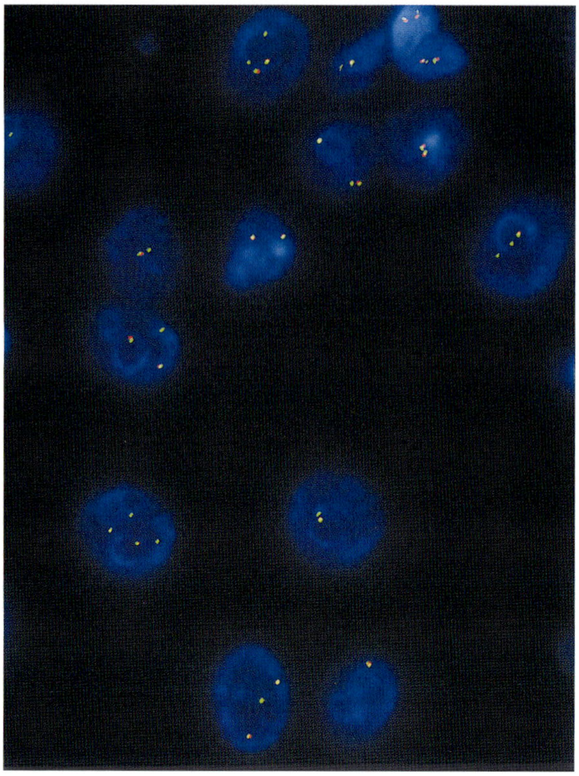

Figure 4-24

FIBROLAMELLAR CARCINOMA

This FISH assay uses a break-apart probe, so normal chromosomes have an adjacent green and red probe, often giving a yellow color. Deletions lead to loss or separation of the red probe from the green probe. Fibrolamellar carcinomas can have polysomy of chromosome 19, so tumor cells can retain normal chromosomes, in addition to chromosomes with the deletion.

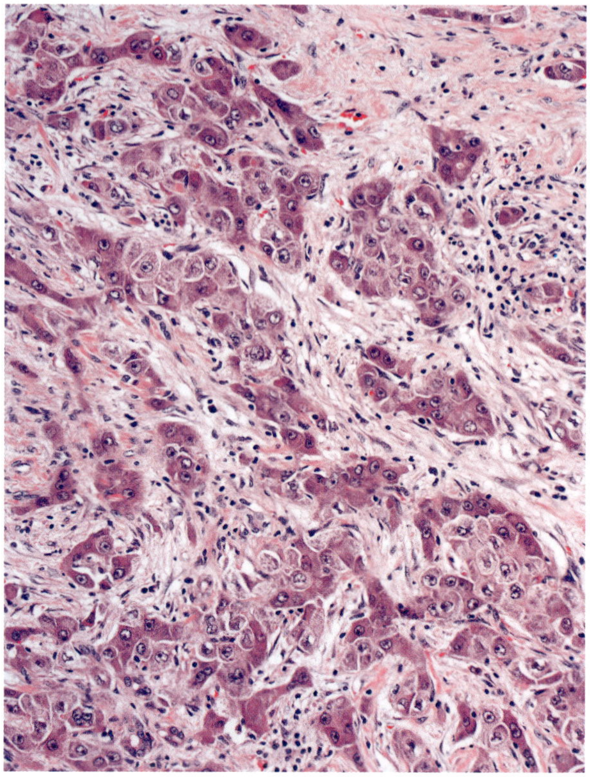

Figure 4-25

SCIRRHOUS HEPATOCELLULAR CARCINOMA

This scirrhous hepatocellular carcinoma mimics fibrolamellar carcinoma.

DNAJB1/PRKACA transcript and fluorescence in situ hybridization (FISH) can detect the DNA deletion that leads to the fusion transcript (fig. 4-24). RT-PCR can be falsely negative in some cases, secondary to RNA degradation, especially in paraffin-embedded tissues, giving advantages to FISH as a routine diagnostic tool.

DIFFERENTIAL DIAGNOSIS

The histologic features of fibrolamellar carcinoma are distinctive but there are several histologic mimics to consider. First, scirrhous hepatocellular carcinomas can closely mimic fibrolamellar carcinomas (fig. 4-25). In fact, in selected microscopic fields, the findings are essentially identical. Examining additional sections can help identify more typical areas of scirrhous hepatocellular carcinoma. The clinical findings (e.g., chronic viral hepatitis, age) can also help distinguish fibrolamellar carcinoma from scirrhous hepatocellular carcinoma, as can examining the background liver for underlying liver disease. Immunostains for CD68 and CK7 or molecular testing can clarify the diagnosis. Another potentially useful clue is weak HepPar1 staining, as all fibrolamellar carcinomas are strongly positive while more than half of scirrhous hepatocellular carcinomas show weak or negative staining (66).

Secondly, the differential diagnosis can include ordinary hepatocellular carcinomas, especially when intratumoral fibrosis is less prominent in the fibrolamellar carcinoma. A subset of hepatocellular carcinomas has large pink cells with prominent nucleoli, the cytologic hallmark of fibrolamellar carcinoma. In some of these cases, the cytology so closely mimics fibrolamellar carcinoma that even expert hepatic pathologists find it challenging to make a definite diagnosis on H&E-stained specimens (67).

Thirdly, the differential can include cholangiocarcinoma when pseudoglands are prominent. Cholangiocarcinoma can be ruled out with HepPar1 or arginase stains, as the pseudoglands in fibrolamellar carcinoma always retain the morphology and immunohistochemical findings of hepatocytic differentiation.

Next, neuroendocrine carcinomas metastatic to the liver can closely mimic fibrolamellar carcinoma, so much so that immunostains are needed to make the correct diagnosis. These diagnostic pitfalls can all be resolved by careful attention to clinical and histologic findings, coupled with additional testing, including immunostains for CD68 and CK7 or molecular testing.

Finally, it may be helpful to consider findings that would strongly argue against a diagnosis of fibrolamellar carcinoma. These include clinical factors such as age extremes or known chronic liver disease. Fibrolamellar carcinomas in individuals younger than 5 years or older than 60 years are very unusual and a diagnosis should be approached cautiously. Likewise, cases with serum AFP levels more than 400 ng/mL or that are positive for AFP by immunohistochemistry are most likely not fibrolamellar carcinoma. In addition, histologic evidence of chronic liver disease would not support a diagnosis of fibrolamellar carcinoma, with the caveat that histologic sections taken at the edge of the tumor often show nonspecific inflammatory changes and fibrosis. Also, the background liver in some cases of fibrolamellar carcinoma can show mild fatty liver disease without advanced fibrosis.

SPREAD AND METASTASES

Lymph nodes are positive for metastatic disease in approximately two thirds of individuals at the time of presentation (1,14,68) and regional lymphadenectomy is recommended for primary tumor resections with curative intent (14). Distant metastatic disease is found at presentation in about 30 percent of individuals (14). The lung is a frequent site of distant metastasis (1). Peritoneal metastasis, which can include abdominal carcinomatosis, is found at presentation in 10 to 15 percent of individuals (1).

After resection with curative intent, recurrent disease develops in 70 to 80 percent of individuals (28). When cancer recurs, about 40 percent of patients have liver recurrence. Extrahepatic recurrent disease is most commonly found in the lungs or peritoneum (69,70).

STAGING

Currently, fibrolamellar carcinomas are staged using the same staging system as typical hepatocellular carcinoma. Vascular invasion is present in 50 to 75 percent of resected fibrolamellar carcinomas (8,29,30,68). Sections taken at the tumor-nontumor interface are usually the best place to find vascular invasion. Tumor staging itself does not strongly predict disease-free survival (68), suggesting that the current staging system, which is modeled on typical hepatocellular carcinoma, could use some revisions, perhaps with a staging system specifically for fibrolamellar carcinoma. The tumor can involve nerves of the large portal tracts and hilum. While perineural growth is not part of the staging system, anecdotal experience suggests this can be a worse prognosis indicator. Likewise, hilar tumors often spread directly into the soft tissue of the liver hilum, a finding that does not readily fit into current tumor staging systems, but anecdotally appears to indicate a worse prognosis.

TREATMENT

Surgical resection with hilar lymph node dissection is the most important treatment option. Aggressive surgical resection of subsequent metastatic disease can also benefit individuals with recurrent disease after primary surgery (13,71). There is limited data on systemic chemotherapy because of the rarity of the tumor. There have been some reports of partial response to platinum base therapy (13) and a case report of complete response to gemcitabine and oxiplatin (72). Overall, however, fibrolamellar carcinomas do not respond any better than typical hepatocellular carcinomas to cisplatin, vincristine, and 5-fluorouracil-based chemotherapy (10). To date, no clear benefit for adjuvant chemotherapy has been identified (2,13,29). Another large study found no benefit from alternating cycles of cisplatin and carboplatin/doxorubicin (73). These pessimistic reports are offset to some degree by rare reports of success, including a case that was successfully down-sized using gemcitabine and oxiplatin, making it resectable

(74). A similar result was achieved in another case using cisplatinum, epirubicin, and 5-fluorouracil combination chemotherapy (75). More recently, aggressive therapy combining surgery and high doses of chemotherapy was successful in one reported case (76). A case report has also documented response to radiotherapy (77).

PROGNOSIS

Resectability is the single most important prognostic finding for patients with fibrolamellar carcinoma (6,10,14,30,68). This is well illustrated by a large study that found a median 5-year survival rate of 76 percent for those who underwent resection, compared to 0 percent for those with unresectable disease (30). For those who undergo surgery, regional lymph node disease and angiolymphatic invasion at the time of resection are the most consistently identified predictors of tumor recurrence (14,28). Many other potential prognostic factors have been identified, but most are weak predictors and have not been reproducibly identified. Also, in most cases, these factors were either not tested in multivariate analysis or were not statistically significant. Nonetheless, possible good prognostic factors include younger age at presentation (6,78), female gender (68), and low tumor stage (6).

Some of the earliest studies reported a good prognosis for fibrolamellar carcinoma when compared to conventional hepatocellular carcinoma. However, when the survival rate in fibrolamellar carcinoma is compared only to conventional hepatocellular carcinomas that arise in the background of noncirrhotic livers, the survival advantage is less apparent, with no survival benefit seen in some series (44,79), although a modest survival benefit is evident in others (29,80,81).

REFERENCES

1. Ang CS, Kelley RK, Choti MA, et al. Clinicopathologic characteristics and survival outcomes of patients with fibrolamellar carcinoma: data from the fibrolamellar carcinoma consortium. Gastrointest Cancer Res 2013;6:3-9.
2. El-Gazzaz G, Wong W, El-Hadary MK, et al. Outcome of liver resection and transplantation for fibrolamellar hepatocellular carcinoma. Transpl Int 2000;13(Suppl 1):S406-409.
3. Niederle IM, Worns MA, Koch S, et al. Clinicopathologic features and prognosis of young patients with hepatocellular carcinoma in a large German cohort. J Clin Gastroenterol 2012;46:775-778.
4. Eggert T, McGlynn KA, Duffy A, Manns MP, Greten TF, Altekruse SF. Fibrolamellar hepatocellular carcinoma in the USA, 2000-2010: A detailed report on frequency, treatment and outcome based on the Surveillance, Epidemiology, and End Results database. United European Gastroenterol J 2013;1:351-357.
5. Kaczynski J, Gustavsson B, Hansson G, Wallerstedt S. Fibrolamellar hepatic carcinoma in an area with a low incidence of primary liver cancer: a retrospective study. Eur J Surg 1996;162:367-371.
6. El-Serag HB, Davila JA. Is fibrolamellar carcinoma different from hepatocellular carcinoma? A US population-based study. Hepatology 2004; 39:798-803.
7. Torbenson M. Fibrolamellar carcinoma: 2012 update. Scientifica (Cairo) 2012;2012:743790.
8. Farhi DC, Shikes RH, Murari PJ, Silverberg SG. Hepatocellular carcinoma in young people. Cancer 1983;52:1516-1525.
9. Klein WM, Molmenti EP, Colombani PM, et al. Primary liver carcinoma arising in people younger than 30 years. Am J Clin Pathol 2005;124:512-8.
10. Katzenstein HM, Krailo MD, Malogolowkin MH, et al. Fibrolamellar hepatocellular carcinoma in children and adolescents. Cancer 2003;97:2006-2012.
11. Allan BJ, Wang B, Davis JS, et al. A review of 218 pediatric cases of hepatocellular carcinoma. J Pediatr Surg 2014;49:166-171; discussion 171.
12. Eggert T, McGlynn KA, Duffy A, Manns MP, Greten TF, Altekruse SF. Epidemiology of fibrolamellar hepatocellular carcinoma in the USA, 2000-10. Gut 2013;62:1667-1668.
13. Maniaci V, Davidson BR, Rolles K, et al. Fibrolamellar hepatocellular carcinoma: prolonged survival with multimodality therapy. Eur J Surg Oncol 2009;35:617-621.

14. Darcy DG, Malek MM, Kobos R, Klimstra DS, DeMatteo R, La Quaglia MP. Prognostic factors in fibrolamellar hepatocellular carcinoma in young people. J Pediatr Surg 2015;50:153-156.
15. Meriggi F, Forni E. [Surgical therapy of hepatic fibrolamellar carcinoma]. Ann Ital Chir 2007;78:53-58. [Italian]
16. Lildballe DL, Nguyen KQ, Poulsen SS, Nielsen HO, Nexo E. Haptocorrin as marker of disease progression in fibrolamellar hepatocellular carcinoma. Eur J Surg Oncol 2011;37:72-79.
17. Wheeler K, Pritchard J, Luck W, Rossiter M. Transcobalamin I as a "marker" for fibrolamellar hepatoma. Med Pediatr Oncol 1986;14:227-229.
18. Evers BM, Rajaraman S, Chung DH, et al. Developmental expression of the neurotensin gene in the rat liver. Ann Surg 1993;218:183-188.
19. Kannangai R, Vivekanandan P, Martinez-Murillo F, Choti M, Torbenson M. Fibrolamellar carcinomas show overexpression of genes in the RAS, MAPK, PIK3, and xenobiotic degradation pathways. Hum Pathol 2007;38:639-644.
20. Malouf GG, Job S, Paradis V, et al. Transcriptional profiling of pure fibrolamellar hepatocellular carcinoma reveals an endocrine signature. Hepatology 2014;59:2228-2237.
21. Soreide O, Czerniak A, Bradpiece H, Bloom S, Blumgart L. Characteristics of fibrolamellar hepatocellular carcinoma. A study of nine cases and a review of the literature. Am J Surg 1986;151:518-523.
22. Terracciano LM, Tornillo L, Avoledo P, Von Schweinitz D, Kuhne T, Bruder E. Fibrolamellar hepatocellular carcinoma occurring 5 years after hepatocellular adenoma in a 14-year-old girl: a case report with comparative genomic hybridization analysis. Arch Pathol Lab Med 2004;128:222-226.
23. Graham RP, Terracciano LM, Meves A, et al. Hepatic adenomas with synchronous or metachronous fibrolamellar carcinomas: both are characterized by LFABP loss. Mod Pathol 2016;29:607-15.
24. Davison FD, Fagan EA, Portmann B, Williams R. HBV-DNA sequences in tumor and nontumor tissue in a patient with the fibrolamellar variant of hepatocellular carcinoma. Hepatology 1990;12:676-679.
25. Dadke D, Jaganath P, Krishnamurthy S, Chiplunkar S. The detection of HBV antigens and HBx-transcripts in an Indian fibrolamellar carcinoma patient: a case study. Liver 2002;22:87-91.
26. Morise Z, Sugioka A, Mizoguchi Y, et al. Fibrolamellar carcinoma of the liver in a Japanese hepatitis B virus carrier. J Gastroenterol Hepatol 2005;20:1136-1138.
27. Oddou S, Vey N, Viens P, et al. Second neoplasms following high-dose chemotherapy and autologous stem cell transplantation for malignant lymphomas: a report of six cases in a cohort of 171 patients from a single institution. Leuk Lymphoma 1998;31:187-194.
28. Herman P, Chagas AL, Perini MV, et al. Surgical treatment of fibrolamellar hepatocellular carcinoma: an underestimated malignant tumor? Hepatobiliary Pancreat Dis Int 2014;13:618-621.
29. Pinna AD, Iwatsuki S, Lee RG, et al. Treatment of fibrolamellar hepatoma with subtotal hepatectomy or transplantation. Hepatology 1997;26:877-883.
30. Stipa F, Yoon SS, Liau KH, et al. Outcome of patients with fibrolamellar hepatocellular carcinoma. Cancer 2006;106:1331-1338.
31. Graham RP, Jin L, Knutson DL, et al. DNAJB1-PRKACA is specific for fibrolamellar carcinoma. Mod Pathol 2015;28:822-829.
32. An T, Ghatak N, Kastner R, Kay S, Lee HM. Hyaline globules and intracellular lumina in a hepatocellular carcinoma. Am J Clin Pathol 1983;79:392-396.
33. Goodman ZD, Ishak KG, Langloss JM, Sesterhenn IA, Rabin L. Combined hepatocellular-cholangiocarcinoma. A histologic and immunohistochemical study. Cancer 1985;55:124-135.
34. Tanaka K, Honna T, Kitano Y, et al. Combined fibrolamellar carcinoma and cholangiocarcinoma exhibiting biphenotypic antigen expression: a case report. J Clin Pathol 2005;58:884-887.
35. Ichikawa T, Federle MP, Grazioli L, Madariaga J, Nalesnik M, Marsh W. Fibrolamellar hepatocellular carcinoma: imaging and pathologic findings in 31 recent cases. Radiology 1999;213:352-361.
36. LeBrun DP, Silver MM, Freedman MH, Phillips MJ. Fibrolamellar carcinoma of the liver in a patient with Fanconi anemia. Hum Pathol 1991;22:396-398.
37. Vecchio FM, Fabiano A, Ghirlanda G, Manna R, Massi G. Fibrolamellar carcinoma of the liver: the malignant counterpart of focal nodular hyperplasia with oncocytic change. Am J Clin Pathol 1984;81:521-526.
38. Imkie M, Myers SA, Li Y, et al. Fibrolamellar hepatocellular carcinoma arising in a background of focal nodular hyperplasia: a report of 2 cases. J Reprod Med 2005;50:633-637.
39. Saxena R, Humphreys S, Williams R, Portmann B. Nodular hyperplasia surrounding fibrolamellar carcinoma: a zone of arterialized liver parenchyma. Histopathology 1994;25:275-278.
40. Saul SH, Titelbaum DS, Gansler TS, et al. The fibrolamellar variant of hepatocellular carcinoma. Its association with focal nodular hyperplasia. Cancer 1987;60:3049-3055.
41. Lloreta J, Vadell C, Fabregat X, Serrano S. Fibrolamellar hepatic tumor with neurosecretory features and systemic deposition of AA amyloid. Ultrastruct Pathol 1994;18:287-292.

42. Garcia de Davila MT, Gonzalez-Crussi F, Mangkornkanok M. Fibrolamellar carcinoma of the liver in a child: ultrastructural and immunohistologic aspects. Pediatr Pathol 1987;7:319-331.
43. Ward SC, Huang J, Tickoo SK, Thung SN, Ladanyi M, Klimstra DS. Fibrolamellar carcinoma of the liver exhibits immunohistochemical evidence of both hepatocyte and bile duct differentiation. Mod Pathol 2010;23:1180-1190.
44. Kakar S, Burgart LJ, Batts KP, Garcia J, Jain D, Ferrell LD. Clinicopathologic features and survival in fibrolamellar carcinoma: comparison with conventional hepatocellular carcinoma with and without cirrhosis. Mod Pathol 2005;18:1417-1423.
45. Chu PG, Ishizawa S, Wu E, Weiss LM. Hepatocyte antigen as a marker of hepatocellular carcinoma: an immunohistochemical comparison to carcinoembryonic antigen, CD10, and alpha-fetoprotein. Am J Surg Pathol 2002;26:978-988.
46. Ross HM, Daniel HD, Vivekanandan P, et al. Fibrolamellar carcinomas are positive for CD68. Mod Pathol 2011;24:390-395.
47. Kojima M, Kunimura T, Inagaki T, et al. A fibrolamellar carcinoma of the liver with a marked solid component. J Gastroenterol 2004;39:905-907.
48. Seitz G, Zimmermann A, Friess H, Büchler MW. Adult-type hepatocellular carcinoma in the center of a fibrolamellar hepatocellular carcinoma. Hum Pathol 2002;33:765-769.
49. Malouf GG, Brugieres L, Le Deley MC, et al. Pure and mixed fibrolamellar hepatocellular carcinomas differ in natural history and prognosis after complete surgical resection. Cancer 2012;118:4981-4990.
50. Cheuk W, Chan JK. Clear cell variant of fibrolamellar carcinoma of the liver. Arch Pathol Lab Med 2001;125:1235-1238.
51. Kaplan JS, Hoda RS. Clear cell variant of fibrolamellar hepatocellular carcinoma: diagnosis of recurrence by fine-needle aspiration. Diagn Cytopathol 2007;35:459-462.
52. Payne CM, Nagle RB, Paplanus SH, Graham AR. Fibrolamellar carcinoma of liver: a primary malignant oncocytic carcinoid? Ultrastruct Pathol 1986;10:539-552.
53. Farhi DC, Shikes RH, Silverberg SG. Ultrastructure of fibrolamellar oncocytic hepatoma. Cancer 1982;50:702-709.
54. Sato S, Masuda T, Oikawa H, et al. Bile canaliculi-like lumina in fibrolamellar carcinoma of the liver: a light- and electron-microscopic study and three-dimensional examination of serial sections. Pathol Int 1997;47:763-768.
55. Caballero T, Aneiros J, Lopez-Caballero J, Gomez-Morales M, Nogales F. Fibrolamellar hepatocellular carcinoma. An immunohistochemical and ultrastructural study. Histopathology 1985;9:445-456.
56. Andreola S, Audisio RA, Lombardi L. A light microscopic and ultrastructural study of two cases of fibrolamellar hepatocellular carcinoma. Tumori 1986;72:609-616.
57. Perez-Guillermo M, Masgrau NA, Garcia-Solano J, Sola-Perez J, de Agustin y de Agustin P. Cytologic aspect of fibrolamellar hepatocellular carcinoma in fine-needle aspirates. Diagn Cytopathol 1999;21:180-187.
58. Sarode VR, Castellani R, Post A. Fine-needle aspiration cytology and differential diagnoses of fibrolamellar hepatocellular carcinoma metastatic to the mediastinum: case report. Diagn Cytopathol 2002;26:95-98.
59. Renshaw AA, Haja J, Wilbur DC, Miller TR; Cytology Committee College of American Pathologists. Fine-needle aspirates of hepatocellular carcinoma that are misclassified as adenocarcinoma: correlating cytologic features and performance in the College of American Pathologists Nongynecologic Cytology Program. Arch Pathol Lab Med 2006;130:19-22.
60. Suen KC. Diagnosis of primary hepatic neoplasms by fine-needle aspiration cytology. Diagn Cytopathol 1986;2:99-109.
61. Mansouri D, Van Nhieu JT, Couanet D, et al. Fibrolamellar hepatocellular carcinoma: a case report with cytological features in a sixteen-year-old girl. Diagn Cytopathol 2006;34:568-571.
62. Kunz G Jr, Chung J, Ali SZ. Hepatocellular carcinoma-fibrolamellar variant: cytopathology of an unusual case. Diagn Cytopathol 2002;26:257-261.
63. Crowe A, Knight CS, Jhala D, Bynon SJ, Jhala NC. Diagnosis of metastatic fibrolamellar hepatocellular carcinoma by endoscopic ultrasound-guided fine needle aspiration. Cytojournal 2011;8:2.
64. Davenport RD. Cytologic diagnosis of fibrolamellar carcinoma of the liver by fine-needle aspiration. Diagn Cytopathol 1990;6:275-279.
65. Honeyman JN, Simon EP, Robine N, et al. Detection of a recurrent DNAJB1-PRKACA chimeric transcript in fibrolamellar hepatocellular carcinoma. Science 2014;343:1010-1014.
66. Krings G, Ramachandran R, Jain D, et al. Immunohistochemical pitfalls and the importance of glypican 3 and arginase in the diagnosis of scirrhous hepatocellular carcinoma. Mod Pathol 2013;26:782-791.
67. Malouf G, Falissard B, Azoulay D, et al. Is histological diagnosis of primary liver carcinomas with fibrous stroma reproducible among experts? J Clin Pathol 2009;62:519-524.

68. Kaseb AO, Shama M, Sahin IH, et al. Prognostic indicators and treatment outcome in 94 cases of fibrolamellar hepatocellular carcinoma. Oncology 2013;85:197-203.
69. Groeschl RT, Miura JT, Wong RK, et al. Multi-institutional analysis of recurrence and survival after hepatectomy for fibrolamellar carcinoma. J Surg Oncol 2014;110:412-415.
70. Do RK, McErlean A, Ang CS, DeMatteo RP, Abou-Alfa GK. CT and MRI of primary and metastatic fibrolamellar carcinoma: a case series of 37 patients. Br J Radiol 2014;87:20140024.
71. Hemming AW, Langer B, Sheiner P, Greig PD, Taylor BR. Aggressive surgical management of fibrolamellar hepatocellular carcinoma. J Gastrointest Surg 1997;1:342-346.
72. Gras P, Truant S, Boige V, et al. Prolonged complete response after gemox chemotherapy in a patient with advanced fibrolamellar hepatocellular carcinoma. Case Rep Oncol 2012;5:169-172.
73. Weeda VB, Murawski M, McCabe AJ, et al. Fibrolamellar variant of hepatocellular carcinoma does not have a better survival than conventional hepatocellular carcinoma—results and treatment recommendations from the Childhood Liver Tumour Strategy Group (SIOPEL) experience. Eur J Cancer 2013;49:2698-2704.
74. Fonseca GM, Varella AD, Coelho FF, Abe ES, Dumarco RB, Herman P. Downstaging and resection after neoadjuvant therapy for fibrolamellar hepatocellular carcinoma. World J Gastrointest Surg 2014;6:107-111.
75. Bower M, Newlands ES, Habib N. Fibrolamellar hepatocellular carcinoma responsive to platinum-based combination chemotherapy. Clin Oncol (R Coll Radiol) 1996;8:331-333.
76. Okur A, Eser EP, Yilmaz G, et al. Successful multimodal treatment for aggressive metastatic and recurrent fibrolamellar hepatocellular carcinoma in a child. J Pediatr Hematol Oncol 2014;36:e328-332.
77. Peacock GJ, Call AJ, Oliver RK. Radiotherapy for metastatic fibrolamellar hepatocellular carcinoma. Rare Tumors 2013;5:e28.
78. Moreno-Luna LE, Arrieta O, Garcia-Leiva J, et al. Clinical and pathologic factors associated with survival in young adult patients with fibrolamellar hepatocarcinoma. BMC Cancer 2005;5:142.
79. Njei B, Konjeti VR, Ditah I. Prognosis of patients with fibrolamellar hepatocellular carcinoma versus conventional hepatocellular carcinoma: a systematic review and meta-analysis. Gastrointest Cancer Res 2014;7:49-54.
80. Houben KW, McCall JL. Liver transplantation for hepatocellular carcinoma in patients without underlying liver disease: a systematic review. Liver Transpl Surg 1999;5:91-95.
81. Mayo SC, Mavros MN, Nathan H, Cosgrove D, Herman JM, Kamel I, et al. Treatment and prognosis of patients with fibrolamellar hepatocellular carcinoma: a national perspective. J Am Coll Surg 2014;218:196-205.
82. Asrani SK, LaRusso NF. Fibrolamellar hepatocellular carcinoma presenting with Budd-Chiari syndrome, right atrial thrombus, and pulmonary emboli. Hepatology 2012;55:977-978.
83. Lamberts R, Nitsche R, de Vivie RE, et al. Budd-Chiari syndrome as the primary manifestation of a fibrolamellar hepatocellular carcinoma. Digestion 1992;53:200-209.
84. Kanai T, Takabayashi T, Kawano Y, Kuramochi S, Miyazawa N. A case of postoperative recurrence of fibrolamellar hepatocellular carcinoma with increased vitamin B12 binding capacity in a young Japanese female. Jpn J Clin Oncol 2004;34:346-351.
85. Knudson JD, Goldberg JF, Ayres NA. Fibrolamellar hepatocellular carcinoma with cardiac spread causing severe inferior vena cava obstruction in a 9-year-old child. Pediatr Cardiol 2012;33:872-873.
86. Sethi S, Tageja N, Singh J, et al. Hyperammonemic encephalopathy: a rare presentation of fibrolamellar hepatocellular carcinoma. Am J Med Sci 2009;338:522-524.
87. Berger C, Dimant P, Hermida L, Paulin F, Pereyra M, Tejo M. [Hyperammonemic encephalopathy and fibrolamellar hepatocellular carcinoma.] Medicina (B Aires). 2012;72:425-427. [Spanish]
88. Sulaiman RA, Geberhiwot T. Fibrolamellar hepatocellular carcinoma mimicking ornithine transcarbamylase deficiency. JIMD Rep 2014;16:47-50.
89. Bender HU, Staudigl M, Schmid I, Führer M. Treatment of paraneoplastic hyperammonemia in fibrolamellar hepatocellular carcinoma with oral sodium phenyl butyrate. J Pain Symptom Manage 2015;49:e8-10.
90. Hashash JG, Thudi K, Malik SM. An 18-year-old woman with a 15-cm liver mass and an ammonia level of 342. Gastroenterology 2012;143:1157, 1401-1402.
91. Tangkijvanich P, Thong-Ngam D, Kullavanijaya P, Suwangool P. Fibrolamellar hepatocellular carcinoma in a Thai man who presented with hypoglycemia: case report and review of literature. J Med Assoc Thai 2000;83:809-816.
92. Dahan MH, Kastell P. Fibrolamellar hepatic carcinoma with a presentation similar to that of septic pregnancy. A case report. J Reprod Med 2002;47:47-49.
93. Soyer P, Roche A, Levesque M. Fibrolamellar hepatocellular carcinoma presenting with obstructive jaundice. A report of two cases. Eur J Radiol 1991;13:196-198.

94. Eckstein RP, Bambach CP, Stiel D, Roche J, Goodman BN. Fibrolamellar carcinoma as a cause of bile duct obstruction. Pathology 1988;20:326-331.
95. Arora R. Fibrolamellar hepatocellular carcinoma presenting as obstructive jaundice: uncommon presentation of a rare entity. Pol J Radiol 2015;80:168-171.
96. De Gaetano AM, Nure E, Grossi U, et al. Fibrolamellar hepatocellular carcinoma with biliary tumor thrombus: an unreported association. Jpn J Radiol 2013;31:706-712.
97. Snook JA, Kelly P, Chapman RW, Jewell DP. Fibrolamellar hepatocellular carcinoma complicating ulcerative colitis with primary sclerosing cholangitis. Gut 1989;30:243-245.
98. Vaideeswar P, Pandit MJ, Deshpande JR, Sivaraman A, Vora IM. Fibrolamellar carcinoma of the liver--an unusual presentation. J Postgrad Med 1993;39:159-161.
99. Gupta P, Dhar S, Strickland NH. Fibrolamellar carcinoma: an unusual clinico-radiological presentation. Eur J Radiol 1999;32:119-123.
100. Debray D, Pariente D, Fabre M, Foucaud P, Valayer J, Bernard O. Fibrolamellar hepatocellular carcinoma: report of a case mimicking a liver abscess. J Pediatr Gastroenterol Nutr 1994;19:468-472.
101. Kutluk MT, Yalcin B, Büyükpamukcu N, Kale G, Büyükpamukcu M. Fibrolamellar hepatocellular carcinoma with skeletal metastases. Pediatr Hematol Oncol 2001;18:273-278.
102. Agarwal VR, Takayama K, Van Wyk JJ, Sasano H, Simpson ER, Bulun SE. Molecular basis of severe gynecomastia associated with aromatase expression in a fibrolamellar hepatocellular carcinoma. J Clin Endocrinol Metab 1998;83:1797-1800.
103. McCloskey JJ, Germain-Lee EL, Perman JA, Plotnick LP, Janoski AH. Gynecomastia as a presenting sign of fibrolamellar carcinoma of the liver. Pediatrics 1988;82:379-382.
104. Hany MA, Betts DR, Schmugge M, et al. A childhood fibrolamellar hepatocellular carcinoma with increased aromatase activity and a near triploid karyotype. Med Pediatr Oncol 1997;28:136-138.
105. Muramori K, Taguchi S, Taguchi T, et al. High aromatase activity and overexpression of epidermal growth factor receptor in fibrolamellar hepatocellular carcinoma in a child. J Pediatr Hematol Oncol 2011;33:e195-197.
106. Al-Matham K, Alabed I, Zaidi SZ, Qushmaq KA. Cold agglutinin disease in fibrolamellar hepatocellular carcinoma: a rare association with a rare cancer variant. Ann Saudi Med 2011;31:197-200.
107. Minutolo V, Licciardello A, Arena M, Minutolo O, Lanteri R, Arena G. Surgical resection of ruptured fibrolamellar hepatocellular carcinoma. Case Rep Surg 2013;2013:679565.
108. Abdul-Al HM, Wang G, Makhlouf HR, Goodman ZD. Fibrolamellar hepatocellular carcinoma: an immunohistochemical comparison with conventional hepatocellular carcinoma. Int J Surg Pathol 2010;18:313-318.
109. Haratake J, Horie A, Lee SD, Huh MH. Fibrolamellar carcinoma of the liver in a middle-aged Korean man. J UOEH 1990;12:349-354.
110. Gornicka B, Ziarkiewicz-Wroblewska B, Wroblewski T, et al. Carcinoma, a fibrolamellar variant—immunohistochemical analysis of 4 cases. Hepatogastroenterology 2005;52:519-523.
111. Van Eyken P, Sciot R, Brock P, Casteels-Van Daele M, Ramaekers FC, Desmet VJ. Abundant expression of cytokeratin 7 in fibrolamellar carcinoma of the liver. Histopathology 1990;17:101-107.
112. Patonai A, Erdelyi-Belle B, Korompay A, et al. Molecular characteristics of fibrolamellar hepatocellular carcinoma. Pathol Oncol Res 2013;19:63-70.
113. Johnson DE, Herndier BG, Medeiros LJ, Warnke RA, Rouse RV. The diagnostic utility of the keratin profiles of hepatocellular carcinoma and cholangiocarcinoma. Am J Surg Pathol 1988;12:187-197.
114. Kannangai R, Sahin F, Torbenson MS. EGFR is phosphorylated at Ty845 in hepatocellular carcinoma. Mod Pathol 2006;19:1456-1461.
115. Buckley AF, Burgart LJ, Kakar S. Epidermal growth factor receptor expression and gene copy number in fibrolamellar hepatocellular carcinoma. Hum Pathol 2006;37:410-414.
116. Zen Y, Vara R, Portmann B, Hadzic N. Childhood hepatocellular carcinoma: a clinicopathological study of 12 cases with special reference to EpCAM. Histopathology 2014;64:671-682.
117. Dhingra S, Li W, Tan D, Zenali M, Zhang H, Brown RE. Cell cycle biology of fibrolamellar hepatocellular carcinoma. Int J Clin Exp Pathol 2010;3:792-797.

5 PEDIATRIC LIVER TUMORS

HEPATOBLASTOMA

Hepatoblastomas are malignant tumors with a range of hepatocellular differentiation, from undifferentiated cells to well-differentiated fetal-type hepatocytes, reflecting the normal developmental stages of the liver. Hepatoblastomas can be purely epithelial but often have a mesenchymal component. An epithelial component is required for a diagnosis of hepatoblastoma.

Clinical Features

Patients usually present with nonspecific signs and symptoms. Some of the common clinical findings include a palpable abdominal mass, abdominal pain, failure to thrive, vomiting, diarrhea, and jaundice (1). Osteopenia is found in about 20 percent of infants at presentation (1). Rarely, patients present with virilization and precocious puberty due to tumor production of human chorionic gonadotropin (2).

Hepatoblastomas have an incidence in the general population of 1.2 to 1.5 cases/million population/year, although the incidence appears to be slowly increasing over time (3). Hepatoblastomas are tumors of the very young and are the most common malignant liver tumor in the pediatric age group, with approximately two thirds of cases presenting before age 2, and 90 percent of cases presenting before age 5 (1). Males are affected at least twice as often as females (1). Hepatoblastomas occasionally arise in older children and rare cases have been reported in adults (4), although many of the putative adult hepatoblastomas are suboptimally documented and may instead be other tumors mimicking hepatoblastomas.

Serum levels of alpha-fetoprotein (AFP) are elevated in nearly all cases and are a useful tool in the primary diagnosis of hepatoblastoma. A tumor with definite hepatocytic differentiation on hematoxylin and eosin (H&E) stain but without an elevated serum AFP, is most likely not a hepatoblastoma. Elevated serum AFP levels are not specific for hepatoblastoma, however, and are also elevated in other benign and malignant pediatric liver diseases, including mesenchymal hamartomas (5) and hepatocellular carcinomas. A small subset of hepatoblastomas has normal or mildly elevated serum AFP levels, correlating with the small cell undifferentiated morphology. Serum levels of AFP are also useful in monitoring for recurrent disease.

Etiology

The etiology of hepatoblastomas is not known, but there are several established risk factors, principally very low birth weight (under 1,500 g) and congenital clinical syndromes. It is unclear whether very low birth weight is a direct risk for the development of hepatoblastoma or whether they instead both share in common an underlying, but unknown, risk factor, one that leads to both low birth weights and hepatoblastomas. Pregnancy with multiple fetuses is another risk factor for hepatoblastomas (6). Parental tobacco use is a proposed risk factor, although the data remain inconclusive (7). In many cases, hepatoblastomas appear to develop in utero, ruling out postnatal environmental risk factors.

Hepatoblastomas are associated with several clinical syndromes, the best established being familial adenomatous polyposis (8) and the Beckwith-Wiedemann syndrome (9). They also develop in individuals with a wide variety of isolated developmental malformations. The strongest association is with congenital abnormalities of the kidney and bladder, but the abnormalities are variable, with no obvious core set of findings. For example, kidney abnormalities range from polycystic kidney disease to kidney failure to ureteral abnormalities (10).

A large number of possible genetic associations have been cited in case reports, but the rarity of these reports makes it challenging

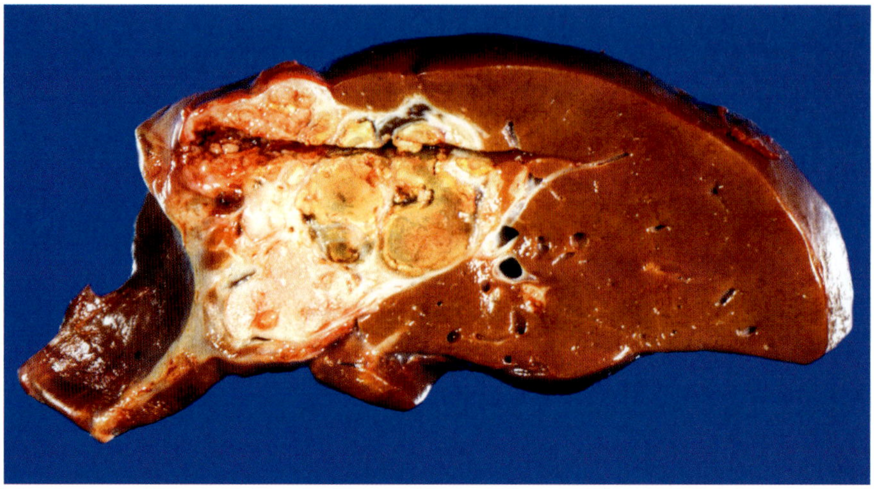

Figure 5-1

HEPATOBLASTOMA

The tumor is multilobulated with varying shades of white and yellow. The background liver is noncirrhotic.

to establish a clear association. Some of these include trisomy 18 and other trisomies (11,12), the Aicardi syndrome (13), and the fragile X syndrome (14).

Gross Findings

Most hepatoblastomas are single lesions and all arise in noncirrhotic livers (fig. 5-1). The tumors have varying colors and textures depending on the subtype and the presence of mesenchymal components. Treated tumors often show extensive necrosis, which can be associated with intratumoral hemorrhage and cystic change. Adequate histologic sampling is important because of tumor heterogeneity and the current guidelines recommend at least one section per centimeter of tumor diameter (15).

Microscopic Findings

The tumor cells in hepatoblastomas range from primitive, undifferentiated cells to well-differentiated epithelial cells that resemble fetal hepatocytes. Mesenchymal components are present in 25 to 40 percent of cases. The mesenchymal component is most commonly undifferentiated fibroblasts. As stated earlier, an epithelial component is needed for the diagnosis of hepatoblastoma.

The epithelial components are currently classified into seven main histologic categories (Table 5-1) (15): small cell undifferentiated, embryonal, pure fetal with low mitotic activity, fetal with mitotic activity, pleomorphic/anaplastic fetal, macrotrabecular, and cholangioblastic. Befitting its name, the small cell undifferentiated pattern shows the least resemblance to mature hepatocytes, while the fetal and macrotrabecular patterns show the greatest resemblance. While the many subtypes can seem somewhat overwhelming, in most cases a diagnosis is rendered comfortably by careful histologic examination and by following the classification guidelines. Of the different epithelial subtypes, the most common are the embryonal and fetal patterns, together making up the majority of tumors. Comparative cytologic findings are seen in figures 5-2 to 5-4, which show small cell undifferentiated, embryonal, and fetal patterns at the same magnification and each with a 10- µm bar in the upper left corner of the image.

The frequency of the different epithelial subtypes of hepatoblastoma varies between studies, but one or more of the fetal patterns are present in 80 to 90 percent of cases. The embryonal pattern is present in about 30 percent of hepatoblastomas and each of the remaining types is seen in 5 percent or fewer cases. Usually, the various epithelial types are admixed within the same tumor and most tumors have two or more epithelial components. The embryonal pattern, for example, is almost never seen alone, but instead is typically accompanied by fetal patterns. When hepatoblastomas do have a single, pure epithelial pattern, the most common pattern is well-differentiated fetal-type hepatoblastoma, found in about 20 percent of cases (3,16). The small cell undifferentiated component is often associated with normal or mild (less than 100 ng/mL) elevations in serum AFP, but at this point there are no other strong correlates between

Table 5-1

CLASSIFICATION OF PEDIATRIC EPITHELIAL MALIGNANCIES

Tumor	Synonym and Notes
Hepatoblastoma	
Small cell undifferentiated	
Positive for INI-1 loss on immunostain	
Negative for INI-1 loss on immunostain	Tumors that show INI-1 or BRG-1 loss should be classified as malignant rhabdoid tumors if they have rhabdoid morphology instead of hepatoblastoma morphology (see chapter 9)
Embryonal	
Pure fetal with low mitotic activity	Synonym (older term): well-differentiated fetal
Mitotically active fetal	Synonym (older term): crowded fetal
Pleomorphic fetal	Synonym (older term): poorly differentiated fetal
Anaplastic fetal	Some classification systems group these with pleomorphic
Macrotrabecular	
Cholangiocellular	Synonym: cholangioblastic
Mixed epithelial and mesenchymal	The hepatoblastoma can have any of the epithelial components; the mesenchymal can be with or without teratoid features
Hepatocellular adenoma	Synonym: hepatic adenoma; adenomas should be subtyped as they are in adults
Hepatocellular carcinoma	
Fibrolamellar carcinoma	Synonym: fibrolamellar hepatocellular carcinoma
Transitional cell tumor	Synonym: hepatocellular neoplasm, NOS
Malignant rhabdoid tumor	
Calcified nested epithelial-stromal tumor	Synonyms (older terms): nested stromal-epithelial tumor; desmoplastic nested spindle cell tumor; nested ossifying stromal-epithelial tumor;
Desmoplastic small round cell tumor	
Peripheral primitive neuroectodermal tumor	

morphologic patterns and demographics, risk factors, serum findings, or imaging findings.

Classic examples of each of the epithelial patterns are readily found and are often used to illustrate talks and books, but in any given case, it is common to find histologic foci that are challenging to classify. As one example, these challenging foci can have features that fall between the classic descriptions of fetal and embryonal patterns. As another example, tumors composed predominately or exclusively of the small cell undifferentiated pattern are generally classified as such by pathologists, but a minor component of the small cell undifferentiated pattern is less reproducibly identified (15).

The most clinically important patterns are the pure fetal pattern with low mitotic activity and the small cell undifferentiated pattern. The pure fetal pattern with low mitotic activity, described below, is generally straightforward to diagnose, but presumes adequate sampling to rule out minor components of other growth patterns. A minor component of the small cell undifferentiated pattern can be particularly challenging to recognize, for example, when occurring in less than 1 percent of the tumor. The use of the INI-1 stain supplements the morphologic findings, although currently the clinical significance is unclear when a tumor contains very small amounts of the small cell undifferentiated pattern with INI-1 retention.

Depending on the treatment protocols of the institution and the pretreatment extent of disease (PRETEXT) stage, many individuals with hepatoblastomas receive chemotherapy prior to resection. The current guidelines recommend pretreatment biopsies to confirm the diagnosis in all cases (15). After chemotherapy, the resected tumors may have an increased mesenchymal component compared to the pretreatment histology. They may also have squamous nests and areas of cholangioblastic differentiation. Treated hepatoblastomas can also

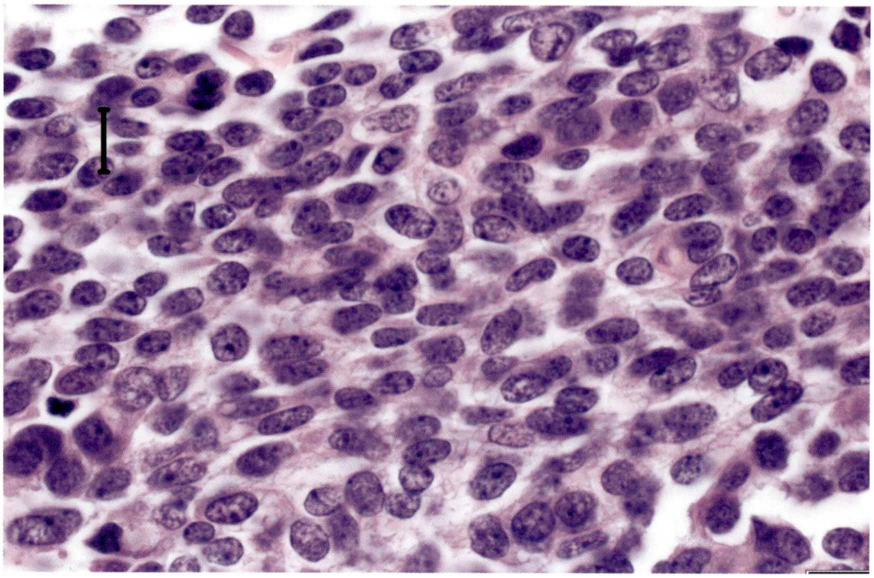

Figure 5-2

HEPATOBLASTOMA: SMALL CELL UNDIFFERENTIATED PATTERN

A solid growth pattern is seen, with immature, undifferentiated tumor cells. Nuclei are round to oval and nucleoli are inconspicuous (bar: 10 µm).

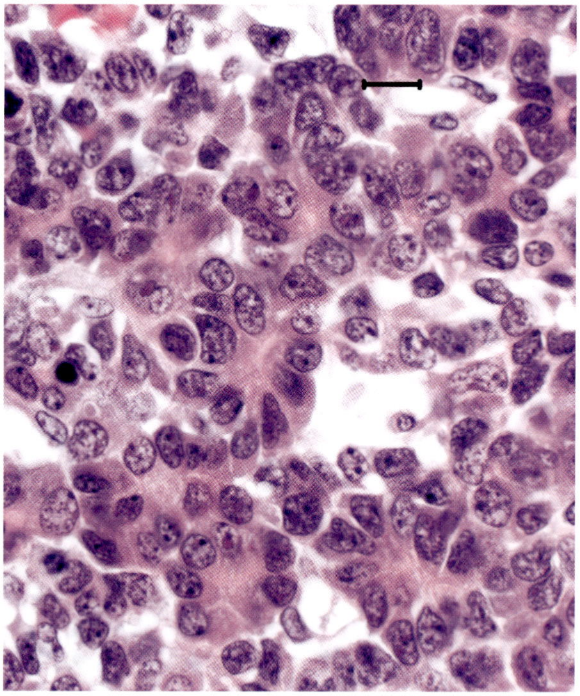

Figure 5-3

HEPATOBLASTOMA: EMBRYONAL PATTERN

The tumor cells show more nuclear angulation and coarser chromatin than those of the small cell undifferentiated pattern. Tumor rosettes are also seen (bar: 10 µm).

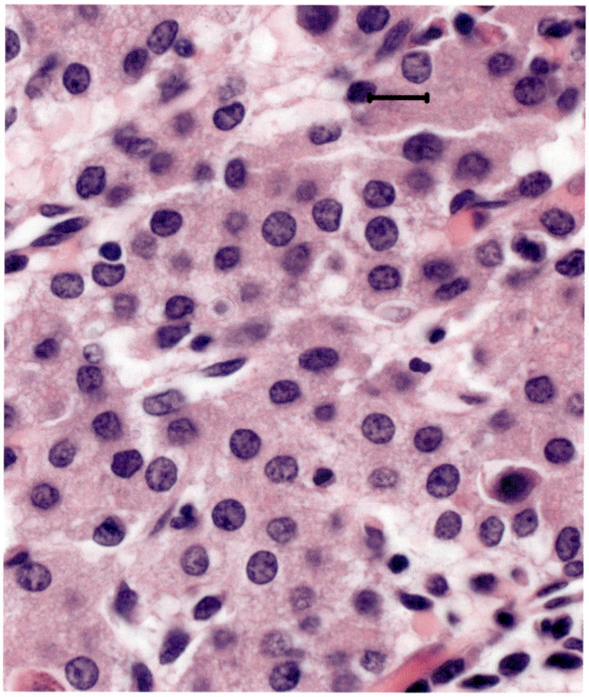

Figure 5-4

HEPATOBLASTOMA: FETAL PATTERN

The tumor cells are clearly hepatoid, with abundant eosinophilic cytoplasm (bar: 10 µm).

show extensive necrosis and cystic change. The percentage of tumor necrosis should be provided in the final pathology report; estimates to the nearest 10 percent are usually adequate.

Histologic Hepatoblastoma Patterns

Small Cell Undifferentiated Pattern. The small cell undifferentiated pattern is defined as small cells (5 to 10 µm) with scant pale to amphophilic cytoplasm, fairly fine nuclear chromatin, and inconspicuous nucleoli. The cells typically grow with a solid or nested pattern and do not show well-defined trabeculae, acini, or pseudoglands. The tumor cells are commonly discohesive (fig. 5-5), in contrast to the other epithelial growth patterns, and can mimic mesenchymal blastemal cells. In some cases, the small cell undifferentiated component has a myxoid background.

The percentage of the tumor showing the small cell undifferentiated pattern varies considerably, from less than 1 percent to the entire tumor (17,18). In about half of cases, this pattern makes up a minor component (less than 10 percent) and is found admixed with the embryonal and fetal patterns.

Cases with the small cell undifferentiated pattern should be stained with INI-1, since loss of INI-1 appears to confer a worse prognosis. However, the data on INI-1 and small cell undifferentiated histology remains incomplete. An initial report found INI-1 loss in all of six cases with a small cell undifferentiated histology (19). Subsequent studies, in contrast, have found mixed results. One study of seven small cell undifferentiated hepatoblastomas found no loss of INI-1 (17), while another study of 12 such tumors found loss in all cases (20). It seems likely that the initial H&E morphologic classification of these tumors is strongly influencing the INI-1 data, but more studies are needed. At this point, tumors that show INI-1 loss should be classified as malignant rhabdoid tumors if they have rhabdoid morphology instead of hepatoblastoma morphology. It is plausible that most if not all INI-1 negative hepatoblastomas are actually rhabdoid tumors with primitive morphology that mimics small cell undifferentiated hepatoblastomas.

Patients with hepatoblastomas with INI-1 loss generally have a worse prognosis (1,18) and typically require more aggressive therapy. In addition, identification of INI-1 loss should prompt genetic testing for germline mutations or deletions in the *SMARCB1/INI-1* gene, as unaffected carriers (e.g., parents, siblings) are also at increased risk for cancer.

Embryonal Pattern. The embryonal pattern is composed of tumor cells that are approximately 10 to 15 µm in size, have a high nuclear/cytoplasmic ratio with angulated nuclei, and have a predominantly solid growth pattern (fig. 5-6), often with areas of pseudoglands or tumor rosettes. The embryonal pattern is often recognizable at low microscopic power as basophilic tumor areas, adjacent to or admixed with the fetal growth pattern.

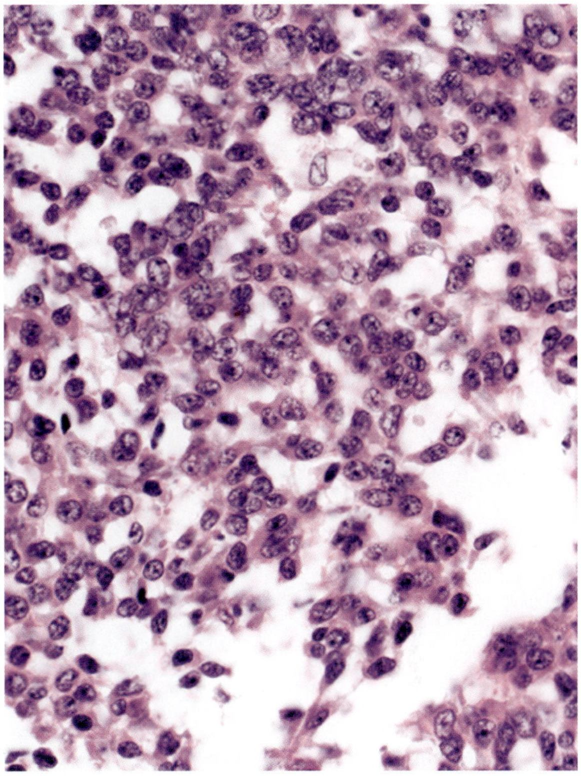

Figure 5-5

HEPATOBLASTOMA: SMALL CELL UNDIFFERENTIATED PATTERN

The tumor cells are poorly cohesive, with round to oval nuclei and scant cytoplasm.

While there can be areas of discohesive growth, overall the tumor cells in the embryonal pattern are more clearly epithelial and more cohesive than areas of small cell undifferentiated growth. Tumor cells in the embryonal pattern have more cytoplasm than in the small cell undifferentiated pattern, but their nuclei are commonly smaller, and at low power the embryonal pattern can appear more basophilic than either the small cell undifferentiated pattern or the fetal pattern. Extramedullary hematopoiesis may be present.

Fetal Pattern. The fetal pattern (fig. 5-7) is the most common histologic pattern in

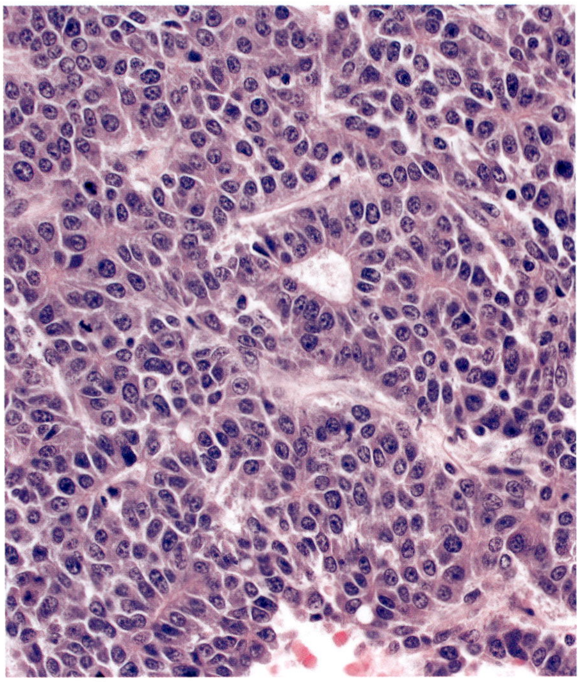

Figure 5-6

HEPATOBLASTOMA: EMBRYONAL PATTERN

The tumor cells have scant to moderate amounts of eosinophilic cytoplasm. A tumor rosette is in the center of the image.

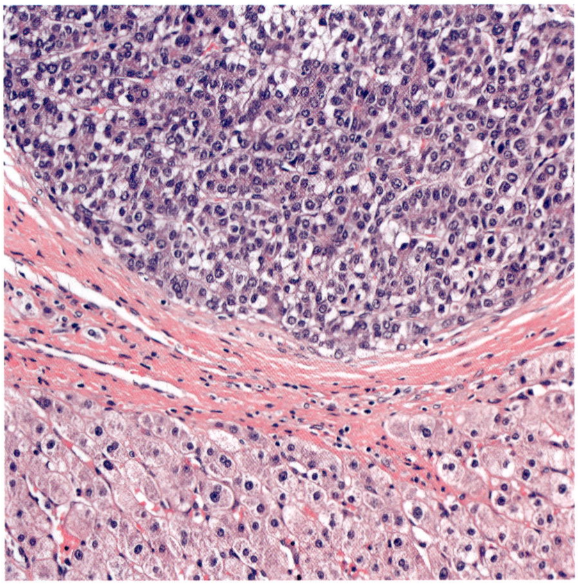

Figure 5-7

HEPATOBLASTOMA: FETAL PATTERN

The tumor at the top can be compared to the adjacent normal liver on the bottom.

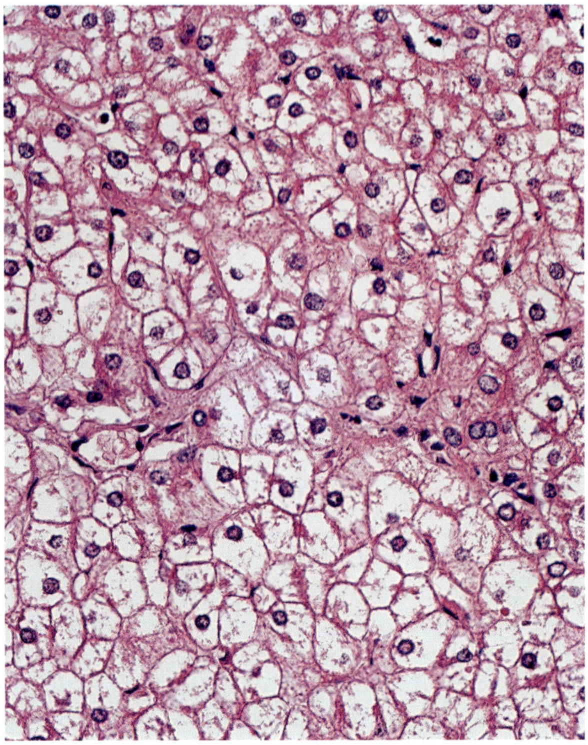

Figure 5-8

HEPATOBLASTOMA: FETAL PATTERN

The tumor cells have abundant clear cytoplasm due to glycogen accumulation.

hepatoblastomas and at least some areas of fetal growth are present in most cases. The fetal-type tumor cells are typically 10 to 20 μm in size, show moderate amounts of eosinophilic to clear cytoplasm, and are recognizable morphologically as having hepatocyte differentiation. The tumor cells grow in solid sheets or as thin trabeculae that are 2 to 3 cells in thickness. The tumor cells in areas of fetal growth can have irregular areas of glycogen accumulation (fig. 5-8) resulting in an alternating "light and dark pattern" at low-power examination (fig. 5-9). They can also be cholestatic (fig. 5-10)

When a tumor is composed only of the fetal growth pattern and the mitotic count is 1 or less in 10 high-power fields, the prognosis is excellent. This tumor is referred to as a *pure fetal hepatoblastoma with low mitotic activity* or with the synonym *well-differentiated fetal hepatoblastoma*. Tumors with a pure fetal growth pattern but with 2 or more mitoses in 10 high-power fields are classified as *mitotically active fetal*

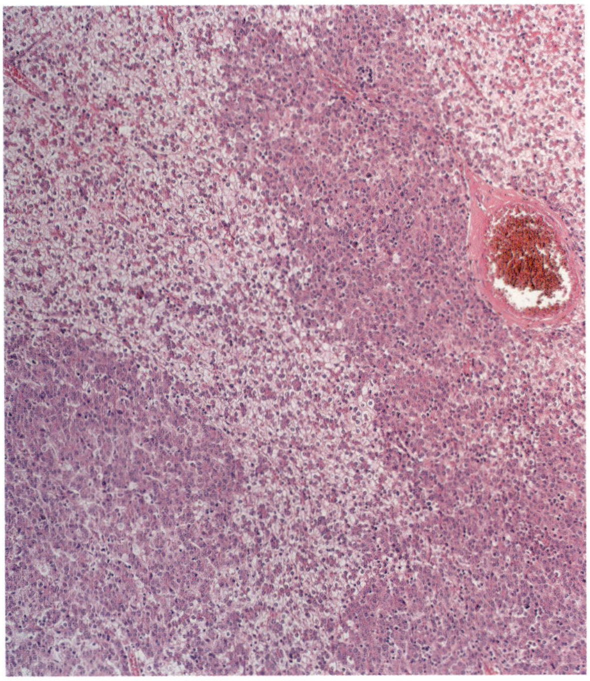

Figure 5-9

HEPATOBLASTOMA: FETAL PATTERN

At low power, a "light and dark" pattern is seen, resulting from irregular bands of fetal cells with abundant glycogen in their cytoplasm alternating with fetal cells with less striking glycogen.

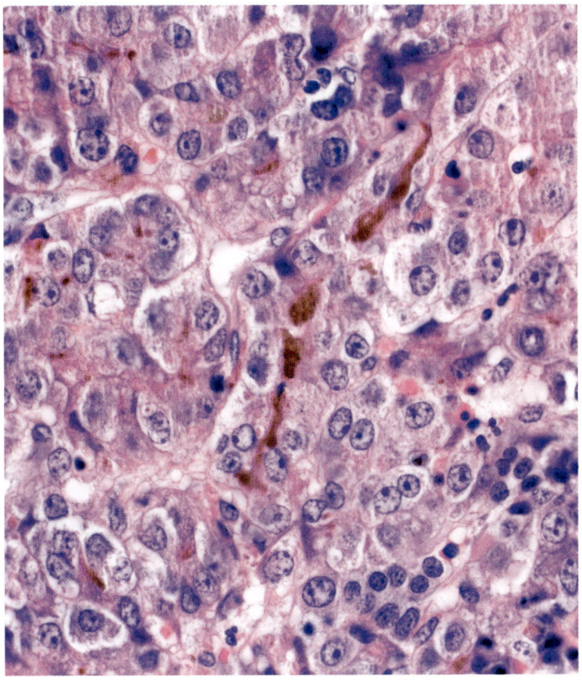

Figure 5-10

HEPATOBLASTOMA: FETAL PATTERN

This hepatoblastoma shows focal cholestasis, located in an area with a fetal growth pattern.

hepatoblastomas, an older term being *crowded fetal hepatoblastoma* (fig. 5-11).

The pleomorphic pattern of fetal hepatoblastoma has also been called *poorly differentiated fetal hepatoblastoma*. This pattern is uncommon, but in many ways resembles an adult hepatocellular carcinoma histologically, with tumor cells showing definite hepatocytic differentiation, but with more striking nuclear atypia than in fetal-type epithelium of hepatoblastomas (fig. 5-12). The atypical features are often patchy but include moderate nuclear pleomorphism with coarse, basophilic chromatin and prominent nucleoli. More typical areas of hepatoblastoma help differentiate this pattern from ordinary hepatocellular carcinoma. Some authors include an "anaplastic" category of fetal hepatoblastomas; these tumors have more striking nuclear enlargement and atypia (fig. 5-13).

As noted above, each of the fetal epithelial subtypes has synonyms, but these are worthwhile using as a first choice: pure fetal with low mitotic activity, mitotically active fetal, pleomorphic fetal.

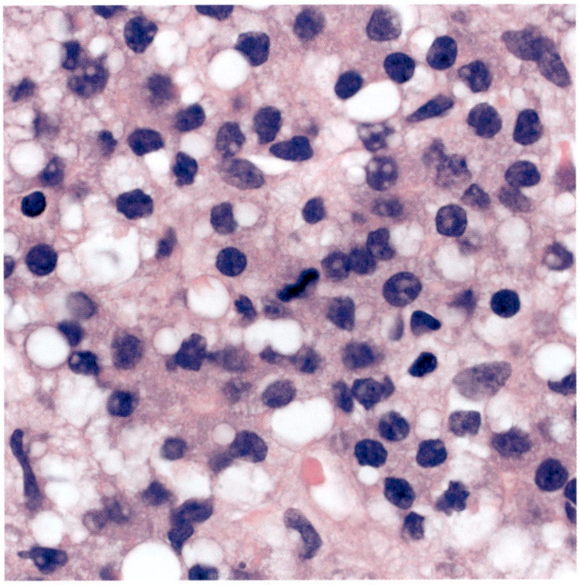

Figure 5-11

HEPATOBLASTOMA: FETAL PATTERN

This hepatoblastoma had a fetal growth pattern with up to 4 mitoses per 10 high-powered fields.

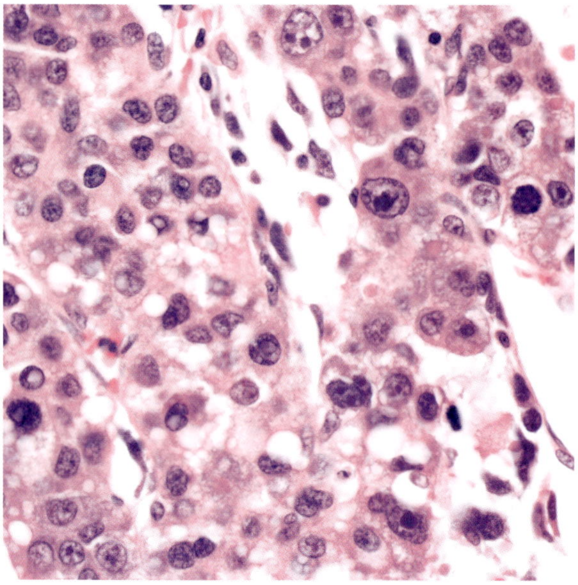

Figure 5-12

HEPATOBLASTOMA: PLEOMORPHIC FETAL PATTERN

The nuclear atypia resembles adult hepatocellular carcinoma.

Macrotrabecular Pattern. The macrotrabecular pattern of tumor growth (fig. 5-14) is defined by tumor cells growing in thickened trabeculae. The trabeculae should be well defined and should be at least 10 cells in thickness (but commonly are greater than 20 cells). A CD34 stain highlights the thick trabeculae (fig. 5-15).

The macrotrabecular pattern can be seen in both hepatoblastomas and adult hepatocellular carcinomas. In fact, the patterns can be essentially identical. In adults, the macrotrabecular pattern is also associated with high serum AFP levels, so AFP levels do not clearly discriminate between these two entities. In hepatoblastoma, the macrotrabecular pattern is most commonly a minor component of a more typical hepatoblastoma; in conventional hepatocellular carcinoma, the macrotrabecular pattern may be the only pattern or may be admixed with other areas of more typical hepatocellular carcinoma. Finding other patterns in the same specimen can resolve the diagnosis in many cases; if a biopsy or resection shows a pure macrotrabecular

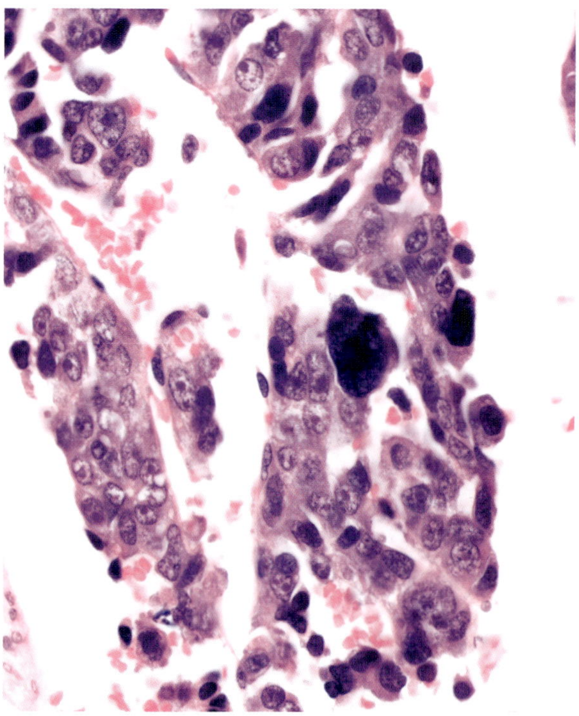

Figure 5-13

HEPATOBLASTOMA: ANAPLASTIC FETAL PATTERN

Nuclear atypia is striking in this case, with scattered anaplastic tumor cells.

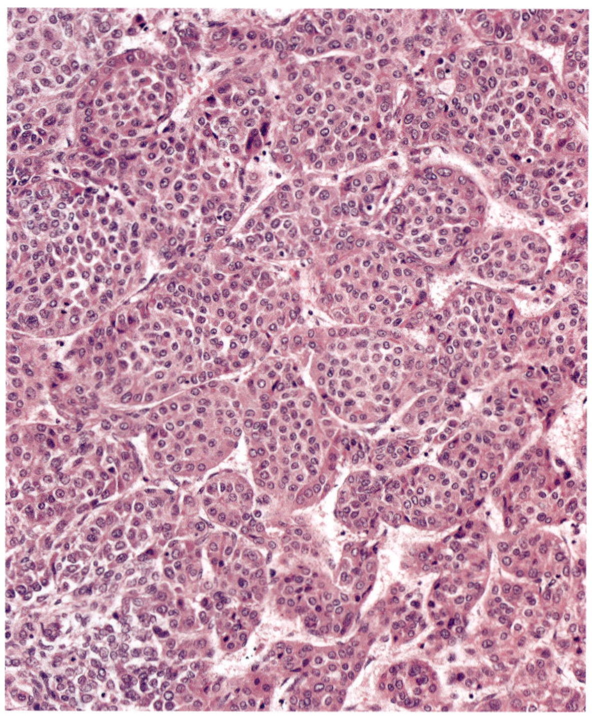

Figure 5-14

HEPATOBLASTOMA: MACROTRABECULAR PATTERN

The tumor is composed of basophilic cells growing in thick trabeculae.

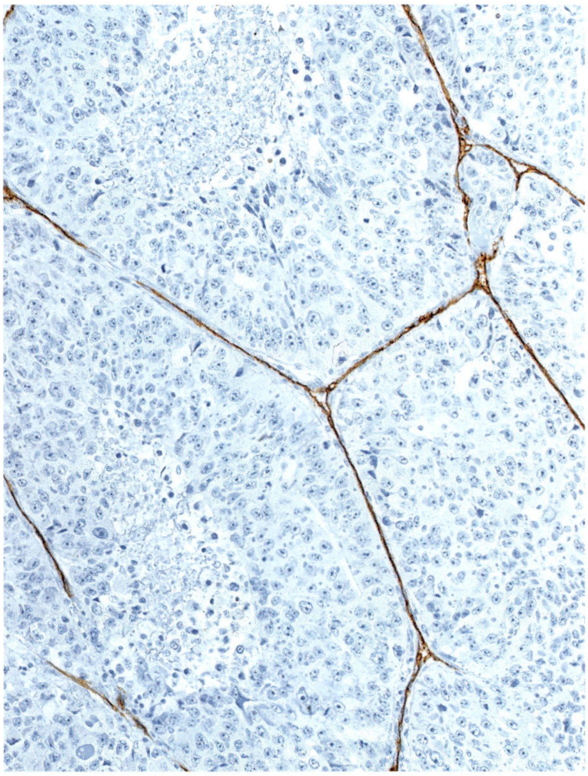

Figure 5-15

HEPATOBLASTOMA: MACROTRABECULAR PATTERN

A CD34 immunostain highlights the thick trabeculae.

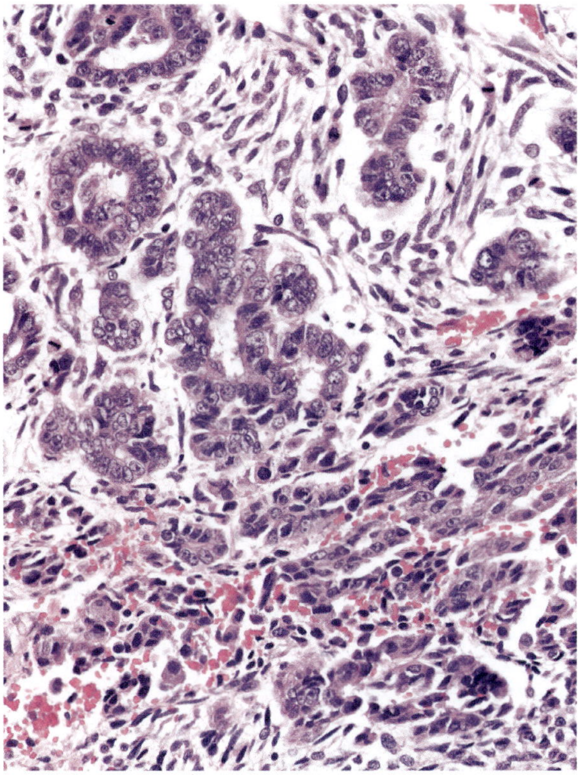

Figure 5-16

HEPATOBLASTOMA: CHOLANGIOCELLULAR PATTERN

This hepatoblastoma has a focal area of glandular growth.

pattern, ordinary hepatocellular carcinoma should be considered as a likely diagnosis, especially in patients 5 years of age or older.

Cholangiocellular Pattern. A cholangiocellular pattern is found in a small subset of hepatoblastomas. In these cases, small, atypical tubular structures are present, resembling ductules (fig. 5-16). In some hepatoblastomas, there is tumor necrosis, especially after treatment, and a reactive bile ductular proliferation can develop at the tumor interface. These benign bile ductules may be difficult to separate from a cholangiocellular pattern in some cases. The location helps distinguish between a reactive or malignant process (at the interface of the tumor versus in the tumor proper), as does a beta-catenin immunostain, which often shows nuclear staining in malignant cells (fig. 5-17) and is always negative in benign, reactive ductular proliferations.

Mesenchymal Component. Twenty to 40 percent of hepatoblastomas have a mesenchymal component, which is commonly composed of

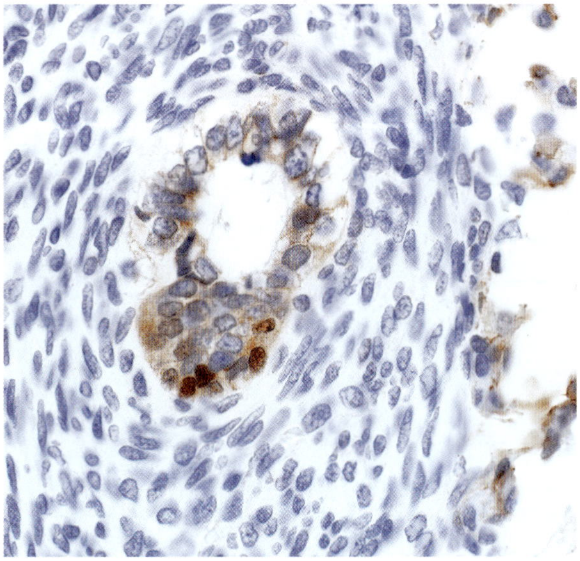

Figure 5-17

HEPATOBLASTOMA: CHOLANGIOCELLULAR PATTERN

An immunostain for beta-catenin shows focal nuclear positivity.

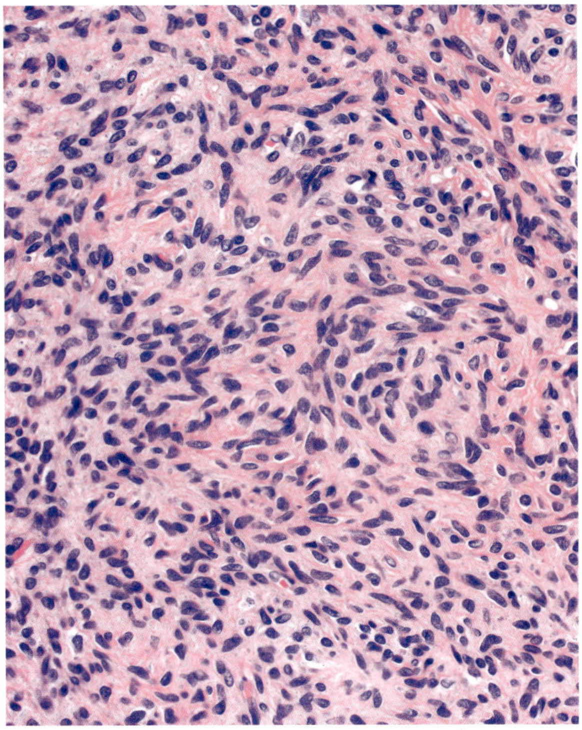

Figure 5-18

HEPATOBLASTOMA: MESENCHYMAL GROWTH

The mesenchymal component shows a cellular proliferation of otherwise nondescript spindled cells.

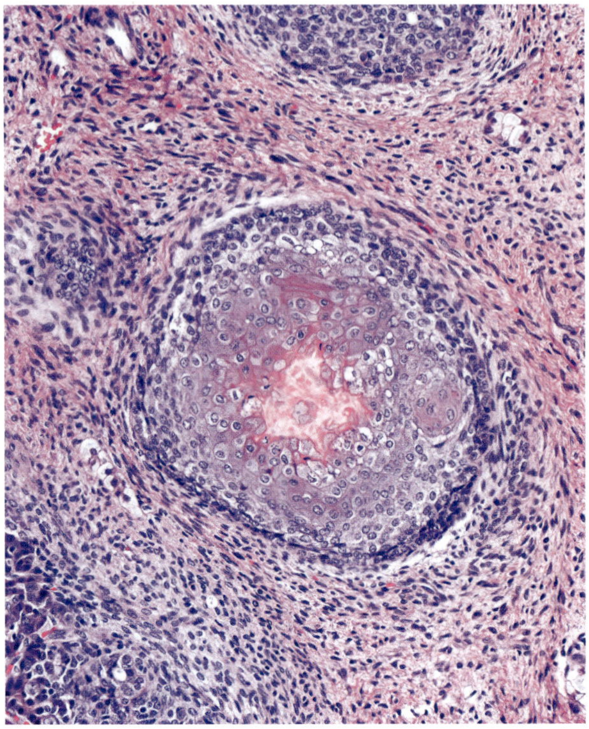

Figure 5-20

HEPATOBLASTOMA: SQUAMOUS DIFFERENTIATION

The nest of tumor cells shows squamous differentiation.

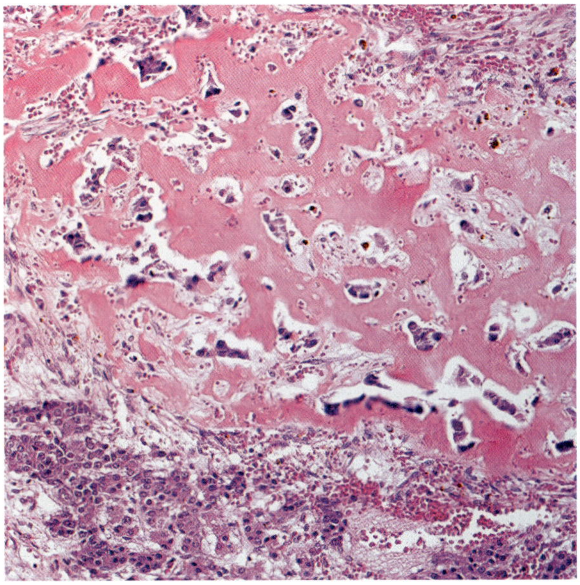

Figure 5-19

HEPATOBLASTOMA: MESENCHYMAL GROWTH

Osteoid production is present in the mesenchymal component of this hepatoblastoma.

nondescript spindled cells (fig. 5-18), but may include skeletal muscle, cartilage, or osteoid material (fig. 5-19). The term "teratoid" is used when sections also show areas with neuroectoderm differentiation, such as neural cells, glial cells, and melanin-containing cells, as well as areas of endoderm differentiation, such as squamous (fig. 5-20), glandular, or mucinous epithelium.

Histologic Grading

Unlike hepatocellular carcinomas, hepatoblastomas are not graded into well-differentiated, moderately differentiated, and poorly differentiated tumors. Instead, the tumors are subtyped as described above.

Immunohistochemical Findings

The results of immunostains in hepatoblastomas depend on the tumor subtype. For example, HepPar1 and arginase are positive in essentially all fetal and embryonal patterns, but are negative in the small cell undifferentiated pattern. Glypican 3 is also positive in the fetal and embryonal

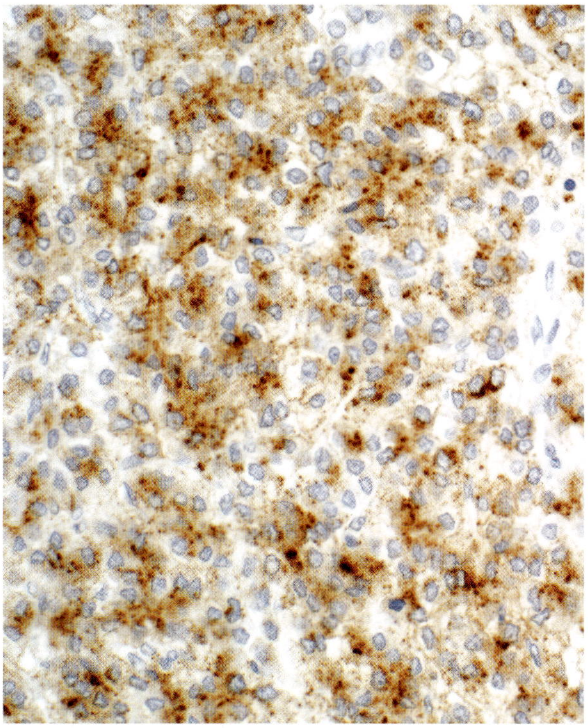

Figure 5-21

HEPATOBLASTOMA: GLYPICAN 3

The fetal pattern shows a finely granular cytoplasmic staining pattern.

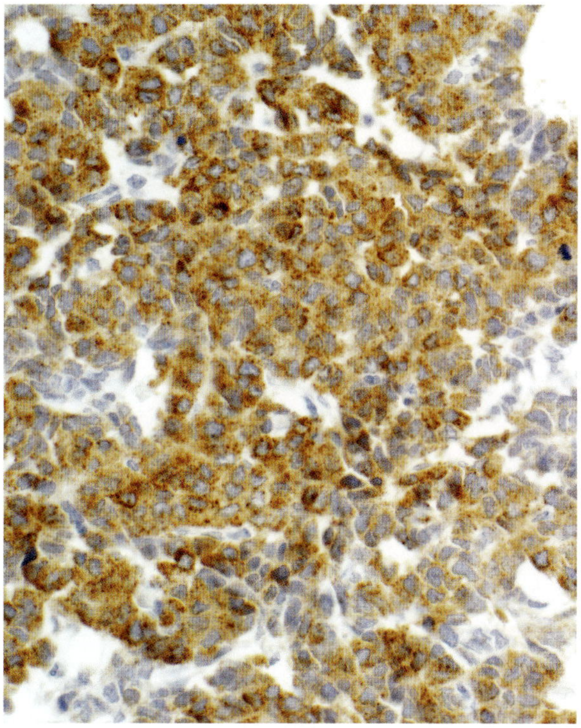

Figure 5-22

HEPATOBLASTOMA: GLYPICAN 3

The embryonal pattern shows a coarse granular staining pattern.

patterns. Some authors (15) report that a fine granular staining pattern for glypican 3 is typical of the well-differentiated fetal pattern (fig. 5-21) and can be useful in separating this pattern from the other patterns, which tend to have coarse cytoplasmic expression (fig. 5-22). However, glypican 3 is probably best used as an adjunct observation and does not trump the H&E findings. In the small cell undifferentiated areas, glypican 3 can be negative (fig. 5-23) or weakly positive, but published data remain limited.

Wnt signaling activation is found in most hepatoblastomas. Beta-catenin is a key protein in the Wnt signaling pathway and its location can be visualized by immunohistochemistry. Benign hepatocytes and bile ducts show a membranous staining pattern, with no nuclear accumulation of beta-catenin. In contrast, hepatoblastomas can show abnormal nuclear staining, especially the embryonal pattern. In the fetal pattern, nuclear staining can be focal and in some cases difficult to find (fig. 5-24); staining is also focal or absent in small cell undifferentiated cases.

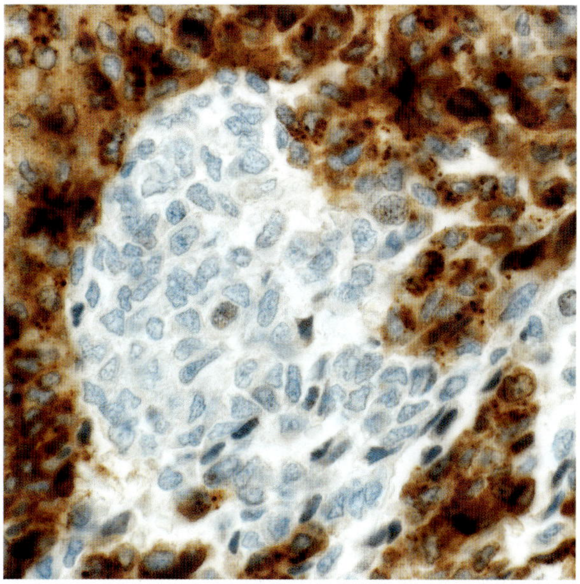

Figure 5-23

HEPATOBLASTOMA: GLYPICAN 3

A focus of small cell undifferentiated pattern is glypican 3 negative, while the adjacent embryonal pattern is positive.

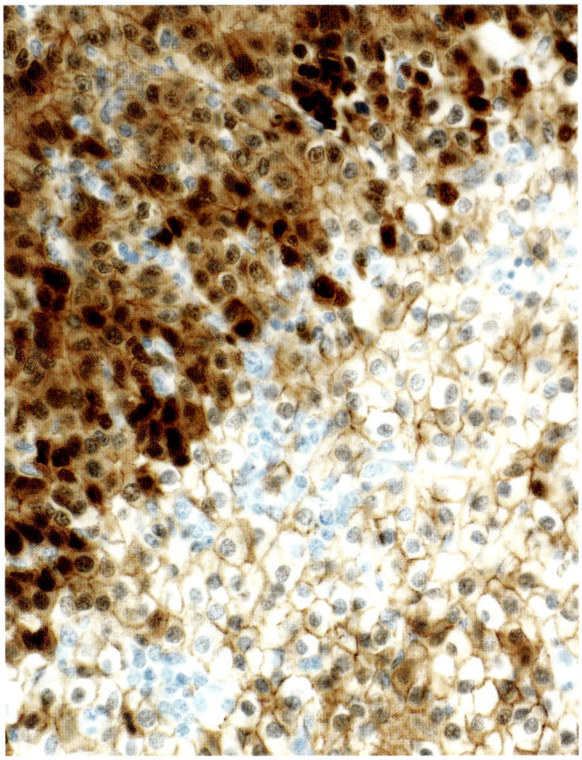

Figure 5-24

HEPATOBLASTOMA: BETA-CATENIN

The embryonal pattern shows strong nuclear and cytoplasmic staining, while the adjacent fetal pattern does not.

Beta-catenin nuclear accumulation is sometimes focally positive in the mesenchymal components of hepatoblastomas. Another abnormal beta-catenin pattern is diffuse cytoplasmic staining. Abnormal diffuse cytoplasmic staining and nuclear staining often coexist. Nevertheless, beta-catenin immunohistochemistry is not useful in diagnosis or subtyping, outside of the rare situation in which pathologists struggle to differentiate a possible area of cholangiocellular growth (often positive for beta-catenin nuclear staining) versus a benign ductular reaction (negative for nuclear staining).

Immunostains for INI-1 should be performed in all cases thought to have a small cell undifferentiated component. In normal liver tissue and in the other patterns of hepatoblastoma, INI-1 shows strong nuclear staining. In contrast, loss of INI-1 expression has been reported in a subset of small cell undifferentiated hepatoblastomas (15). These cases may require more aggressive chemotherapy and, in patients with an extensive loss of tumor staining, genetic counseling to rule out a germline defect, since family members may also be at increased risk for various malignancies.

Ultrastructural Findings

Electron microscopy currently does not play a diagnostic role in hepatoblastoma evaluation. The ultrastructural findings parallel the light microscopic findings, with fetal tumor epithelial components showing abundant mitochondria, lysosomes, and glycogen, while the embryonal cells show scant cytoplasmic organelles, mostly rough endoplasmic reticulum and mitochondria (21).

Cytologic Findings

The cytology findings in a fine-needle aspirate generally parallel the epithelial findings found in biopsy or resection specimens. Typically, the smears are highly cellular with populations of small to intermediate-sized cells. Trabecular growth and acinar formation may be seen with fetal and embryonal growth patterns. Extramedullary hematopoiesis is common. Mesenchymal tissue is often absent in the smears, even if the resection shows a mixed epithelial and mesenchymal hepatoblastoma. The cytology of small cell undifferentiated tumors resembles that of small round blue cell tumors, with small cells showing scant to moderate amounts of cytoplasm and no clear evidence of differentiation. Cytology often does not allow adequate distinction between an ordinary hepatocellular carcinoma and hepatoblastoma. Also, the cytologic features of the small cell undifferentiated pattern and the embryonal pattern show significant overlap (22). For these reasons, fine-needle aspirates are not encouraged for primary diagnosis.

Molecular Genetic Findings

There is a reasonably large body of literature on the molecular findings of hepatoblastomas, but the numerous observations do not paint a clear picture of the molecular pathology driving tumor formation. Karyotype abnormalities are common, with structural defects (various deletions and translocations) frequently involving chromosome 1q (23), a finding that is also true for fibrolamellar carcinoma and hepatocellular carcinoma, indicating that an important oncogene or tumor suppressor gene is likely located on chromosome

1q. Numerical abnormalities are also common, including trisomy 20, 2, and 8, but consistent findings have not been identified and hepatoblastomas demonstrate a confusing potpourri of gains, losses, and translocations.

Whole genome sequencing has shown that hepatoblastomas have few mutations, with the beta-catenin (*CTNNB1*) gene the most common target (24). Tumors can have either large deletions or point mutations in exon 3. These mutations can lead to abnormal nuclear accumulation of beta-catenin, which is demonstrated by immunostaining, but the correlation between mutation status and immunostain findings is not perfect. In contrast to adult hepatocellular carcinoma, mutations in the telomerase reverse transcriptase (*TERT*) gene promoter are rare (24). There is a large list of other pathways dysregulated in hepatoblastomas, including the Notch signaling pathway and the Hedgehog pathway, but to date a consistent molecular picture has not emerged, and genetic alterations that can be targeted for diagnosis or therapy have not been identified.

Differential Diagnosis

The morphologic patterns present in a given hepatoblastoma determine the differential diagnosis. For specimens with a predominately or exclusively fetal growth pattern, the differential includes conventional hepatocellular carcinoma. The presence of underlying liver disease or age over 5 years also strongly favors conventional hepatocellular carcinoma. In contrast, the presence of other hepatoblastoma morphologies helps establish the diagnosis of hepatoblastoma, including morphologies such as a mesenchymal growth pattern.

Normal or mildly elevated serum AFP levels are seen almost exclusively with the small cell undifferentiated variant of hepatoblastoma, typically when that is the predominant component. A normal or mildly elevated serum AFP level would be unusual for a hepatoblastoma with fetal or embryonal growth and would suggest a diagnosis of hepatocellular carcinoma. In contrast, elevated serum AFP levels are found in both hepatoblastomas and ordinary hepatocellular carcinomas and are not useful in distinguishing these two tumors. There are no immunostains useful for differentiating hepatocellular carcinoma from hepatoblastoma, including nuclear expression of beta-catenin. Instead, the distinction is based on morphologic findings.

For cases with the small cell undifferentiated pattern, the differential diagnosis includes small round blue cell tumors. Since most hepatoblastomas with the small cell undifferentiated pattern also have either fetal or embryonal patterns, additional sampling of the tumor is helpful. In cases with a pure small cell undifferentiated pattern, immunostains are useful in excluding entities such as Ewing sarcoma (positive for CD99), lymphoma (positive with lymphoid markers), and Wilms tumor (postive for WT1). Some cases of small cell undifferentiated hepatoblastoma and all cases of rhabdoid tumors of the liver show INI-1 loss, but they can be separated by their very different morphologies.

Some hepatoblastomas have glandular foci, raising the differential of a reactive bile ductular proliferation or a cholangiocellular growth pattern. This problem seems to arise more often in treated tumors. The morphology of the glandular cells and their location allow distinction in most cases cases: ductular reactions are found at the tumor and nontumor interface, whereas the cholangiocellar pattern can be found anywhere within the tumor. Morphologically, the cells in the cholangiocellar pattern appear more primitive and show more atypia than benign reactive ductules. The cholangiocellar component is also commonly nuclear beta-catenin positive, while the ductular reaction is not.

Spread and Metastases

Hepatoblastomas spread most commonly to the lungs (25), with about 20 percent of individuals having metastases to the lung at the time of presentation (26). Metastases to the brain and bone are less common, but well reported (25). After complete remission, the relapse rate for hepatoblastoma is about 10 percent, with disease recurring most commonly in the liver, lungs, or both organs. Other sites of recurrence include the peritoneum and brain (25,27). The median time to recurrence is about 12 months (27).

Staging

Hepatoblastomas are commonly staged by the pretreatment extent of disease (PRETEXT) system, which divides the liver into four sections, and stages the tumor based on the number of

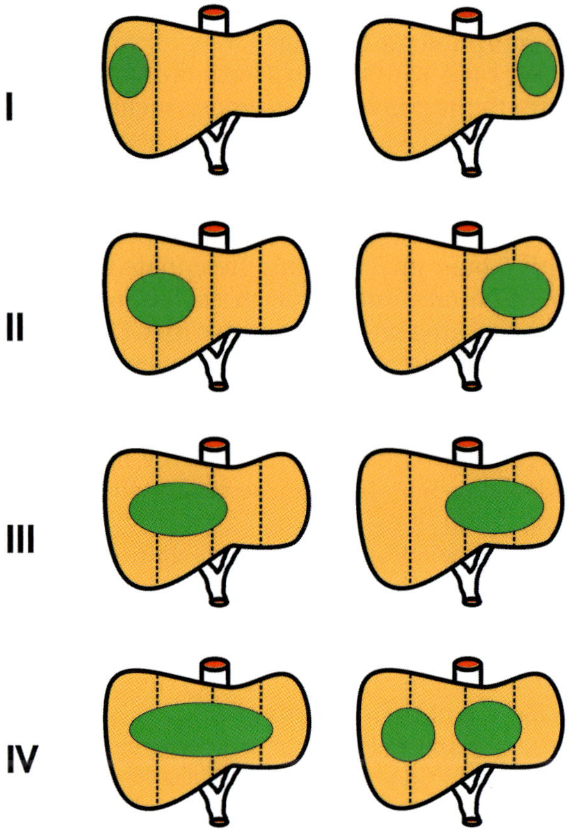

Figure 5-25

PRETREATMENT EXTENT OF DISEASE (PRETEXT) STAGING SYSTEM

The liver is divided into four sections. The boundaries are the right and middle hepatic veins and the umbilical fissure. Stage I is defined by three contiguous disease-free sections; stage II by two contiguous disease-free sections; stage III by one disease free section; stage IV by no disease-free sections. If the hepatoblastoma is multifocal, then additional combinations are possible (not illustrated) for stages II and III. This system can also be used after therapy and is then called the POST-TEXT.

sections involved (fig. 5-25). Any of these four PRETEXT groups can involve the inferior vena cava or hepatic veins (V+), involve the main portal vein or both right and left branches of the portal vein (both branches are needed; P+), have extrahepatic disease by direct extension (E+), involve the caudate lobe (C+), have nodal disease (N+), or have metastatic disease other than nodal disease and direct extension (M+). The V and P scores are further annotated as V 1-3 and P 1-3 as follows: 1 = tumor touching; 2 = tumor compressing or distorting; and 3 = tumor ingrowth, encasement, or thrombus. The E score is further annotated as follows: E1 = direct extension into adjacent organs or the diaphragm; E2 = peritoneal nodules; and E2 with ascites = peritoneal nodules with ascites. For nodal disease: N1= abdominal lymph node disease only; N2= any extra-abdominal lymph node disease.

Table 5-2

TRADITIONAL CHILDREN'S ONCOLOGY GROUP (COG) STAGING SYSTEM FOR HEPATOBLASTOMA

COG Stage	Description
I	Tumor is completely resected with negative margins
II	Tumor is completely resected grossly, but the microscopic margins are positive
III	Biopsy only at diagnosis Or residual gross disease at resection Or tumor spill at time of resection Or complete gross resection with node positive disease
IV	Metastatic disease at diagnosis

Individuals with standard risk have PRETEXT stages I, II, or III, while high risk is defined by any of these findings: PRETEXT IV, AFP level less than 100 ng/mL at diagnosis, metastasis at diagnosis, or small cell undifferentiated histology.

The traditional Children's Oncology Group (COG) staging system of hepatoblastomas is shown in Table 5-2. An updated COG risk classification system is shown in Table 5-3.

Treatment

Treatment for hepatoblastomas is now largely based on protocols developed by several major study groups, such as the COG, the International Childhood Liver Tumors Strategy Group (SIOPEL), the German Society for Pediatric Oncology (GPOH), and the Japanese Study Group for Pediatric Liver Tumors (JPLT). While they have many similarities, one major difference is that SIOPEL recommends preoperative chemotherapy in all cases, while the COG recommends surgical resection in hepatoblastomas classified as PRETEXT I or PRETEXT II, when the surgeon can obtain clean vascular margins. If histologic examination shows pure well-differentiated fetal histology, then resection is curative and no chemotherapy is needed.

Table 5-3

CURRENT CHILDREN'S ONCOLOGY GROUP (COG) RISK CATEGORY[a]

Risk Category	Description
Very low risk	PRETEXT [b] stage I or II with pure fetal histology and successful primary resection
Low risk	PRETEXT stage I or II and successful primary resection
Intermediate risk	PRETEXT stage II, III, or IV that is unresectable and/or any of the following: small cell undifferentiated histology, V+, P+, E+
High risk	Any PRETEXT that is M+ and/or AFP <100 ng/mL at diagnosis

[a](http://www.cancer.gov/types/liver/hp/child-liver-treatment-pdq#link/_740_toc)
[b]PRETEXT = pretreatment extent of disease; AFP = alpha-fetoprotein.

The specific chemotherapeutic agents used to treat hepatoblastomas are likely to change as new agents become available. At this time, all protocols are cisplatin based. As one example, the current COG protocol has carboplatin, 5-fluoracil, and vincristine as a foundation, with added agents, such as doxorubicin, for higher-risk tumors.

Prognosis

The prognosis for patients with hepatoblastoma has improved dramatically in the past 50 years, from a 5-year survival rate of about 30 percent to up to 90 percent (28–33). This striking improvement is the result of better surgical techniques and better chemotherapy. Many of the improvements have been driven by large multicenter study groups, pooling patients' data to generate sufficient numbers for statistical analysis, establishing standard treatment protocols, and enrolling patients in new study trials.

Clinical findings such as low birth weight, low platelet count, and other significant comorbidities are unfavorable prognostic findings. Tumor-specific adverse prognostic findings revolve around tumor size and spread. Patients with multifocal liver disease (30,34), metastatic disease at diagnosis (28,34,35), unresectable vessel involvement, positive surgical margins, or tumor rupture have a worse prognosis.

Laboratory and histologic findings are also key prognostic indicators. Serum AFP levels indicate a bad prognosis when they are very low or extremely high (34,35). Serum levels of less than 100 ng/mL in untreated patients are strongly associated with small cell undifferentiated histology and confer a worse prognosis (33). Serum levels of greater than 1,000,000 ng/mL are associated with larger tumors that involve both lobes of the liver, with multifocal disease, vascular invasion, and distant metastases. Individuals with high AFP levels who do not have a large early decrease in serum AFP following therapy have an increased risk for recurrence (36,37).

As noted in the section on treatment, some treatment protocols call for all individuals with hepatoblastomas to receive chemotherapy prior to surgery. In this setting, the prognostic value of histologic findings after chemotherapy is less clear, but in untreated individuals, several key observations have prognostic relevance. Small cell undifferentiated histology appears to be an important unfavorable prognostic factor. At this point, however, much remains unclear, including the relevance of small amounts of small cell undifferentiated histology. For example, is 1 percent clinically relevant? Does a case with 50 percent small cell undifferentiated histology have a worse prognosis than a case with 5 percent? In some cases, the small cell undifferentiated component shows loss of INI-1 by immunohistochemistry (15). This is generally thought to confer a worse prognosis than cases with retained expression of INI-1, but the added prognostic value of INI-1 loss has not been thoroughly established. To evaluate for INI-1 loss, the entire tumor focus in question should show loss of nuclear staining. Occasional or scattered tumor cells that do not have INI-1 staining, admixed with clearly positive tumor cells, should not be scored as INI-1 loss. It is important to check that retained nuclear staining is not in admixed stromal or inflammatory cells.

Despite these uncertainties, it is important to carefully look for small cell undifferentiated histology, as its presence changes management. Currently, hepatoblastomas that are COG stages I and II, which are classified as very low risk and low risk, respectively, are upgraded to intermediate risk if a small cell undifferentiated histology is present, regardless of the extent of the small cell undifferentiated component or INI-1 status. In contrast, patients with hepatoblastomas with a pure well-differentiated fetal

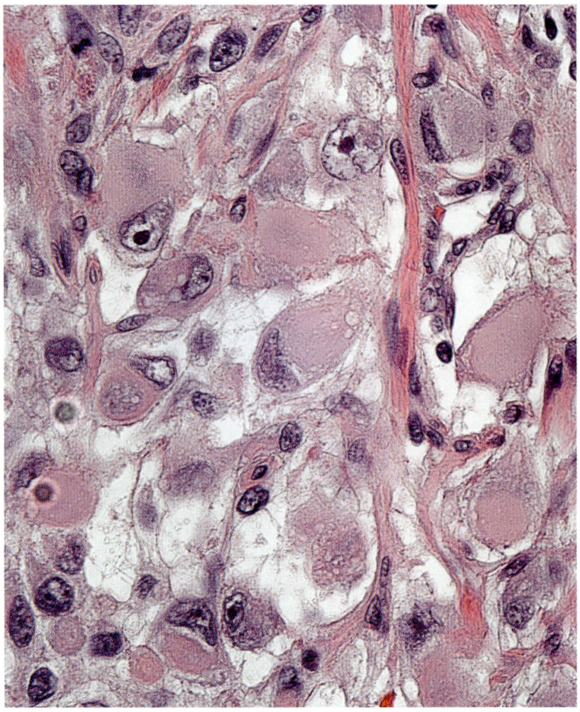

Figure 5-26

MALIGNANT RHABDOID TUMOR

The tumor cells are epithelioid, with abundant cytoplasm, often with a large perinuclear inclusion.

histology with low mitotic activity have an excellent prognosis (25,33,34,38) and can be treated exclusively by surgical resection (39).

MALIGNANT RHABDOID TUMOR

Malignant rhabdoid tumors of the liver are defined by their rhabdoid cytologic features and either loss of nuclear INI-1 expression or molecular testing showing mutations/deletions in the *SMARCB1/INI-1* gene on chromosome 22q11.2. Rare cases can show BRG1 loss.

Clinical Features

In reviews of published cases, the median age of presentation is 8 months (40,41) and the average age at presentation is 2 years (42). Nevertheless, individuals can present into their teenage years (40).

Spontaneous tumor rupture has been reported by several authors as a dramatic clinical presentation (41,43–45). In most cases, however, the clinical findings are nonspecific, such as a palpable mass or hepatomegaly. Systemic symptoms are also common, but show no clear pattern. These may include fever, lethargy, and anorexia. No clear demographic correlates have been identified to date, including gender or ethnicity (40).

In most cases, serum AFP levels are normal or mildly elevated, but there have been reports of cases with levels up to 13,000 ng/mL (41). Other laboratory abnormalities are nonspecific but include hypercalcemia, anemia, and thrombocytosis.

Up to 30 percent of individuals have germline mutations in the *SMARCB1* gene (41). No other etiologic risk factors have been identified to date.

Gross and Microscopic Findings

Most rhabdoid tumors are very large. They can be multifocal and occupy most of the liver. They often show hemorrhage and necrosis and may have areas of cystic degeneration. Their borders range from well-defined and fibrotic to ill-defined and infiltrative.

Malignant rhabdoid tumors are composed of large tumor cells with a fairly uniform appearance (fig. 5-26). The tumor cells are epithelioid, with abundant eosinophilic cytoplasm, and often have an eccentrically located nucleus, leading to a plasmacytoid or rhabdoid appearance. A PAS-positive perinuclear inclusion is found in some cases. The cells grow in slightly discohesive sheets, but occasionally show foci of trabecular or nested growth. In some areas, the tumor cells can show a more spindled pattern. The tumor cell nuclei have vesicular chromatin and prominent nucleoli. In areas adjacent to necrosis, the tumors may have heavy infiltrates of lymphocytes and macrophages, which can sometimes obscure the true nature of the tumor.

Malignant rhabdoid tumors are not graded in the traditional manner, as all are poorly differentiated tumors. No histologic subtypes are recognized in malignant rhabdoid tumor.

Immunohistochemical Findings

By definition, malignant rhabdoid tumors show loss of INI-1 or BRG-1 nuclear expression by immunohistochemistry (fig. 5-27). They also are strongly positive for vimentin, with diffuse cytoplasmic staining that may highlight the perinuclear inclusion. Cytokeratin stains are typically positive, although there can be variability in the pattern of expression (46–49).

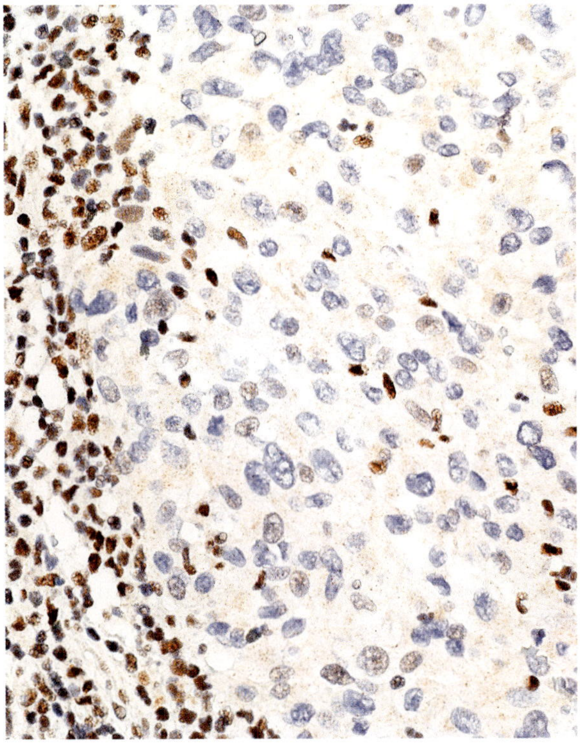

Figure 5-27

MALIGNANT RHABDOID TUMOR: INI-1

An immunostain for INI-1 is negative in the tumor cells.

Overall, CK8 appears to the most commonly expressed cytokeratin. Other stains can also be positive, but tend to be more variable in expression, are not diagnostically helpful, and in fact are commonly a source of diagnostic confusion. These stains include S-100 protein, CD99, neuron-specific esterase (NSE), synaptophysin, CD34, and smooth muscle actin. Immunostains for skeletal muscle differentiation are negative (myogenin, myo-D1). HepPar1 and arginase 1 are negative. Glypican 3 is positive in about two thirds of cases (50,51), and can tempt a pathologist into a misdiagnosis of hepatoblastoma or hepatocellular carcinoma.

Ultrastuctural Findings

By electron microscopy, the perinuclear inclusion is composed of whorls of intermediate filaments (46–48,52). The cells also show prominent rough endoplasmic reticulum and ribosomes. Some lipid droplets may be present, but glycogen is not prominent (47).

Cytologic Findings

Because of the rarity of the tumor, published experience concerning cytology is sparse (53). Aspirates typically show medium-sized tumor cells with the same vesicular nuclear chromatin and prominent nucleoli seen in biopsy and resection specimens. The cytoplasm on smears shows dense perinuclear inclusions in some cases.

Molecular Genetic Findings

Molecular data on primary hepatic malignant rhabdoid tumors is very limited because of the rarity of the tumor. However, looking at malignant rhabdoid tumors from all sites, approximately one third of individuals have an underlying germline *SMARCB1* alteration. Germline mutations also suggest that the patient's parents and siblings may be at increased risk for malignancies and genetic counselling can be helpful (54).

SMARCB1 encodes a protein that is part of the SWI/SNF complex, a multi-subunit chromatin remodeling complex that serves as tumor suppressor. Mutations have also been reported in genes encoding other subunits of the SWI/SNF complex, including *SMARCA2, PBRM1, SMARCA4,* and *ARID1a* (55). Mutations in CK8 have not been studied in malignant rhabdoid tumors of the liver, but have been reported in malignant rhabdoid tumors from other sites and from cell lines, and may explain the perinuclear inclusions, which are composed of intermediate filaments (52).

Differential Diagnosis

In infants and young children, the differential diagnosis for malignant rhabdoid tumors of the liver includes hepatoblastomas with small cell undifferentiated morphology. Some of these hepatoblastomas have INI-1 loss (19). The histology of these hepatoblastomas has not been described in detail, other than that they were initially classified as small cell undifferentiated hepatoblastomas. At this point, hepatoblastomas with small cell undifferentiated morphology and INI-1 loss are best diagnosed as such, and should not be considered as identical to malignant rhabdoid tumors.

Other entities in the differential diagnosis include tumors with a small blue round cell morphology, such as lymphoma, Ewing sarcoma/primitive neuroectodermal tumors (PNET), and rhabdomyosarcoma. INI-1 and BRG-1 staining is a major diagnostic tool in this setting, but these possibilities can be further excluded by immunostains for CD45 and other lymphocyte markers (to exclude lymphomas), CD99 and FLI-1 (to exclude Ewing sarcoma/PNET), and myogenin and myo-D1 (to exclude rhabdomyosarcoma).

Spread and Metastases

Metastatic disease is present in about three fourths of individuals at the time of clinical presentation (40). The lungs are the most common metastatic site (65 percent of cases), followed by lymph nodes (35 percent) and the central nervous system (10 percent) (40). Many other sites are involved to a lesser degree, including, skin, bone, adrenal gland, peritoneum, retroperitoneum, mesentery, and pleura. Because of the rarity of the tumor, a staging system for malignant rhabdoid tumors of the liver has not been developed.

Treatment and Prognosis

Complete surgical resection is performed when possible. No chemotherapy or radiotherapy regiment has emerged as the preferred therapy for malignant rhabdoid tumors, but the most common chemotherapy agents are doxorubicin, vincristine, etoposide, cisplatin, carboplatin, ifosfamide, and cyclophosphamide (40,41).

Malignant rhabdoid tumors are very aggressive and the prognosis is poor, with few long-term survivors. In one review of the literature, there was a single survivor from 35 individuals who had metastatic disease at presentation (40). Of 11 who had complete resections and no metastatic disease, 3 survived. For those who died of disease, the overall median survival period was 1.5 months. Findings associated with a better overall survival rate were age over 1 year at presentation, complete surgical resection, and no metastatic disease at presentation (40,41).

CALCIFIED NESTED STROMAL-EPITHELIAL TUMOR

This rare primary tumor of the liver is composed of both epithelial and stromal elements, but the epithelial elements do not show hepatic differentiation and the stromal elements are not neoplastic, as would be seen in hepatoblastoma. This distinctive tumor appears to have been described first in the 2001 edition of the Armed Forces Institute of Pathology (AFIP) liver Fascicle (56), using the term "ossifying stromal-epithelial tumor." Currently, this tumor is referred to as *calcifying nested stromal-epithelial tumor* or *nested stromal-epithelial tumor*.

General Features

Calcified nested stromal-epithelial tumors affect children and young adults, with an age range of 2 to 33 years (57). The tumor primarily affects teenage women. Most tumors are identified as incidental lesions (58). In one case, the tumor was present since childhood, diagnosed initially as calcified hemangioma by radiology (57).

In one series, two of six individuals had Cushing syndrome that resolved with tumor resection (58). In another series, one of nine individuals had Cushing syndrome (57). Other case reports have also documented Cushing syndrome in association with this tumor (59–61). There are reports of other possible associations, but because of the tumor's rarity, it is unclear how strong these associations are. For example, isolated cases of calcified nested stromal-epithelial tumors were followed by a subsequent diagnosis of nephroblastomatosis or Wilms tumor (58). Another case of calcified nested stromal-epithelial tumors was reported in the setting of Beckwith-Wiedemann syndrome (62). No other strong demographic or clinical correlates have been reported, but this may change over time as more cases are studied and reported.

Serum AFP levels are normal. Adrenocorticotropic hormone (ACTH) levels are elevated in some but not all individuals and no consistent serum markers have been identified to date. The elevated ACTH levels presumably explain the clinical presentations with Cushing syndrome.

The etiology is unknown. The tumor is not associated with underlying chronic liver disease or other known genetic syndromes.

Gross and Microscopic Findings

Calcified nested stromal-epithelial tumors are most commonly located in the right hepatic lobe (57), but can be found in the left lobe as well (58). The tumors are grossly well demarcated but not encapsulated (fig. 5-28). They can be unifocal, composed of an aggregate of separate but adjacent nodules, or multifocal. Tumor size ranges from 4 to 30 cm in diameter (58). The tumors

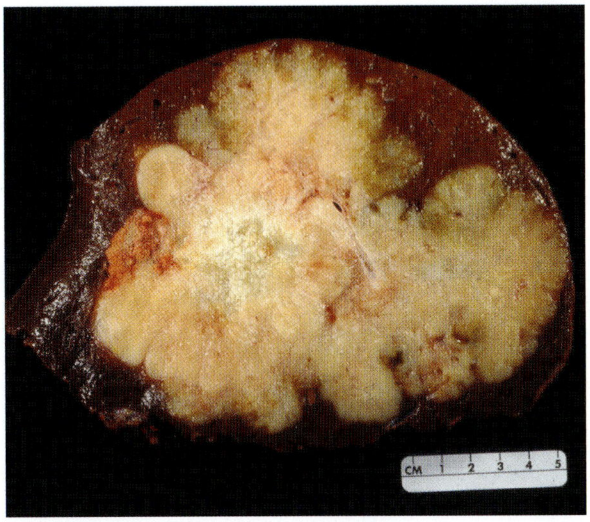

Figure 5-28

CALCIFIED NESTED STROMAL-EPITHELIAL TUMOR

The tumor is yellow-tan and lobulated.

range from tan to pink in color and may have areas of calcification as well as cystic changes.

The main histologic pattern is that of irregular but well-defined nests of bland-appearing epithelial cells surrounded by bands of desmoplastic stroma (fig. 5-29). In the epithelial areas, tumor cells grow in broad sheets, with no gland formation and no well-formed trabeculae. In some cases, bile ducts are found, presumably entrapped within the growing tumor nests (fig. 5-30). In the center of the tumor, the stroma surrounding the epithelial nests is often densely collagenized, in contrast to the periphery of the tumor, where the stroma is typically more loose and myxoid. While the epithelium in the tumor nests is clearly neoplastic, the collagenous stroma appears to be reactive.

In some tumor nests, the epithelial cells are more spindled; in others, there is central necrosis and areas of cystic change (fig. 5-31). In addition, calcification and ossification are commonly found in the epithelial nests. The calcification and ossification can be focal, involving scattered epithelial nests, or can be diffuse, involving most of the epithelial nests. Often, the epithelial cells take on a clear cell morphology in areas of calcification (fig. 5-32). The mitotic activity in epithelial nests typically ranges from 1 to 5 mitoses/10 high-power fields. Vascular invasion from the epithelial component is occasionally identified (fig. 5-33).

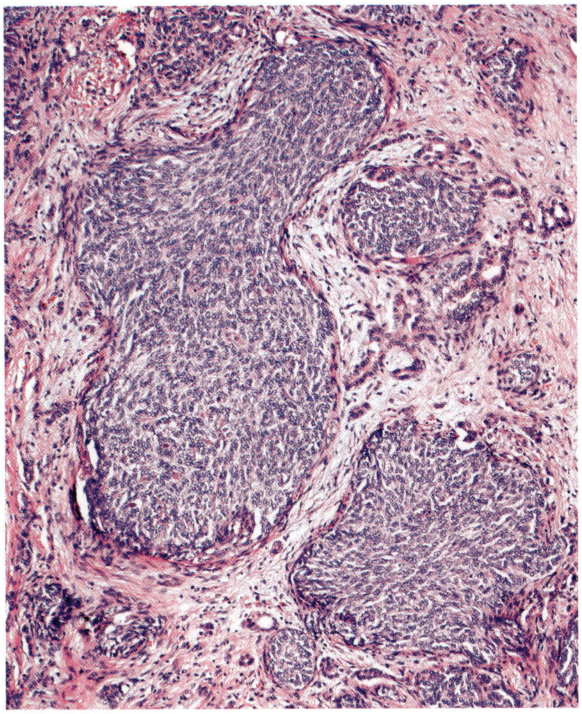

Figure 5-29

CALCIFIED NESTED STROMAL-EPITHELIAL TUMOR

Tumor cells grow in irregular nests, cuffed by a desmoplastic response and ductular reaction.

The overall morphologic pattern can show variation from the edges of the tumor to the center. The edges often have an infiltrative growth pattern (fig. 5-34), with tumor nests extending irregularly into the nontumor hepatic parenchyma. At the tumor/nontumor interface, tumor nests are often surrounded by a ductular reaction, which diminishes steadily toward the center of the tumor. In addition, the center areas of larger tumors can be dominated by prominent ossification and collagen formation (fig. 5-35), with only occasional residual epithelial nests.

Rare cases have nodules of tumor de-differentiation, with small epithelial cells growing in sheets and ribbons. In this setting, the poorly differentiated cells often lose their beta-catenin nuclear expression and the diagnosis can only be made after finding areas with the more typical morphology of calcified nested stromal-epithelial tumors.

The cytologic atypia in most cases is mild. Tumors, however, are not graded in the usual fashion of well to poorly differentiated. There are no recognized histologic subtypes.

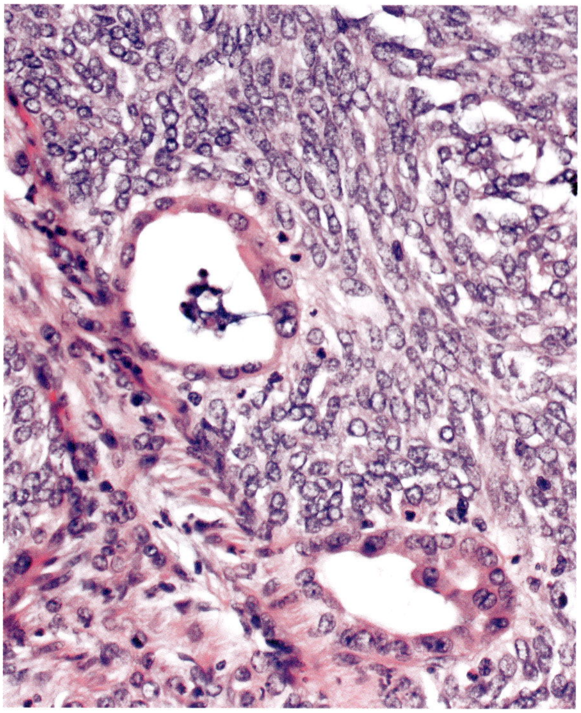

Figure 5-30

CALCIFIED NESTED STROMAL-EPITHELIAL TUMOR

Several well-formed bile ducts are present within this tumor nest.

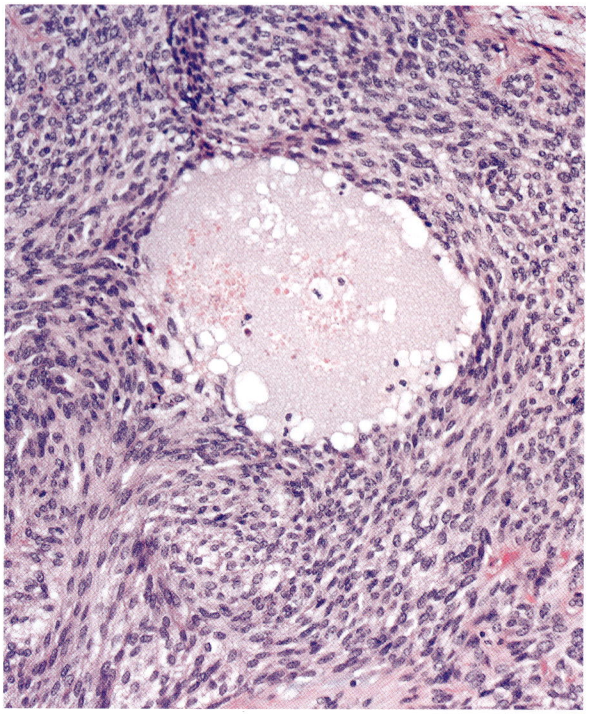

Figure 5-31

CALCIFIED NESTED STROMAL-EPITHELIAL TUMOR

The center of this tumor nest has undergone cystic degeneration.

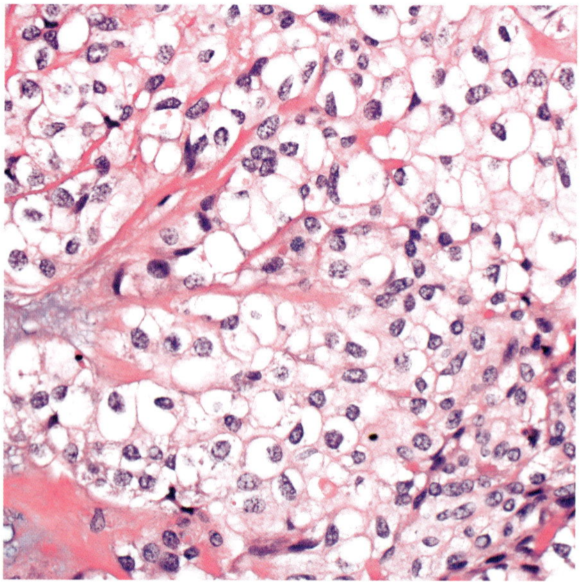

Figure 5-32

CALCIFIED NESTED STROMAL-EPITHELIAL TUMOR

The tumor cells show clear cell morphology adjacent to an area of calcification.

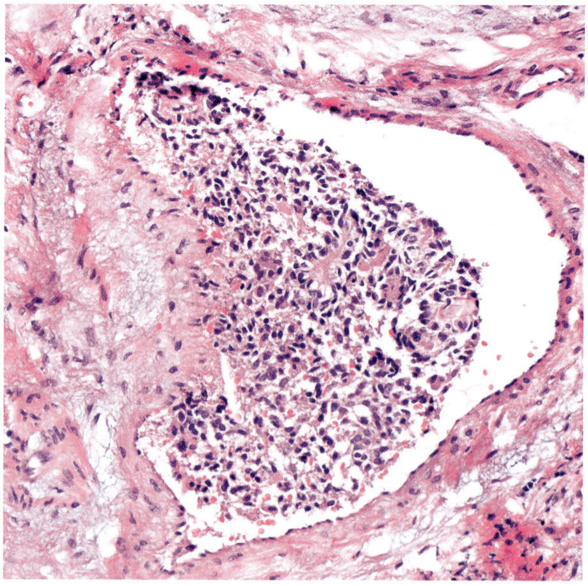

Figure 5-33

CALCIFIED NESTED STROMAL-EPITHELIAL TUMOR

A focus of vascular invasion is seen.

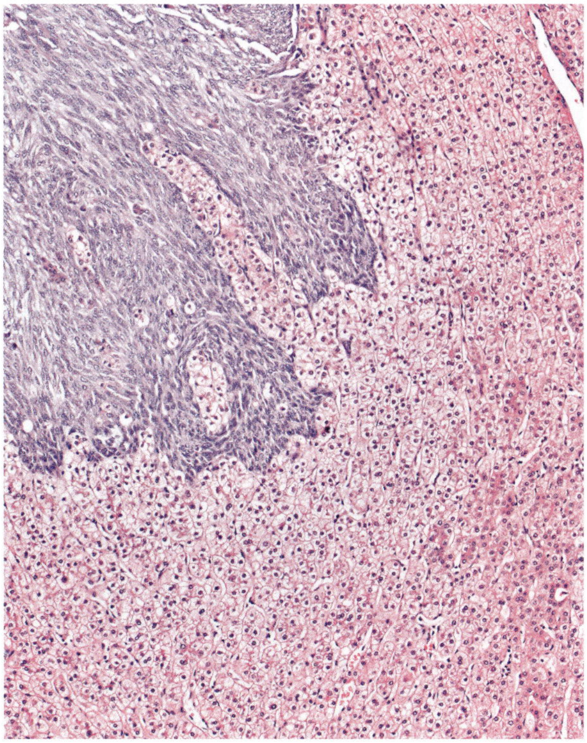

Figure 5-34

CALCIFIED NESTED STROMAL-EPITHELIAL TUMOR

The tumor shows an infiltrative growth pattern at the interface of the tumor with the background liver.

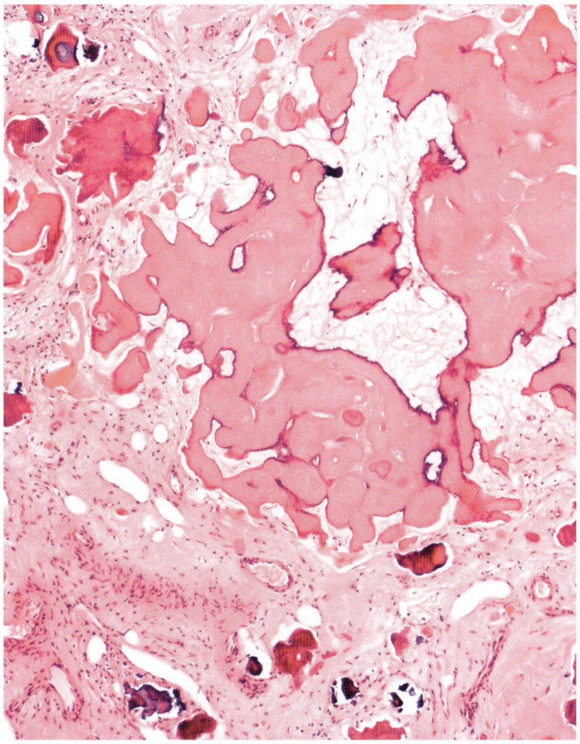

Figure 5-35

CALCIFIED NESTED STROMAL-EPITHELIAL TUMOR

The tumor center is dominated by fibrosis and ossification.

Immunohistochemical Findings

The epithelial nests are keratin positive (57,58,63,64): cytokeratin AE1/AE3 is positive in most cases and CAM5.2 is also typically positive. CK7, CK8, and CK19 are positive in a variable number of cases, while CK20 is negative. EMA tends to show focal or absent staining. NSE, WT1, and vimentin are positive in nearly 100 percent of cases (57,58,63). Nuclear beta-catenin accumulation is found in all reported cases stained for beta-catenin (62,65), but cytoplasmic staining also occurs (fig. 5-36). Hepatocytic markers are consistently negative (57,58,63,64), including the absence of a canalicular staining pattern on polyclonal CEA, and negative staining for HepPar1, AFP, and albumin in situ hybridization. CD56 is positive in most reported cases , but chromogranin and synaptophysin are negative (57,58,63,66). CD99 can show focal weak staining, but is generally negative. Estrogen receptor (ER) staining is negative, while occasional tumors show some progesterone receptor (PR) positivity. ACTH is positive in about one fourth of cases (57,58). S-100 protein can show focal staining, particularly in areas undergoing ossification (57,63,64,66). C-KIT is positive in the epithelial nests of occasional cases (62). The reactive stromal cells can show smooth muscle actin staining, but desmin and myogenin are negative.

Ultrastructural and Cytologic Findings

Data are limited, but by electron microscopy, the tumor cells show abundant rough endoplasmic reticulum and mitochondria, with no evidence of neuroendocrine differentiation (60,65). Cytology findings have not been described because of tumor rarity.

Molecular Genetic Findings

While only a few cases have been studied, calcified nested stromal-epithelial tumors have deletions in the *β-catenin* gene, which in turn

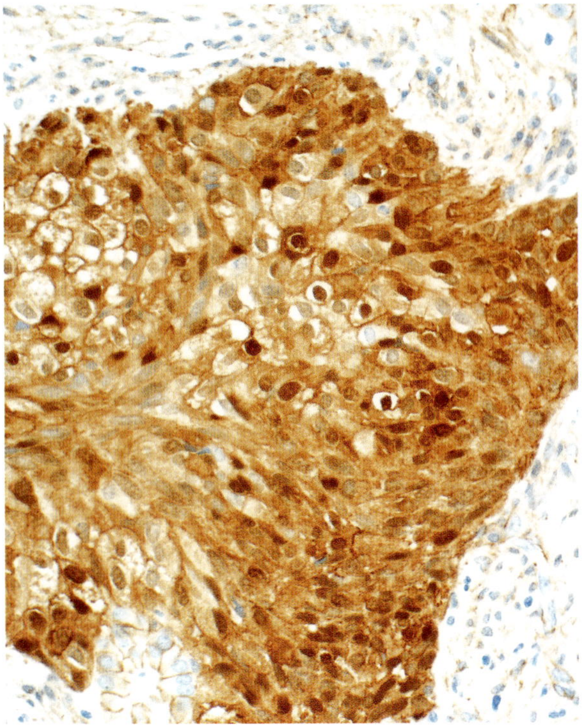

Figure 5-36

CALCIFIED NESTED STROMAL-EPITHELIAL TUMOR: BETA-CATENIN

The tumor shows strong nuclear and cytoplasmic staining.

leads to nuclear accumulation of β-catenin as seen by immunohistochemistry (fig. 5-36) (65). Studies for the *EWS-WT1* fusion, which is found in desmoplastic small round cell tumors, have been largely negative using both fluorscence in situ hybridization (FISH) and polymerase chain reaction (PCR) (57,63,66). In addition, PCR testing for the *SYT-SSX* fusion product, which is found in synovial sarcomas, is negative (63). Testing is negative for *FGFR2* translocations (found in some cholangiocarcinomas) and for the *DNAJB1-PRKACA* translocation (found in fibrolamellar carcinoma).

Differential Diagnosis

The histologic findings are very distinctive, with few real histologic overlaps. Before this entity was described, some cases were classified as hepatoblastoma for lack of a better tumor category, but even then they were recognized as being atypical for hepatoblastoma. Overall, calcified nested stromal epithelial tumors have too much cytoplasm to be a good fit for small cell undifferentiated hepatoblastomas and the complete lack of hepatocytic differentiation helps separate this entity from embryonal and fetal patterns of hepatoblastoma. The differential diagnosis includes a desmoplastic small round cell tumor, and testing for *EWS-WT1* fusion (positive in desmoplastic small round cell tumors) is helpful in difficult cases.

Spread and Metastases

Because of the tumor's rarity and the overall indolent behavior, the patterns of tumor spread are not clear, but lymph node metastases and lung metastases have been reported (60,67). No staging system has been developed.

Treatment and Prognosis

The primary form of treatment is resection. The overall prognosis appears to be favorable. Cases do recur, however, and there can be lymph node and lung metastases, which can lead to patient death (60,67,68).

TRANSITIONAL CELL TUMORS

Some liver carcinomas in older children and teenaged individuals have many histologic findings consistent with hepatocellular carcinoma, and would be called hepatocellular carcinoma in adults, but because of the patients' ages and focal areas that resemble hepatoblastomas, the question arises as to their proper classification. These cases can be challenging to classify and have been called *transitional cell tumors* (69). Most are predominately hepatocellular carcinomas on histologic examination, with focal areas that suggest hepatoblastoma (fig. 5-37). Macrotrabecular growth patterns are fully acceptable in conventional hepatocellular carcinomas, as either major or minor components, and do not suggest a transitional cell tumor in isolation.

To date, transitional cell tumors have been studied in only a single case series (69) and much remains unknown about the best classification for these tumors, including the best way to formally define them at the histologic level. Because the histologic criteria have not been well defined, it may be tempting to overuse this category. However, this tumor classification does not fit into most protocols for patient care and guidance by pathology is important for patient management. Thus, a reasonable approach is to use the predominant histologic patterns to classify these tumors as either hepatoblastomas or hepatocellular carcinomas. In order to flag these cases for future studies and clinical management decisions, the comment section of the pathology report can be used to indicate that the tumor has some features of a transitional cell tumor.

Because the proper classification for these tumors remains uncertain, a recent consensus paper on the classification of pediatric liver tumors has suggested replacing the term "transitional cell tumor" with the term "hepatocellular malignant neoplasm, not otherwise specified (NOS)" (15). This latter term, however, will likely be unpopular and confusing to many groups, including families, treating physicians, and pathologists. For this reason, the approach outlined above has the advantage of being practical and useful for clinical care, while recognizing that some tumors have a "transitional" type morphology and are hard to classify in a completely satisfactory manner using the binary system of hepatoblastoma and hepatocellular carcinoma. The term hepatocellular malignant neoplasm, NOS could have its uses in research studies, but does not have any clear advantages over the original term of transitional cell tumor.

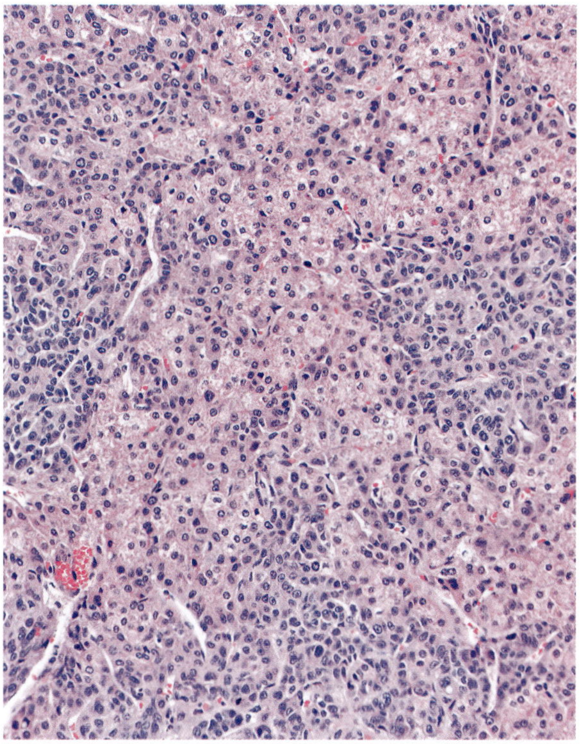

Figure 5-37

TRANSITIONAL CELL CARCINOMA

Most of this tumor showed findings of typical hepatocellular carcinoma, but a focal area in this field suggested the embryonal pattern of hepatoblastoma, admixed with ordinary hepatocellular carcinoma.

PEDIATRIC FOCAL NODULAR HYPERPLASIA

Focal nodular hyperplasia is a mass-forming lesion that is not a neoplasm in the classic sense, but instead is a benign proliferation of mature hepatocytes resulting from a focal vascular shunt.

Clinical Features

Focal nodular hyperplasias are uncommon in children. In most cases, no etiology is evident, but studies estimate that 30 percent of cases have a potential identifiable cause, such as biliary atresia, prior chemotherapy for malignancies, inherited abnormalities in the hepatic vasculature, and glycogen storage diseases (70–72). Focal nodular hyperplasias that develop following chemotherapy are multifocal in 80 to 90 percent of cases, while those arising in other settings tend to be unifocal (70,71). Focal nodular hyperplasias develop in about 5 percent of children who receive chemotherapy, but the lag time from chemotherapy to a diagnosis of focal nodular hyperplasia is long, with a median interval of about 8 to 10 years (71).

Microscopic Findings

The histologic findings in focal nodular hyperplasia are exactly the same in children as they are in adults. Lesions are composed of benign, mature hepatocytes with no atypia, growing in nodules that are separated by fibrous bands. The fibrous bands contain a mild ductular reaction and in the larger lesions, the fibrosis bands often coalesce into central scars. The central scars commonly show abnormal vessels, with eccentrically thickened walls. In smaller lesions, however, the nodularity and fibrous bands tend to be less developed and sometimes absent. The hepatocytes next to the fibrous bands can show cholate stasis changes and mild copper accumulation.

The lesion is not encapsulated and the background liver is noncirrhotic. The hepatocytes in focal nodular hyperplasia can sometimes show fatty changes, including steatohepatitis. In these cases, the background liver also typically shows fatty liver disease.

Differential Diagnosis

The differential diagnosis includes hepatocellular adenoma and hepatocellular carcinoma. The distinction between these entities is made in the same manner as it is in adults. Briefly, focal nodular hyperplasia tends to have fibrous bands and a ductular reaction within the lesion, which are not present in hepatocellular carcinomas. The nodules of proliferating hepatocytes in focal nodular hyperplasias can have aberrant arteries in the parenchyma and show diffuse, or near diffuse CD34 staining, so these features should not be used to distinguish focal nodular hyperplasia from hepatocellular carcinoma. The hepatocytes in focal nodular hyperplasia lack cytologic atypia and a reticulin stain demonstrates a normal reticulin pattern.

The inflammatory subtype of hepatocellular adenoma can show some histologic overlap with focal nodular hyperplasia. Findings that favor focal nodular hyperplasia are well-defined lesion nodularity, resulting from dissecting fibrous bands, as well as aberrant, thick-walled vessels in the fibrous bands. Glutamine synthetase shows a map-like staining pattern in focal nodular hyperplasia, with broad chunky areas of staining that spare the hepatocytes lining the fibrous bands. In contrast, inflammatory adenomas show zone 3 staining around central draining vessels, or in about 10 percent of cases, a diffuse staining pattern indicating beta-catenin activation. Inflammatory adenomas are also positive for C-reactive protein (CRP) and serum amyloid A. In focal nodular hyperplasia, the CRP stain often shows patchy staining so diffuse and strong staining is the pattern that would suggest an inflammatory adenoma. Copper stains do not help in this differential, as copper accumulation is found in both lesions.

PEDIATRIC HEPATOCELLULAR ADENOMAS

Hepatocellular adenomas are benign neoplasms composed of mature hepatocytes. *Pediatric hepatocellular adenomas* are rare but occur in several settings. In contrast to adult adenomas, most of the pediatric cases are not associated with excess estrogen or androgen exposure. Instead, most occur in the setting of glycogen storage disease type I, type III, and less commonly, type VI (73–75). Familial adenomatosis polyposis is another known risk factor. In addition, case reports and small case series have documented a wide range of conditions associated with pediatric hepatocellular adenomas (Table 5-4). In most cases, a predisposing risk factor is identified, but rare exceptions have been reported (76–79). Interestingly, the adenomas without known predisposing factors tend to be very large, and many of the published case reports use the term "giant" to describe them.

The histologic findings and the overall diagnostic approach are the same as for adult hepatocellular adenomas. The tumors are composed of well-differentiated mature hepatocytes growing in trabeculae and broad sheets. There should be no significant cytologic atypia, no architectural atypia, and no reticulin loss. Ki-67 shows a low proliferate rate, typically less than 1 percent.

The adenomas can be subtyped using the same panel of markers used for adult hepatocellular adenomas. In patients with glycogen storage diseases, most adenomas are of the inflammatory type (fig. 5-38) or are unclassified (80). Type 1 adenomas, with loss of LFABP1 protein expression and *HNF1-alpha* mutations, were not found in one large study of glycogen storage disease-associated adenomas (81). Some cases can show a striking steatohepatitic morphology with balloon cells and Mallory hyaline, neutrophilic inflammation, and intertumoral fibrosis. About one third of adenomas show beta-catenin activation (81). Rare cases of malignant transformation have been reported (82).

The differential diagnosis includes focal nodular hyperplasias, which also occur in children, and should be distinguished from hepatocellular adenomas in the same way as they are in adults, using morphology and immunohistochemistry. Focal nodular hyperplasia is typically composed of nodules of benign hepatocytes separated by fibrous septa containing a mild ductular reaction. The fibrous septa may also contain abnormal thick-walled vessels and often coalesce into central scars. Glutamine synthetase shows a map-like staining pattern. Hepatocellular

Table 5-4

RISK FACTORS FOR PEDIATRIC HEPATOCELLULAR ADENOMAS

Risk Factor	Comment and/or Reference
Inherited metabolic diseases	
Glycogen storage disease type I	Adenomas are inflammatory, beta-catenin activated, or unclassified; (80, 81) *HNF1A* inactivated tumors are rare
Glycogen storage disease type III	(73)
Glycogen storage disease type IV	(74)
Glycogen storage disease type VI	The adenoma was not confirmed histologically (106)
Glycogen storage disease type IX	(107)
Hurler syndrome	(108)
Other inherited diseases	
Alpha-1-antitrypsin deficiency	(109)
Carney syndrome	(110)
Familial adenomatous polyposis	(111,112)
Microvillus inclusion disease	(113)
Maturity onset diabetes of the young, type 3	(114)
Prader-Willi syndrome	(115)
Severe combined immunodeficiency	(108)
Turcot syndrome	(116)
Wolf-Hirschhorn syndrome	Syndrome is caused by deletion of chromosome 4p16.3 (117)
Hormone-related tumors	
Androgen related	Examples include androgen use for medical treatments (108,
Estrogen related	118) and body building
Polycystic ovarian syndrome	(119)
Turner syndrome with human growth hormone therapy	(120)
Precocious puberty treated with cyproterone acetate	(121)
Other Associations	
Obesity	(122)
Vascular abnormalities	For example, following Fontan procedure (123,124)
Oxcarbazepinetherapy	Anti-seizure medication (125)
Biliary atresia	(126)

carcinomas should be distinguished from hepatocellular adenomas by their cytologic atypia, architectural atypia, and loss of reticulin.

PEDIATRIC HEPATOCELLULAR CARCINOMA

Hepatocellular carcinomas are rare in the pediatric population but do occur (Table 5-5). In most cases, presenting symptoms and signs are vague and nonspecific, such as abdominal pain, swelling, anorexia, and weight loss. Thrombocytosis can be seen in about 20 percent of individuals at presentation (83).

The frequency of underlying liver disease ranges considerably, from 30 to 80 percent, with higher frequencies found with perinatal transmission of chronic hepatitis B (83–85). In patients with chronic liver disease, the frequency of background liver fibrosis depends on the specific underlying liver disease and the patient's age. For patients less than 10 years of age who develop hepatocellular carcinoma, the three most common causes of cirrhosis are biliary atresia, glycogen storage disorders, and primary disorders of bile acid synthesis/transport such as MDR3 deficiency (86). For older children/young adults, perinatally acquired chronic hepatitis B is an important risk factor for cirrhosis and hepatocellular carcinoma (85,87).

Hepatocellular carcinomas also develop in noncirrhotic livers. Hepatitis B is the most commonly identified risk factor (85), but other risk factors include portal vein loss in Abernathy malformation (88). Rare hepatocellular carcinomas also develop by malignant transformation of hepatocellular adenomas (83,89). Fibrolamellar carcinomas may arise in children and are discussed in chapter 4.

The morphologic findings of pediatric hepatocellular carcinomas (fig. 5-39) are essentially the same as those seen in adult cases; the same

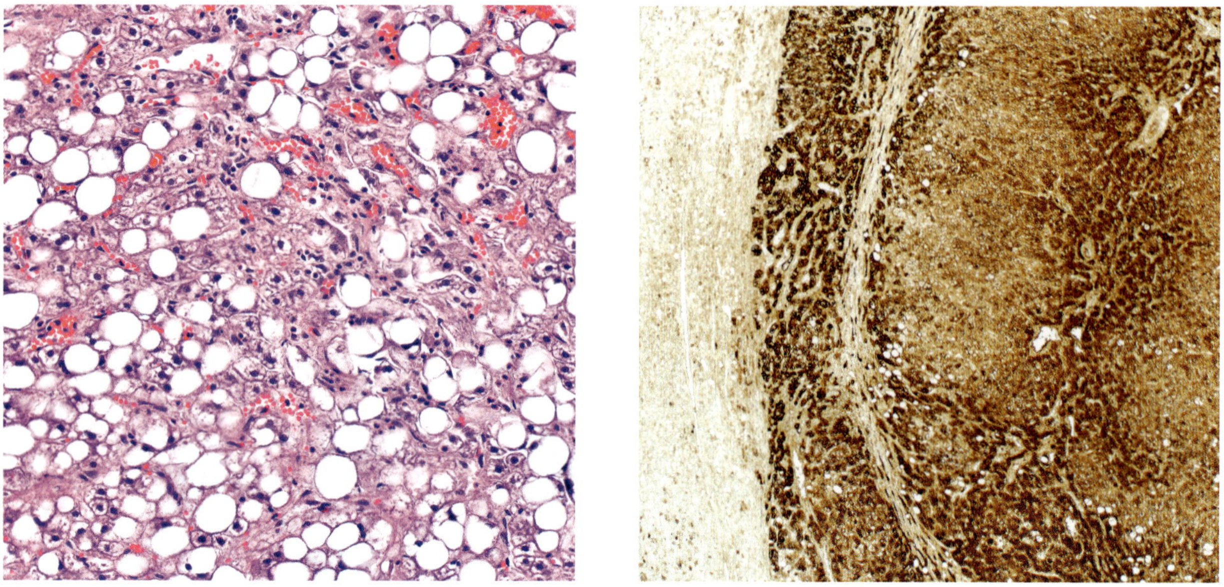

Figure 5-38

HEPATOCELLULAR ADENOMA

Left: This adenoma developed in the setting of type I glycogen storage disease. The adenoma has abundant fat, but immunostains showed it to be an inflammatory adenoma.

Right: An immunostain for C-reactive protein (CRP) is strongly positive.

Table 5-5

RISK FACTORS FOR PEDIATRIC HEPATOCELLULAR CARCINOMAS

Clinical Setting	Comment and/or Reference
Chronic viral hepatitis	
Hepatitis B	Occurs in cirrhotic and noncirrhotic livers (127)
Hepatitis C	Very rare, cirrhotic livers (128)
Inherited diseases	
Tyrosinemia type 1	Livers are typically cirrhotic (129–131)
Arginase deficiency	Noncirrhotic liver (132)
Wilson disease	Cirrhotic liver (92)
PFIC 1 (*ATP8B1* mutation)	(92)
PFIC 2 (*ABCB11* mutation; BSEP deficiency)	Cirrhotic and noncirrhotic livers (130,133,134)
PFIC 3 (*ABCB4* mutation; MDR3 deficiency)	(86)
Tight-junction protein 2 deficiency	Cirrhotic livers (135)
Glycogen storage disease, type Ia	(75)
Glycogen storage disease, type IV	(130,136)
Glycogen storage disease, type VI	(75)
Vascular diseases	
Cardiac cirrhosis	(137)
Congenital absence of portal vein	(138)
Other	
Biliary atresia	(130,139)
Allagile syndrome	(140)
Prolonged TPN therapy	Noncirrhotic liver (141)
Turner syndrome	(138,142)
Status postradiation therapy for Wilms tumor	Noncirrhotic liver (83)

histologic findings and histochemical techniques are used to make the diagnosis. Pediatric hepatocellular carcinomas appear to have a higher frequency of CK7 staining than adult tumors (90), but no other significant differences have been reported to date. While there is a relative paucity of data on the immunohistochemical findings in pediatric versus adult hepatocellular carcinomas, it is generally believed they have similar staining profiles with HepPar1, arginase 1, and reticulin.

Subtypes of hepatocellular carcinoma have not been well defined in the pediatric age group. As one possible exception, several reports have described pediatric hepatocellular carcinomas characterized by numerous tumor syncytial giant cells (83,91).

Metastatic disease is found in about 30 percent of individuals at presentation, most commonly involving the lungs (84,92), but other sites include the bone and adrenal glands (85).

The main entity in the differential diagnosis of pediatric hepatocellular carcinoma is the fetal type of hepatoblastoma. Perhaps counterintuitive, serum AFP levels are not helpful with this differential when they are elevated. In contrast, a diagnosis of hepatocellular carcinoma is favored over hepatoblastoma when serum AFP levels are normal or borderline elevated in a tumor showing clear hepatocellular differentiation. In terms of other clinical findings, none are absolute, but malignant hepatocellular tumors in those less than 3 years of age are almost always hepatoblastomas. Tumors in individuals over age 5 are much more likely to be hepatocellular carcinoma.

Underlying chronic liver disease, even if there is no cirrhosis, strongly favors hepatocellular carcinoma. If there is cirrhosis, the best diagnosis will essentially never be hepatoblastoma. In order to properly apply this guideline, tissue for examining the background liver must be taken far enough away from the tumor to avoid peritumoral changes, which can have sufficient chronic inflammation and fibrosis to closely mimic underlying liver disease. The general rule is to try to get a section of tissue at least 1 cm away from the tumor. In biopsy specimens, the radiologist can separately sample the background liver, away from the tumor. Histologically, finding an embryonal pattern of growth or finding mesenchymal components can help secure the diagnosis of hepatoblastoma. In fetal areas of growth, the classic "light and dark" morphology of fetal hepatoblastoma somewhat favors hepatoblastoma but is not highly sensitive or specific.

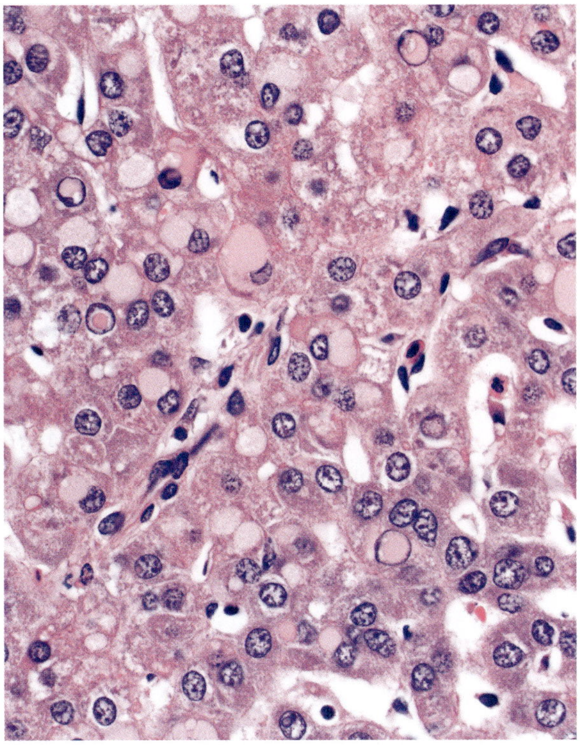

Figure 5-39

HEPATOCELLULAR CARCINOMA

This hepatocellular carcinoma arose in the setting of tyrosinemia. Pale bodies can be seen in the cytoplasm of some of the tumor cells.

While some cases are truly challenging to classify, most are comfortably classified as hepatoblastoma or hepatocellular carcinoma if the above guidelines are followed. Many times the problem of classification arises because of a tendency to try to "force" a diagnosis of hepatoblastoma on a liver tumor because of a patient's young age and high AFP levels, even though the histology is not typical for hepatoblastoma. Overall, if the patient is older than age 5 years and the tumor cytology is consistent with ordinary hepatocellular carcinoma, then that is almost always the best diagnosis.

Calcified nested stromal-epithelial tumors can be separated from hepatocellular carcinomas by their lack of hepatocytic differentiation. While

Table 5-6

RISK FACTORS FOR PEDIATRIC CHOLANGIOCARCINOMA

Clinical Setting	Comment and/or Reference
Primary sclerosing cholangitis	(143)
Small duct sclerosing cholangitis	(144)
Caroli disease	
Choledochal cyst	
Congenital biliary dilatation	(145,146)
Biliary atresia	(126)
HIV	(147)
De novo, following liver transplant	Post-transplant course with recurrent high-grade biliary strictures; the cholangiocarcinoma had a papillary morphology (148)
PFIC 2 (*ABCB11* mutation; BSEP deficiency)	(149)
Wilson disease	(150)
No identifiable risk factors	(151)

the tumors show clear epithelial differentiation by keratin stains, there is no evidence of hepatocytic differentiation by polyclonal CEA, HepPar1, arginase, or albumin in situ hybridization.

PEDIATRIC CHOLANGIOCARCINOMA

Cholangiocarcinomas in the pediatric population are very rare. Risk factors include various chronic biliary tract diseases, such as Caroli disease, and primary sclerosing cholangitis (Table 5-6). Pediatric cholangiocarcinomas have been studied mostly at the epidemiologic and treatment levels, and there is a paucity of good morphologic and immunohistochemical data. Nonetheless, pediatric cholangiocarcinomas are broadly similar to adult cholangiocarcinomas in both morphology (fig. 5-40) and immunohistochemistry.

PEDIATRIC HEPATIC GERM CELL TUMORS

Primary hepatic germ cell tumors are rare and show the same morphology as germ cell tumors in other organs. They are classified as pure yolk sac tumors, choriocarcinomas, embryonal carcinomas, teratomas, and mixed germ cell tumors. Their frequency in the pediatric population is not well defined, but they are much less common than hepatoblastomas and are considerably less common than typical hepatocellular carcinomas.

The age at presentation of germ cell tumors ranges from infancy to teenage years. The clinical findings generally include vague symptoms as well as a liver mass. Serum studies show elevated levels of AFP or beta-human chorionic gonadotropin (HCG), depending on the tumor morphology. The microscopic findings are essentially the same in primary hepatic germ cell tumors as they are in germ cell tumors from other sites. There are no good data on which subtype of primary germ cell tumor of the liver is most common.

Yolk sac tumors in the pediatric population have been reported in a number of case studies (93–97). One case involved primarily the falciform ligament (98). Yolk sac tumors show a microvesicular/reticular pattern of growth, characterized by thin-walled cysts of variable size that are lined by epithelial cells; the epithelial cells resemble endothelial cells, often with scant cytoplasm and flattened morphology. Hyaline globules may also be found in tumor cytoplasm.

In the *hepatoid pattern* of yolk sac tumor, tumor cells resemble hepatocytes, with moderately abundant eosinophilic cytoplasm. The *endodermal sinus pattern* of growth shows a thin-walled central blood vessel surrounded by cuboidal to columnar epithelial cells, a pattern also called Schiller-Duval bodies. In other areas, there can be *solid, myxomatous, sarcomatoid,* and *polyvesicular vitelline growth patterns.* In many cases, multiple patterns of growth are found, often merging into each other without sharp borders.

While not specific, intracytoplasmic hyaline globules are seen in a subset of yolk sac tumors and can be a helpful diagnostic clue. The cytoplasmic globules are positive for alpha-1-antitrypsin in approximately 50 percent of cases. Yolk sac tumors are also keratin positive and typically positive for AFP and/or glypican 3. Immunostains for CD30 are typically negative.

Choriocarcinomas are characterized by malignant cells with trophoblastic differentiation, including cytotrophoblastic and syncytiotrophoblastic elements in juxtaposition (99,100). The tumors may be very hemorrhagic. Tumor cells are positive for keratins and beta-HCG. In very young infants, correlation with placental findings may be important to rule out metastases from a placental primary (101). Because beta-HCG is positive in about 2 percent of hepatocellular carcinomas (102,103), 15 to 20 percent of cholangiocarcinomas (102,103), and occasional hepatoblastomas (104,105), elevated serum HCG levels are not diagnostic for a specific tumor type.

Embyronal carcinomas are composed of pleomorphic cells growing in sheets and cords, sometimes with papillary structures. The tumor cells have abundant amphophilic to basophilic cytoplasm and vesiculated nuclear chromatin, often with prominent nucleoli. The tumor cells can also be positive for both AFP and beta-HCG if there is a yolk sac or choriocarcinoma component.

Teratomas are defined as tumors with immature or mature types of tissue that are not found in the normal liver. The tissue can be immature or normal in its microscopic appearance, showing elements with differentiation toward all of the three germ cell layers (endoderm, mesoderm, and ectoderm). Common tissue types include gastrointestinal, respiratory, squamous, cartilaginous, and bony tissue.

The differential diagnosis for germ cell tumors depends on the subtype. Teratomas are typically easy to recognize. The most important task is to section well enough to ensure that the teratoma is not part of a hepatoblastoma. Choriocarcinomas lack hepatocytic differentiation and have mononuclear cytotrophoblast cells, often with larger multinuclear syncytiotrophoblast cells at the periphery. Embryonal carcinomas are poorly differentiated and a rhabdoid tumor may be suggested, but immunostains for INI-1 and beta-HCG will quickly sort out these two possibilities. Many times, the hardest part of diagnosing embryonal carcinoma is to remember it in the list of differential diagnoses.

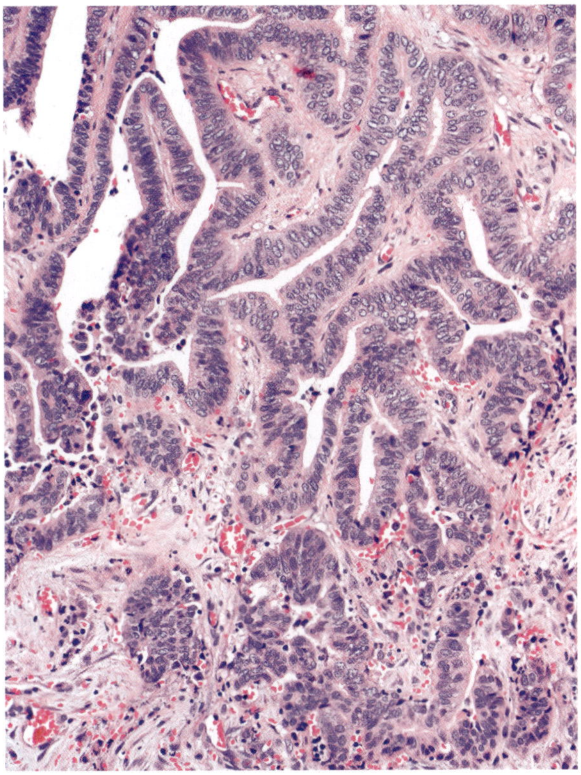

Figure 5-40

CHOLANGIOCARCINOMA

This hilar cholangiocarcinoma shows the typical morphology of an adenocarcinoma embedded within a desmoplastic stroma.

Yolk sac tumors can mimic hepatoblastomas or hepatocellular carcinomas, especially when they have a solid pattern growth pattern with hepatoid differentiation. Finding other areas of more typical hepatoblastoma or more typical yolk sac tumor leads to the proper diagnosis in most cases. In difficult cases, molecular testing for isochromosome 12p is helpful, because isochromosome 12p is found in most germ cell tumors (97).

REFERENCES

1. Lack EE, Neave C, Vawter GF. Hepatoblastoma. A clinical and pathologic study of 54 cases. Am J Surg Pathol 1982;6:693-705.
2. Eren E, Demirkaya M, Cakir ED, Sevinir B, Saglam H, Tarim O. A rare cause of precocious puberty: hepatoblastoma. J Clin Res Pediatr Endocrinol 2009;1:281-283.
3. Czauderna P, Lopez-Terrada D, Hiyama E, Haberle B, Malogolowkin MH, Meyers RL. Hepatoblastoma state of the art: pathology, genetics, risk stratification, and chemotherapy. Curr Opin Pediatr 2014;26:19-28.
4. Wang YX, Liu H. Adult hepatoblastoma: systemic review of the English literature. Dig Surg 2012;29:323-330.
5. Unal E, Koksal Y, Akcoren Z, Tavl L, Gunel E, Kerimoglu U. Mesenchymal hamartoma of the liver mimicking hepatoblastoma. J Pediatr Hematol Oncol 2008;30:458-440.
6. Heck JE, Meyers TJ, Lombardi C, et al. Case-control study of birth characteristics and the risk of hepatoblastoma. Cancer Epidemiol 2013;37:390-395.
7. Johnson KJ, Williams KS, Ross JA, et al. Parental tobacco and alcohol use and risk of hepatoblastoma in offspring: a report from the children's oncology group. Cancer Epidemiol Biomarkers Prev 2013;22:1837-1843.
8. Giardiello FM, Petersen GM, Brensinger JD, et al. Hepatoblastoma and APC gene mutation in familial adenomatous polyposis. Gut 1996;39:867-869.
9. DeBaun MR, Tucker MA. Risk of cancer during the first four years of life in children from The Beckwith-Wiedemann Syndrome Registry. J Pediatr 1998;132:398-400.
10. Venkatramani R, Spector LG, Georgieff M, et al. Congenital abnormalities and hepatoblastoma: a report from the Children's Oncology Group (COG) and the Utah Population Database (UPDB). Am J Med Genet A 2014;164A:2250-2255.
11. Maruyama K, Ikeda H, Koizumi T. Hepatoblastoma associated with trisomy 18 syndrome: a case report and a review of the literature. Pediatr Int 2001;43:302-305.
12. Tan ZH, Lai A, Chen CK, Chang KT, Tan AM. Association of trisomy 18 with hepatoblastoma and its implications. Eur J Pediatr 2014;173:1595-1598.
13. Kamien BA, Gabbett MT. Aicardi syndrome associated with hepatoblastoma and pulmonary sequestration. Am J Med Genet A 2009;149A:1850-1852.
14. Wirojanan J, Kraff J, Hawkins DS, et al. Two boys with fragile x syndrome and hepatic tumors. J Pediatr Hematol Oncol 2008;30:239-241.
15. Lopez-Terrada D, Alaggio R, de Davila MT, et al. Towards an international pediatric liver tumor consensus classification: proceedings of the Los Angeles COG liver tumors symposium. Mod Pathol 2014;27:472-491.
16. Meyers RL, Maibach R, Hiyama E, et al. Risk-stratified staging in paediatric hepatoblastoma: a unified analysis from the Children's Hepatic tumors International Collaboration. Lancet Oncol 2017;18:122-31.
17. Zhou S, Gomulia E, Mascarenhas L, Wang L. Is INI1-retained small cell undifferentiated histology in hepatoblastoma unfavorable? Hum Pathol 2015;46:620-624.
18. Haas JE, Muczynski KA, Krailo M, et al. Histopathology and prognosis in childhood hepatoblastoma and hepatocarcinoma. Cancer 1989;64:1082-1095.
19. Trobaugh-Lotrario AD, Tomlinson GE, Finegold MJ, Gore L, Feusner JH. Small cell undifferentiated variant of hepatoblastoma: adverse clinical and molecular features similar to rhabdoid tumors. Pediatr Blood Cancer 2009;52:328-334.
20. Vokuhl C, Oyen F, Haberle B, von Schweinitz D, Schneppenheim R, Leuschner I. Small cell undifferentiated hepatoblastomas (SCUD): all malignant rhabdoid tumors? Genes Chromosomes Cancer 2016;55:925-931.
21. Abenoza P, Manivel JC, Wick MR, Hagen K, Dehner LP. Hepatoblastoma: an immunohistochemical and ultrastructural study. Hum Pathol 1987;18:1025-1035.
22. Sola Perez J, Perez-Guillermo M, Bas Bernal AB, Mercader JM. Hepatoblastoma. An attempt to apply histologic classification to aspirates obtained by fine needle aspiration cytology. Acta Cytol 1994;38:175-182.
23. Tomlinson GE, Douglass EC, Pollock BH, Finegold MJ, Schneider NR. Cytogenetic evaluation of a large series of hepatoblastomas: numerical abnormalities with recurring aberrations involving 1q12-q21. Genes Chromosomes Cancer 2005;44:177-184.
24. Eichenmuller M, Trippel F, Kreuder M, et al. The genomic landscape of hepatoblastoma and their progenies with HCC-like features. J Hepatol 2014;61:1312-1320.
25. Feusner JH, Krailo MD, Haas JE, Campbell JR, Lloyd DA, Ablin AR. Treatment of pulmonary metastases of initial stage I hepatoblastoma in childhood. Report from the Childrens Cancer Group. Cancer 1993;71:859-864.

26. Brown J, Perilongo G, Shafford E, et al. Pretreatment prognostic factors for children with hepatoblastoma—results from the International Society of Paediatric Oncology (SIOP) study SIOPEL 1. Eur J Cancer 2000;36:1418-1425.
27. Semeraro M, Branchereau S, Maibach R, et al. Relapses in hepatoblastoma patients: clinical characteristics and outcome—experience of the International Childhood Liver Tumour Strategy Group (SIOPEL). Eur J Cancer 2013;49:915-922.
28. Hishiki T, Matsunaga T, Sasaki F, et al. Outcome of hepatoblastomas treated using the Japanese Study Group for Pediatric Liver Tumor (JPLT) protocol-2: report from the JPLT. Pediatr Surg Int 2011;27:1-8.
29. Tannuri AC, Cristofani LM, Teixeira RA, Odone Filho V, Tannuri U. New concepts and outcomes for children with hepatoblastoma based on the experience of a tertiary center over the last 21 years. Clinics (Sao Paulo) 2015;70:387-392.
30. Saettini F, Conter V, Provenzi M, et al. Is multifocality a prognostic factor in childhood hepatoblastoma? Pediatr Blood Cancer 2014;61:1593-1597.
31. Hiyama E, Ueda Y, Onitake Y, et al. A cisplatin plus pirarubicin-based JPLT2 chemotherapy for hepatoblastoma: experience and future of the Japanese Study Group for Pediatric Liver Tumor (JPLT). Pediatr Surg Int 2013;29:1071-1075.
32. Haeberle B, Schweinitz D. Treatment of hepatoblastoma in the German cooperative pediatric liver tumor studies. Front Biosci (Elite Ed) 2012;4:493-498.
33. Meyers RL, Rowland JR, Krailo M, Chen Z, Katzenstein HM, Malogolowkin MH. Predictive power of pretreatment prognostic factors in children with hepatoblastoma: a report from the Children's Oncology Group. Pediatr Blood Cancer 2009;53:1016-1022.
34. Maibach R, Roebuck D, Brugieres L, et al. Prognostic stratification for children with hepatoblastoma: the SIOPEL experience. Eur J Cancer 2012;48:1543-1549.
35. Sakamoto S, Kasahara M, Mizuta K, et al. Nationwide survey of the outcomes of living donor liver transplantation for hepatoblastoma in Japan. Liver Transpl 2014;20:333-346.
36. Fukuzawa H, Urushihara N, Fukumoto K, et al. Can we predict the prognosis of resectable hepatoblastoma from serum alpha-fetoprotein response during preoperative chemotherapy? Pediatr Surg Int 2012;28:887-891.
37. Koh KN, Park M, Kim BE, et al. Prognostic implications of serum alpha-fetoprotein response during treatment of hepatoblastoma. Pediatr Blood Cancer 2011;57:554-560.
38. Fuchs J, Rydzynski J, Von Schweinitz D, et al. Pretreatment prognostic factors and treatment results in children with hepatoblastoma: a report from the German Cooperative Pediatric Liver Tumor Study HB 94. Cancer 2002;95:172-182.
39. Malogolowkin MH, Katzenstein HM, Meyers RL, et al. Complete surgical resection is curative for children with hepatoblastoma with pure fetal histology: a report from the Children's Oncology Group. J Clin Oncol 2011;29:3301-3306.
40. Oita S, Terui K, Komatsu S, et al. Malignant rhabdoid tumor of the liver: a case report and literature review. Pediatr Rep 2015;7:5578.
41. Trobaugh-Lotrario AD, Finegold MJ, Feusner JH. Rhabdoid tumors of the liver: rare, aggressive, and poorly responsive to standard cytotoxic chemotherapy. Pediatr Blood Cancer 2011;57:423-428.
42. Martelli MG, Liu C. Malignant rhabdoid tumour of the liver in a seven-month-old female infant: a case report and literature review. Afr J Paediatr Surg 2013;10:50-54.
43. Kachanov D, Teleshova M, Kim E, et al. Malignant rhabdoid tumor of the liver presented with initial tumor rupture. Cancer Genet 2014;207:412-414.
44. Clairotte A, Ringenbach F, Laithier V, Aubert D, Kantelip B. [Malignant rhabdoid tumor of the liver with spontaneous rupture: a case report]. Ann Pathol 2006;26:122-125. [French]
45. Ravindra KV, Cullinane C, Lewis IJ, Squire BR, Stringer MD. Long-term survival after spontaneous rupture of a malignant rhabdoid tumor of the liver. J Pediatr Surg 2002;37:1488-1490.
46. Yuri T, Danbara N, Shikata N, et al. Malignant rhabdoid tumor of the liver: case report and literature review. Pathol Int 2004;54:623-629.
47. Scheimberg I, Cullinane C, Kelsey A, Malone M. Primary hepatic malignant tumor with rhabdoid features. A histological, immunocytochemical, and electron microscopic study of four cases and a review of the literature. Am J Surg Pathol 1996;20:1394-1400.
48. Foschini MP, Van Eyken P, Brock PR, et al. Malignant rhabdoid tumour of the liver. A case report. Histopathology 1992;20:157-165.
49. Hunt SJ, Anderson WD. Malignant rhabdoid tumor of the liver. A distinct clinicopathologic entity. Am J Clin Pathol 1990;94:645-648.
50. Kohashi K, Nakatsura T, Kinoshita Y, et al. Glypican 3 expression in tumors with loss of SMARCB1/INI1 protein expression. Hum Pathol 2013;44:526-533.
51. Chan ES, Pawel BR, Corao DA, et al. Immunohistochemical expression of glypican-3 in pediatric tumors: an analysis of 414 cases. Pediatr Dev Pathol 2013;16:272-277.

52. Shiratsuchi H, Saito T, Sakamoto A, et al. Mutation analysis of human cytokeratin 8 gene in malignant rhabdoid tumor: a possible association with intracytoplasmic inclusion body formation. Mod Pathol 2002;15:146-153.
53. Pogacnik A, Zidar N. Malignant rhabdoid tumor of the liver diagnosed by fine needle aspiration cytology. A case report. Acta Cytol 1997;41:539-543.
54. Eaton KW, Tooke LS, Wainwright LM, Judkins AR, Biegel JA. Spectrum of SMARCB1/INI1 mutations in familial and sporadic rhabdoid tumors. Pediatr Blood Cancer 2011;56:7-15.
55. Rao Q, Xia QY, Wang ZY, et al. Frequent co-inactivation of the SWI/SNF subunits SMARCB1, SMARCA2 and PBRM1 in malignant rhabdoid tumours. Histopathology 2015;67:121-129.
56. Ishak KG, Goodman ZD, Stocker JT. Tumors of the liver and intrahepatic bile ducts. Atlas of Tumor Pathology, Third Series, Fascicle 31; Washington DC: American Registry of Pathology; 2001.
57. Makhlouf HR, Abdul-Al HM, Wang G, Goodman ZD. Calcifying nested stromal-epithelial tumors of the liver: a clinicopathologic, immunohistochemical, and molecular genetic study of 9 cases with a long-term follow-up. Am J Surg Pathol 2009;33:976-983.
58. Heerema-McKenney A, Leuschner I, Smith N, Sennesh J, Finegold MJ. Nested stromal epithelial tumor of the liver: six cases of a distinctive pediatric neoplasm with frequent calcifications and association with cushing syndrome. Am J Surg Pathol 2005;29:10-20.
59. Geramizadeh B, Foroutan H, Foroutan A, Bordbar M. Nested stromal epithelial tumor of liver presenting with Cushing syndrome: a rare case report. Indian J Pathol Microbiol 2012;55:253-255.
60. Brodsky SV, Sandoval C, Sharma N, et al. Recurrent nested stromal epithelial tumor of the liver with extrahepatic metastasis: case report and review of literature. Pediatr Dev Pathol 2008;11:469-473.
61. Rod A, Voicu M, Chiche L, et al. Cushing's syndrome associated with a nested stromal epithelial tumor of the liver: hormonal, immunohistochemical, and molecular studies. Eur J Endocrinol 2009;161:805-810.
62. Malowany JI, Merritt NH, Chan NG, Ngan BY. Nested stromal epithelial tumor of the liver in Beckwith-Wiedemann syndrome. Pediatr Dev Pathol 2013;16:312-317.
63. Hill DA, Swanson PE, Anderson K, et al. Desmoplastic nested spindle cell tumor of liver: report of four cases of a proposed new entity. Am J Surg Pathol 2005;29:1-9.
64. Grazi GL, Vetrone G, d'Errico A, et al. Nested stromal-epithelial tumor (NSET) of the liver: a case report of an extremely rare tumor. Pathol Res Pract 2010;206:282-286.
65. Assmann G, Kappler R, Zeindl-Eberhart E, et al. β-Catenin mutations in 2 nested stromal epithelial tumors of the liver—a neoplasia with defective mesenchymal-epithelial transition. Hum Pathol 2012;43:1815-1827.
66. Oviedo Ramirez MI, Bas Bernal A, Ortiz Ruiz E, Bermejo J, De Alava E, Hernandez T. Desmoplastic nested spindle cell tumor of the liver in an adult. Ann Diagn Pathol 2010;14:44-49.
67. Hommann M, Kaemmerer D, Daffner W, et al. Nested stromal epithelial tumor of the liver—liver transplantation and follow-up. J Gastrointest Cancer 2011;42:292-295.
68. Heywood G, Burgart LJ, Nagorney DM. Ossifying malignant mixed epithelial and stromal tumor of the liver: a case report of a previously undescribed tumor. Cancer 2002;94:1018-1022.
69. Prokurat A, Kluge P, Kosciesza A, Perek D, Kappeler A, Zimmermann A. Transitional liver cell tumors (TLCT) in older children and adolescents: a novel group of aggressive hepatic tumors expressing beta-catenin. Med Pediatr Oncol 2002;39:510-518.
70. Cha DI, Yoo SY, Kim JH, Jeon TY, Eo H. Clinical and imaging features of focal nodular hyperplasia in children. AJR Am J Roentgenol 2014;202:960-965.
71. Smith EA, Salisbury S, Martin R, Towbin AJ. Incidence and etiology of new liver lesions in pediatric patients previously treated for malignancy. AJR Am J Roentgenol 2012;199:186-191.
72. Ma IT, Rojas Y, Masand PM, et al. Focal nodular hyperplasia in children: an institutional experience with review of the literature. J Pediatr Surg 2015;50:382-387.
73. Labrune P, Trioche P, Duvaltier I, Chevalier P, Odievre M. Hepatocellular adenomas in glycogen storage disease type I and III: a series of 43 patients and review of the literature. J Pediatr Gastroenterol Nutr 1997;24:276-279.
74. Alshak NS, Cocjin J, Podesta L, et al. Hepatocellular adenoma in glycogen storage disease type IV. Arch Pathol Lab Med 1994;118:88-91.
75. Manzia TM, Angelico R, Toti L, et al. Glycogen storage disease type Ia and VI associated with hepatocellular carcinoma: two case reports. Transplant Proc 2011;43:1181-1183.
76. Vaithianathan R, Philipchandran, Selvambigai G, Jayaganesh P. Spontaneous hepatocellular adenoma in paediatric age group - case report. J Clin Diagn Res 2013;7:2962-2963.
77. Ronaldi AE, Hairston FJ, Giles HW, Nowicki MJ. Giant hepatocellular adenoma in a child. Dig Liver Dis 2014;46:287.

78. von Riedenauer WB, Shanti CM, Abouljoud MS. Resection of giant liver adenoma in a 17-year-old adolescent boy using venovenous bypass, total hepatic vascular isolation, and in situ cooling. J Pediatr Surg 2007;42:E23-27.
79. Morris MW, Berch B, Westmoreland T, Sawaya DE, Blewett CJ. Resection of a giant hepatic adenoma in an eight-year-old girl. Am Surg 2013;79:889-890.
80. Sakellariou S, Al-Hussaini H, Scalori A, et al. Hepatocellular adenoma in glycogen storage disorder type I: a clinicopathological and molecular study. Histopathology 2012;60:E58-65.
81. Calderaro J, Labrune P, Morcrette G, et al. Molecular characterization of hepatocellular adenomas developed in patients with glycogen storage disease type I. J Hepatol 2013;58:350-357.
82. Toiyama Y, Inoue Y, Yasuda H, et al. Hepatocellular adenoma containing hepatocellular carcinoma in a male patient with familial adenomatous polyposis coli: report of a case. Surg Today 2011;41:1442-1446.
83. Lack EE, Neave C, Vawter GF. Hepatocellular carcinoma. Review of 32 cases in childhood and adolescence. Cancer 1983;52:1510-1515.
84. Czauderna P, Mackinlay G, Perilongo G, et al. Hepatocellular carcinoma in children: results of the first prospective study of the International Society of Pediatric Oncology group. J Clin Oncol 2002;20:2798-2804.
85. Zhang XF, Liu XM, Wei T, et al. Clinical characteristics and outcome of hepatocellular carcinoma in children and adolescents. Pediatr Surg Int 2013;29:763-770.
86. Vij M, Safwan M, Shanmugam NP, Rela M. Liver pathology in severe multidrug resistant 3 protein deficiency: a series of 10 pediatric cases. Ann Diagn Pathol 2015;19:277-282.
87. Malik S, Dekio F, Wen JW. Liver transplantation in a child with multifocal hepatocellular carcinoma hepatitis C and management of post-transplant viral recurrence using boceprevir. Pediatr Transplant 2014;18:E64-68.
88. Lisovsky M, Konstas AA, Misdraji J. Congenital extrahepatic portosystemic shunts (Abernethy malformation): a histopathologic evaluation. Am J Surg Pathol 2011;35:1381-1390.
89. Turan A, Unlu HA, Karakus E, Yazal Erdem A, Yakut ZI. Atypical [b]-catenin activated child hepatocellular tumor. Pediatr Gastroenterol Hepatol Nutr 2015;18:144-148.
90. Klein WM, Molmenti EP, Colombani PM, et al. Primary liver carcinoma arising in people younger than 30 years. Am J Clin Pathol 2005;124:512-518.
91. Atra A, Al-Asiri R, Wali S, Al-Husseini H, Al-Bassas A, Zimmermann A. Hepatocellular carcinoma, syncytial giant cell: a novel variant in children: a case report. Ann Diagn Pathol 2007;11:61-63.
92. Yu SB, Kim HY, Eo H, et al. Clinical characteristics and prognosis of pediatric hepatocellular carcinoma. World J Surg 2006;30:43-50.
93. Littooij AS, McHugh K, McCarville MB, Sebire NJ, Bahrami A, Roebuck DJ. Yolk sac tumour: a rare cause of raised serum alpha-foetoprotein in a young child with a large liver mass. Pediatr Radiol 2014;44:18-22.
94. Verma M, Agarwal S, Mohta A. Primary mixed germ cell tumour of the liver—a case report. Indian J Pathol Microbiol 2003;46:658-659.
95. Hart WR. Primary endodermal sinus (yolk sac) tumor of the liver. First reported case. Cancer 1975;35:1453-1458.
96. Abramson LP, Pillai S, Acton R, Melin-Aldana H, Superina R. Successful orthotopic liver transplantation for treatment of a hepatic yolk sac tumor. J Pediatr Surg 2005;40:1185-1187.
97. Gilbert KL, Bergman S, Dodd LG, Volmar KE, Creager AJ. Cytomorphology of yolk sac tumor of the liver in fine-needle aspiration: a pediatric case. Diagn Cytopathol 2006;34:421-423.
98. Atkinson JB, Foster CE 3rd, Lally KP, Isaacs H, Siegel SE. Primary endodermal sinus (yolk sac) tumor of the falciform ligament. J Pediatr Surg 1992;27:105-107.
99. Hongo T, Fujii Y, Fukuoka T, et al. Long-term treatment in infantile choriocarcinoma. Acta Paediatr Jpn 1992;34:52-59.
100. Szavay PO, Wermes C, Fuchs J, Schrappe M, Flemming P, von Schweinitz D. Effective treatment of infantile choriocarcinoma in the liver with chemotherapy and surgical resection: a case report. J Pediatr Surg 2000;35:1134-1135.
101. Kishkurno S, Ishida A, Takahashi Y, et al. A case of neonatal choriocarcinoma. Am J Perinatol 1997;14:79-82.
102. Nonomura A, Mizukami Y, Matsubara F, et al. Human chorionic gonadotropin and alpha-fetoprotein in cholangiocarcinoma in relation to the expression of ras p21: an immunohistochemical study. Liver 1989;9:205-215.
103. Nakanuma Y, Unoura M, Noto H, Ohta G. Human chorionic gonadotropin in primary liver carcinoma in adults. An immunohistochemical study. Virchows Arch A Pathol Anat Histopathol 1986;409:365-373.
104. Marino S, Caruso M, Magro G, et al. Hepatoblastoma presenting as precocious puberty: a case report. J Pediatr Endocrinol Metab 2015;28:429-432.
105. Morinaga S, Yamaguchi M, Watanabe I, Kasai M, Ojima M, Sasano N. An immunohistochemical study of hepatoblastoma producing human chorionic gonadotropin. Cancer 1983;51:1647-1652.

106. Roscher A, Patel J, Hewson S, et al. The natural history of glycogen storage disease types VI and IX: Long-term outcome from the largest metabolic center in Canada. Mol Genet Metab 2014;113:171-176.
107. Bali DS, Goldstein JL, Fredrickson K, et al. Variability of disease spectrum in children with liver phosphorylase kinase deficiency caused by mutations in the PHKG2 gene. Mol Genet Metab 2014;111:309-313.
108. Resnick MB, Kozakewich HP, Perez-Atayde AR. Hepatic adenoma in the pediatric age group. Clinicopathological observations and assessment of cell proliferative activity. Am J Surg Pathol 1995;19:1181-1190.
109. McDaniel JD, Kukreja K, Ristagno RL, Yazigi N, Nathan JD, Tiao G. Radiofrequency ablation of a large hepatic adenoma in a child. J Pediatr Surg 2013;48:E19-22.
110. Terracciano LM, Tornillo L, Avoledo P, Von Schweinitz D, Kuhne T, Bruder E. Fibrolamellar hepatocellular carcinoma occurring 5 years after hepatocellular adenoma in a 14-year-old girl: a case report with comparative genomic hybridization analysis. Arch Pathol Lab Med 2004;128:222-226.
111. Bala S, Wunsch PH, Ballhausen WG. Childhood hepatocellular adenoma in familial adenomatous polyposis: mutations in adenomatous polyposis coli gene and p53. Gastroenterology 1997;112:919-922.
112. Gupta A, Sheridan RM, Towbin A, Geller JI, Tiao G, Bove KE. Multifocal hepatic neoplasia in 3 children with APC gene mutation. Am J Surg Pathol 2013;37:1058-1066.
113. Burgis JC, Pratt CA, Higgins JP, Kerner JA. Multiple hepatic adenomas in a child with microvillus inclusion disease. Dig Dis Sci 2013;58:2784-2788.
114. Willson JS, Godwin TD, Wiggins GA, Guilford PJ, McCall JL. Primary hepatocellular neoplasms in a MODY3 family with a novel HNF1A germline mutation. J Hepatol 2013;59:904-907.
115. Takayasu H, Motoi T, Kanamori Y, et al. Two case reports of childhood liver cell adenomas harboring beta-catenin abnormalities. Hum Pathol 2002;33:852-855.
116. Hamilton SR, Liu B, Parsons RE, et al. The molecular basis of Turcot's syndrome. N Engl J Med 1995;332:839-847.
117. Prunotto G, Cianci P, Cereda A, et al. Two cases of hepatic adenomas in patients with Wolf-Hirschhorn syndrome: a new rare complication? Am J Med Genet A 2013;161A:1759-1762.
118. Kumar AR, Wagner JE, Auerbach AD, et al. Fatal hemorrhage from androgen-related hepatic adenoma after hematopoietic cell transplantation. J Pediatr Hematol Oncol 2004;26:16-18.
119. Triantafyllopoulou M, Whitington PF, Melin-Aldana H, Benya EC, Brickman W. Hepatic adenoma in an adolescent with elevated androgen levels. J Pediatr Gastroenterol Nutr 2007;44:640-642.
120. Espat J, Chamberlain RS, Sklar C, Blumgart LH. Hepatic adenoma associated with recombinant human growth hormone therapy in a patient with Turner's syndrome. Dig Surg 2000;17:640-643.
121. Watanabe S, Cui Y, Tanae A, et al. Follow-up study of children with precocious puberty treated with cyproterone acetate. Ad hoc Committee for CPA. J Epidemiol 1997;7:173-178.
122. Rosencrantz RA, Wu Y, Sonke PY, Yusuf Y. Giant hepatocellular adenoma in a previously obese thirteen-year-old boy. Ann Hepatol 2015; 14:559-563.
123. Ghaferi AA, Hutchins GM. Progression of liver pathology in patients undergoing the Fontan procedure: Chronic passive congestion, cardiac cirrhosis, hepatic adenoma, and hepatocellular carcinoma. J Thorac Cardiovasc Surg 2005;129:1348-1352.
124. Babaoglu K, Binnetoglu FK, Aydogan A, et al. Hepatic adenomatosis in a 7-year-old child treated earlier with a Fontan procedure. Pediatr Cardiol 2010;31:861-864.
125. Lautz TB, Finegold MJ, Chin AC, Superina RA. Giant hepatic adenoma with atypical features in a patient on oxcarbazepine therapy. J Pediatr Surg 2008;43:751-754.
126. Yoon HJ, Jeon TY, Yoo SY, et al. Hepatic tumours in children with biliary atresia: single-centre experience in 13 cases and review of the literature. Clin Radiol 2014;69:e113-119.
127. Lanier AP, Holck P, Ehrsam Day G, Key C. Childhood cancer among Alaska Natives. Pediatrics 2003;112:e396.
128. Gonzalez-Peralta RP, Langham MR Jr, Andres JM, et al. Hepatocellular carcinoma in 2 young adolescents with chronic hepatitis C. J Pediatr Gastroenterol Nutr 2009;48:630-635.
129. van Ginkel WG, Gouw AS, van der Jagt EJ, de Jong KP, Verkade HJ, van Spronsen FJ. Hepatocellular carcinoma in tyrosinemia type 1 without clear increase of AFP. Pediatrics 2015;135:e749-752.
130. Romano F, Stroppa P, Bravi M, et al. Favorable outcome of primary liver transplantation in children with cirrhosis and hepatocellular carcinoma. Pediatr Transplant 2011;15:573-579.
131. Bahador A, Dehghani SM, Geramizadeh B, et al. Liver transplant for children with hepatocellular carcinoma and hereditary tyrosinemia type 1. Exp Clin Transplant 2015;13:329-332.

132. Schlune A, Vom Dahl S, Haussinger D, Ensenauer R, Mayatepek E. Hyperargininemia due to arginase I deficiency: the original patients and their natural history, and a review of the literature. Amino Acids 2015;47:1751-1762.
133. Vilarinho S, Erson-Omay EZ, Harmanci AS, et al. Paediatric hepatocellular carcinoma due to somatic CTNNB1 and NFE2L2 mutations in the setting of inherited bi-allelic ABCB11 mutations. J Hepatol 2014;61:1178-1183.
134. Knisely AS, Strautnieks SS, Meier Y, et al. Hepatocellular carcinoma in ten children under five years of age with bile salt export pump deficiency. Hepatology 2006;44:478-486.
135. Zhou S, Hertel PM, Finegold MJ, et al. Hepatocellular carcinoma associated with tight-junction protein 2 deficiency. Hepatology 2015;62:1914-1916.
136. de Moor RA, Schweizer JJ, van Hoek B, Wasser M, Vink R, Maaswinkel-Mooy PD. Hepatocellular carcinoma in glycogen storage disease type IV. Arch Dis Child 2000;82:479-480.
137. Yamada K, Shinmoto H, Kawamura Y, et al. Transarterial embolization for pediatric hepatocellular carcinoma with cardiac cirrhosis. Pediatr Int 2015;57:766-770.
138. Morotti RA, Killackey M, Shneider BL, Repucci A, Emre S, Thung SN. Hepatocellular carcinoma and congenital absence of the portal vein in a child receiving growth hormone therapy for turner syndrome. Semin Liver Dis 2007;27:427-431.
139. Kim JM, Lee SK, Kwon CH, Joh JW, Choe YH, Park CK. Hepatocellular carcinoma in an infant with biliary atresia younger than 1 year. J Pediatr Surg 2012;47:819-821.
140. Bhadri VA, Stormon MO, Arbuckle S, Lam AH, Gaskin KJ, Shun A. Hepatocellular carcinoma in children with Alagille syndrome. J Pediatr Gastroenterol Nutr 2005;41:676-678.
141. Patterson K, Kapur SP, Chandra RS. Hepatocellular carcinoma in a noncirrhotic infant after prolonged parenteral nutrition. J Pediatr 1985;106:797-800.
142. Zhao X, Wang Z, Cao L, et al. Hyperfibrinogenemia and prolonged clotting times in a Turner syndrome patient with hepatocellular carcinoma. Blood Coagul Fibrinolysis 2010;21:398-405.
143. Liu R, Cox K, Guthery SL, et al. Cholangiocarcinoma and high-grade dysplasia in young patients with primary sclerosing cholangitis. Dig Dis Sci 2014;59:2320-2324.
144. Lai J, Taouli B, Iyer KR, et al. Cholangiolocellular carcinoma in a pediatric patient with small duct sclerosing cholangitis: a case report. Semin Liver Dis 2012;32:360-366.
145. Saikusa N, Naito S, Iinuma Y, Ohtani T, Yokoyama N, Nitta K. Invasive cholangiocarcinoma identified in congenital biliary dilatation in a 3-year-old boy. J Pediatr Surg 2009;44:2202-2205.
146. Tanaka S, Kubota M, Yagi M, et al. An 11-year-old male patient demonstrating cholangiocarcinoma associated with congenital biliary dilatation. J Pediatr Surg 2006;41:e15-19.
147. Mangeya N, Mafukidze AT, Pascoe M, et al. Cholangiocarcinoma presenting in an adolescent with vertically acquired HIV infection. Int J STD AIDS 2008;19:717-718.
148. Channabasappa N, Johnson-Welch S, Mittal N. De novo cholangiocarcinoma after liver transplantation in a pediatric patient. Pediatr Transplant 2010;14:E110-114.
149. Scheimann AO, Strautnieks SS, Knisely AS, Byrne JA, Thompson RJ, Finegold MJ. Mutations in bile salt export pump (ABCB11) in two children with progressive familial intrahepatic cholestasis and cholangiocarcinoma. J Pediatr 2007;150:556-559.
150. Walshe JM, Waldenstrom E, Sams V, Nordlinder H, Westermark K. Abdominal malignancies in patients with Wilson's disease. QJM 2003;96:657-662.
151. Hall C, Mamlok V, Al-Khalil I. A sporadic case of advanced metastatic cholangiocarcinoma in a child: a case report and review of literature. J Pediatr Hematol Oncol 2015;37:e333-335.

6 BENIGN AND BORDERLINE BILIARY NEOPLASMS AND TUMOR-LIKE LESIONS

INTRADUCTAL PAPILLARY NEOPLASM

Definition. *Intraductal papillary neoplasm of the bile duct* (IPNB) consists of neoplastic epithelium arranged in a well-organized papillary architecture along delicate fibrovascular stalks and often produces abundant amounts of mucin (1–3). This entity covers previous categories including biliary papilloma, biliary papillomatosis, and mucin-producing bile duct tumors (1,4). Before the concept of IPNB was proposed, some cases of IPNB were diagnosed as papillary cholangiocarcinoma or biliary cystadenoma and cystadenocarcinoma that lack an ovarian-like stroma (5). Although the distinction between IPNB and papillary cholangiocarcinoma remains debatable, IPNB typically shows a more organized papillary structure. When IPNB progresses to invasive adenocarcinoma, it is called *IPNB with an associated invasive carcinoma*.

General Features. IPNB has been widely accepted as a biliary counterpart of intraductal papillary mucinous neoplasm (IPMN) of the pancreas based on their histologic similarities (1,6,7). These two conditions, however, are not identical. The most significant difference is the degree of malignancy. More than 50 percent of pancreatic neoplasms correspond to low-grade dysplasia, with no surgical intervention being required, while approximately 90 percent of IPNBs have at least high-grade dysplasia, including carcinoma in situ (8,9). The overproduction of mucin is more common in pancreatic IPMN, while an associated invasive carcinoma is more frequently detected in IPNB (8,9).

Earlier cases of IPNB were mainly reported in East Asia (10,11). Korean and Taiwanese single-institute studies identified and examined up to 100 patients with IPNB (12,13), in contrast to the largest Western study, in which only 45 patients were collected from 6 institutions in Europe (14). A recent international collaborative study involving three medical centers in Seattle, London, and Seoul revealed that IPNB accounted for 4.4 percent of primary hepatobiliary malignancies surgically resected in Seoul, while its proportions were less than 1 percent in the American and British cohorts (15). The higher incidence of IPNB in Korea is less likely due to genetic susceptibility because IPNB patients diagnosed in Seattle and London were all non-Asian in ancestry in spite of the large number of Asian people living in these cities. Hepatolithiasis and liver flukes appear to be the main predisposing factors contributing to the higher incidence of IPNB in Asia, given that approximately 50 percent of Korean patients with IPNB have at least one of these conditions (12,13,15,16).

Primary sclerosing cholangitis (PSC) is known to increase the risk of cholangiocarcinoma, but typically follows a biliary intraepithelial neoplasia (BilIN)-cholangiocarcinoma sequence independent of IPNB. Papillomucinous cholangiocarcinoma sometimes develops against the background of PSC; however, most cases do not fit with IPNB because of the markedly complex papillotubular histologic architecture (17). To date, we have encountered only one case of IPNB associated with PSC.

A caveat is that universally accepted diagnostic criteria for IPNB are not available. The separation between IPNB and papillary cholangiocarcinoma clearly requires further discussion. Some pathologists consider almost all grossly papillary neoplasms to be IPNB, while others use this diagnostic term in selected cases. In previous studies on IPNB, the prevalent anatomic location, proportion of invasive cases, and incidence of mucin overproduction differed widely, which may have been due to the different diagnostic criteria applied. We suggest discriminating IPNB from papillary cholangiocarcinoma based on the histologic architecture (fig. 6-1). IPNB has

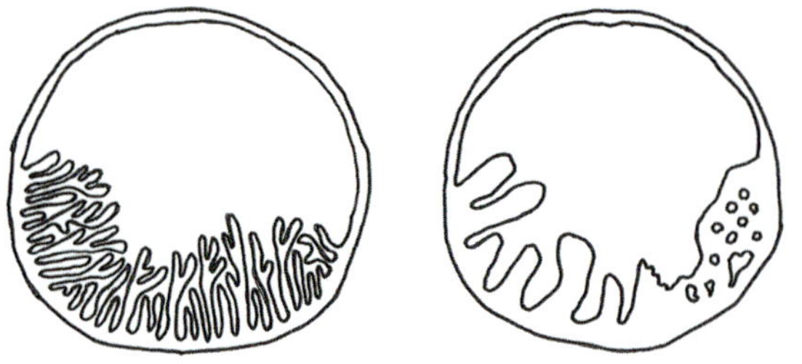

Figure 6-1

INTRADUCTAL PAPILLARY NEOPLASM OF BILE DUCT (IPNB) AND PAPILLARY CHOLANGIOCARCINOMA

The papillary architecture is more organized in IPNB, while the cribriform or solid growth in the intraductal components is often seen in papillary cholangiocarcinoma.

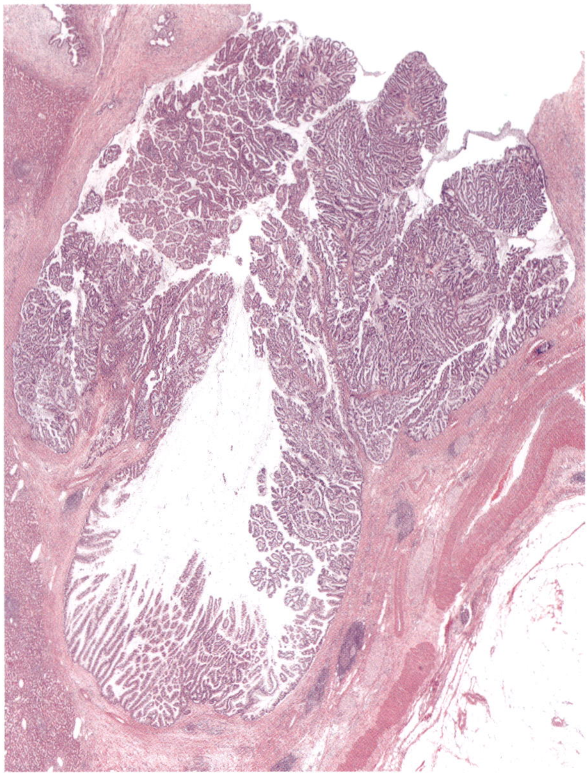

Figure 6-2

INTRADUCTAL PAPILLARY NEOPLASM OF THE BILE DUCT

The papillary architecture is well organized, with thin fibrous stalks.

well-organized papillary projections with delicate thin fibrovascular stalks, as described in the World Health Organization (WHO) classification (fig. 6-2) (3). If the papillary architecture is more complex, with thick fibrovascular stalks, solid tubular areas, or comedo-type necrosis, papillary cholangiocarcinoma may be a more appropriate diagnostic term (fig. 6-3) (17a).

Based on these stringent criteria, one third of biliary papillary tumors are classified as IPNB, with the remaining two thirds being papillary cholangiocarcinoma (17a). These two categories appear to differ in some clinicopathologic parameters. Most IPNBs are located in the liver (60 percent), followed by the hilar ducts (35 percent) and extrahepatic bile ducts (5 percent). These proportions are completely opposite in papillary cholangiocarcinoma because the majority of tumors develop in either the extrahepatic (80 percent) or hilar (15 to 20 percent)bile ducts, and intrahepatic papillary cholangiocarcinoma is uncommon (less than 5 percent) (17a). Approximately 50 percent of IPNBs are noninvasive, while papillary cholangiocarcinoma is usually associated with an invasive carcinoma at the time of diagnosis. The overproduction of mucin is more common in IPNB than in papillary cholangiocarcinoma (72 versus 7 percent) (17a).

Clinical Features. Patients are typically more than 40 years of age; however, in occasional cases, particularly those with hepatolithiasis or liver flukes, patients have been diagnosed with IPNB in their 30s (12,13). IPNB occurs more frequently in men than in women, with a male to female ratio of 2 to 1. Common presenting manifestations include abdominal pain, jaundice, fever, and elevations in liver function tests. CA19-9 is elevated in approximately 50 percent of patients, including in noninvasive (35 percent) and invasive cases (60 percent). Although carcinoembryonic antigen (CEA) is elevated in only 16 percent of patients, this increase is more specific to invasive IPNB (12).

The imaging features of IPNB include an intraductal papillary mass, bile duct dilatation, and mucobilia (18). Intraductal papillary masses, which are detectable in most cases (19), range from a small localized lesion to a widespread tumor involving multiple segments of the liver (fig. 6-4). Dilatation of the affected bile ducts is a nearly consistent feature (19). Some

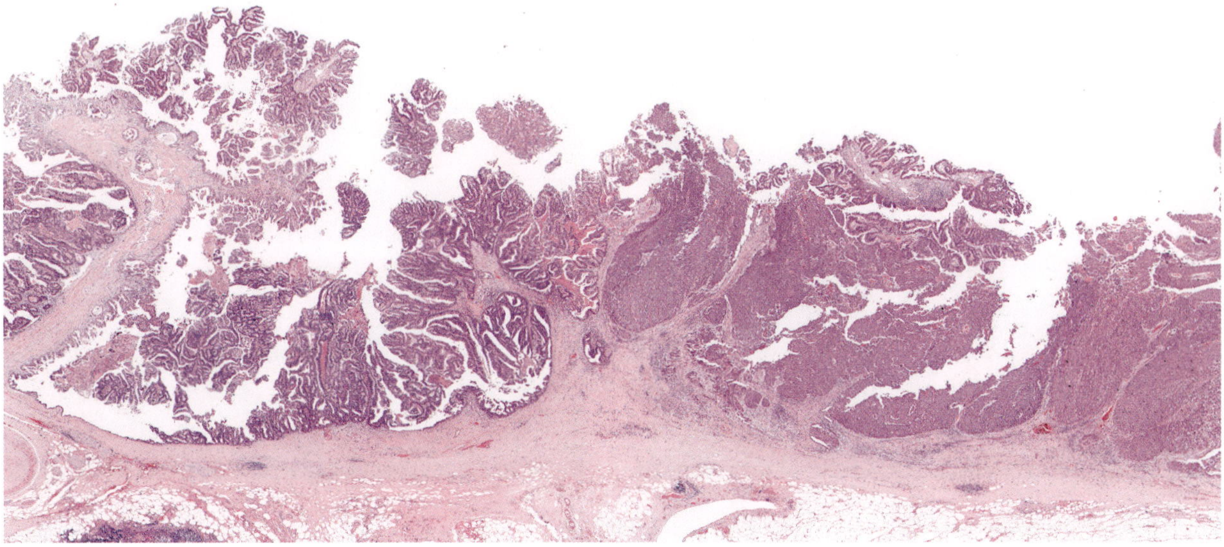

Figure 6-3

PAPILLARY CHOLANGIOCARCINOMA

The papillary architecture is complex, with cribriform or solid foci.

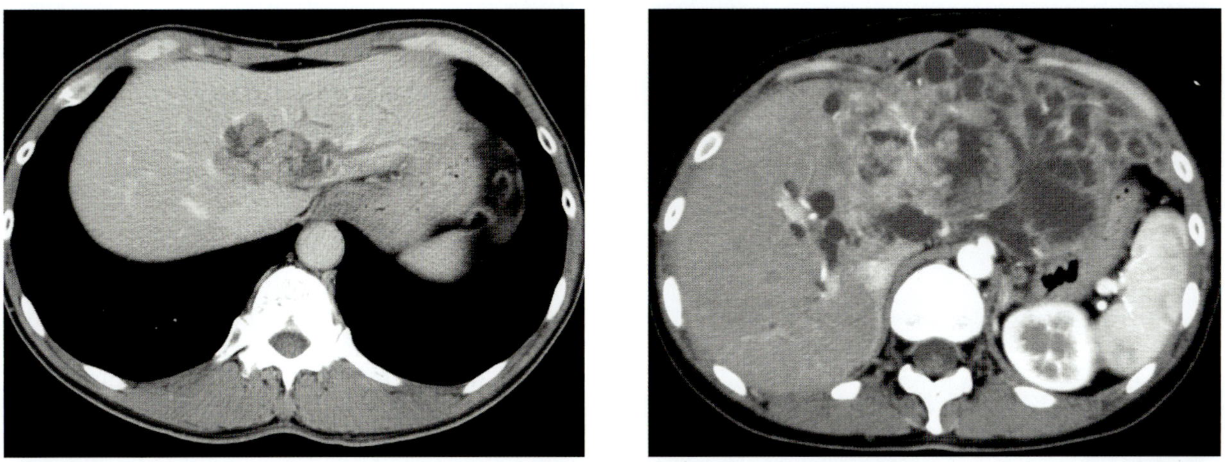

Figure 6-4

INTRADUCTAL PAPILLARY NEOPLASM OF THE BILE DUCT

Left: On computerized tomography (CT) imaging, the large bile ducts are dilated by an intraductal papillary tumor. Right: The bile ducts in the left lobe show extensive dilatation with intraductal papillary masses.

cases show large cystic dilatation of the affected ducts (cystic IPNB), often leading to the imaging diagnosis of a cystic neoplasm (fig. 6-5) (20). Radiologic evidence of bile duct communication contributes to the differentiation of IPNB from mucinous cystic neoplasm (MCN) because the latter typically forms a cystic mass independent of the biliary tree (fig. 6-6) (21,22). Amorphous floating filling defects, consistent with thick mucin, are often noted in the bile duct (23). In some cases, mucin extrudes from the ampulla of Vater, similar to cases of pancreatic IPMN. The presence of a solid or mucinous nodular mass in the liver parenchyma suggests an association with an invasive malignancy.

Multiple lesions rarely occur simultaneously or metachronously in the biliary tree (1). In rare cases, in which papillary tumors develop in the

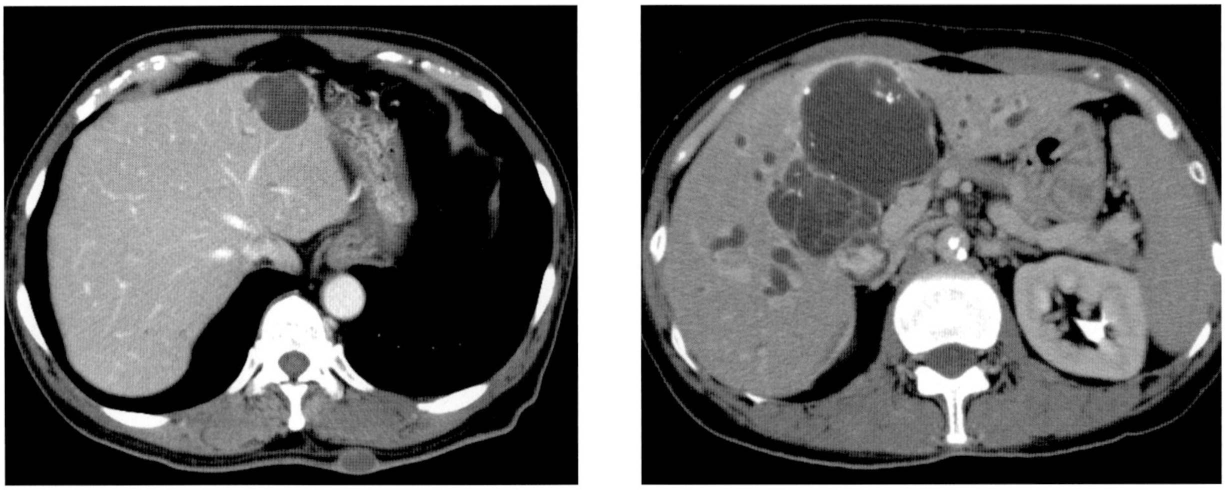

Figure 6-5

INTRADUCTAL PAPILLARY NEOPLASM OF THE BILE DUCT

Left: On CT, localized cystic dilatation of the bile duct by a papillary tumor is noted. Right: The extensive cystic dilatation of the bile ducts resembles a cystic neoplasm.

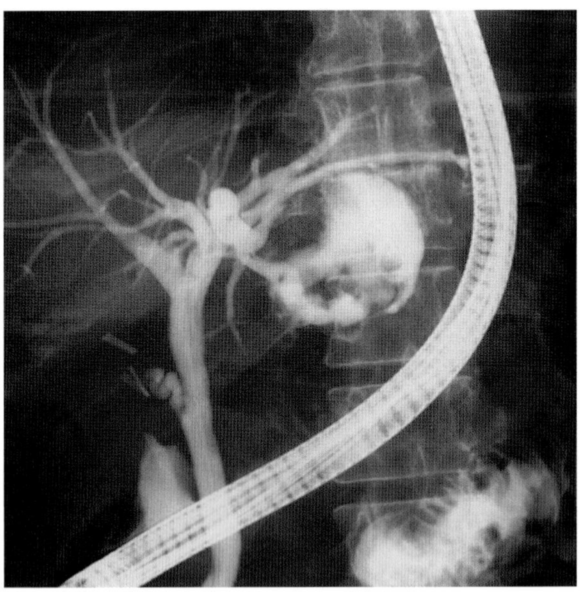

Figure 6-6

INTRADUCTAL PAPILLARY NEOPLASM OF THE BILE DUCT

Endoscopic retrograde cholangiogram confirms the luminal communication between the bile duct and the cystic space.

residual biliary mucosa several years after complete resection of the primary IPNB, difficulties are still associated with determining whether the second tumor is another primary IPNB or intraductal metastasis/dissemination of the original tumor (23a). Tissue comparisons with immunohistochemical and genetic analyses may be useful, but sometimes lead to inconclusive results. IPNB generally develops from the surface lining epithelium of the large bile ducts, but also rarely occurs in the peribiliary glands (fig. 6-7) (24,25).

Gross Findings. IPNB ranges in size from 1 to 15 cm, with a median size of approximately 4 cm. IPNB may be grossly appreciated as a delicate papillary tumor filling the bile duct lumen (fig. 6-8). Its papillary projections are thin and fragile. Mucin may be present on the tumor surface or inside the dilated bile ducts (fig. 6-9). In addition to high papillary main tumors, lower granular projections may be present on the adjacent mucosa, suggesting lateral spread (22). When multiple papillary masses are present, extensive sampling is required in order to establish whether they are true separate neoplasms or a continuous lesion. In cases of cystic IPNB (fig. 6-10), it is important to identify bile duct communication for a differentiation from MCN; however, it is often challenging to grossly prove a connection to the adjacent bile ducts.

Similar to conventional cholangiocarcinoma, invasive adenocarcinomas that develop in IPNB create a solid fibrous mass involving the liver parenchyma or periductal connective tissue (fig. 6-11). Muconodular tumors are detected in cases of IPNB associated with an invasive mucinous carcinoma (fig. 6-12). Invasive nodular masses are typically present in the duct wall or adjacent liver parenchyma, but are also sometimes observed inside the papillary nodule (fig. 6-13).

Microscopic Findings. IPNB is characterized by a papillary proliferation of neoplastic epithelium along thin fibrovascular stalks (fig. 6-14). Although the pattern of proliferation varies among cases, it is relatively uniform among different areas of the same case. At least some neoplastic cells have intracytoplasmic mucin, which is highlighted by mucicarmine, high-iron diamine (HID), Alcian blue, and periodic acid–Schiff (PAS) after digestion with diastase stains (fig. 6-15). This is also true for cases that lack grossly visible mucin. Necrosis is rarely noted, even in noninvasive IPNB, and this may be due to preoperative intraductal interventions (i.e., stents).

In most cases, bile duct communication is demonstrated by a histologic transition from the non-neoplastic biliary epithelium to neoplastic cells. However, it may be less obvious, particularly in cystic IPNB. In these cases, the presence of peribiliary glands in the cyst wall suggests that the origin of the cyst is the dilated

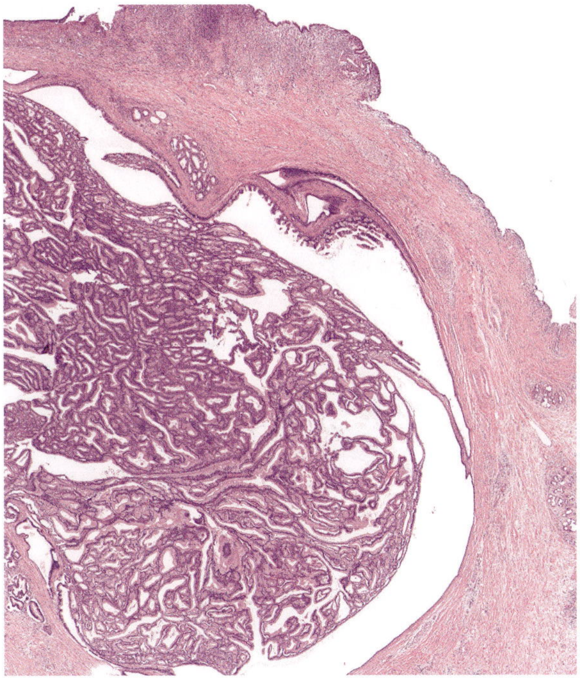

Figure 6-7

INTRADUCTAL PAPILLARY NEOPLASM OF THE BILE DUCT ARISING FROM PERIBILIARY GLANDS

The tumor is located within the duct wall. The surface mucosa of the bile duct (top) is not affected by the tumor.

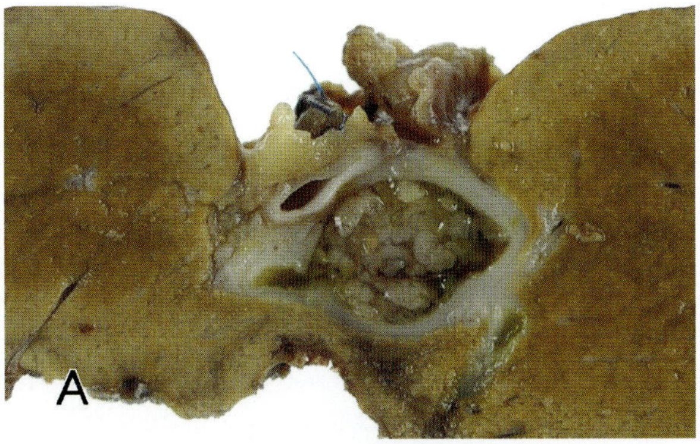

Figure 6-8

INTRADUCTAL PAPILLARY NEOPLASM OF THE BILE DUCT

A: The dilated bile duct contains a papillary tumor and abundant mucin.

B: Some of the dilated ducts are filled with papillary tumors.

C: A granular papillary tumor is noted in the dilated hilar bile duct.

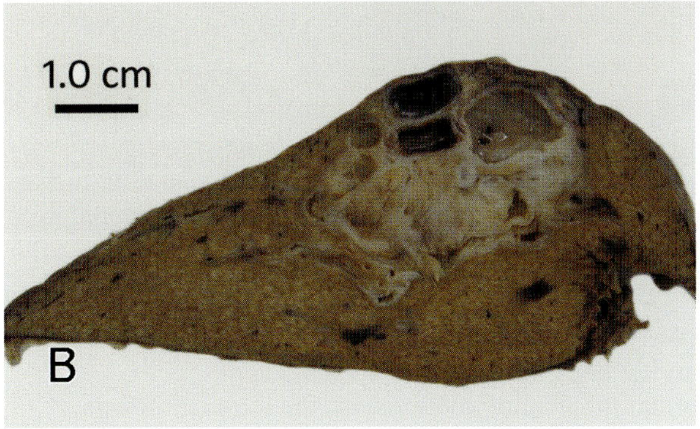

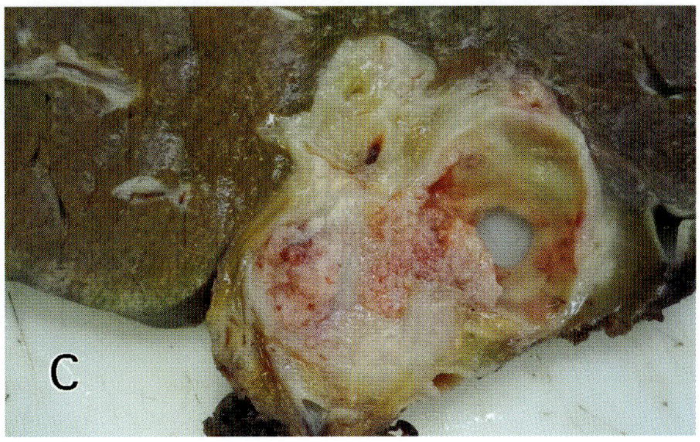

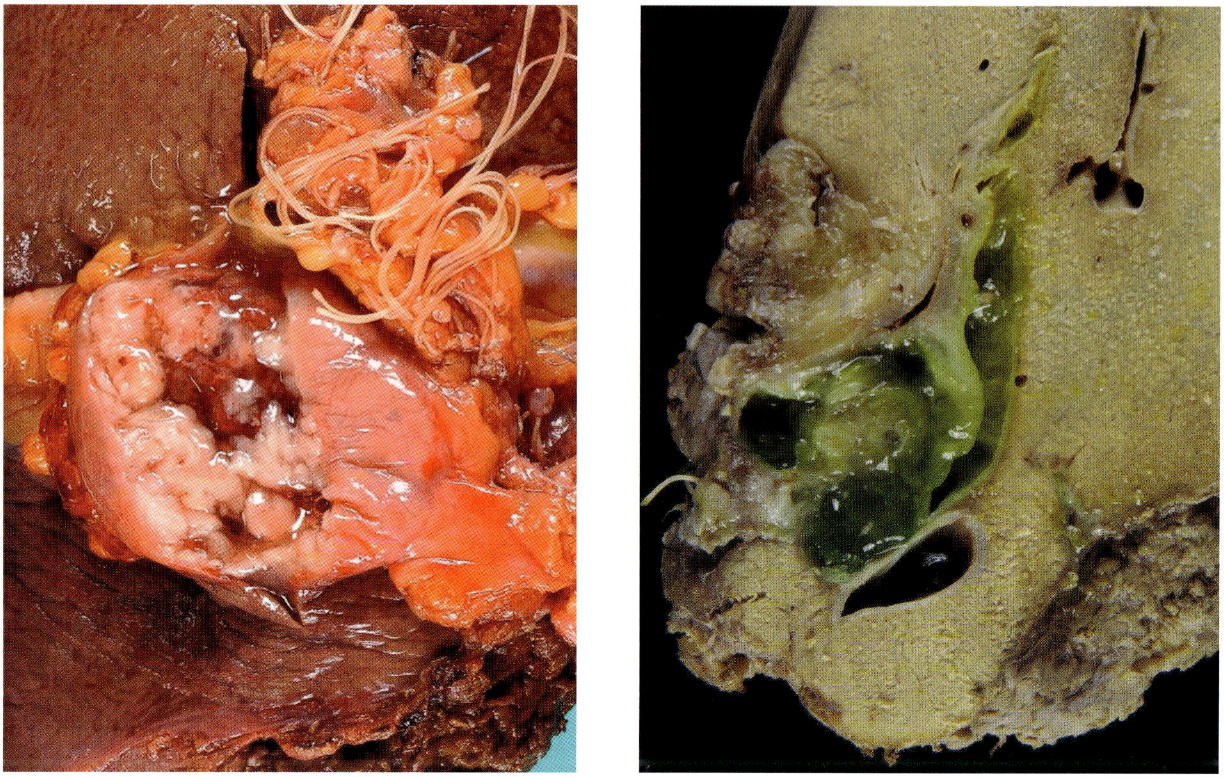

Figure 6-9

INTRADUCTAL PAPILLARY NEOPLASM OF THE BILE DUCT

Left: Abundant mucin is present around the tumor.
Right: Thick mucin is noted around the papillary tumor.

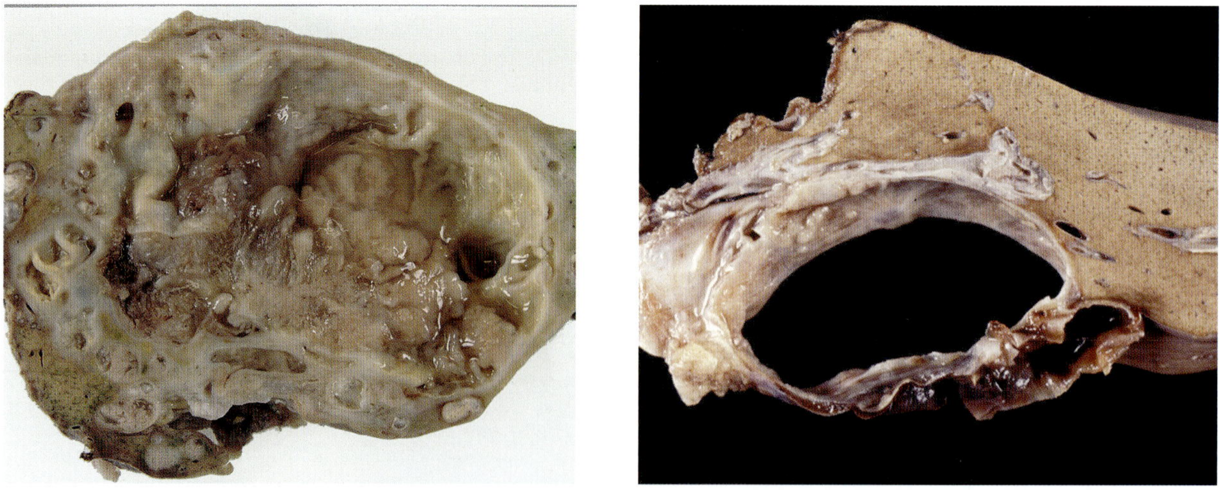

Figure 6-10

INTRADUCTAL PAPILLARY NEOPLASM OF THE BILE DUCT

Left: Papillary masses and abundant mucin are present in the cystically dilated bile ducts.
Right: The tumor is a unilocular cystic lesion. Small granular projections are noted on the luminal surface.

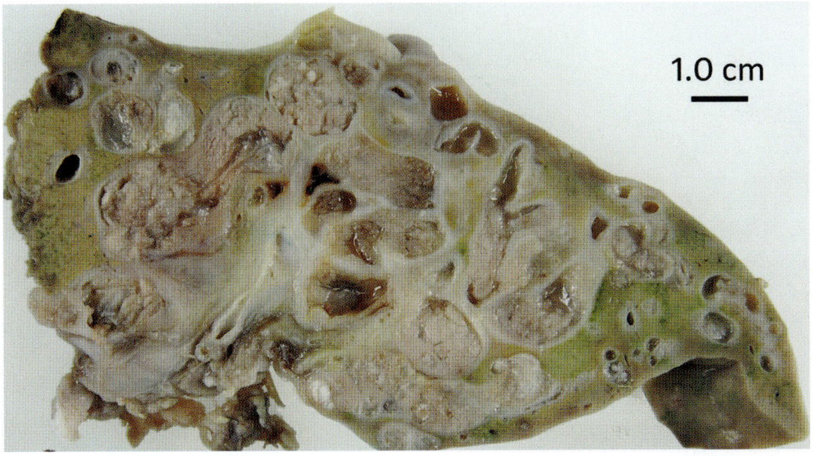

Figure 6-11

INTRADUCTAL PAPILLARY NEOPLASM OF THE BILE DUCT WITH INVASIVE CARCINOMA

A widespread papillary tumor is present within the bile ducts. Infiltrative adenocarcinoma was found in the fibrotic periductal connective tissue by microscopic examination.

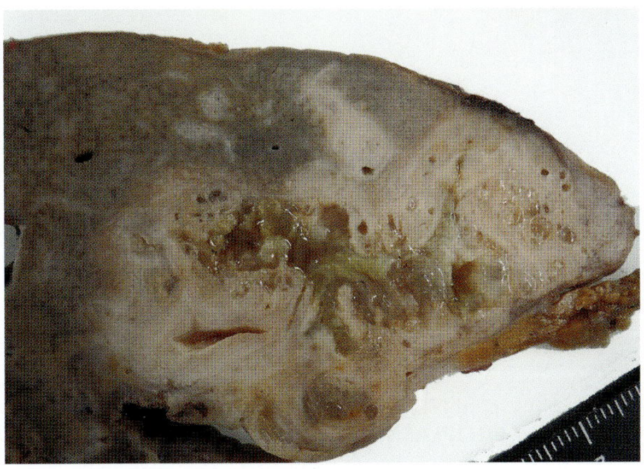

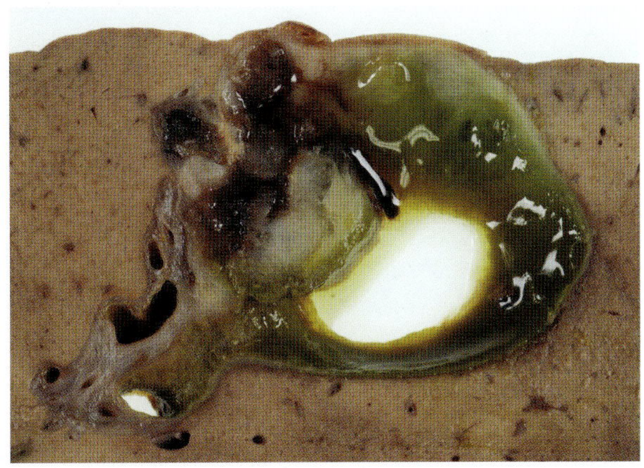

Figure 6-12

INTRADUCTAL PAPILLARY NEOPLASM OF THE BILE DUCT WITH INVASIVE MUCINOUS CARCINOMA

Muconodular areas around the dilated duct represent the invasive carcinoma.

Figure 6-13

INTRADUCTAL PAPILLARY NEOPLASM OF THE BILE DUCT WITH INVASIVE CARCINOMA

The invasive cancer was found in the intraductal mass by histologic examination.

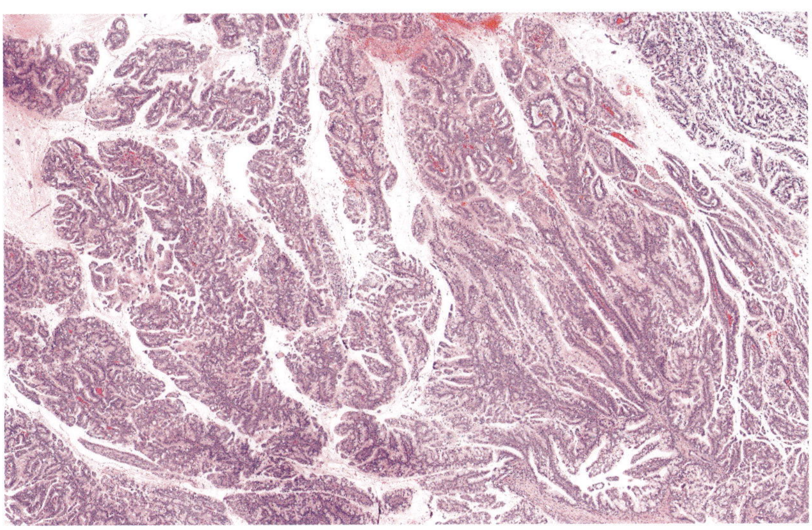

Figure 6-14

INTRADUCTAL PAPILLARY NEOPLASM OF THE BILE DUCT

The tumor cells are arranged in a high papillary architectural pattern with delicate fibrovascular stalks.

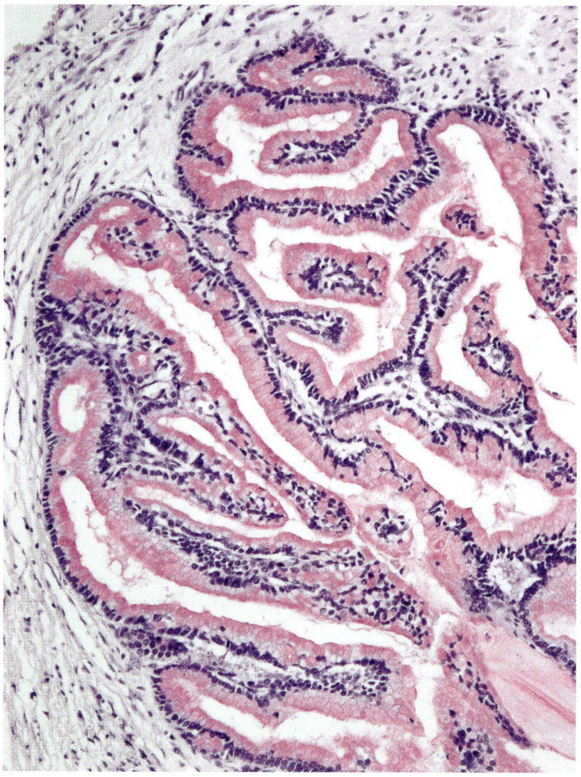

Figure 6-15

INTRADUCTAL PAPILLARY NEOPLASM OF THE BILE DUCT

The cytoplasm of the tumor cells is positive for mucin (mucicarmine stain).

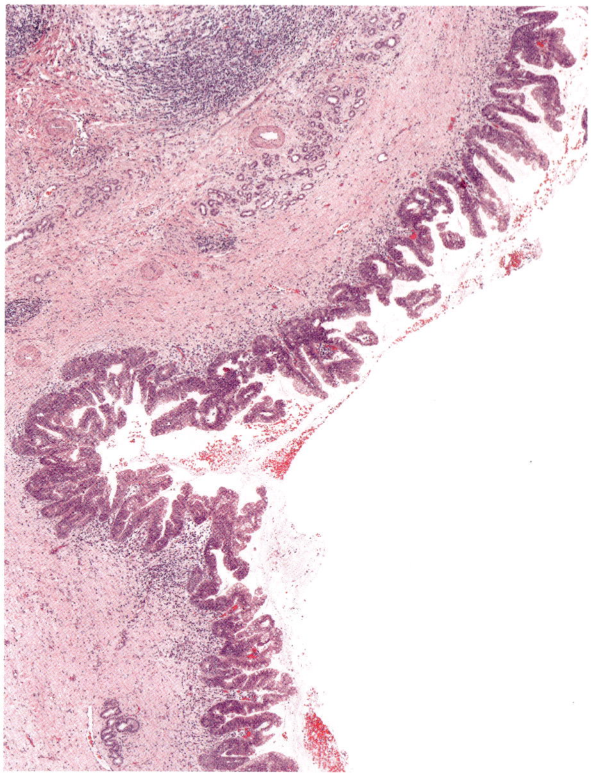

Figure 6-16

INTRADUCTAL PAPILLARY NEOPLASM OF THE BILE DUCT

Peribiliary glands are present in the cyst wall.

bile ducts (fig. 6-16) (5). Liver parenchyma entrapped in fibrous interlocular septa may be another histologic finding suggesting luminal communication to the bile duct (fig. 6-17).

IPNB has been classified into four types based on cellular differentiation, and the histologic types correlate with tumor grading (Table 6-1) (1,4,13,14). Although a grading system has not yet been established for IPNB, the classification scheme for pancreatic IPMN is generally used for the biliary counterpart (26). Noninvasive IPNB is graded into *low-*, *intermediate-*, or *high-grade dysplasia* based on structural and cellular atypia (Table 6-2) (3). As described above, most cases of IPNB have at least high-grade dysplasia, while low-grade dysplasia is less common.

The *pancreatobiliary type* is the most common (about 40 percent) and is characterized by the papillary proliferation of cuboidal or columnar neoplastic cells with round nuclei and eosinophilic cytoplasm (fig. 6-18A). Its cytologic features are similar to those of non-neoplastic biliary epithelium and conventional cholangiocarcinoma, and the degree of cellular atypia is generally less than that expected in invasive cholangiocarcinoma (fig. 6-18B). Fibrovascular stalks sometimes become edematous (fig. 6-18C). This change is commonly, but not exclusively, observed in the pancreatobiliary type. Foci of gastric foveolar or pyloric-gland differentiation may be present. Most cases of pancreatobiliary IPNB have at least high-grade dysplasia.

The *intestinal type* is the second most common histologic type (about 30 percent). Intestinal-type IPNB consists of columnar epithelium with elongated nuclei, nuclear stratification, and eosinophilic cytoplasm (fig. 6-19). Goblet cells are occasionally present. The proliferation pattern is high papillary and long villous, and its overall appearance is reminiscent of villous

Table 6-1

INCIDENCE, GRADE, AND IMMUNOPHENOTYPE OF FOUR HISTOLOGIC TYPES OF INTRADUCTAL PAPILLARY NEOPLASM OF THE BILE DUCT (IPNB)

	Incidence	Histologic Grade of Dysplasia			Immunohistochemistry			
		High	Intermed	Low	MUC1	MUC2	MUC5AC	MUC6
Pancreatobiliary	40%	100%	-	-	+	-	+	+
Intestinal	30%	90%	10%	-	-	+	+	-
Gastric	20%	70%	20%	10%	-	-	+	+/-
Oncocytic	10%	100%	-	-	+	-	+	+

Table 6-2

HISTOLOGIC GRADING OF INTRADUCTAL PAPILLARY NEOPLASM OF THE BILE DUCT

Low-grade dysplasia:
Papillary proliferation of the well-polarized single-layered epithelium. The cells have small uniform nuclei with only mild pleomorphism and rare mitoses.

Intermediate-grade dysplasia:
Well-organized papillary architecture, but the cells show nuclear stratification, crowding, and loss of polarity. The nuclei are enlarged and moderately hyperchromatic.

High-grade dysplasia:
Severe cytologic atypia. The cells lack polarity, and the nuclei are enlarged, hyperchromatic, and irregular in shape. Mitoses are frequently found.

adenoma of the colon. This type has a slightly lower histologic grade than the pancreatobiliary type, with cases occasionally classified as intermediate-grade dysplasia.

The *gastric type* (about 20 percent) is characterized by cellular differentiation similar to gastric foveolar epithelium. Histologically, differentiation is recognized by abundant intracytoplasmic mucin and basally located nuclei (fig. 6-20, left). In addition to the papillary architecture, the arrangement of tumor cells may be tubular, potentially representing pyloric-gland differentiation. The degree of cellular atypia is the least conspicuous among the four histologic types, with some cases graded as low-grade dysplasia. A transition from low-grade to high-grade areas can be found in individual cases (fig. 6-20, right).

The *oncocytic type* (about 10 percent) has unique cytologic features including abundant eosinophilic cytoplasm and centrally located round nuclei. The proliferation pattern of oncocytic IPNB is more complex than that of other histologic types (fig. 6-21, left). Cells are arranged in arborizing papillae, cribriform patterns, and solid nests (fig. 6-21, right). Despite the complex histologic architecture, oncocytic IPNB is regarded as a noninvasive neoplasm, unless convincing stromal invasion is identified

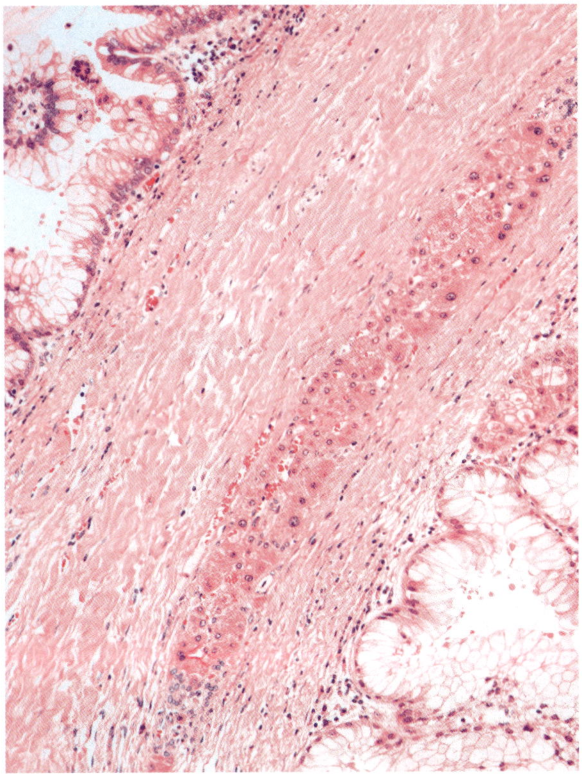

Figure 6-17

INTRADUCTAL PAPILLARY NEOPLASM OF THE BILE DUCT

The liver parenchyma is entrapped in the fibrous septum between neoplastic cystic spaces.

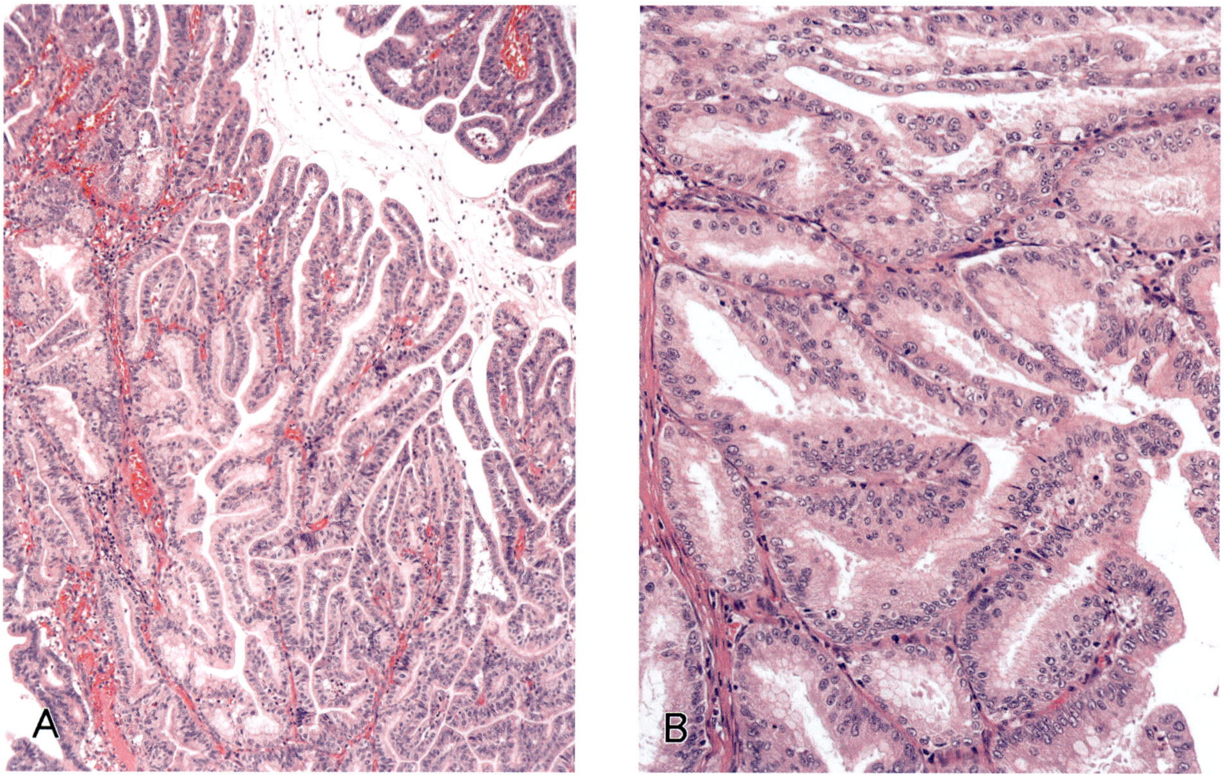

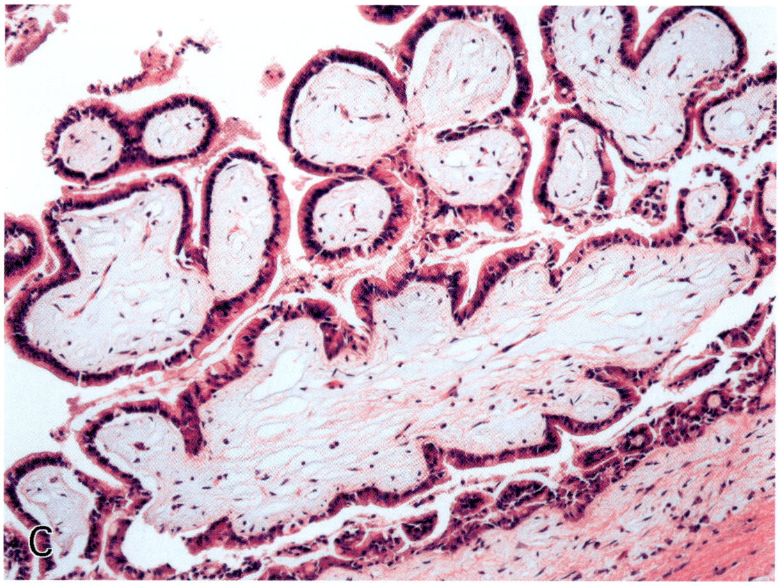

Figure 6-18

INTRADUCTAL PAPILLARY NEOPLASM OF THE BILE DUCT OF PANCREATOBILIARY TYPE

A: Columnar tumor cells with eosinophilic cytoplasm are arranged in a papillary architecture.

B: The tumor cells have eosinophilic cytoplasm and round nuclei.

C: Thick and edematous fibrovascular stalks are present.

in the bile duct wall. Although its histologic architecture is complex, this tumor has been categorized as IPNB since the extensive oncocytic change is not a feature of conventional cholangiocarcinoma. There may be coexisting components of other classic histologic types, typically pancreatobiliary or gastric types, which is another reason why this tumor belongs to the spectrum of IPNB. Similar to the pancreatobiliary type, the oncocytic type displays sufficient cytoarchitectural atypia to be regarded as high-grade dysplasia.

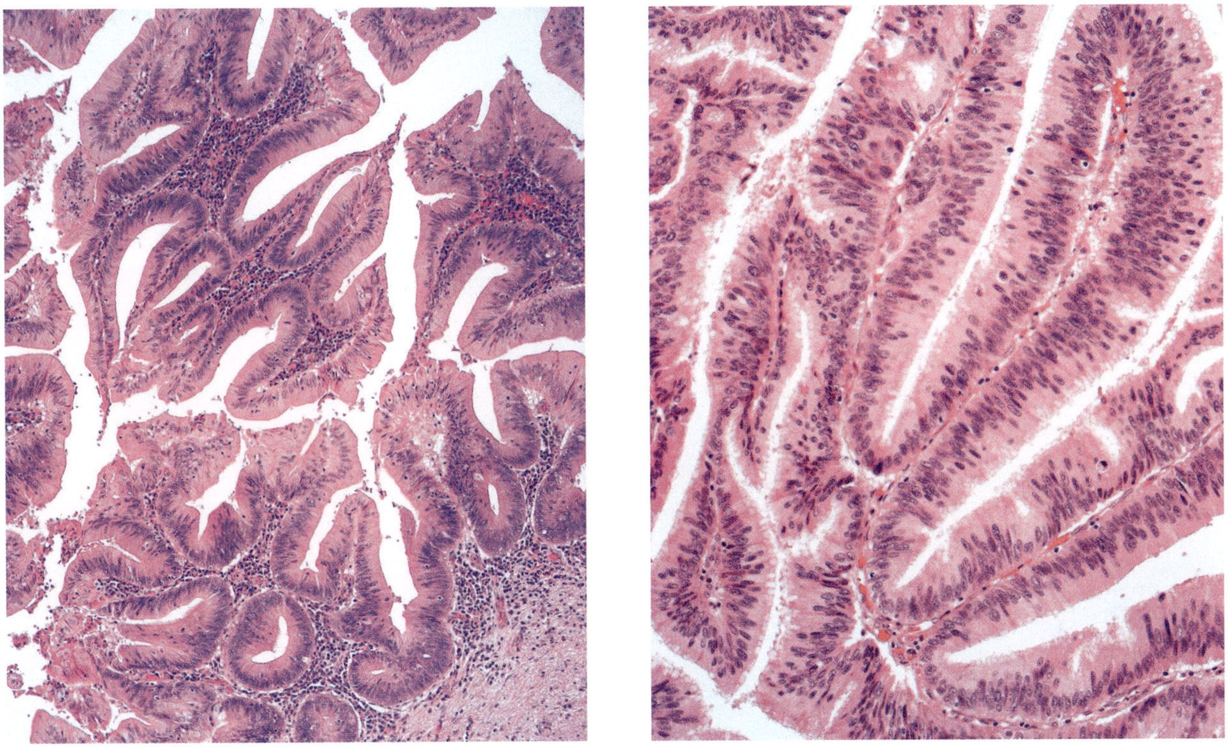

Figure 6-19

INTRADUCTAL PAPILLARY NEOPLASM OF THE BILE DUCT OF INTESTINAL TYPE

Left: The tumor resembles villous adenoma of the colon.
Right: The tumor cells are columnar, with elongated nuclei and nuclear stratification.

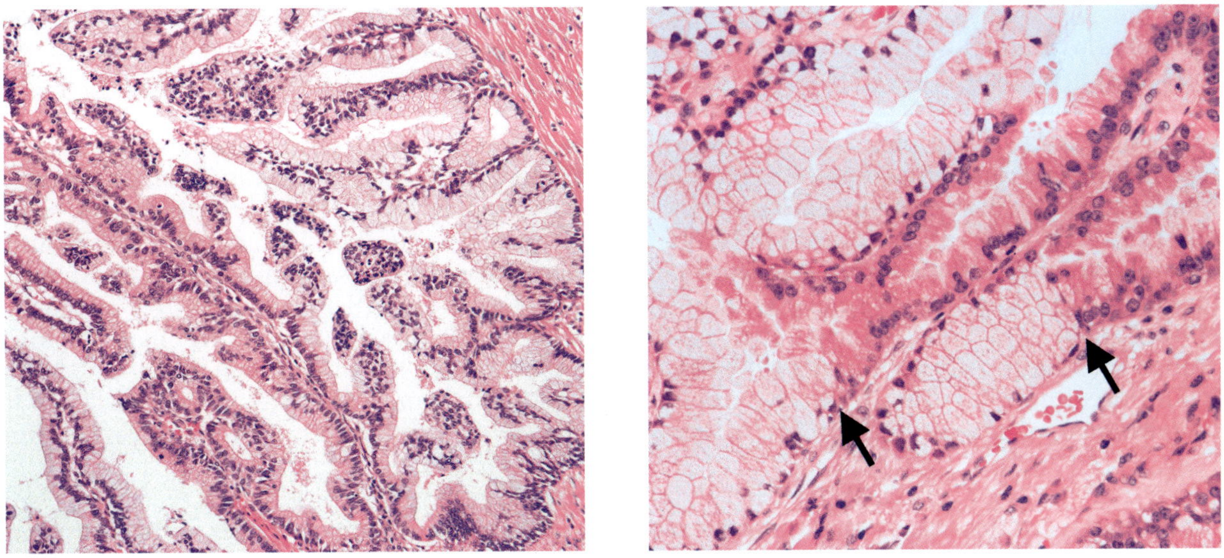

Figure 6-20

INTRADUCTAL PAPILLARY NEOPLASM OF THE BILE DUCT OF GASTRIC TYPE

Left: Mucinous tumor cells are arranged in a papillary architecture.
Right: The tumor cells have abundant intracytoplasmic mucin. A transition from low-grade to high-grade dysplasia is seen (arrows).

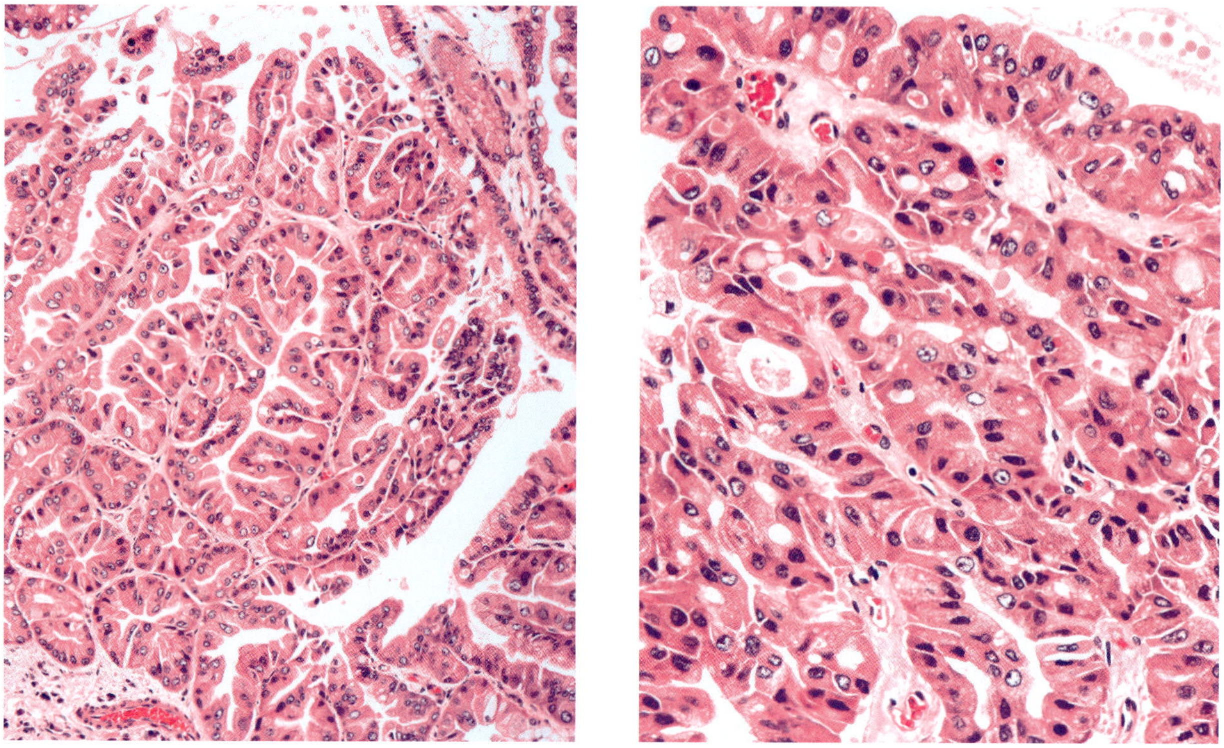

Figure 6-21

INTRADUCTAL PAPILLARY NEOPLASM OF THE BILE DUCT OF ONCOCYTIC TYPE

Left: The cuboidal tumor cells with eosinophilic cytoplasm are arranged in a tubulopapillary architecture. Right: The tumor cells have eosinophilic cytoplasm and centrally located nuclei.

In previous studies, the proportion of IPNBs associated with invasive cancer ranged from 31 to 74 percent (1,2,4,9,12–14,27). Approximately 50 percent have an associated invasive adenocarcinoma at the initial presentation. The two types of invasive cancer that develop in IPNB are tubular adenocarcinoma and mucinous carcinoma (1,2,4,9,12–14,27). Progression in the former is more common, and the histologic features of invasive cancers are basically similar to those of conventional cholangiocarcinoma (fig. 6-22). Tumor cells form irregular tubules embedded in fibrotic stroma and show infiltrative growth. Progression to mucinous carcinoma is frequently observed in intestinal-type IPNB. In the invasive area, tumor cells float in extracellular mucin (fig. 6-23). Mucinous carcinoma should be distinguished from acellular mucin ("mucous lake"), which reflects the spillage of mucin into the stroma due to the rupture of ducts. Tubular and mucinous adenocarcinomas are intermixed in some cases.

Frozen Sections. A frozen section diagnosis is often considered for patients with suspected IPNB for several reasons. One reason is establishing a diagnosis. Difficulties are commonly associated with determining whether an intraductal mass is neoplastic prior to surgery, particularly when the patient has chronic cholangiopathy (i.e., intrahepatic stones and liver flukes). A gross examination is important, with the most suspicious area being sampled. In addition to the sample from the "mass" lesion, sections from the transitional area to the adjacent mucosa are also useful sometimes. Even if the degree of cellular atypia is not severe, the high-papillary architecture favors a neoplastic nature over a hyperplastic process.

Another common scenario is that a frozen section diagnosis is requested for cystic lesions, for which cystic IPNB, MCN, and degenerated simple cysts are included in the differential diagnosis. In these cases, the internal surface with preserved mucosa needs to be sampled because

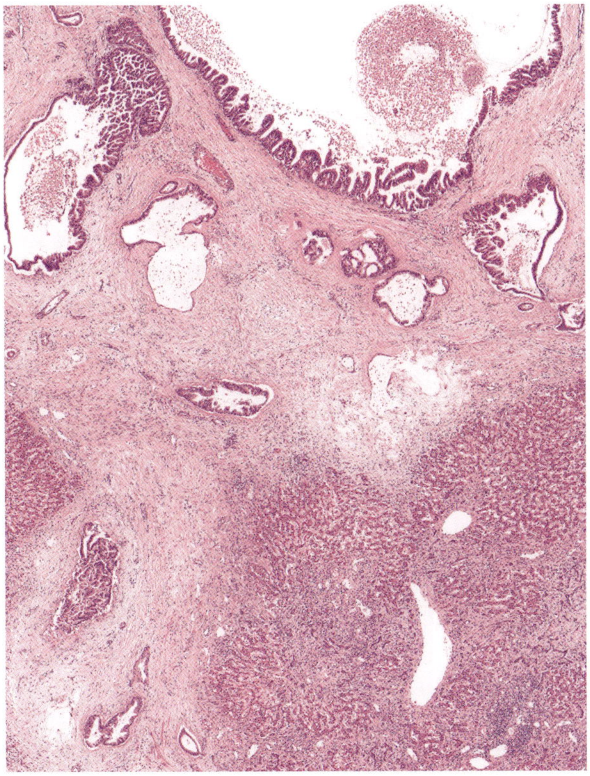

Figure 6-22

INTRADUCTAL PAPILLARY NEOPLASM OF THE BILE DUCT WITH INVASIVE TUBULAR ADENOCARCINOMA

A tubular adenocarcinoma infiltrates along the periportal connective tissue.

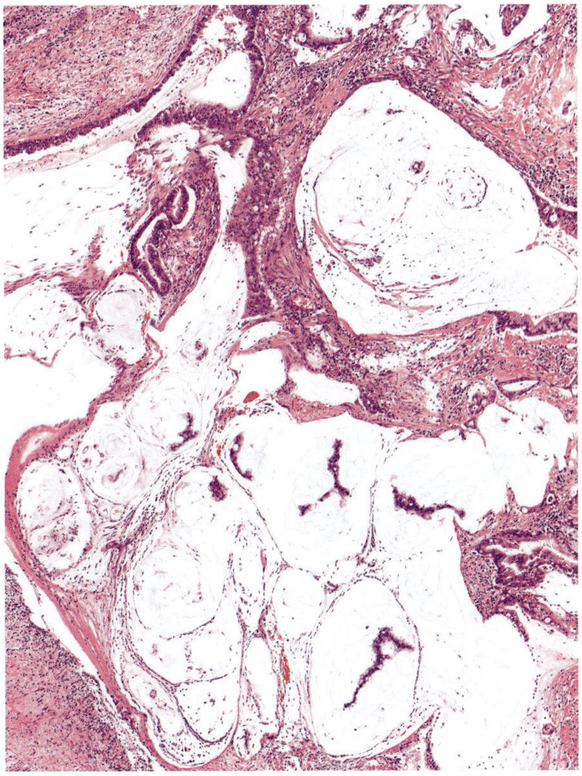

Figure 6-23

INTRADUCTAL PAPILLARY NEOPLASM OF THE BILE DUCT WITH INVASIVE MUCINOUS CARCINOMA

The tumor cells produce abundant mucin, and some of the cells float in the mucin.

erosive areas are often not diagnostic. The histologic features that are useful in this setting are described below (Differential Diagnosis).

It may be more challenging to assess the presence or absence of an invasive malignancy in patients with IPNB from a frozen section examination. Multiple samples need to be taken from the dominant mass. Even if there is no conclusive evidence of an invasive malignancy in the sections, sampling errors are always a possibility because of small invasive foci. It is also important to note that IPNB commonly shows lateral spread along the biliary tree (fig. 6-24). At the spreading ends, the proliferation pattern may become low-papillary or even flat. Therefore, a microscopic examination at the bile duct margin may be required during surgery in some cases.

Immunohistochemical Findings. Most cases of IPNB diffusely express cytokeratins and label with CAM5.2 and AE1/AE3. Although biliary cytokeratins such as CK7, CK8, CK18, and CK19 are also typically positive, their expression may be weak and focal (1,6). CK20, an intestinal-type molecule, can be expressed focally, particularly in intestinal-type IPNB (6).

Immunostaining for mucin core proteins (MUCs) is useful for determining histologic type. MUC2 as well as CDX2 are commonly expressed in the intestinal type (Table 6-1) (4, 6,14). Intestinal-type IPNB rarely consists predominantly of goblet cells, and its appearance is somewhat resembles the gastric type (fig. 6-25, left). In these cases, immunostaining for MUC2 is useful for proving intestinal differentiation (fig. 6-25, right). MUC1 is detected in 30 to 40 percent of IPNBs, typically invasive cases (4,6,14). MUC5AC, a gastric mucin, is expressed in 90 percent of cases, irrespective of histologic type (fig. 6-26); therefore, the expression of MUC5AC alone is not sufficient for identifying gastric differentiation.

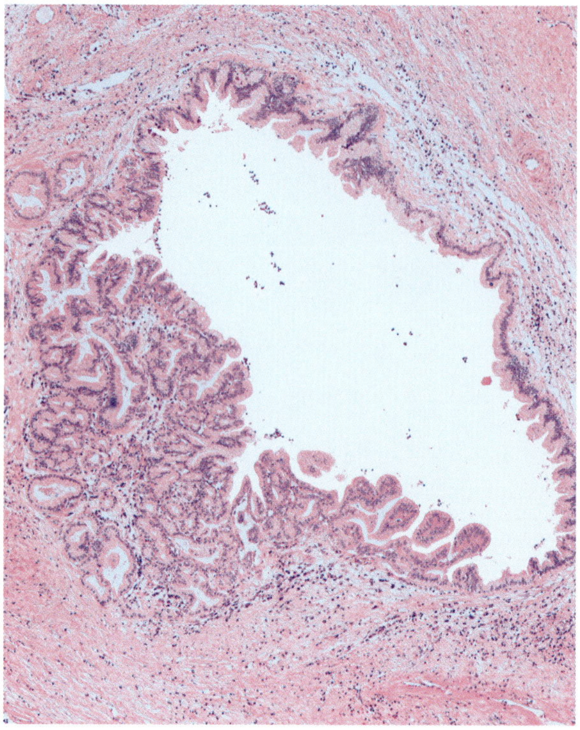

Figure 6-24

INTRADUCTAL PAPILLARY NEOPLASM OF THE BILE DUCT

A tumor extending into the septal bile duct shows a low-papillary architecture.

Ultrastructural Findings. Neoplastic cells are tightly connected by junctional complexes. These cells have microvilli and also contain apical and cytoplasmic mucin. In oncocytic IPNB, numerous mitochondria are packed in the cytoplasm. Ultrastructural examinations are rarely considered for the diagnosis of IPNB.

Cytologic Findings. Cytologic samples are obtained by biliary brushing or bile cytology. Difficulties are associated with establishing a specific diagnosis of IPNB based on cytologic findings because neither the papillary architecture nor mucin production is specific for IPNB. However, the presence of a mucinous epithelium against the background of abundant amounts of mucin suggests IPNB over conventional cholangiocarcinoma in appropriate clinical settings (fig. 6-27). Radiologic and pathologic correlation is also useful, given that most cases of IPNB have a papillary mass in dilated bile ducts, which is an uncommon imaging feature in conventional cholangiocarcinoma.

Approximately 90 percent of IPNBs have at least high-grade dysplasia. Cellular atypia can be easily appreciated in most cases. Cells arranged in large papillae, small clusters, or individual cells display nuclear crowding, the loss of polarity with piled-up nuclei, and

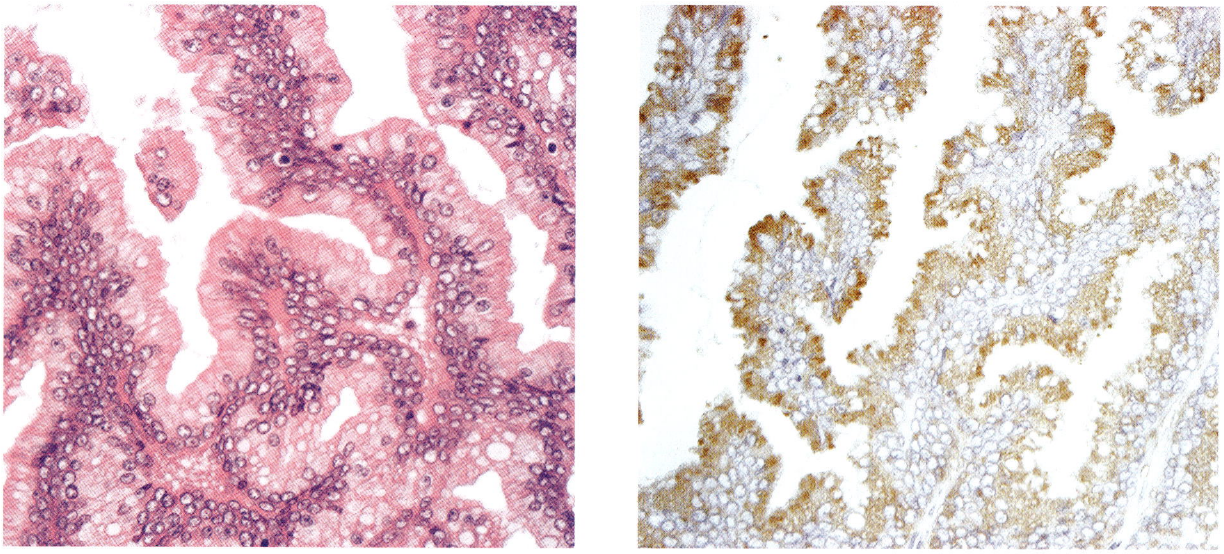

Figure 6-25

INTRADUCTAL PAPILLARY NEOPLASM OF THE BILE DUCT OF INTESTINAL TYPE

Left: The tumor consists of many mucous cells, an appearance reminiscent of the gastric type. Right: MUC2 expression in mucinous tumor cells is consistent with the intestinal differentiation.

hyperchromasia (figs. 6-28–6-30). The presence of necrosis may suggest an association with an invasive malignancy.

Molecular Genetic Findings. *KRAS* mutations have been confirmed in up to 30 percent of IPNB cases (14,28–30). This genetic alteration is also observed to a similar extent in histologic types other than the oncocytic type, in which *KRAS* is generally the wild type (14). Since *GNAS* mutations at codon 201 have been identified as a genetic event highly specific to IPMN among pancreatic neoplasms (31,32), previous studies examined the *GNAS* status in IPNB. However, the findings obtained have been highly controversial. Two studies from the United States and Europe showed *GNAS* mutations in a single case each (2 to 3 percent of all cases) (14,29), while two Asian studies suggested that *GNAS* was mutated in 30 to 50 percent of IPNB cases, particularly intestinal-type cases (28,30). Although differences in underlying etiopathogenetic factors such as incidence of hepatolithiasis and liver

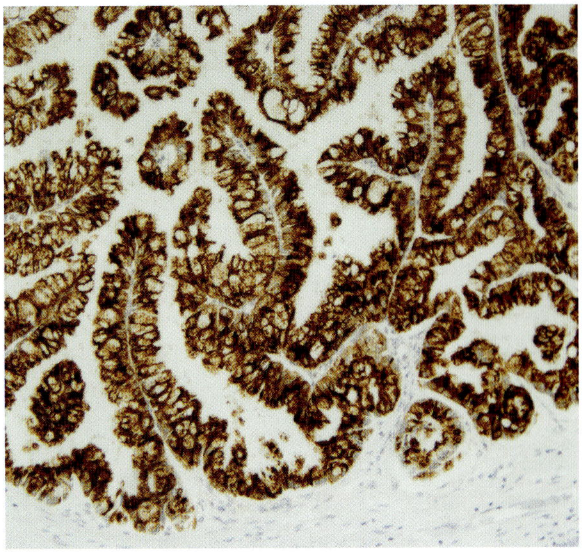

Figure 6-26

INTRADUCTAL PAPILLARY NEOPLASM OF THE BILE DUCT

MUC5AC is diffusely expressed in tumor cells.

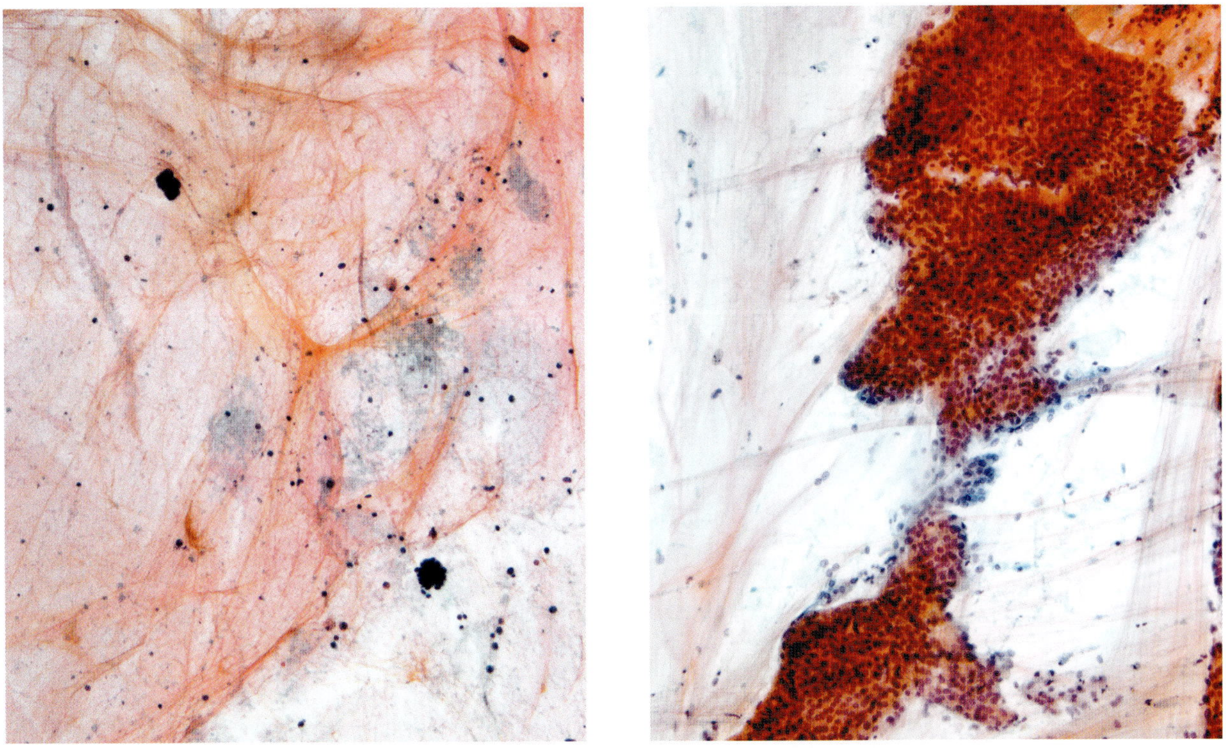

Figure 6-27

INTRADUCTAL PAPILLARY NEOPLASM OF THE BILE DUCT

Left: Epithelial clusters are present against the abundant mucin (bile cytology).
Right: Large epithelial clusters are present in abundant mucin (biliary brushing).

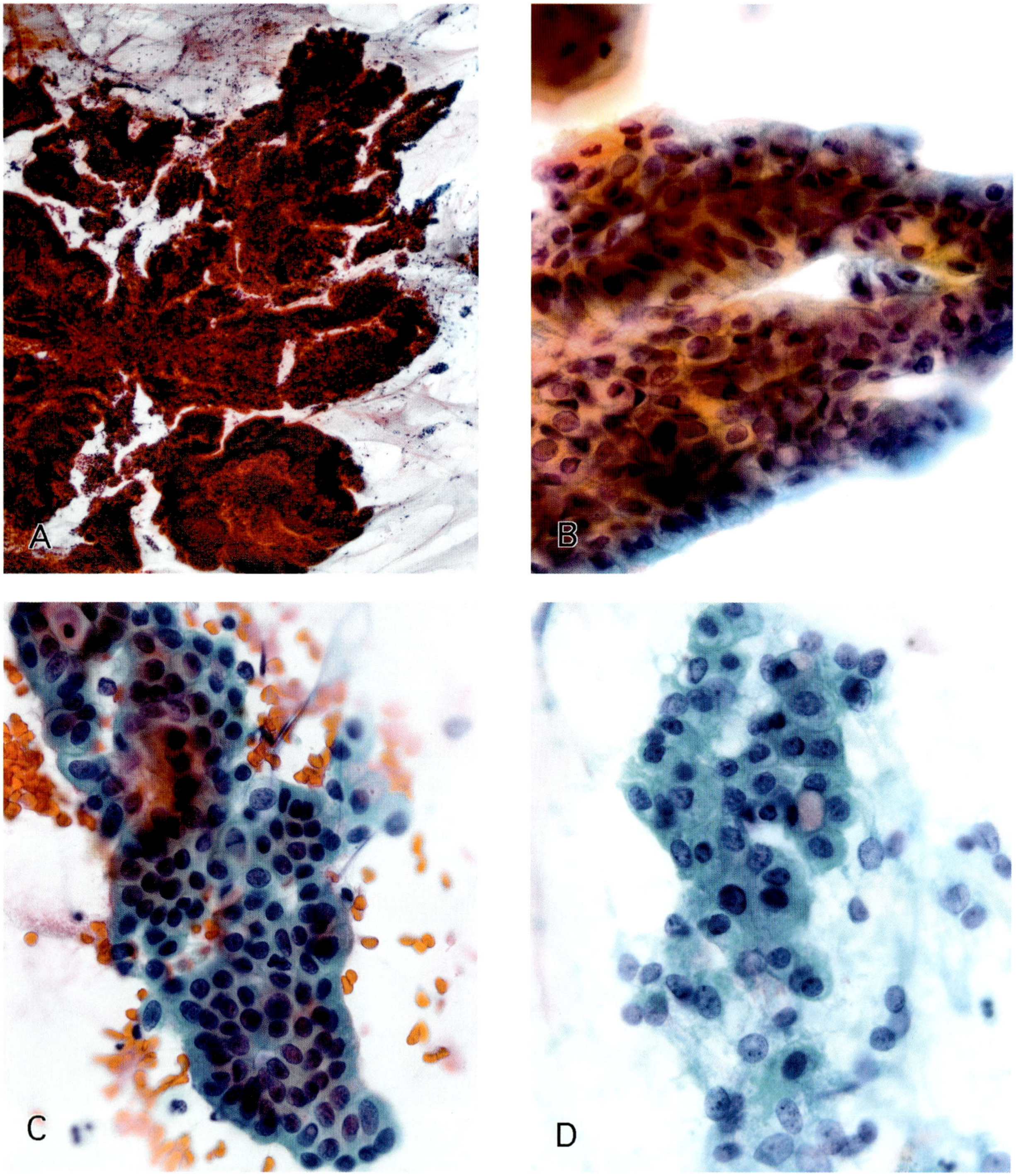

Figure 6-28

INTRADUCTAL PAPILLARY NEOPLASM OF THE BILE DUCT WITH HIGH-GRADE DYSPLASIA

A: A large papillary epithelial cluster is present (biliary brushing).

B: The atypical cells show increased cellularity, enlarged nuclei, and intracytoplasmic mucin (biliary brushing).

C: The cells display hyperchromasia, nuclear enlargement, and slight disturbance of cellular polarity (biliary brushing).

D: The cells show moderate disturbance of cellular polarity. Some of the cells have intracytoplasmic mucin (biliary brushing).

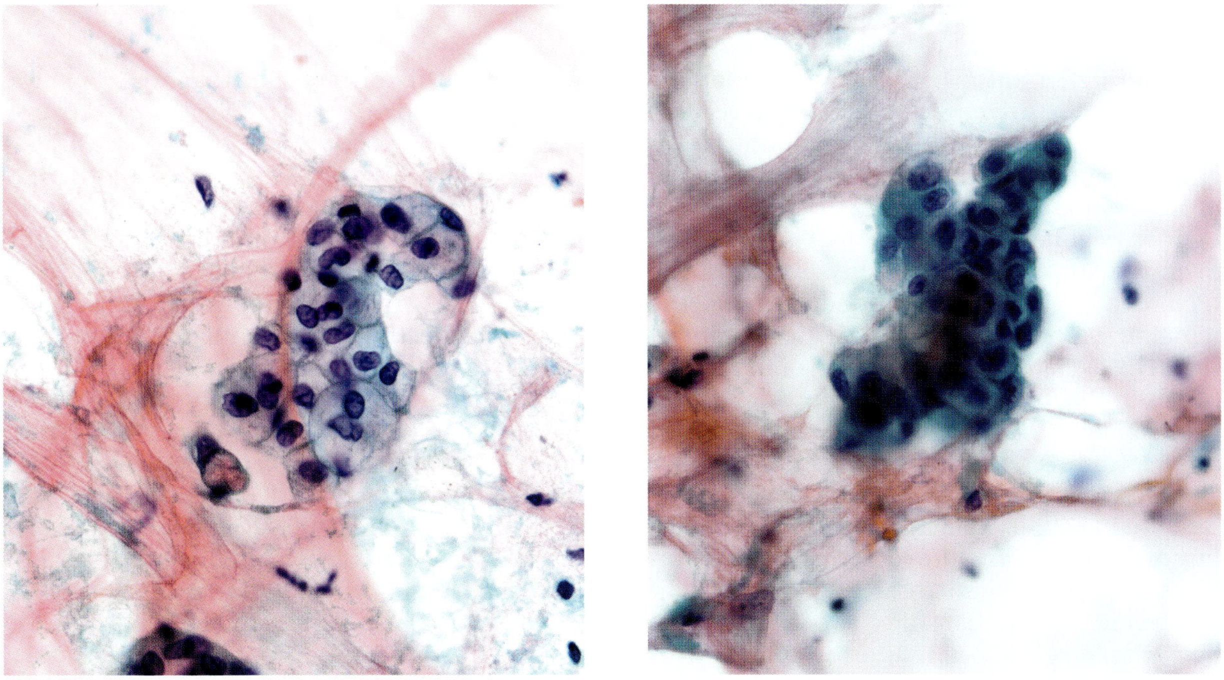

Figure 6-29

INTRADUCTAL PAPILLARY NEOPLASM OF THE BILE DUCT WITH HIGH-GRADE DYSPLASIA

Left: The dysplastic cells with loss of polarity are found against the background of mucin (biliary brushing).

Right: The cells have nuclear crowding, hyperchromasia, and moderate pleomorphism. Occasional cells have intracytoplasmic mucin (biliary brushing).

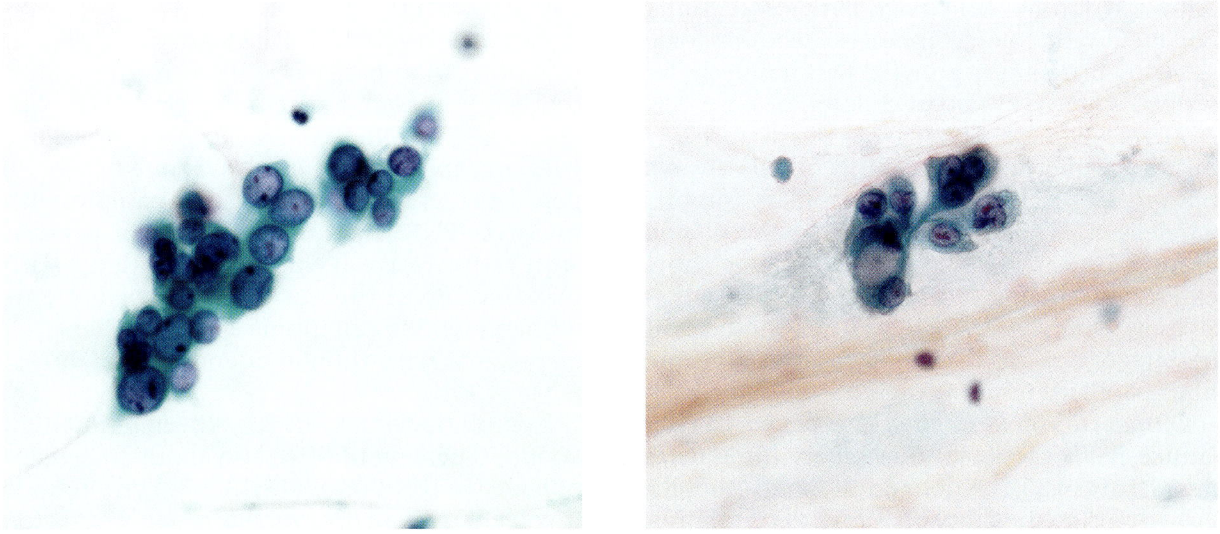

Figure 6-30

INTRADUCTAL PAPILLARY NEOPLASM OF THE BILE DUCT WITH HIGH-GRADE DYSPLASIA

Left: The small epithelial cluster shows nuclear clearing and irregularity in nuclear size. The appearance is similar to conventional cholangiocarcinoma (bile cytology).

Right: Slightly degenerated atypical cells have an irregular nuclear membrane and intracytoplasmic mucin (bile cytology).

flukes between the regions may partly explain this discrepancy, further studies are needed in order to determine whether *GNAS* mutations are among the driver genetic events in IPNB.

The expression of p21, p53, and cyclin D1 is gradually upregulated during the progression of IPNB, whereas that of SMAD/DPC4 and p16 is downregulated (33). The loss of p16 and overexpression of p53 are early events in the IPNB-cholangiocarcinoma sequence, while the remaining molecules show step-wise alterations (14). The overall alteration pattern of these molecules in IPNB is similar to that in the progression model of BilIN; the early overexpression of p53, however, is not detected in BilIN (33).

A previous study revealed high-level microsatellite instability (allelic shifts in at least two out of five microsatellite loci) in 12 percent of cases and low-level microsatellite instability in 35 percent (34). In that study, two cases of IPNB had extensive microsatellite instability, with allelic shifts in five out of the five and four out of the five microsatellite markers examined. Although the same microsatellite markers were shifted in the intraductal and invasive components, the pattern of allelic shifts was not always identical, suggesting significant genetic heterogeneity within these neoplasms (34).

Differential Diagnosis. IPNB needs to be discriminated from papillary cholangiocarcinoma and metastatic colorectal cancer predominantly showing intrabiliary growth. This has been described above and also in chapter 7.

Micropapillary BilIN. Another histologic mimic is micropapillary BilIN. IPNB always has grossly visible dominant papillary tumors, whereas BilIN consists basically of microscopic lesions. Unusual examples of BilIN may show extensive intraepithelial spread with no invasive malignancy (35). These cases should still be categorized as BilIN unless a grossly visible high-papillary tumor is present.

Intraductal tubulopapillary neoplasm (ITPN). Unlike IPNB, ITPN, another biliary intraductal neoplasm (36,37), predominantly shows tubular growth inside the duct. MUC5AC is commonly expressed in IPNB, while ITPN lacks such expression by definition (36,37). Gross mucin is not a feature of ITPN. However, it may be difficult to discriminate these two neoplasms using small biopsy samples.

Mucinous Cystic Neoplasm (MCN). Cystic IPNB needs to be discriminated from MCN. Features useful for this differential diagnosis include histologic evidence of an ovarian-like stroma and bile duct communication. A general rule is that IPNB lacks an ovarian-like stroma and has biliary connections, while MCN has an ovarian-like stroma and no communication to the bile ducts (5,38). The presence or absence of an ovarian-like stroma is more important than a biliary connection because biliary communication is sometimes difficult to prove in IPNB and may be rarely observed in MCN due to inflammation or preoperative biliary intervention (i.e., drainage). In most MCN cases, cystic spaces are lined by a completely flat epithelium, but papillary tumors resembling IPNB may occasionally develop in MCN with high-grade dysplasia or an associated invasive carcinoma (38).

Treatment and Prognosis. Although rare examples of IPNB have only low-grade dysplasia, surgery needs to be considered in view of the high risk of malignant transformation. Approximately 50 percent of IPNBs are noninvasive at the time of diagnosis. In cases of unresectable or recurrent tumors, the treatment strategy needs to follow the guidelines for conventional cholangiocarcinoma. However, inoperable diseases at initial presentation are very uncommon in patients with IPNB.

Patients with IPNB have a significantly better prognosis than patients with conventional intrahepatic cholangiocarcinoma (1). Those with noninvasive IPNB have an excellent prognosis, with an expected 5-year survival rate of over 90 percent (12,13). The prognosis of patients with invasive IPNB is poorer than that of patients with noninvasive IPNB. Among patients with invasive IPNB, the survival rate of patients with mucinous carcinoma is better than that of patients with tubular adenocarcinoma (fig. 6-31) (1,4).

Lymph node metastasis has been reported in about 10 percent of IPNB and about 20 percent of invasive IPNB cases (12,13,27). Lymph node involvement is an unfavorable prognostic factor. Other poor prognostic factors include a positive surgical margin, deep invasion beyond the duct wall, and immunoreactivity to MUC1 (4,13,27). No significant difference has been reported in patient survival among histologic types.

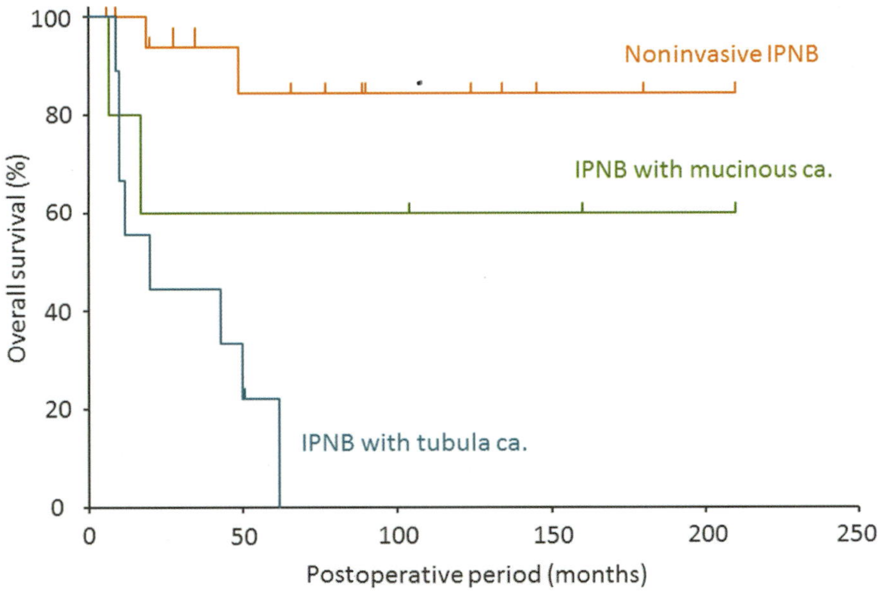

Figure 6-31

PROGNOSIS OF PATIENTS WITH INTRADUCTAL PAPILLARY NEOPLASM OF THE BILE DUCT

Patients with noninvasive IPNB have a better prognosis than those with invasive IPNB. IPNB patients with mucinous carcinoma have better prognosis than those with tubular adenocarcinoma. Abbreviation: ca = carcinoma.

INTRADUCTAL TUBULOPAPILLARY NEOPLASM

Definition. *Intraductal tubulopapillary neoplasm* (ITPN) of the bile duct is a primary biliary neoplasm consisting predominantly of a tubular proliferation of epithelial tumor cells within the dilated bile duct. The papillary architecture may be focally present, but never becomes dominant. MUC5AC is always negative and serves as a negative diagnostic marker (36). Gross mucin is also not detected.

ITPN is classified into two categories: *ITPN with high-grade dysplasia* and *ITPN with an associated invasive carcinoma* (37). To date, ITPN with low-grade dysplasia has not been documented. This recently proposed entity is currently designated as the biliary counterpart of pancreatic ITPN because of their clinicopathologic and molecular similarities (36,39). Although only a small number of studies is currently available, ITPN appears to be rare, with an expected frequency of less than 1 percent of all primary biliary neoplasms and 15 percent of intraductal neoplasms of the bile duct (37). A synonym is *intraductal tubular neoplasm* of the bile duct (40).

Clinical Features. Patients are typically more than 40 years of age, with a median age of 60 to 65 years (37,40). Women are more likely to be affected, with a male to female ratio of 1 to 2. Although ITPN develops anywhere in the biliary tree, 80 percent of cases occur in the liver, with the remainder located at either the hilar or extrahepatic bile duct (37,40).

The presenting symptoms are similar to those in patients with conventional cholangiocarcinoma, with jaundice and abdominal pain being the most commonly reported. Most patients do not have a history of hepatobiliary disorders or chronic cholangiopathies.

Imaging reveals dilated bile ducts almost entirely packed with the solid mass (fig. 6-32) (40). Unlike IPNB, cystic dilatation of the affected bile duct is an uncommon manifestation.

Gross Findings. The tumor size varies widely (subcentimeter to 15 cm). Tumor masses predominantly grow within the bile ducts (fig. 6-33). In some cases, the duct lumens are almost entirely filled by intraductal tumors, obscuring the duct wall contour (fig. 6-34) (37). Therefore, it may be difficult to appreciate that the nodules are truly intraductal. Invasive foci typically display fibrotic solid nodules in the liver parenchyma. Macroscopic mucin hypersecretion or a muconodular mass is absent. If present, another diagnosis, such as IPNB, is suggested.

Microscopic Findings. ITPN forms well-circumscribed exophytic nodules with a fairly smooth surface (fig. 6-35). These nodules are histologically composed of small, back-to-back tubular units with only minimal or no visible stroma (fig. 6-36) (36,37,40,41). In some cases, less differentiated components with solid

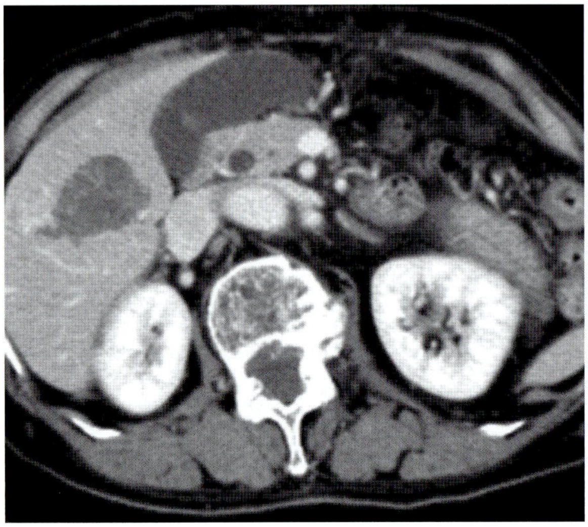

Figure 6-32

INTRADUCTAL TUBULOPAPILLARY NEOPLASM (ITPN)

In this CT image, the bile duct in the right lobe shows localized dilatation with an intraductal mass.

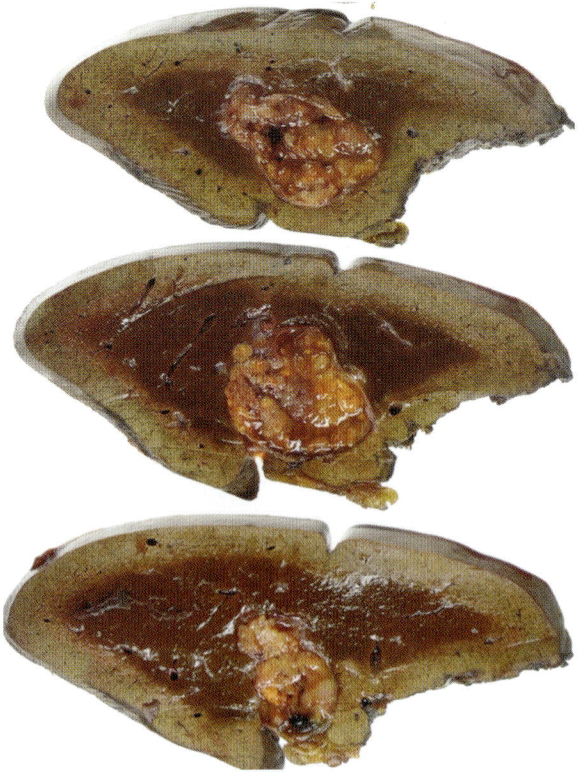

Figure 6-33

INTRADUCTAL TUBULOPAPILLARY NEOPLASM

The dilated bile duct is filled with a yellowish solid mass.

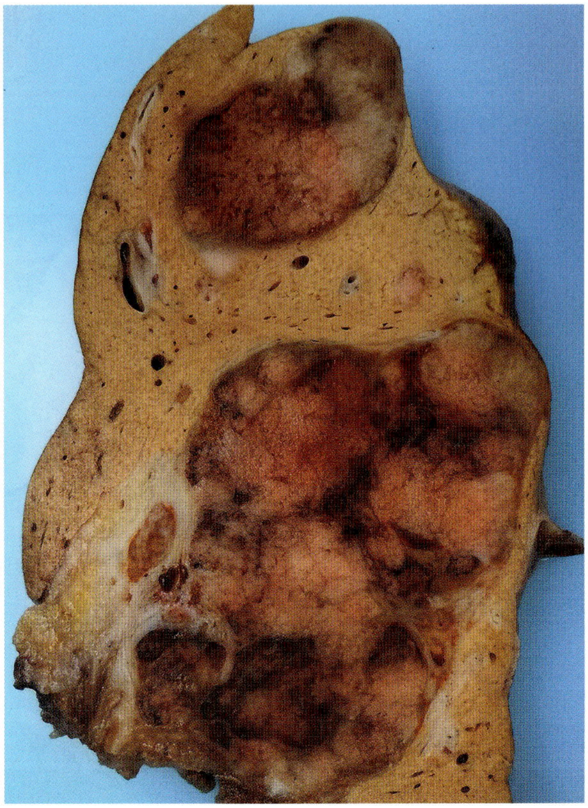

Figure 6-34

INTRADUCTAL TUBULOPAPILLARY NEOPLASM

The nodular mass in the liver may be difficult to grossly appreciate as an intraductal tumor.

growth coexist. Papillary architecture may be present in up to 50 percent of cases, but generally occupies less than 30 percent of the entire tumor.

Neoplastic cells have cellular features of the pancreatobiliary type (fig. 6-37). Although clear cell or eosinophilic changes may be present, differentiation to gastric or intestinal epithelium (i.e., goblet cells) is absent. Microscopic mucin may be present within some tubules, but should be very focal. Spotty necrosis and comedo-type necrosis are common (fig. 6-38). The neoplastic cells have enlarged nuclei, distinct nucleoli, and distorted cellular polarity, with cytoarchitectural atypia of high-grade dysplasia. In some cases, ITPN is closely associated with peribiliary cysts, suggesting that this intraductal neoplasm may arise from the peribiliary gland epithelium (36).

Seventy to 80 percent of cases harbor invasive carcinomas that infiltrate the liver parenchyma

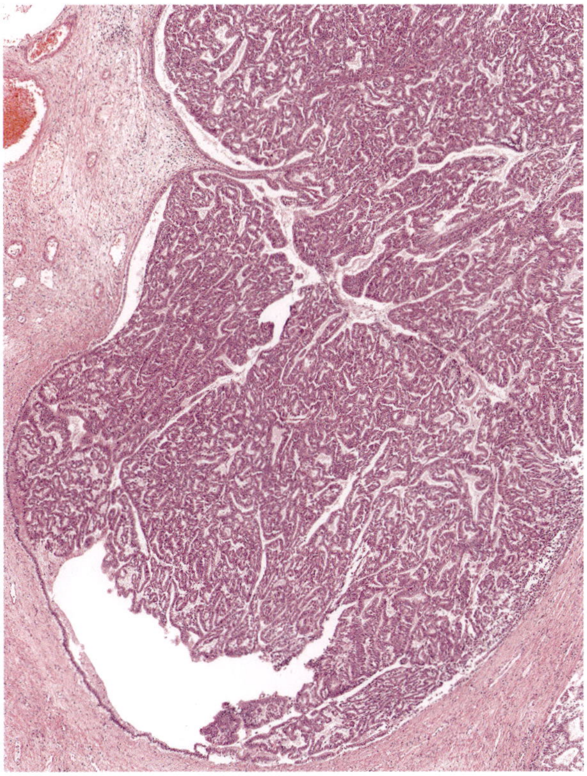

Figure 6-35

INTRADUCTAL TUBULOPAPILLARY NEOPLASM

This is an intraductal tumor, with tumor cells arranged in a tubular pattern.

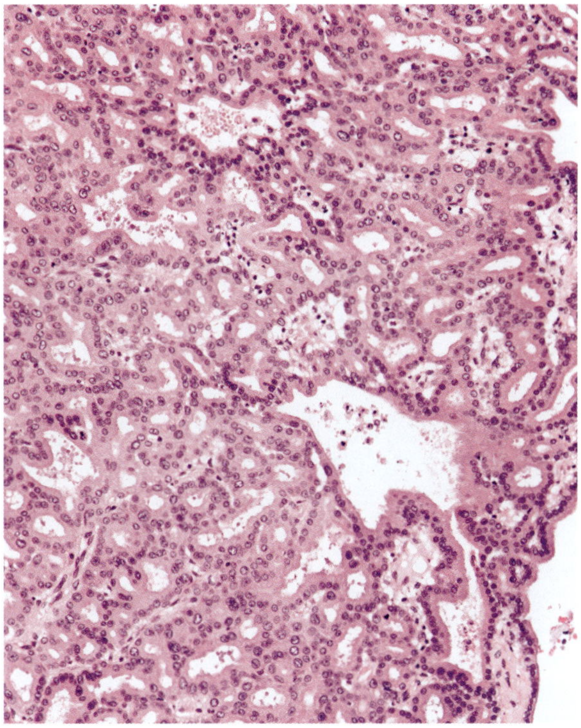

Figure 6-36

INTRADUCTAL TUBULOPAPILLARY NEOPLASM

The tumor cells are arranged predominantly in a tubular architecture.

or bile duct wall (37,40). Cytologic features in the invasive areas are similar to those in the noninvasive components; however, a fibrotic desmoplastic stroma appears to be more prominent in the invasive foci. In most patients with invasive cancer, tubular adenocarcinoma similar to conventional cholangiocarcinoma is at least focally present. Other invasive growth patterns include solid or cribriform nests with comedo necrosis and a tubulocystic architecture (fig. 6-39) (37). The former is sometimes difficult to recognize as an invasive component because a similar pattern may also occur in the intraductal area. Tubulocystic foci are similar to invasive tubulocystic carcinoma, a variant of conventional intrahepatic cholangiocarcinoma (see chapter 7) (42).

Immunohistochemical Findings. Biliary cytokeratins, including CK7 and CK19, are diffusely positive (fig. 6-40). ITPN commonly expresses MUC1 (about 80 percent) and MUC6

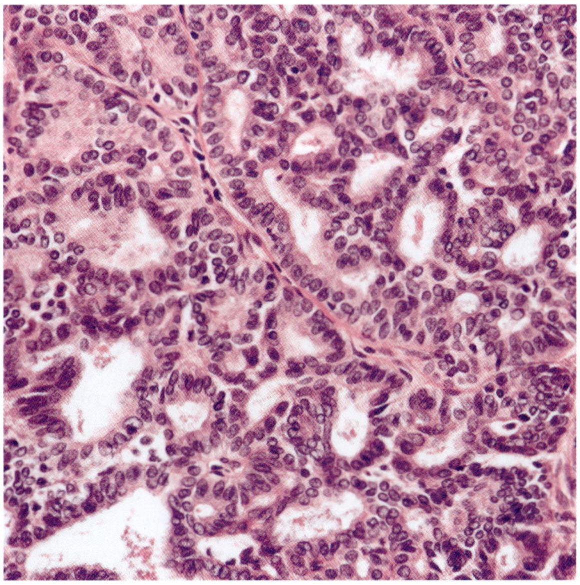

Figure 6-37

INTRADUCTAL TUBULOPAPILLARY NEOPLASM

The tumor cells have eosinophilic cytoplasm with round nuclei, in keeping with the pancreatobiliary type.

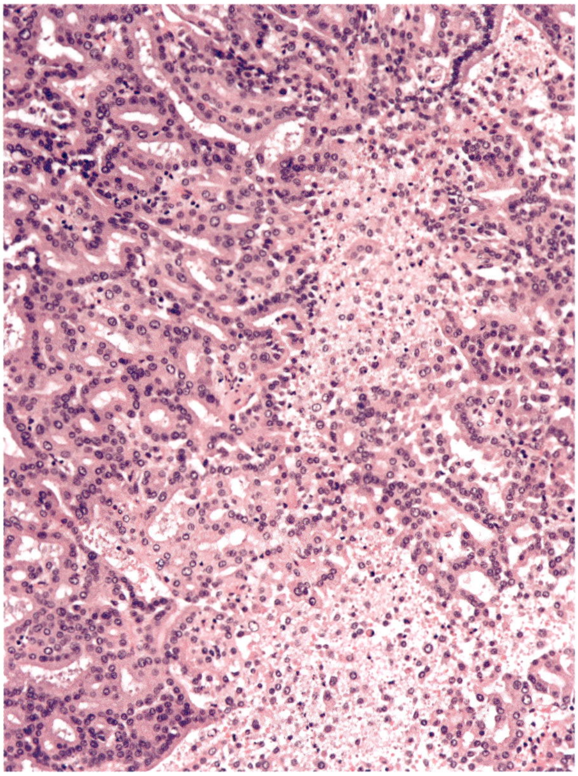

Figure 6-38

INTRADUCTAL TUBULOPAPILLARY NEOPLASM

A necrotic focus is seen in the noninvasive intraductal component.

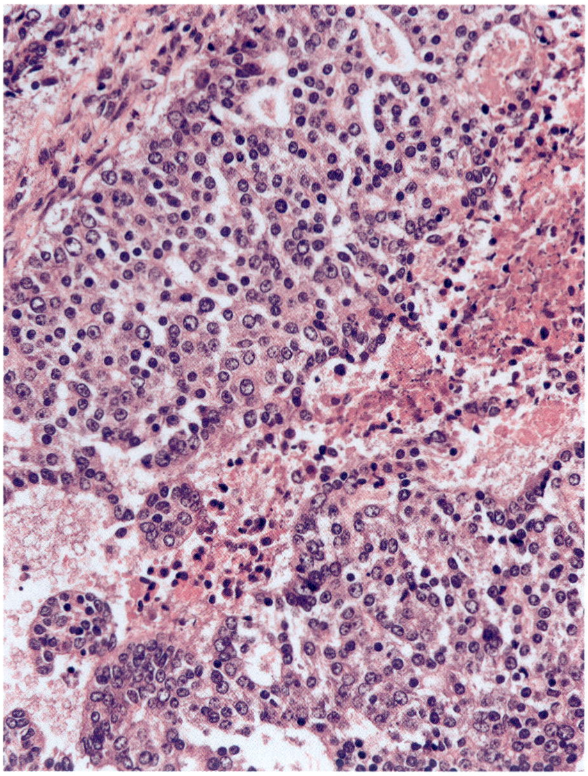

Figure 6-39

INTRADUCTAL TUBULOPAPILLARY NEOPLASM WITH INVASIVE CANCER

The invasive component shows solid growth with comedo-type necrosis.

(about 40 percent), but is generally negative for MUC2 and CDX2. MUC5AC is always negative because its expression is currently considered to be an exclusion criterion. HepPar1, synaptophysin, and chromogranin are negative.

Molecular Genetic Findings. Genetic alterations in *KRAS*, *GNAS*, and *BRAF* are uncommon, with only rare cases confirmed to harbor *KRAS* mutations (36,37). Except for the loss of p16 expression, which has been reported in 40 percent of ITPNs, other tumor-related genes (i.e., *p53*, *SMAD4/CDK4*, *IDH1/2*, *β-catenin*, *HER2*, and *EGFR*) commonly examined in biliary neoplasms are only rarely mutated in ITPN (37). Although *PIK3CA* is known to be mutated in 30 percent of pancreatic ITPNs (43), its mutation is rare (6 percent) in the biliary equivalent (37). Therefore, no common driver mutations in biliary ITPN have been identified to date.

Differential Diagnosis. *IPNB*. ITPN may be discriminated from IPNB in most cases by the predominant proliferation pattern (Table 6-3). The lack of expression of MUC5AC is also helpful in this setting; however, MUC5AC is negative in approximately 10 percent of IPNBs and 60 percent of conventional intrahepatic cholangiocarcinomas (1). The mass-forming type of intrahepatic cholangiocarcinoma sometimes invades the large bile ducts, and may exhibit intraductal tubular growth (fig. 6-41). Although the histologic features of the intraductal components are similar to ITPN, the large volume of the tumor is located within the liver parenchyma, which is unusual for ITPN.

Other Intraductal Tumors. We have encountered a few unusual intraductal tumors that do not match IPNB or ITPN. These tumors showed intraductal tubular growth with no invasive components, which were morphologic findings consistent with ITPN. However, MUC5AC was widely expressed. The current classification

Table 6-3

PATHOLOGIC COMPARISON OF INTRADUCTAL PAPILLARY NEOPLASM OF THE BILE DUCT AND INTRADUCTAL TUBULOPAPILLARY NEOPLASM

	IPNB	ITPN
Pathologic Features		
Gross appearance	Papillary mass in the dilated bile duct	Relatively solid mass in the bile duct
Mucin overproduction	Frequent	None
Histologic architecture	Predominantly papillary	Predominantly tubular
MUC5AC expression	90%	Negative
Invasive malignancy	50%	70-80%
Patterns of invasive growth	Tubular or mucinous	Tubular, solid, cribriform, or tubulocystic
Molecular Features		
KRAS mutations	~30%	Rare
GNAS mutations	0-30%	None
Associated Conditions	Hepatolithiasis Liver flukes	None

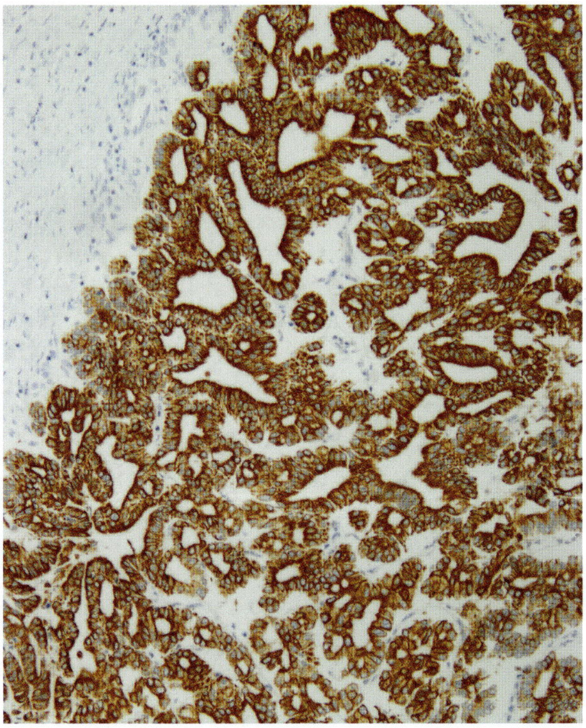

Figure 6-40

INTRADUCTAL TUBULOPAPILLARY NEOPLASM

The cells are diffusely positive for CK19 (immunohistochemical stain).

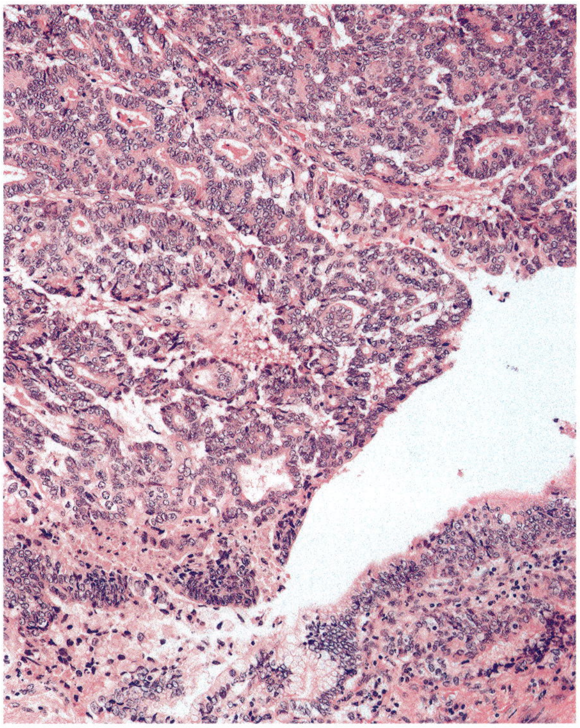

Figure 6-41

INTRAHEPATIC CHOLANGIOCARCINOMA

The mass-forming cholangiocarcinoma sometimes invades the large duct and forms an intraductal mass, the appearance of which may be reminiscent of ITPN.

system may not cover all intraductal neoplasms of the bile duct.

Treatment and Prognosis. Surgical resection is the treatment of choice for ITPN. Lymph node metastasis has been reported in about 15 percent of invasive cases (37,40). Although 70 to 80 percent of cases have invasive malignancies at the time of diagnosis, prognosis appears to be favorable, with an expected 5-year overall survival rate of 90 percent (37). Some patients, however, may develop late recurrence years after the initial surgery (40).

MUCINOUS CYSTIC NEOPLASM

Definition. *Mucinous cystic neoplasm* (MCN) is a cyst-forming tumor lined by cuboidal to columnar epithelium with subepithelial cellular stroma mimicking ovarian connective tissue ("ovarian-like stroma") (38,44). Based on the degree of cytoarchitectural atypia in the lining epithelium, cystic neoplasms are graded into *low-*, *intermediate-*, and *high-grade dysplasia*. When a component of invasive cancer is present, the lesion is designated as *MCN with an associated invasive carcinoma*. Most MCNs occur in the liver, but rare examples in the extrahepatic biliary system have also been documented (45). Synonyms include *biliary cystadenoma* and *cystadenocarcinoma* (46,47).

Until 2010, when an ovarian-like stroma was required for a histologic diagnosis (44), the definition of this entity had been less stringent. In retrospect, other cyst-forming lesions, such as cystic IPNB and biliary hamartomas, were supposedly included in this group (47,48). This needs to be considered when interpreting the literature on this condition, particularly in studies published before 2010.

General Features. Although MCN of the liver is histologically nearly identical to MCN of the pancreas, their biologic behaviors differ. Approximately 10 percent of pancreatic MCNs have an associated invasive carcinoma at initial presentation (49,50), whereas malignant transformation is less common in the hepatic equivalent (38). This may be related to the earlier detection or inherently lower malignant potential of hepatic MCN. Since MCN of the liver is significantly larger than the pancreatic equivalent, the possibility of lower malignant potential may be more likely (38).

Although the actual incidence of MCN currently remains unknown, it may be more common in Western countries than in Asia. MCN accounts for 2 to 3 percent of surgical cases of primary hepatobiliary neoplasm in the United States and Europe, but is less common (less than 1 percent) in Korea and Japan (15). No epidemiologic data are available in other countries. Since MCN typically develops in normal livers with no known risk factors, differences in incidences between countries may represent various genetic susceptibilities among ethnic groups.

Clinical Features. MCN occurs almost exclusively in women (38,51,52). Patient ages vary widely from 20 to 80 years of age, with a median age of approximately 50 years. Patients commonly present with nonspecific symptoms such as abdominal pain or discomfort. When the biliary tree is obstructed by a tumor, jaundice may develop. In some patients, an incidental cystic tumor is found on imaging. An uncommon, but critical presentation is spontaneous rupture (53).

Approximately 55 percent of MCNs develop in the left medial segment (segment IV) of the liver, while 20 percent each develop in the right lobe and left lateral segment, with the remaining 5 percent occurring in the caudate lobe (15,38). The imaging appearance is a unilocular (10 percent) or multilocular cyst with internal septation or a cyst-in-cyst appearance (90 percent) (fig. 6-42) (38). The cyst wall is variably thick. The presence of an intracystic papillary tumor suggests at least high-grade dysplasia. Organized hematoma within the cyst is sometimes detected as an enhancing mass, leading to its misinterpretation as a papillary mural nodule (54,55). There is no communication to the biliary tree.

Gross Findings. MCN ranges from 2 to 25 cm, with a median diameter of 11 cm (38). Tumors form large cystic masses with thick fibrotic walls. Although the name of the entity includes "mucinous," the intracystic contents are not always mucinous. Thick mucin is rare, with watery, serous, or hemorrhagic fluid being more common.

Sectioning of the cyst wall reveals multiple small mural cysts. The cystic space may be subdivided by fibrous septa (fig. 6-43). The internal surface is generally flat, with slight irregularities in low-grade lesions, and extensive erosion is often noted (fig. 6-44). Papillary or solid nodules are present in higher-grade lesions (fig. 6-45) (38). MCN is typically located in the liver parenchyma, but rarely involves perihilar connective tissue. Another rare, but known manifestation, is protrusion of the cystic mass into a large bile duct. We have also encountered extreme examples showing a cyst-containing intraductal polypoid mass without involvement of the liver parenchyma. Even in these cases, there is no luminal communication between the bile duct and cyst.

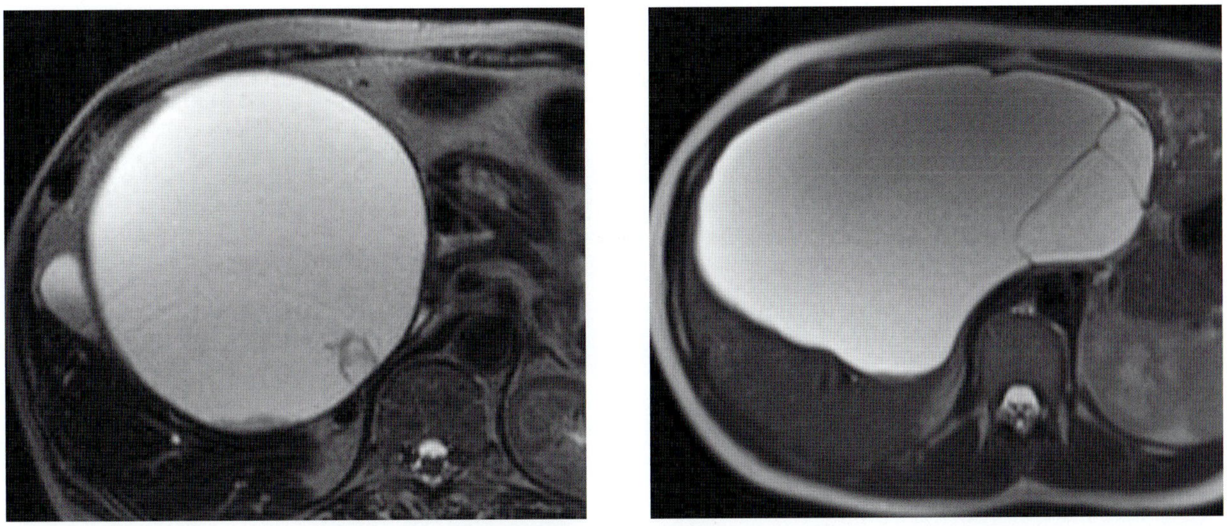

Figure 6-42

MUCINOUS CYSTIC NEOPLASM (MCN)

Left: The large cystic tumor has a cyst-in-cyst appearance on magnetic resonance imaging (MRI). Right: The tumor is a multilocular cyst with septation.

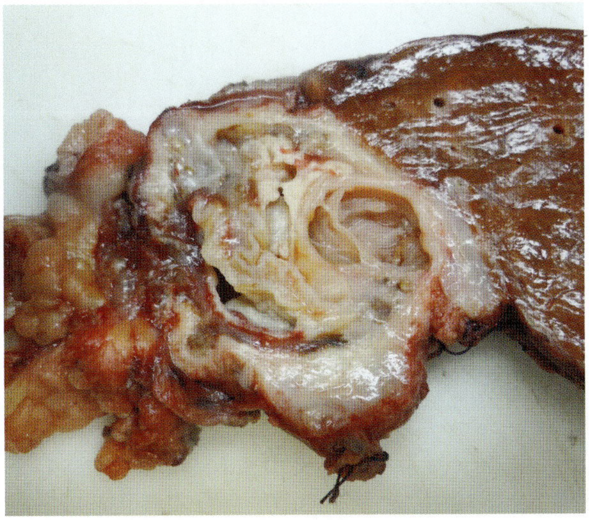

Figure 6-43

MUCINOUS CYSTIC NEOPLASM WITH LOW-GRADE DYSPLASIA

The cystic tumor has a fibrous wall and intracystic septa.

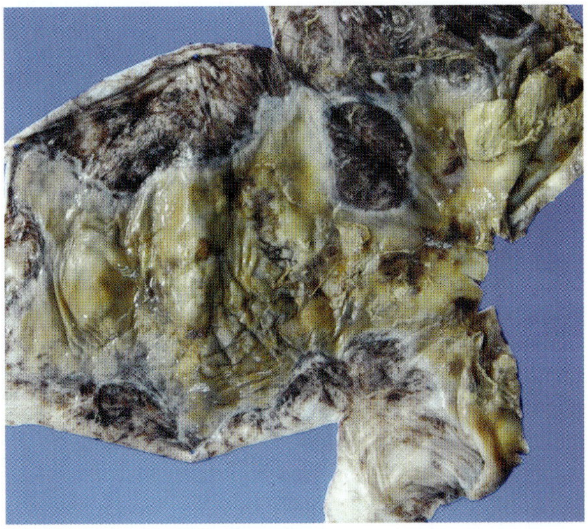

Figure 6-44

MUCINOUS CYSTIC NEOPLASM WITH LOW-GRADE DYSPLASIA

The luminal surface of the cystic tumor sometimes shows extensive erosion.

Microscopic Findings. MCN has a single-layer lining epithelium supported by an ovarian-like stroma (38,52). In MCN with low-grade dysplasia, the lining epithelium consists of bland-looking columnar or cuboidal cells (fig. 6-46). Mucous cells are focally noted (fig. 6-47). In MCN with intermediate-grade dysplasia, there are occasional foci of enlarged nuclei, nuclear stratification, and an increased nuclear/cytoplasm ratio (fig. 6-48). These dysplastic foci are histologically flat or micropapillary, and generally found incidentally in microscopic examinations; extensive sampling is needed. In

Figure 6-45

MUCINOUS CYSTIC NEOPLASM WITH HIGH-GRADE DYSPLASIA

A: Papillary mural nodules are present on the cyst wall.

B: The cyst was partially resected previously. There is a residual papillary mural nodule in the cyst wall.

C: The solid mural nodule represents invasive carcinoma.

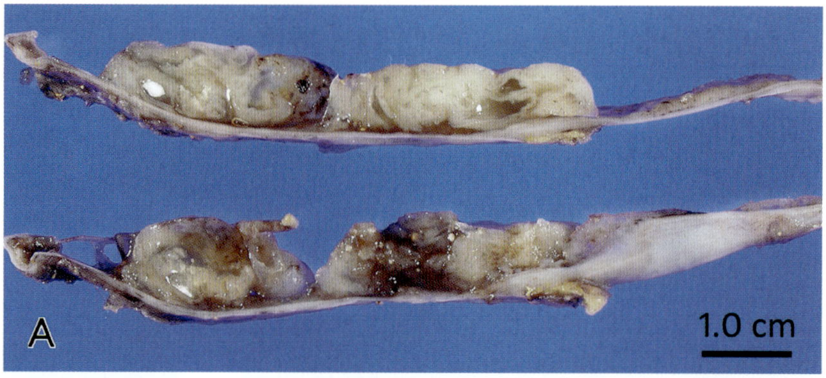

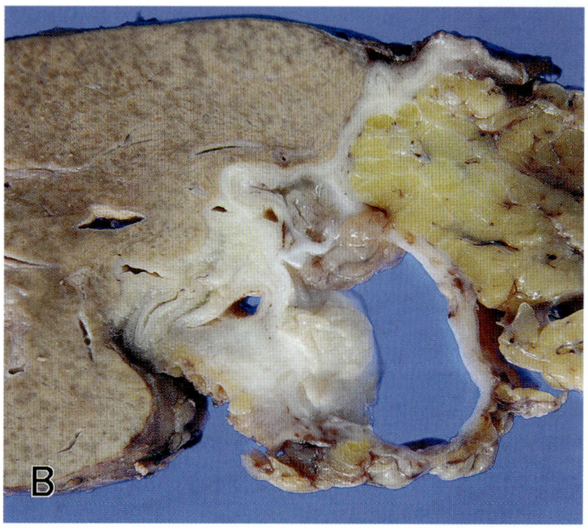

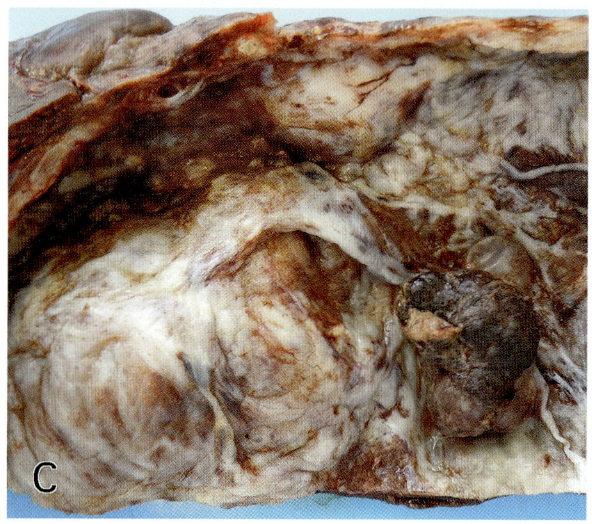

MCN with high-grade dysplasia, atypical cells with increased cellularity, nuclear pleomorphism, and occasional mitotic figures are arranged in a complex papillotubular architecture (fig. 6-49). In MCN with low-grade dysplasia, neoplastic cells are the pancreatobiliary type in morphology, while intestinal differentiation, as evidenced by the presence of goblet cells, nuclear stratification, and a brush border, has been reported in higher-grade lesions (38).

Invasive carcinomas arising in MCN display the histologic features of tubular adenocarcinoma (fig. 6-50). Small foci of mucinous carcinoma may coexist (fig. 6-51). Although pancreatic MCN is known to progress to other types of invasive malignancies, including undifferentiated carcinoma (56), it currently remains unknown whether this is also the case in hepatic MCN because only a limited number of cases of invasive MCN with a histology-proven ovarian-like stroma have been reported.

Since different histologic grades have been detected in different areas of the same case (fig. 6-52), MCN needs to be graded at the most atypical focus and extensive sampling is required. Most cases are graded as MCN with low-grade dysplasia (90 percent) or MCN with intermediate-grade dysplasia (5 to 10 percent) (15,38). Less than 5 percent of cases have high-grade dysplasia or invasive carcinoma (15,38). The histologic grade correlates well with the macroscopic appearance. MCN with low- or intermediate-grade dysplasia lacks papillary mural nodules, while MCN with high-grade dysplasia or an associated carcinoma generally has grossly visible solid or papillary nodules (38). Nevertheless, an invasive cancer arising from the flat mucosa, as observed in pancreatic MCN, is expected.

An ovarian-like stroma consisting of plump spindle cells and small blood vessels is easily observed in most cases (fig. 6-53). The thickness of the stroma and cellularity of the mesenchymal

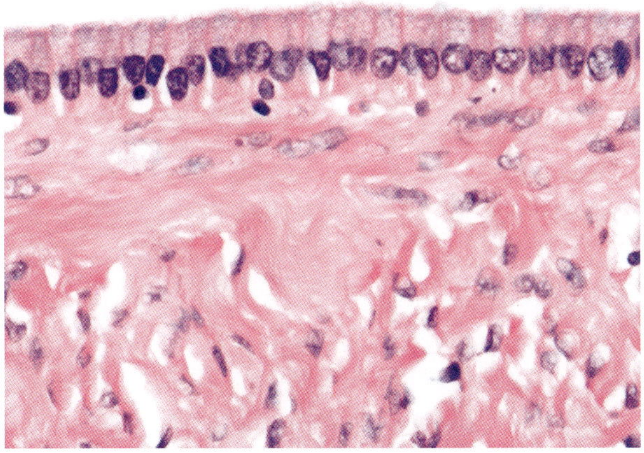

Figure 6-46

MUCINOUS CYSTIC NEOPLASM WITH LOW-GRADE DYSPLASIA

The cyst is lined by biliary type epithelium with little cytologic atypia.

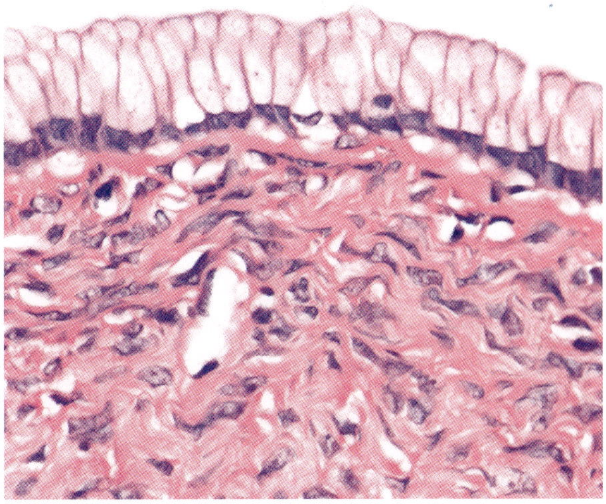

Figure 6-47

MUCINOUS CYSTIC NEOPLASM WITH LOW-GRADE DYSPLASIA

The tumor cells contain intracytoplasmic mucin. The subepithelial cellular stroma consists of plump spindle cells (ovarian-like stroma).

cells vary (fig. 6-54) (38). The stroma may show luteinization. In MCN with high-grade dysplasia, an ovarian-like stroma may be observed in the fibrovascular cores of papillary components (fig. 6-55). Secondary changes, including the deposition of hemosiderin, cholesterol clefts, and small foci of calcification, are commonly detected in the cyst wall (fig. 6-56). Large veins are also present, and smooth muscle fibers of the vascular wall are irregularly embedded in the cyst wall. This should not be interpreted as a muscle layer, as observed in ciliated foregut cysts.

Frozen Sections. The most common reason for a frozen section examination in patients with suspected MCN is to establish whether the cystic liver lesion is truly MCN or something else, particularly a simple cyst. Grossly, a thick fibrous wall and the presence of mural cysts or septation suggest MCN over a simple cyst. However, simple cysts with secondary degenerative changes such as hemorrhage and organization may mimic MCN by gross examination. Histologic evidence of an ovarian-like stroma is critical for this differential diagnosis. Since the diagnostic stroma may be focal, a frozen section diagnosis requires multiple samples, at least five from different areas, particularly those with thick walls. This approach also contributes to determining the degree of dysplasia. Erosive

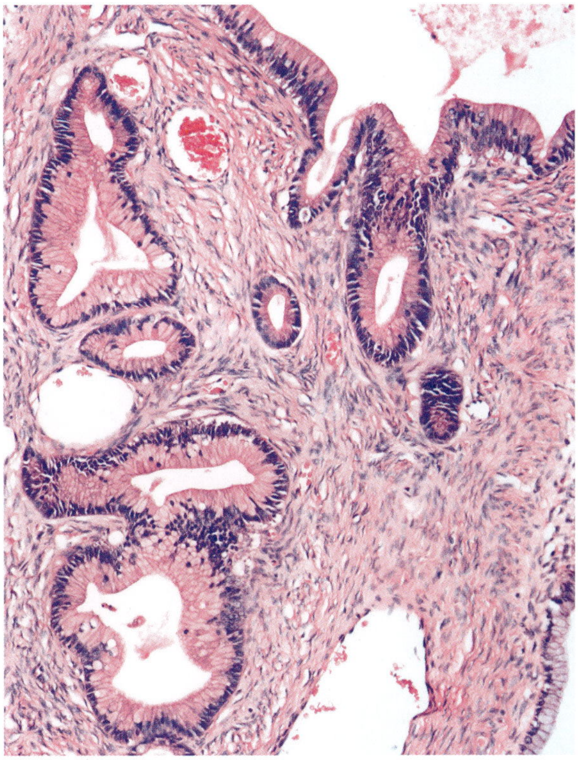

Figure 6-48

MUCINOUS CYSTIC NEOPLASM WITH INTERMEDIATE-GRADE DYSPLASIA

The cells show nuclear stratification and piled-up nuclei.

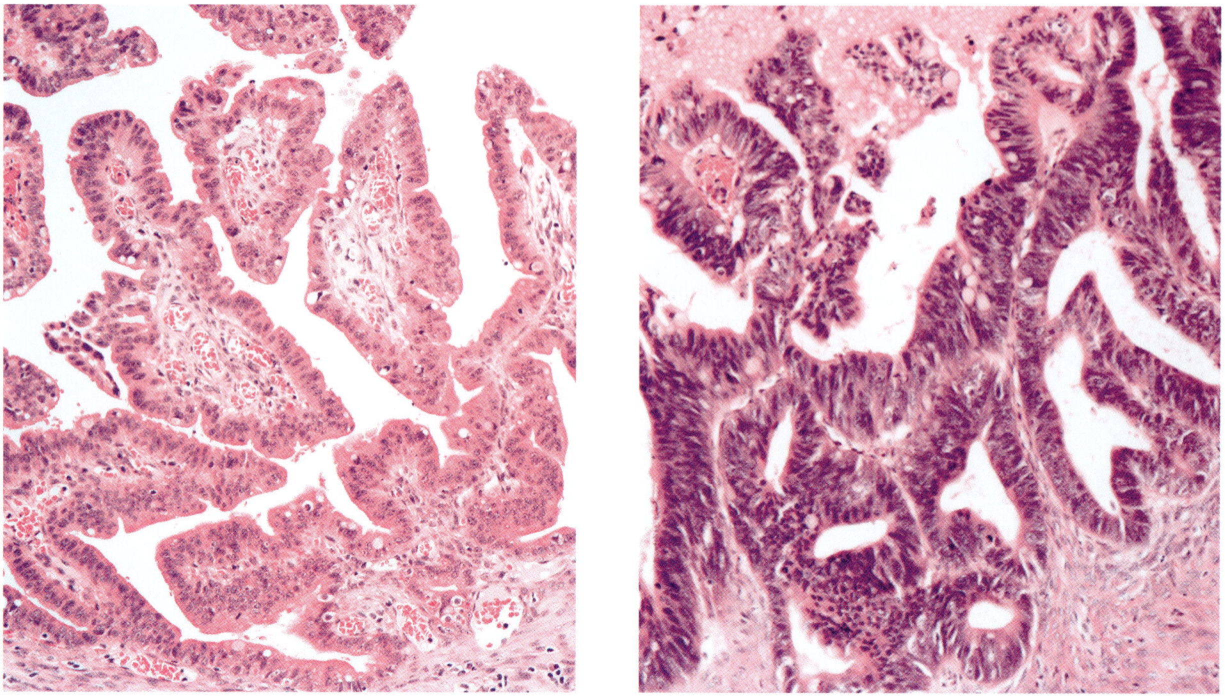

Figure 6-49

MUCINOUS CYSTIC NEOPLASM WITH HIGH-GRADE DYSPLASIA

Left: The lining cells show a high-papillary proliferation. There is also severe cellular atypia such as nuclear pleomorphism and loss of polarity.

Right: Dysplastic features such as increased cellularity, hyperchromasia, and nuclear stratification are obvious.

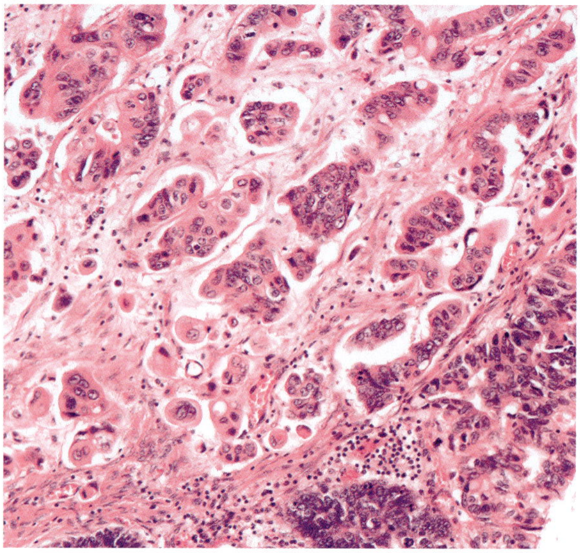

Figure 6-50

MUCINOUS CYSTIC NEOPLASM WITH INVASIVE CARCINOMA

Poorly differentiated carcinoma is seen in the cyst wall.

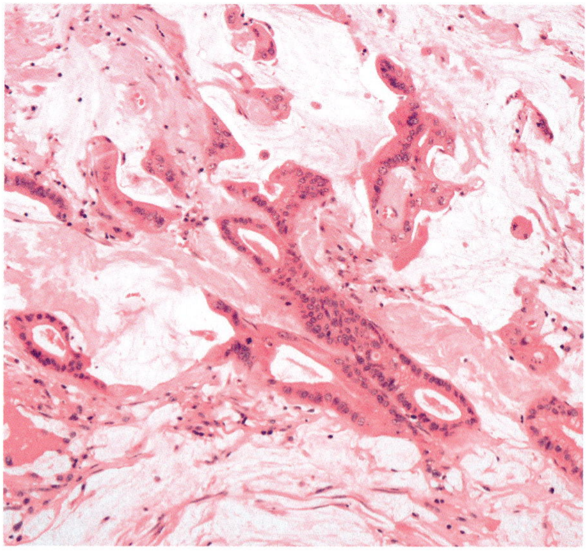

Figure 6-51

MUCINOUS CYSTIC NEOPLASM WITH INVASIVE CARCINOMA

The invasive component shows features of mucinous carcinoma.

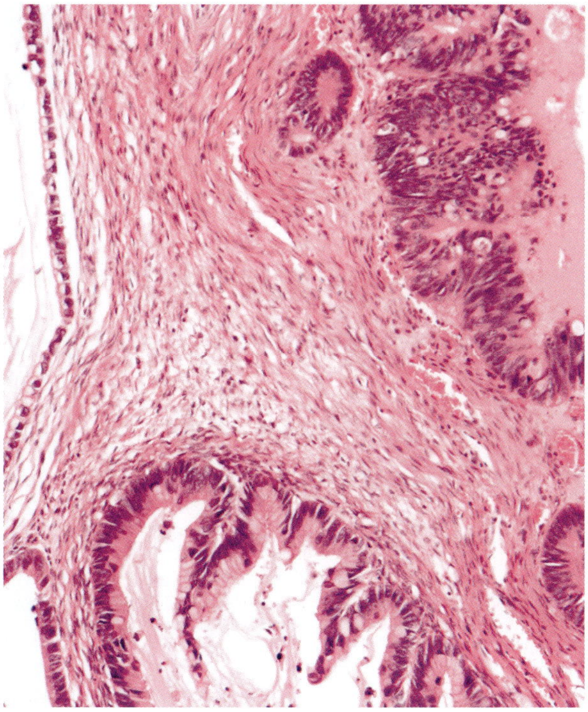

Figure 6-52

MUCINOUS CYSTIC NEOPLASM

Different degrees of dysplasia are seen in this image.

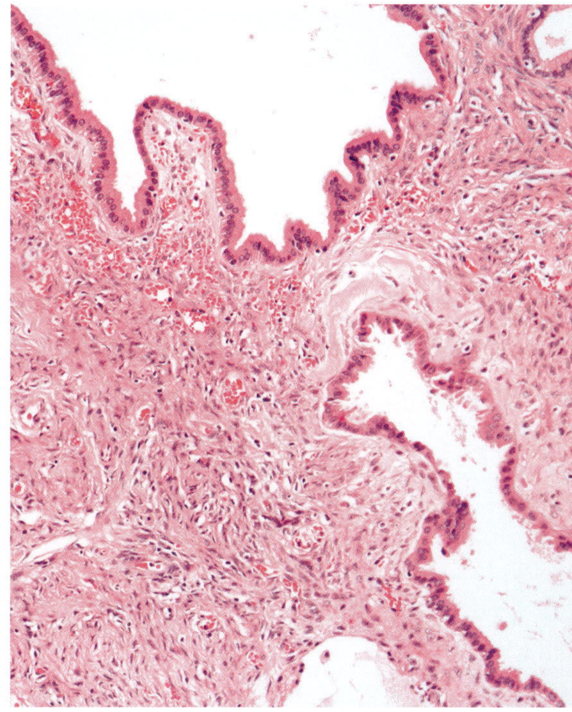

Figure 6-53

MUCINOUS CYSTIC NEOPLASM

The cellular ovarian-like stroma consists of plump spindle cells with small blood vessels.

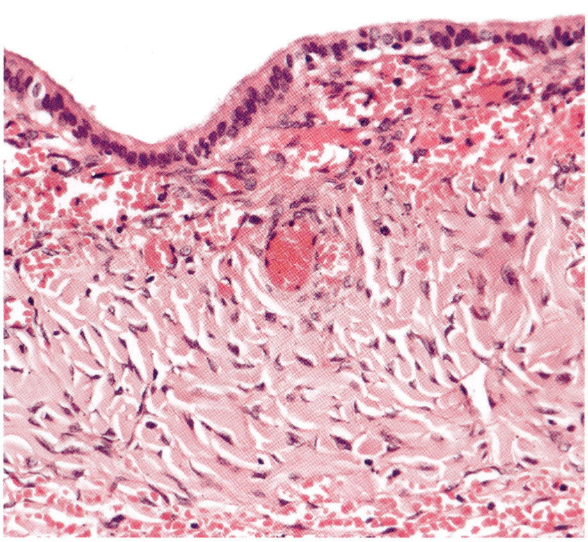

Figure 6-54

MUCINOUS CYSTIC NEOPLASM

The stroma appears to be less cellular with hyalinization than typically seen (fig. 6-53) or in a normal ovary.

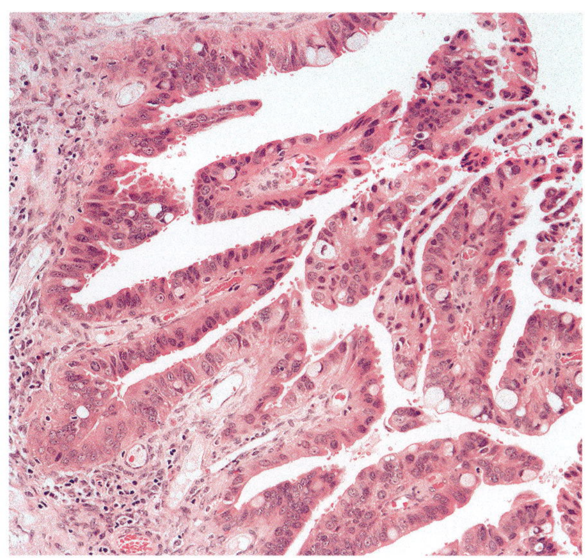

Figure 6-55

MUCINOUS CYSTIC NEOPLASM WITH HIGH-GRADE DYSPLASIA

The ovarian-like stroma is sometimes found in the papillary mural nodule.

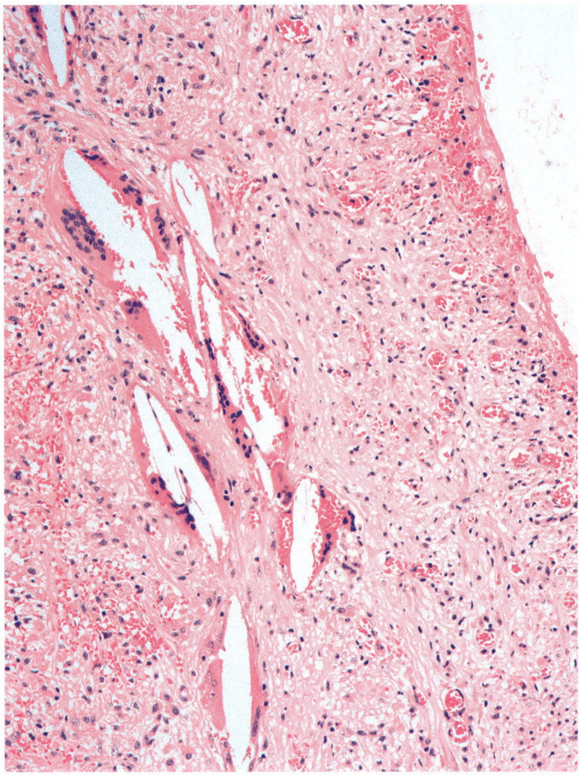

Figure 6-56

MUCINOUS CYSTIC NEOPLASM

The cyst wall is degenerative and contains cholesterol clefts.

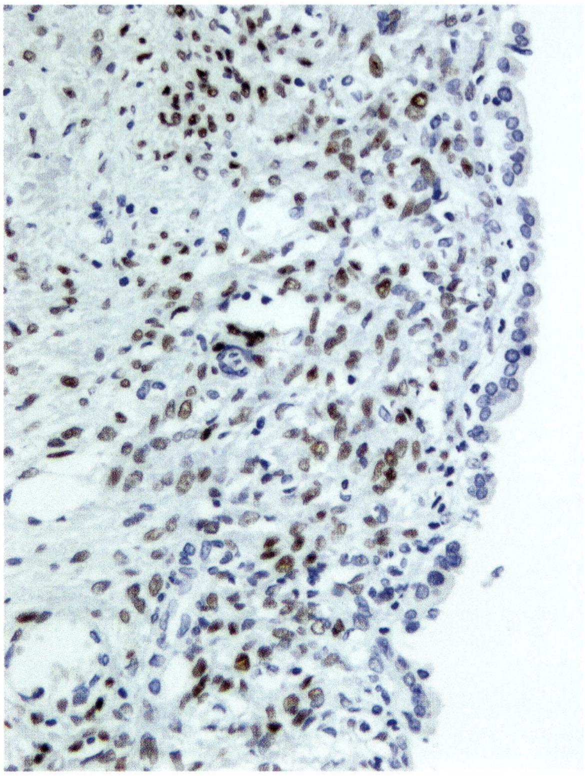

Figure 6-57

MUCINOUS CYSTIC NEOPLASM

Estrogen receptor is positive in the nuclei of spindle cells in an ovarian-like stroma (immunohistochemical stain).

areas are not suitable for this diagnosis because inflammation and fibrosis may obscure the diagnostic stroma and a lining epithelium for histologic grading does not exist. A papillary or solid nodule also needs to be sampled if present.

Immunohistochemical Findings. Immunostaining for estrogen receptor (ER) and progesterone receptor (PR) is helpful for the detection and confirmation of an ovarian-like stroma. PR is positive in more than 90 percent of cases and ER in 70 percent (fig. 6-57) (38). Inhibin-alpha is also expressed in 20 percent of cases, particularly in the luteinized stroma (fig. 6-58). The lining epithelium is negative for ER and PR.

The immunophenotype of the lining epithelium changes during tumor progression. Neoplastic cells in MCN with low-grade dysplasia are generally positive for CK7 and CK19, and negative for CK20, MUC1, MUC2, MUC5AC, and MUC6, which is consistent with the biliary phenotype (38). Gastrointestinal markers including CK20, MUC2, MUC5AC, and MUC6 are increasingly expressed in higher-grade lesions (38). MUC1 only becomes positive in MCN with high-grade dysplasia or an associated invasive carcinoma.

Cytologic Findings. Aspiration specimens from cysts contain occasional aggregates of cuboidal or columnar epithelial cells, which are occasionally arranged in papillary clusters, in a background of chronic inflammation (57). Epithelial cells are bland in MCN with low-grade dysplasia, while varying degrees of cytologic atypia such as nuclear enlargement, pleomorphism, and an increased nuclear/cytoplasmic ratio, are seen in MCN with intermediate-grade or high-grade dysplasia. The inflammatory background may be due to erosion of the internal mucosa.

The diagnosis of MCN cannot be established based purely on cytologic grounds because a diagnostic ovarian-like stroma is not identified. A more important reason for collecting cytology samples from patients with suspected MCN is excluding the possibility of overt malignancy.

Differential Diagnosis. MCN needs to be discriminated from other cyst-forming lesions including simple cysts, multicystic biliary hamartoma, and cystic IPNB (Table 6-4). Hybrid cysts should also be considered in the differential.

Simple Cysts. Most simple cysts are unilocular, while the majority of MCNs are multilocular with septation or mural cysts (19,58). Clinical information regarding the presence or absence of cysts elsewhere in the liver may be beneficial because MCN is typically solitary, and multiplicity is more common in simple cysts. A solitary lesion, suspicious intracystic components, septation, and biliary dilatation are regarded as imaging features suggestive of MCN more than simple cysts (59). The diagnostic sensitivity of these imaging findings is high (about 90 percent), whereas specificity is poor (about 50 percent) because degenerated simple cysts show complex imaging abnormalities (60).

Multicystic Biliary Hamartoma. This rare hamartomatous condition displays a honeycomb-like multicystic appearance (61,62), which is an uncommon presentation in MCN. Although the lining epithelium of the cyst is similar to that in MCN with low-grade dysplasia,

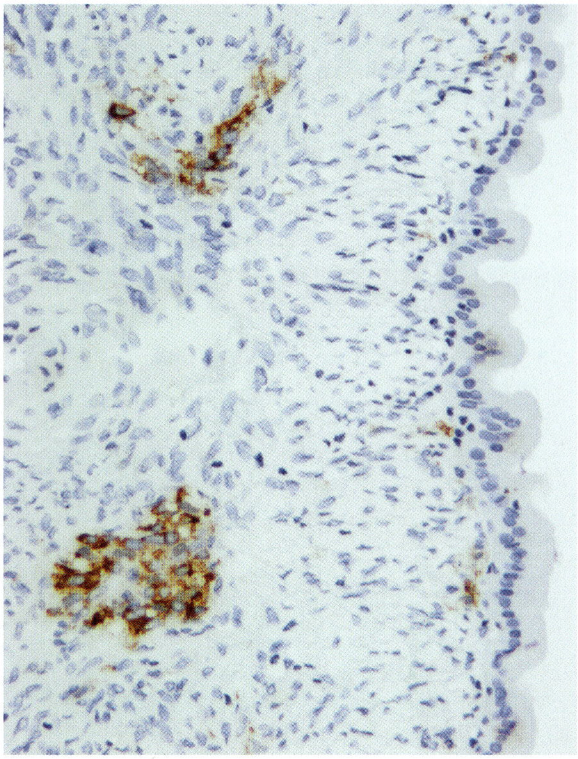

Figure 6-58

MUCINOUS CYSTIC NEOPLASM

Inhibin-alpha is focally expressed in the stroma (immunohistochemical stain).

Table 6-4

DIFFERENTIAL FEATURES OF CYST-FORMING HEPATOBILIARY LESIONS

	MCN[a]	Cystic IPNB	Simple cyst	Multicystic Biliary Hamartoma	Endometriotic Cyst	Localized Duct Dilatation
Age (years)	20 to 80	40 to 80	any age	30 to 70	30 to 60	adult
Gender	female	male>female	male>female	male>female	female	both
Shape of the cyst	multilocular cyst with mural cysts or septation	grape-like appearance with solid or papillary mural nodule and biliary communication	usually unilocular but complex appearance with mural nodules and septation in degenerated cysts	honeycomb-like appearance	complex solid and cystic mass; endometriosis at other sites other sites in the abdomen	cystic dilatation of of the bile duct; mural inflammatory nodule may be present
Histology	epithelial lining with subepithelial ovarian-like stroma	papillary proliferation of the neoplastic cells along delicate fibrovascular cores	lining of the biliary-type epithelium	dilated hamartomatous bile ducts embedded in fibrous stroma	endometrial tissue consisting of glands and cellular stroma	nonspecific bile duct dilatation with chronic, focally xanthogranulomatous inflammation

[a]MCN = mucinous cystic neoplasm; IPNB = intraductal papillary neoplasm of the bile duct.

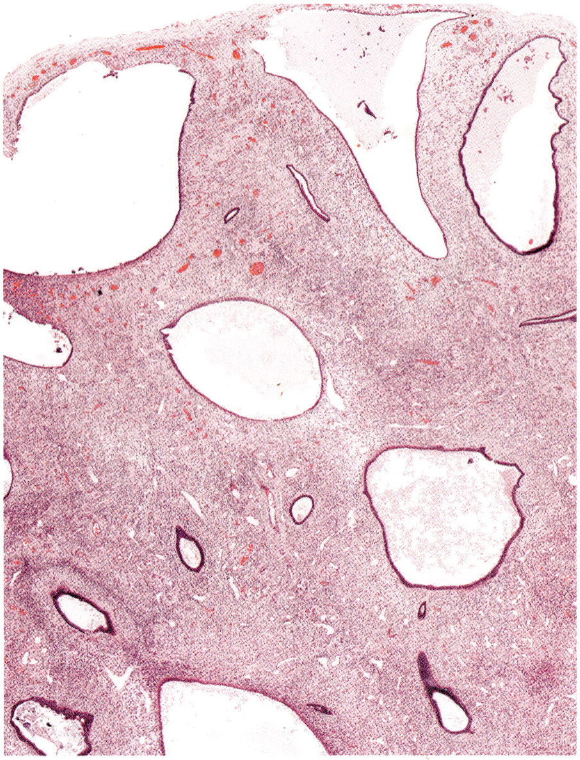

Figure 6-59

ENDOMETRIOTIC CYST

Endometriosis forms a solid and cystic mass. The combination of epithelial cysts and cellular stroma may resemble MCN.

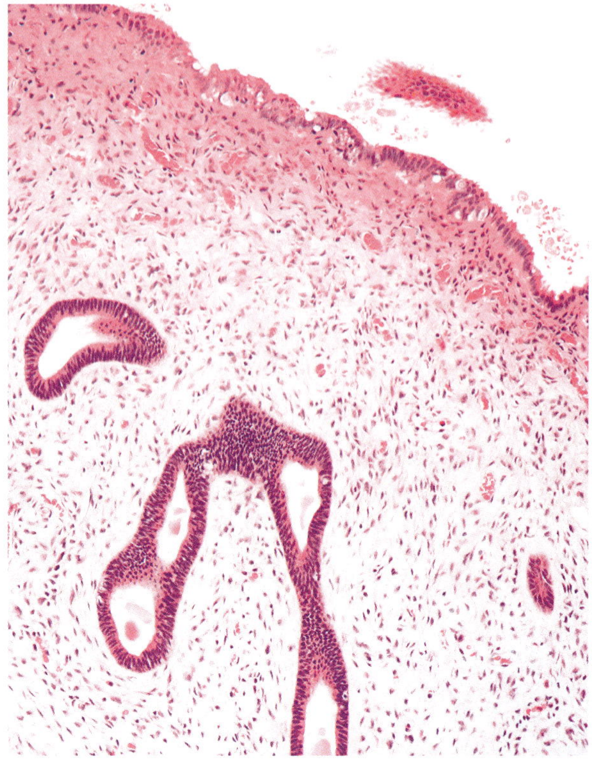

Figure 6-60

ENDOMETRIOTIC CYST

The epithelial component comprises the surface lining and deep glands.

an ovarian-like stroma is never present in this hamartomatous condition. More details of this condition are described below.

IPNB. Unlike MCN, cystic IPNB has bile duct communication (5,22). Solid or papillary mural nodules are present in most cases of cystic IPNB, whereas they only appear in MCN with high-grade dysplasia or an associated invasive carcinoma (less than 5 percent of MCNs) (38). Although gross and imaging appearances are helpful for differentiation, the presence or absence of ovarian-like stroma is crucial for discrimination.

Endometriotic Cysts. These rarely occur in the liver but may mimic MCN, particularly on frozen sections (fig. 6-59) (63). Most patients have endometriosis at other sites. Unlike MCN, in which the epithelium is present on the luminal surface, endometriotic cysts may have glandular elements in the deep stroma (fig. 6-60). ER and PR are positive in the epithelium and stromal cells in endometriotic cysts, whereas they are only positive in the stromal cells of MCN (63). CD10 is positive in the endometrial stroma, but negative in the ovarian-like stroma of MCN.

Bile Duct Dilation. Another rare condition that may mimic MCN is localized bile duct dilatation, which usually occurs at the hepatic hilum. Ducts may dilate up to 5 cm, and have chronic, focally xanthogranulomatous inflammation in their walls (fig. 6-61). This condition has not been described well in the literature. Since all the patients we have encountered were adults, this is likely an acquired condition distinct from choledochal cysts or Caroli disease. There is no evidence of congenital hepatic fibrosis in the liver.

Hydatid Cysts. Hydatid cysts are caused by infestation with *Echinococcus. Echinococcus granulosus* causes a unilocular hydatid cyst, while *Echinococcus multilocularis* causes multilocular, necrotic, and cystic cavities (64–66). Histologically, the cysts contain a laminated membrane or protoscolices, but no epithelial lining. Therefore, its histologic discrimination

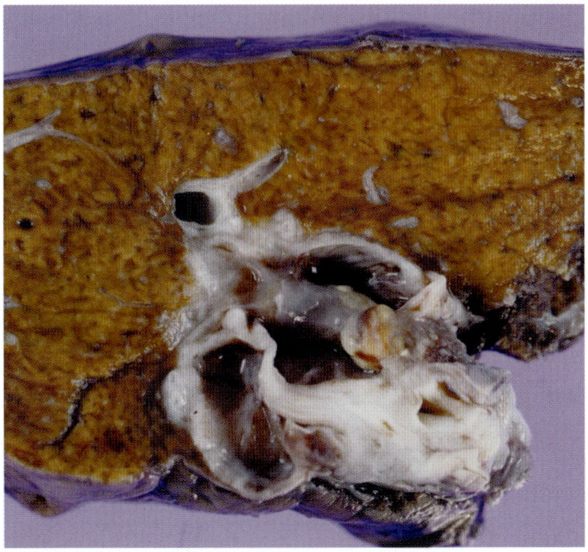

Figure 6-61

LOCALIZED BILE DUCT DILATATION

The large bile duct shows localized cystic dilatation. The yellowish mural nodule represents xanthogranulomatous inflammation.

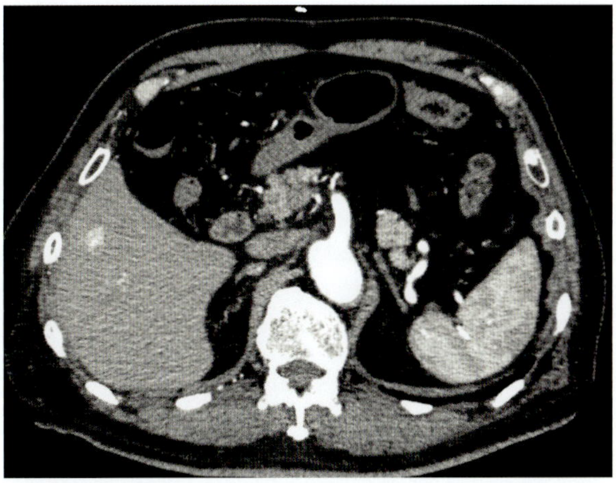

Figure 6-62

BILE DUCT ADENOMA

The tumor is an enhanced nodule in the right lobe.

from MCN is straightforward. Most hydatid cysts can be diagnosed based on imaging features in conjunction with serology (64,65).

Treatment and Prognosis. Complete resection is the standard treatment for MCN of the liver. Tumors involving the hepatic lobes or perihilar connective tissue may result in incomplete resection. Generally, prognosis is excellent, with an expected 5-year overall survival rate of over 95 percent (15). Although the lining tumor cells in MCN with low-grade dysplasia are bland-looking and similar in appearance to non-neoplastic biliary epithelium, they have neoplastic potential. We encountered a patient who initially had fenestration for a suspected large simple cyst. The residual lesion was completely excised after the pathologic diagnosis of MCN. Although the tumor showed low-grade dysplasia, the patient eventually developed the complication of peritoneal dissemination several years later.

BILE DUCT ADENOMA/PERIBILIARY GLAND HAMARTOMA

Definition. This is a small nodular lesion consisting of uniformly distributed, bland-looking tubules and surrounding fibrotic stroma. The diagnostic term *bile duct adenoma* is widely used, but this entity is also called *peribiliary gland hamartoma* based on previous findings in which tubules have the phenotype of normal peribiliary glands (67).

Clinical Features. Bile duct adenoma develops almost equally in males and females. Most patients are adults: an Armed Forces Institute of Pathology (AFIP) series of 152 cases only contained 2 pediatric cases (1 and 12 years of age) (68). No clinical signs or symptoms have been attributed to the lesion. Multiple lesions have been reported in 15 percent of patients. Bile duct adenoma is almost exclusively found incidentally during intra-abdominal surgery, at autopsy, or by pathologic examination of livers resected for other reasons. We recently observed a 7-mm bile duct adenoma that was discovered by imaging analysis (fig. 6-62).

Gross Findings. Bile duct adenoma is grossly well circumscribed, round, and whitish on cut section (fig. 6-63). No fibrous capsule is present. Lesions that are incidentally found during surgery are subcapsular in location, while intraparenchymal lesions are commonly identified during gross examination of livers resected for other conditions. The tumor size is less than 1 cm in most cases (90 percent).

Microscopic Findings. Bile duct adenoma consists of branching and anastomosing tubules and fibrous stroma, which may be reminiscent of

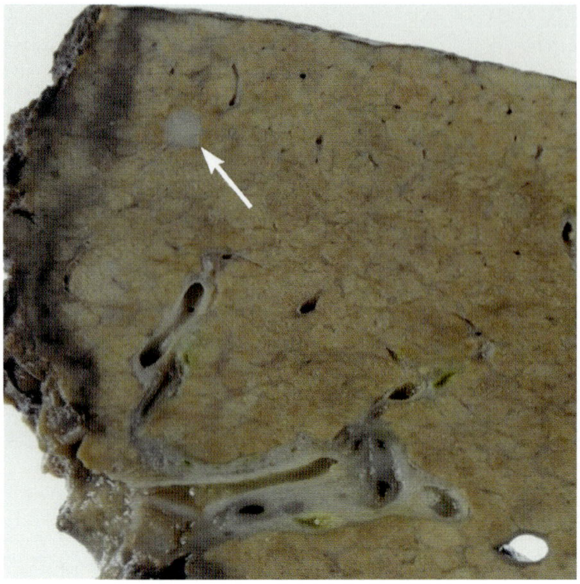

Figure 6-63

BILE DUCT ADENOMA

A whitish well-circumscribed nodule (arrow) is present in the liver parenchyma.

a ductular reaction (fig. 6-64A). The tubules have inconspicuous narrow lumens in most cases (fig. 6-64B), but are slightly dilated in rare cases (fig. 6-64C). If dilatation is conspicuous and irregular in shape, another diagnosis, such as von Meyenburg complexes, is suggested (fig. 6-65). The tubules are lined by a single-layered cuboidal epithelium with no or minimal dysplastic features. No mitotic figures are noted. The background stroma is variably fibrotic and may be associated with an inflammatory infiltrate (fig. 6-66). The proportion of tubules and stroma varies among cases, but is fairly uniform within the same lesion. Portal tracts are often entrapped within the nodules (fig. 6-64A).

Rare examples of bile duct adenoma show extensive clear cell changes, regarded as the *clear cell type* (69,70). Another variant is *oncocytic bile duct adenoma*, in which the lesional cells have an abundant eosinophilic cytoplasm and centrally located round nuclei (fig. 6-67) (71–73). Unlike the classic type, oncocytic bile duct adenoma consists of dilated tubules (72,73).

Frozen Sections. Bile duct adenoma is often encountered in frozen section specimens. A common scenario is that a nodule beneath the hepatic capsule incidentally found during surgery is submitted in order to exclude a metastatic deposit. Bile duct adenoma becomes the main benign differential diagnosis in that clinical setting. The size of the lesion is important because bile duct adenoma is unlikely to be larger than 1.5 cm.

Histologically, bile duct adenoma typically shows a relatively uniform distribution of tubules in contrast to metastatic adenocarcinomas, in which neoplastic tubules/ducts are more irregular in distribution and shape. Cytologic atypia is expected to be more pronounced in adenocarcinomas; however, difficulties are associated with assessing cytologic features in frozen sections (fig. 6-68). The presence of mitotic figures or necrosis suggests that malignancy is more likely. In bile duct adenoma, the interface between the lesion and liver parenchyma is well circumscribed with no obvious tissue destruction, whereas adenocarcinomas may display hepatocyte necrosis at the interface due to the invasive nature of the lesion.

Immunohistochemical Findings. Bile duct adenoma has a biliary phenotype, as evidenced by immunopositivity for CK7, CK8, CK18, CK19, and epithelial membrane antigen (EMA) (74). Furthermore, MUC5AC and MUC6 are positive in approximately 90 percent of cases (75). HepPar1 is always negative. CD56 may be focally expressed in 70 percent of cases (76). The Ki-67 index is low, generally less than 5 percent. The expression of p53 and MUC1, which are often positive in cholangiocarcinoma, is weak and heterogeneous, if present (77). Unlike cholangiocarcinoma, in which the expression of p16 is lost in approximately 80 percent of cases, bile duct adenoma preserves the expression of p16 in 80 percent of cases (78). The clear cell and oncocytic variants have a similar immunophenotype (69,70).

Differential Diagnosis. *Adenocarcinoma.* The main differential diagnosis of bile duct adenoma is adenocarcinoma, both primary (cholangiocarcinoma) and metastatic. Morphologic features helpful in this setting are described in the section, Frozen Sections in chapter 7. In most cases, differentiation is achieved based purely on the morphologic features, whereas immunohistochemistry may be required for equivocal cases. Commonly used markers include Ki-67, p53, p16, and MUC1.

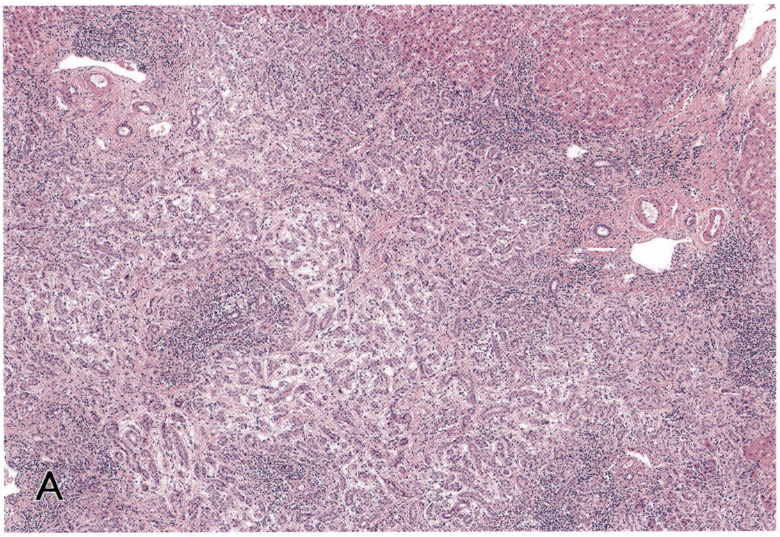

Figure 6-64

BILE DUCT ADENOMA (PERIBILARY GLAND HAMARTOMA)

A: The tumor consists of anastomosing tubules embedded in the fibrous stroma, with or without an inflammatory infiltrate. The pattern of growth is fairly uniform.

B: The tubules show inconspicuous lumens and minimal cellular atypia.

C: The tubules are slightly dilated.

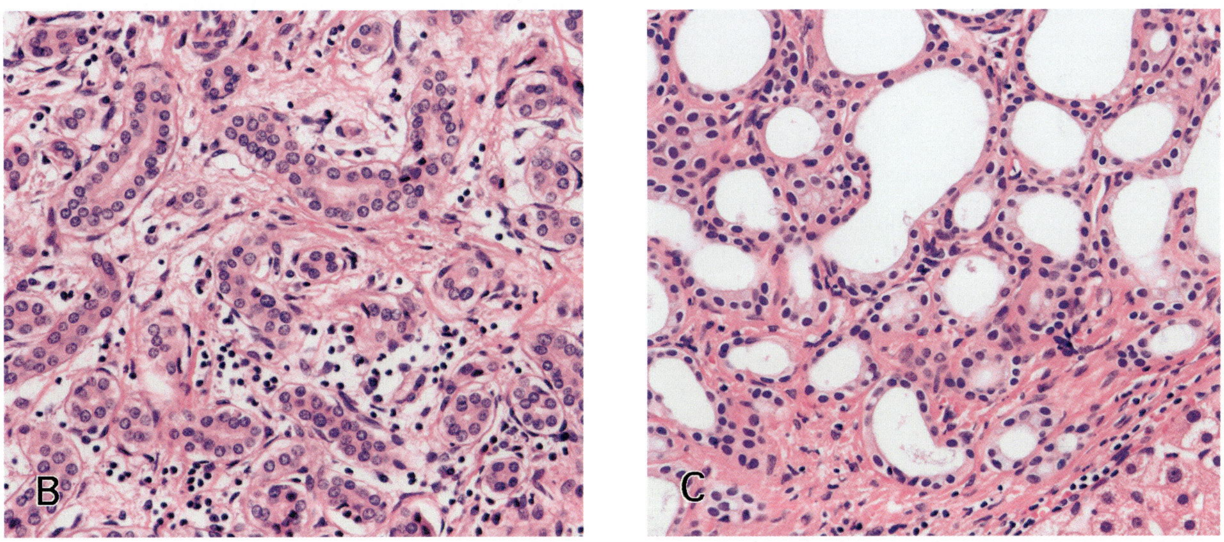

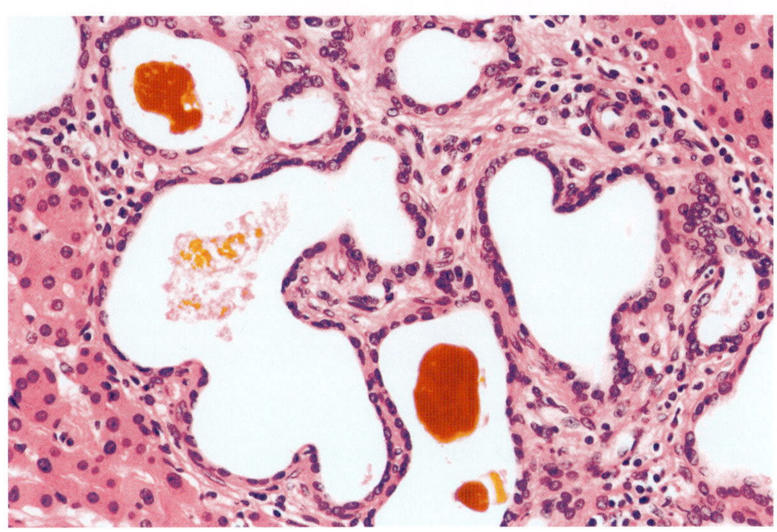

Figure 6-65

VON MEYENBURG COMPLEX

Bile contents are present in irregularly dilated ducts.

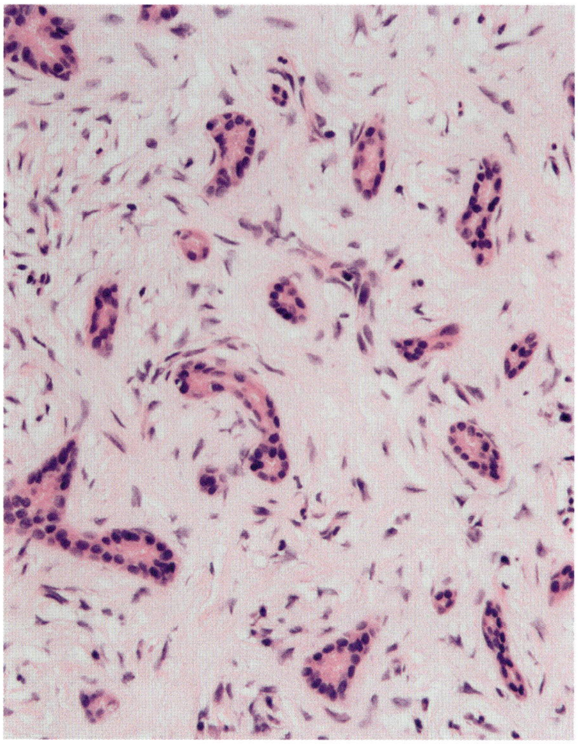

Figure 6-66

BILE DUCT ADENOMA

The stroma is fibrotic.

Immunostaining for CEA using a monoclonal antibody is often positive in metastatic adenocarcinoma but typically negative for bile duct adenoma (74).

Von Meyenburg Complexes. Bile duct adenoma differs from von Meyenburg complexes in that the tubular lumen of bile duct adenoma is narrow with no intraluminal bile contents (79,80). Von Meyenburg complexes are smaller than bile duct adenomas (less than 5 mm), and the lining epithelium is more attenuated.

Ductular Reaction. When bile duct adenoma develops against the background of chronic liver disease, it is important to discriminate it from ductular reactions. The nodular shape of the lesions suggests that duct adenoma is more likely because a ductular reaction is typically present in stellate-shaped portal tracts (81).

Treatment and Prognosis. Once bile duct adenoma is excised, the tumor does not recur. If a recurrent tumor develops, the original diagnosis of bile duct adenoma will be questioned. The risk of malignant transformation was previously considered to be very low (82); however, a recent study revealed that *BRAF* mutations are present in 50 percent of bile duct adenomas, suggesting

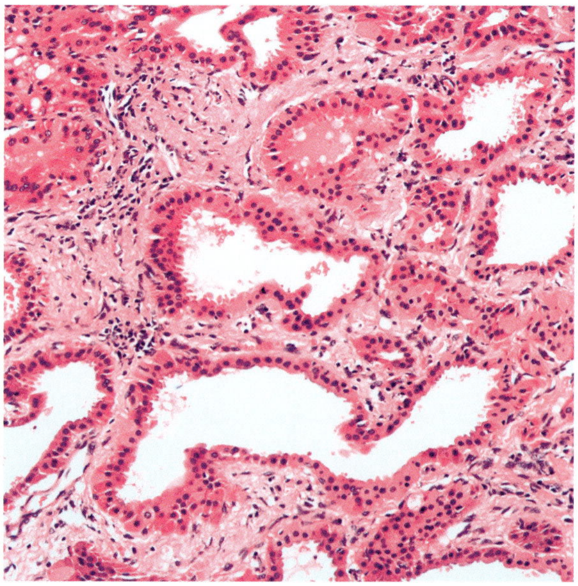

Figure 6-67

ONCOCYTIC BILE DUCT ADENOMA

The cells show oxyphilic change and form dilated tubules.

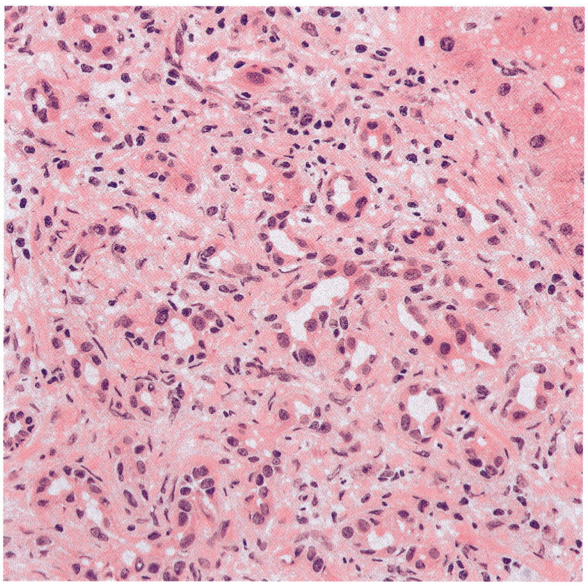

Figure 6-68

BILE DUCT ADENOMA

Nuclear enlargement and irregularity of tubular architecture may become conspicuous on frozen section.

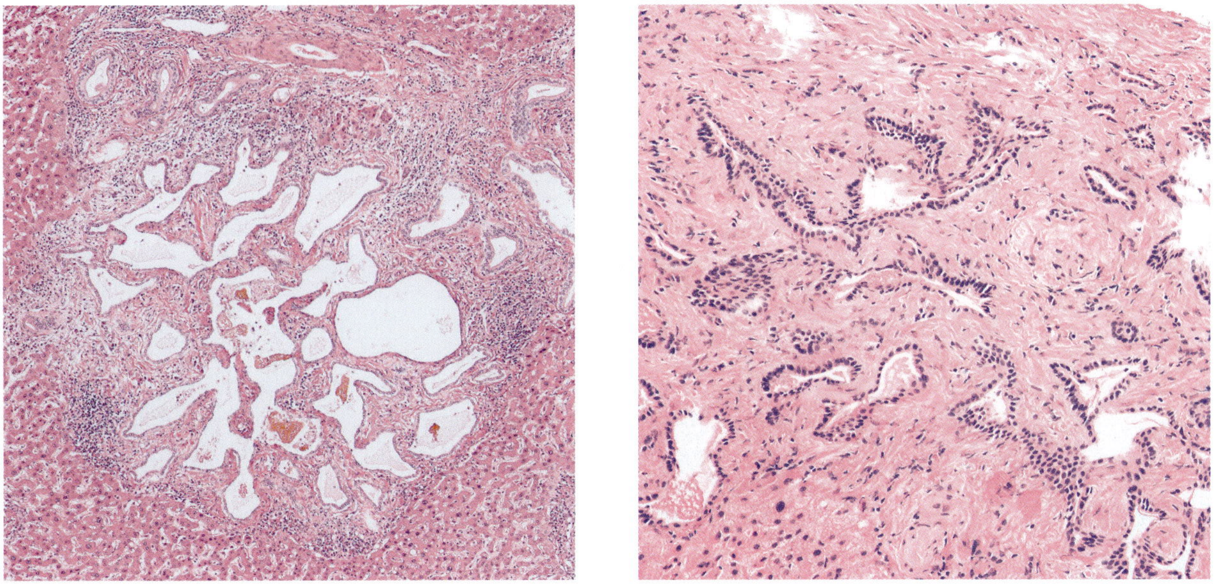

Figure 6-69

VON MEYENBURG COMPLEX

Left: A minute nodular lesion consisting of irregularly shaped, dilated ducts and a fibrotic stroma is present next to the small portal tract (right upper field). Bile-stained secretions are observed in ductal lumens.

Right: In this frozen section, a subcapsular lesion is made of irregularly shaped, bile-containing ducts embedded in a fibrotic stroma, leading to the diagnosis of von Meyenburg complex.

a possible link to *BRAF*-mutated intrahepatic cholangiocarcinoma (83). This progression model requires further examination.

VON MEYENBURG COMPLEX

Definition. *Von Meyenburg complex* is a microscopic hamartoma consisting of irregularly shaped dilated ducts and fibrotic stroma. It is suspected to represent a developmental remnant of embryonic ductal plates. The von Meyenburg complex is also called *biliary microhamartoma* (84).

Clinical Features. Von Meyenburg complex is common, with the prevalence at 5.6 percent based on an autopsy series (80). It is considerably more common in patients with other liver or kidney diseases of ductal plate malformation (e.g., polycystic liver and kidney). Its association with solitary biliary cysts also raises the possibility that some of the liver cysts may arise from dilatation of von Meyenburg complex (85). The microhamartomas are often multiple, particularly in cases associated with other fibrocystic diseases. In extreme examples, numerous small nodules with microcysts may suggest metastatic deposits on imaging (86–88). Similar to bile duct adenoma, subcapsular von Meyenburg complex is sometimes identified during surgery and is submitted for pathologic examination in order to rule out metastatic malignancy.

Gross Findings. The von Meyenburg complex is typically found incidentally at microscopic examination. A minute white nodule may be appreciated by close gross examination. Individual lesions are usually less than 5 mm (typically 1 to 2 mm).

Microscopic Findings. The von Meyenburg complex is commonly observed next to small portal tracts or in the subcapsular area (fig. 6-69). The lesions consist of dilated ductal structures and a surrounding fibrotic stroma (fig. 6-69, left). Irregular branching or papillary folding suggestive of ductal plate malformation may be observed. Ducts are lined by attenuated cuboidal epithelium with no dysplastic change (fig. 6-70). Bile-stained proteinaceous secretions are present in some ductal lumens (fig. 6-65). Inflammation is not conspicuous. These lesions may incidentally be found in medical liver biopsies (fig. 6-71).

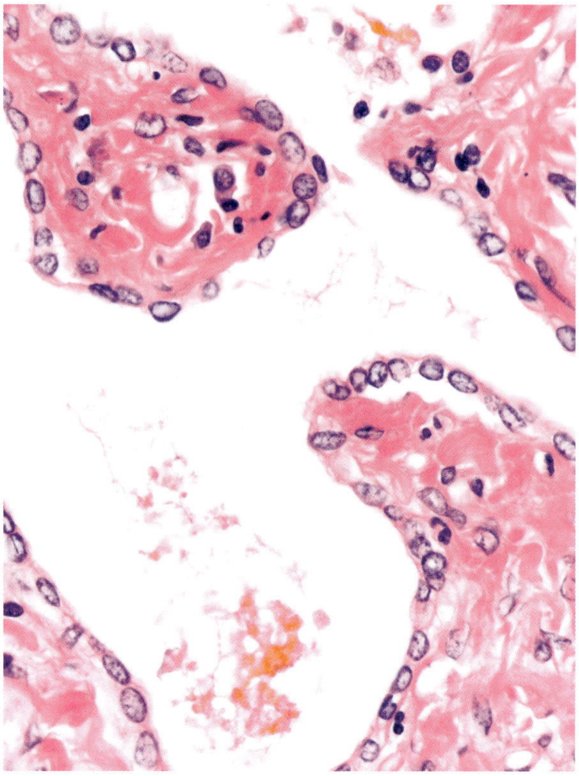

Figure 6-70

VON MEYENBURG COMPLEX

The lining epithelium is flattened and not dysplastic. Nuclei are round and hypochromatic.

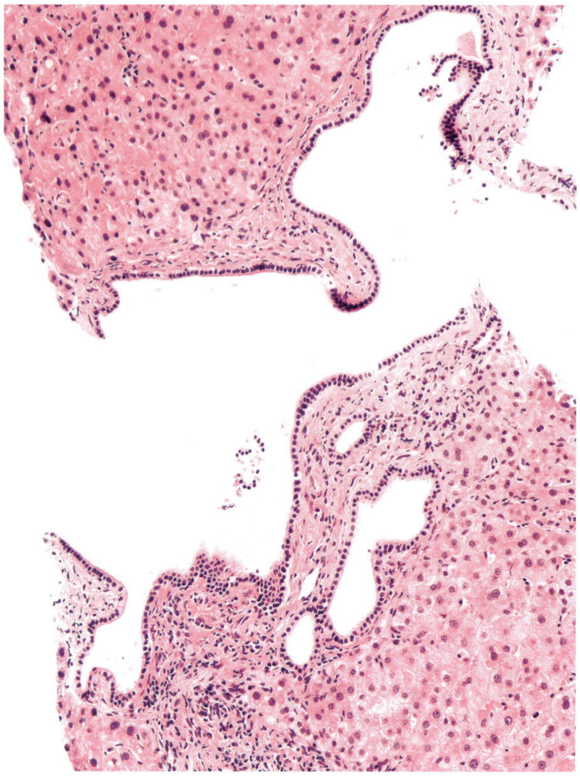

Figure 6-71

VON MEYENBURG COMPLEX

A part of the lesion is incidentally sampled in a liver needle biopsy. Abnormal dilated ducts surrounded by fibrous connective tissue raises the possibility of von Meyenburg complex.

The lining epithelium is positive for CK7, CK8, CK18, CK19, and EMA, in keeping with the biliary immunophenotype. Proliferative activity (e.g., MIB-1) is low (about 1 percent) (89).

Differential Diagnosis. *Bile Duct Adenoma.* The main entity in the differential diagnosis is bile duct adenoma, because the histologic appearance of tubules/ducts embedded in a fibrotic stroma is somewhat similar. Incidental identification is also a common scenario for both. The irregular shape of ducts, luminal dilatation, and presence of bile-stained secretion suggest von Meyenburg complex (84,90).

Ductal Plate Malformation-Type Intrahepatic Cholangiocarcinoma. This distinction may be challenging, particularly in biopsy samples. The uncommon subtype of cholangiocarcinoma shows dilated, irregularly shaped ductal structures and occasionally intraluminal bile (fig. 6-72) (91). The presence or absence of cellular atypia is crucial for this discrimination. The lining epithelium of von Meyenburg complex is flattened with small round nuclei (fig. 6-70), while ductal plate malformation-type intrahepatic cholangiocarcinoma is composed of columnar cells with atypical enlarged nuclei (fig. 6-73). Although the MIB-1 index is low (less than 5 percent) in the latter (91), von Meyenburg complex is less proliferating, with the index usually less than 1 percent (89). Both conditions are negative for p53.

Cholangiocarcinoma. There are some reports of cholangiocarcinoma arising from von Meyenburg complex (89,92), but this association has not been completely proven and requires further studies. Some of the reported cases may represent ductal plate malformation-type cholangiocarcinoma.

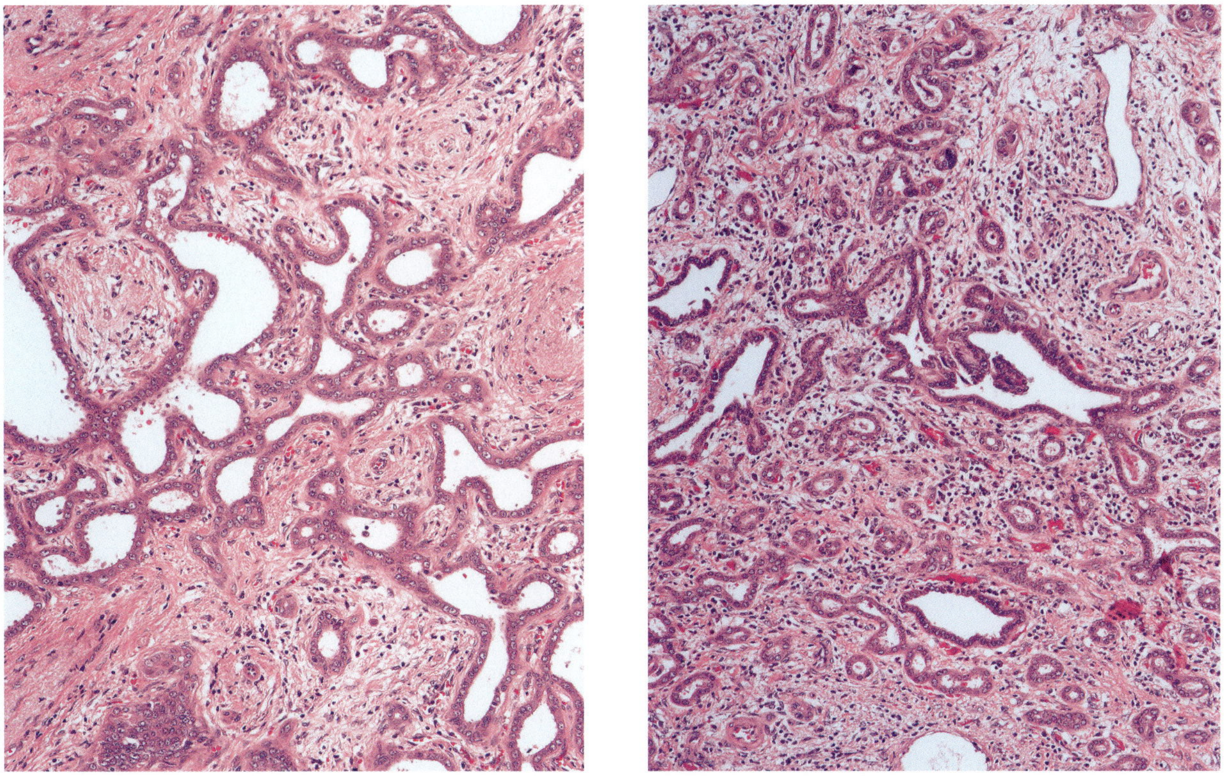

Figure 6-72

DUCTAL PLATE MALFORMATION-TYPE INTRAHEPATIC CHOLANGIOCARCINOMA

Left: Tumor cells are arranged in irregularly dilated ducts with papillary folding, resembling ductal plate malformation. The microscopic appearance may partly resemble von Meyenburg complex.

Right: Tumor cells form focally dilated tubules, some containing bile. This uncommon form of cholangiocarcinoma may be mistaken for von Meyenburg complex.

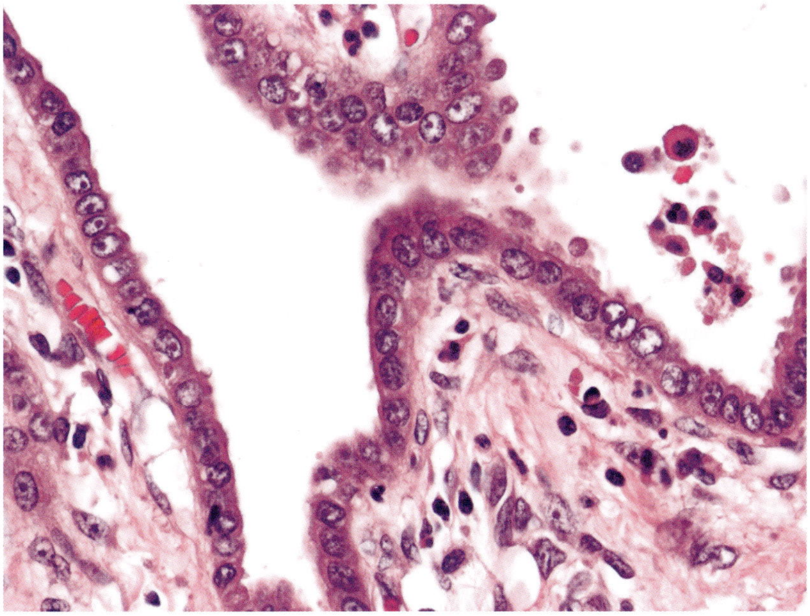

Figure 6-73

DUCTAL PLATE MALFORMATION-TYPE INTRAHEPATIC CHOLANGIOCARCINOMA

The lining epithelium has enlarged nuclei with distinct nucleoli, an appearance that is clearly more atypical than that in von Meyenburg complex (see fig. 6-70).

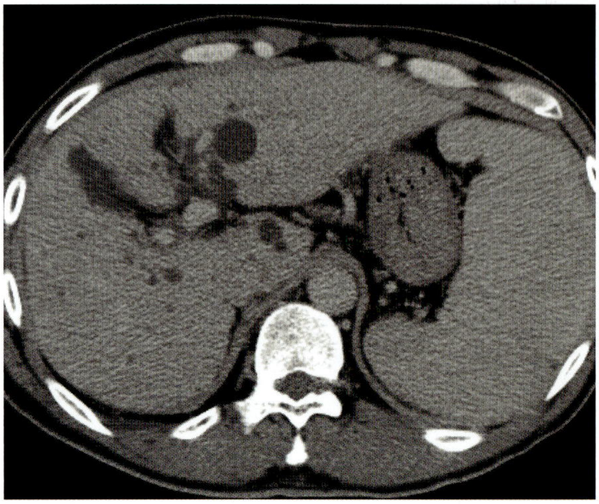

Figure 6-74

PERIBILIARY CYSTS

Multiple cysts around the perihilar bile ducts are seen in this CT scan.

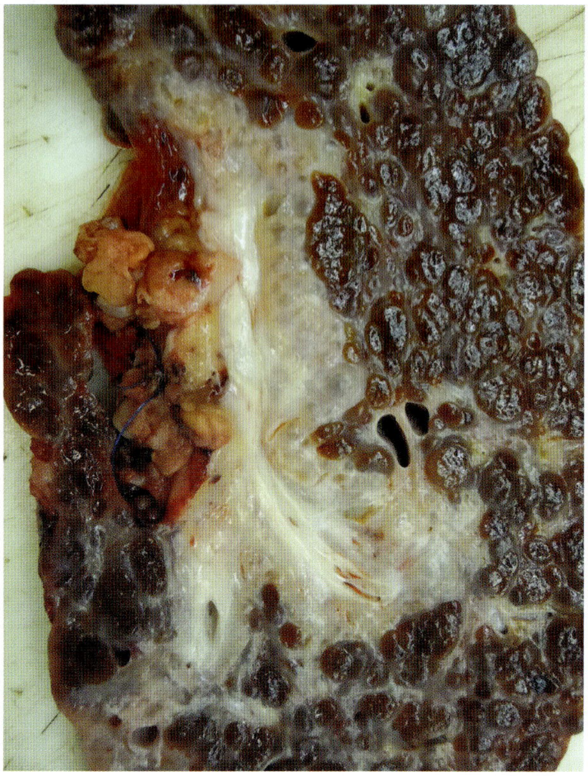

Figure 6-75

PERIBILIARY CYSTS

Multiple small cysts are located in the perihilar connective tissue.

OTHER BENIGN BILIARY LESIONS

Peribiliary Cysts. Peribiliary cysts are characterized by cystic dilatation of the peribiliary glands or their conduits (fig. 6-74). Although they usually develop at a perihilar location, extensive cases also involve extrahepatic bile ducts. They may be solitary and multiple. Cysts are typically found incidentally by imaging analysis. Many patients with peribiliary cysts have chronic liver disease, particularly alcoholic liver disease. If multiple cysts are compressing the bile duct, imaging shows irregular biliary strictures reminiscent of cholangiocarcinoma or PSC.

Grossly, the cysts around the large bile ducts range in diameter from 0.2 to 2.0 cm and contain serous, sometimes mucinous fluid (fig. 6-75). Histologically, the cysts are lined by flattened cuboidal epithelium surrounded by fibrous connective tissue (fig. 6-76, left). The lining epithelium may focally show mucinous metaplasia, and dysplasia is uncommon. The presence of peribiliary glands nearby is a diagnostic clue for determining the origin of the cysts (fig. 6-76, right). Although few studies have described biliary neoplasms potentially arising from peribiliary cysts (fig. 6-77), the risk of neoplastic transformation appears to be very low (24).

Ciliated Foregut Cysts. These have been suggested to arise from a remnant of the embryonic foregut (93). The most prevalent site is the subcapsular area of segment IV, but they may also develop elsewhere in the liver (94). They generally form unilocular cysts less than 5 cm in diameter; however, larger lesions up to 19 cm in diameter have been reported (95). Their contents are fluid that is slightly mucinous, clear, or milky.

The classic histologic appearance of these lesions consists of four layers: an inner epithelial lining, loose connective tissue, smooth muscle, and a fibrous capsule (fig. 6-78) (95,96). The lining is ciliated, pseudostratified columnar epithelium resembling the bronchial mucosa. Squamous or gastric metaplasia is observed in up to 20 percent of cases (95,97). Malignant transformation is rare, and all reported cases of associated carcinoma have exhibited squamous differentiation (95,98–102).

Multicystic Biliary Hamartoma. This was originally described as a protruding mass around the falciform ligament (61); however, additional

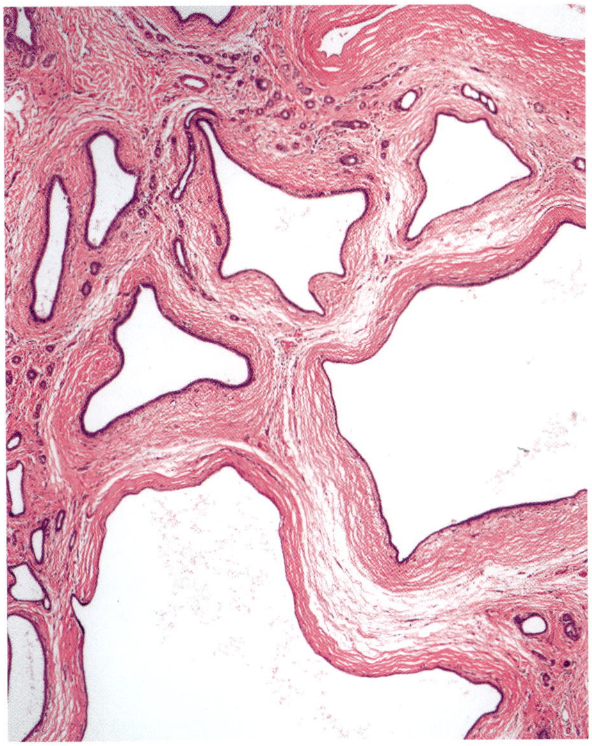

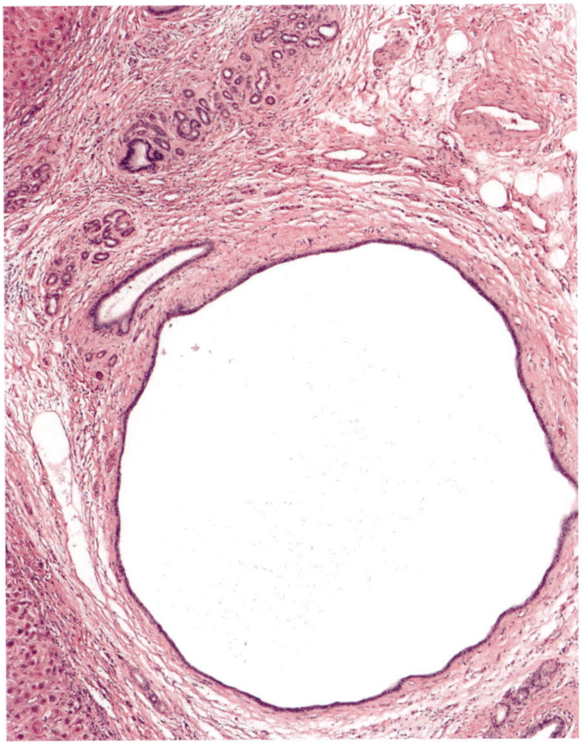

Figure 6-76

PERIBILIARY CYSTS

Left: The cysts are lined by the flat attenuated epithelium. Nondilated glands are present around the cysts. Right: The presence of glands around the cyst suggests a peribiliary gland origin.

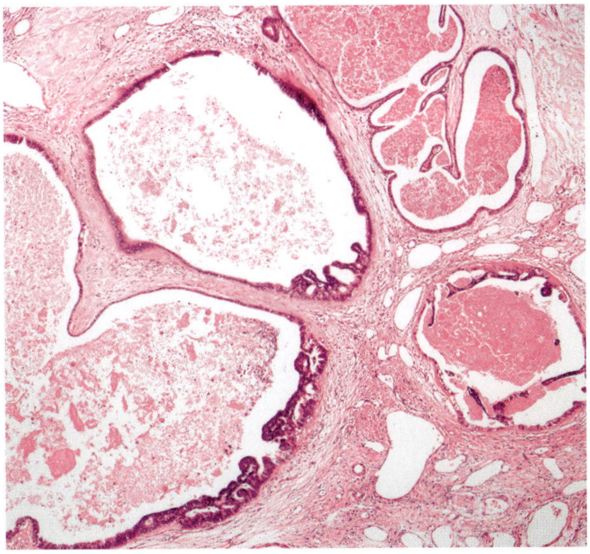

Figure 6-77

CARCINOMA ARISING IN PERIBILIARY CYSTS

The lining epithelium shows micropapillary proliferation and cellular atypia.

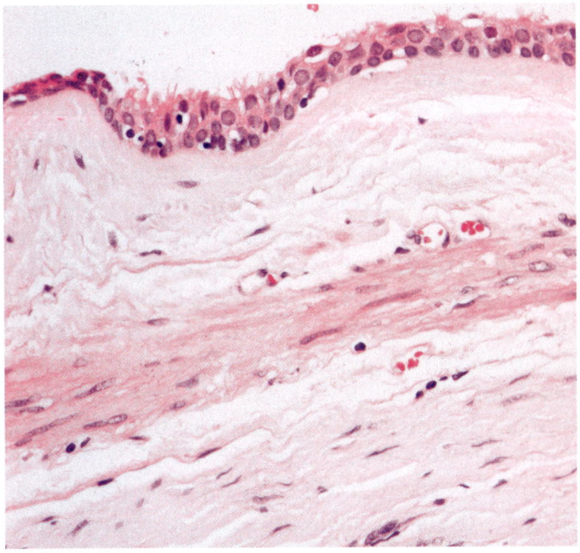

Figure 6-78

CILIATED FOREGUT CYST

The lining epithelium is composed of ciliated columnar cells. A muscular layer is present in the cyst wall.

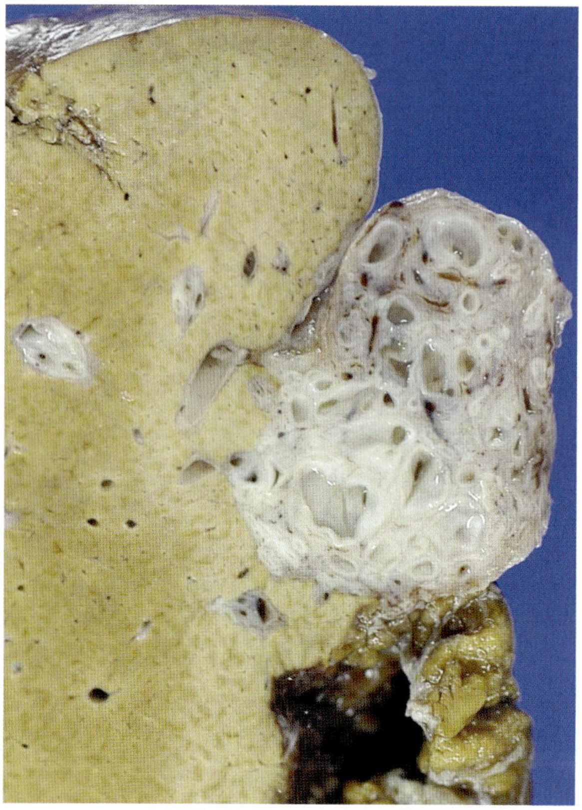

Figure 6-79

MULTICYSTIC BILIARY HAMARTOMA

A protruding mass has a honeycomb-like appearance on cut section.

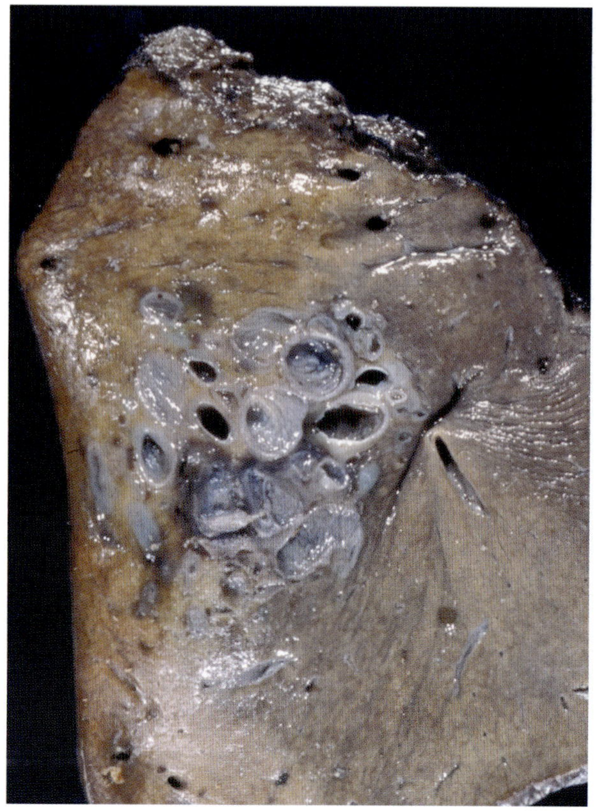

Figure 6-80

MULTICYSTIC BILIARY HAMARTOMA

Large ducts are aggregated in the liver parenchyma.

studies suggested that this hamartomatous lesion can develop within the liver parenchyma of any segment. A characteristic gross feature is a honeycomb-like appearance on cut section (fig. 6-79) (62,103,104). Multiple cysts that are relatively similar in size are present in the fibrotic stroma (fig. 6-80). Histologically, the cysts consist of dilated bile ducts lined by a nondysplastic columnar epithelium (fig. 6-81). Liver parenchyma or peribiliary glands are present between the ducts. Similar to other hamartomatous conditions, the fibrous obliteration of small ducts may be noted (fig. 6-82). Although its appearance may mimic monolobular Caroli disease, there are no features of congenital hepatic fibrosis in the background liver.

Biliary Adenofibroma. This is a rare neoplasm that has not been characterized in detail because only sporadic single case reports are available (105–110). The pathologic features of the reported cases are not consistent: some cases show a solid mass with sponge-like microcysts (105), while others display a cystic mass containing multiple large cysts (107). Due to the lack of a clear definition, this diagnostic term may have been used for various benign-appearing lesions (i.e., unusual hamartoma and low-grade carcinoma) that contain glandular and stromal components and do not fit with other known entities.

The clinicopathologic features of cases reported as "biliary adenofibroma" are summarized as follows. Patients are all adults, with the youngest being 20 years of age. Tumor size ranges from 6 to 20 cm (108). The tumors show a sponge-like or solid and cystic appearance on cut section. The lesions consist of tubulocystic glandular components and surrounding fibrous connective tissue (108). Glands are irregular in shape, with intraglandular papillary projections reminiscent of ductal plate malformation

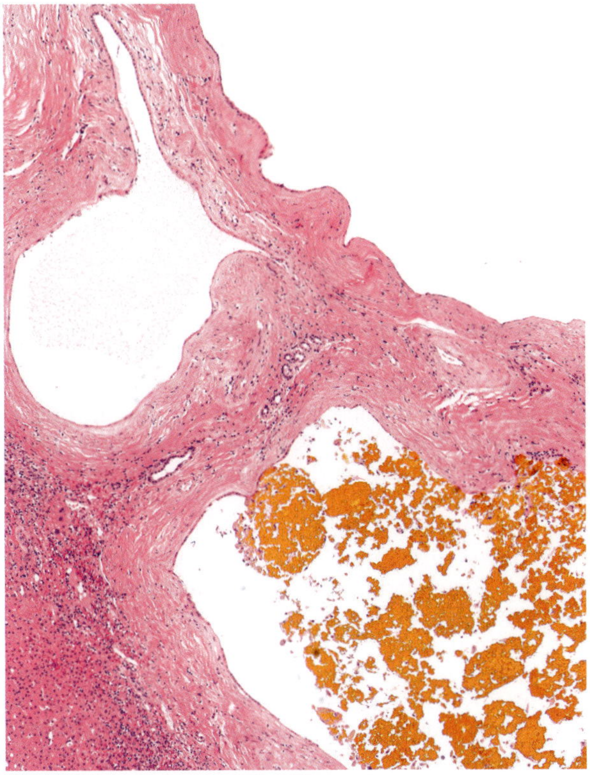

Figure 6-81

MULTICYSTIC BILIARY HAMARTOMA

The cysts are lined by the flat cuboidal epithelium. Bile may be present in the cysts. Small glands are seen in the periductal fibrous connective tissue.

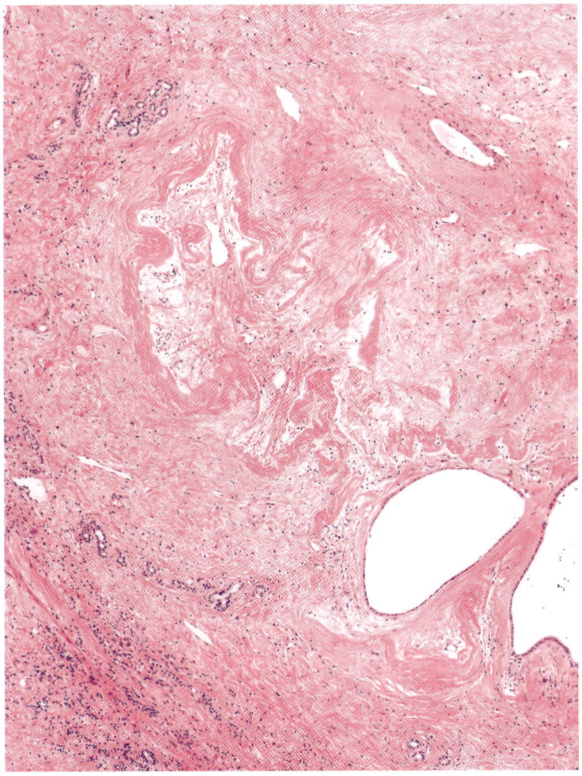

Figure 6-82

MULTICYSTIC BILIARY HAMARTOMA

There is fibrous obliteration of the duct.

(106,108). The lining is single-layered cuboidal epithelium with no goblet cells. Many "apocrine snouts" are detected (105). The epithelial cells are bland; however, 4 out of the 9 cases reported had malignant transformation of the epithelial components (107–109,111).

REFERENCES

1. Zen Y, Fujii T, Itatsu K, et al. Biliary papillary tumors share pathological features with intraductal papillary mucinous neoplasm of the pancreas. Hepatology 2006;44:1333-1343.
2. Ohtsuka M, Kimura F, Shimizu H, et al. Similarities and differences between intraductal papillary tumors of the bile duct with and without macroscopically visible mucin secretion. Am J Surg Pathol 2011;35:512-521.
3. Nakanuma Y, Curado MP, Franceschi S, Gores G, Paradis V, Sripa B. Intrahepatic cholangiocarcinoma. In: Bosman FT, Carneiro F, Hruban RH, Theise ND, eds. WHO classification of tumours of the digestive system. Lyon: IARC; 2010:217-224.
4. Shibahara H, Tamada S, Goto M, et al. Pathologic features of mucin-producing bile duct tumors: two histopathologic categories as counterparts of pancreatic intraductal papillary-mucinous neoplasms. Am J Surg Pathol 2004;28:327-338.
5. Zen Y, Fujii T, Itatsu K, et al. Biliary cystic tumors with bile duct communication: a cystic variant of intraductal papillary neoplasm of the bile duct. Mod Pathol 2006;19:1243-1254.

6. Zen Y, Sasaki M, Fujii T, et al. Different expression patterns of mucin core proteins and cytokeratins during intrahepatic cholangiocarcinogenesis from biliary intraepithelial neoplasia and intraductal papillary neoplasm of the bile duct—an immunohistochemical study of 110 cases of hepatolithiasis. J Hepatol 2006;44:350-358.
7. Kloppel G, Kosmahl M. Is the intraductal papillary mucinous neoplasia of the biliary tract a counterpart of pancreatic papillary mucinous neoplasm? J Hepatol 2006;44:249-250.
8. Minagawa N, Sato N, Mori Y, Tamura T, Higure A, Yamaguchi K. A comparison between intraductal papillary neoplasms of the biliary tract (BT-IPMNs) and intraductal papillary mucinous neoplasms of the pancreas (P-IPMNs) reveals distinct clinical manifestations and outcomes. Eur J Surg Oncol 2013;39:554-558.
9. Kloek JJ, van der Gaag NA, Erdogan D, et al. A comparative study of intraductal papillary neoplasia of the biliary tract and pancreas. Hum Pathol 2011;42:824-832.
10. Chen TC, Nakanuma Y, Zen Y, et al. Intraductal papillary neoplasia of the liver associated with hepatolithiasis. Hepatology 2001;34(Pt 1):651-658.
11. Kim HJ, Kim MH, Lee SK, et al. Mucin-hypersecreting bile duct tumor characterized by a striking homology with an intraductal papillary mucinous tumor (IPMT) of the pancreas. Endoscopy 2000;32:389-393.
12. Yeh TS, Tseng JH, Chen TC, et al. Characterization of intrahepatic cholangiocarcinoma of the intraductal growth-type and its precursor lesions. Hepatology 2005;42:657-664.
13. Jung G, Park KM, Lee SS, Yu E, Hong SM, Kim J. Long-term clinical outcome of the surgically resected intraductal papillary neoplasm of the bile duct. J Hepatol 2012;57:787-793.
14. Schlitter AM, Born D, Bettstetter M, et al. Intraductal papillary neoplasms of the bile duct: stepwise progression to carcinoma involves common molecular pathways. Mod Pathol 2014;27:73-86.
15. Zen Y, Jang KT, Ahn S, et al. Intraductal papillary neoplasms and mucinous cystic neoplasms of the hepatobiliary system: demographic differences between Asian and Western populations, and comparison with pancreatic counterparts. Histopathology 2014;65:164-173.
16. Jang KT, Hong SM, Lee KT, et al. Intraductal papillary neoplasm of the bile duct associated with Clonorchis sinensis infection. Virchows Arch 2008;453:589-598.
17. Zen Y, Quaglia A, Heaton N, Rela M, Portmann B. Two distinct pathways of carcinogenesis in primary sclerosing cholangitis. Histopathology 2011;59:1100-1110.
17a. Fujikura K, Fukumoto T, Ajiki T, et al. Comparative clinicopathological study of biliary intraductal papillary neoplasms and papillary cholangiocarcinomas. Histopathology 2016;69:950-961.
18. Liu Y, Zhong X, Yan L, Zheng J, Liu Z, Liang C. Diagnostic performance of CT and MRI in distinguishing intraductal papillary neoplasm of the bile duct from cholangiocarcinoma with intraductal papillary growth. Eur Radiol 2015;25:1967-1974.
19. Kim HJ, Yu ES, Byun JH, et al. CT differentiation of mucin-producing cystic neoplasms of the liver from solitary bile duct cysts. AJR Am J Roentgenol 2014;202:83-91.
20. Lim JH, Zen Y, Jang KT, Kim YK, Nakanuma Y. Cyst-forming intraductal papillary neoplasm of the bile ducts: description of imaging and pathologic aspects. AJR Am J Roentgenol 2011;197:1111-1120.
21. Takanami K, Yamada T, Tsuda M, et al. Intraductal papillary mucininous neoplasm of the bile ducts: multimodality assessment with pathologic correlation. Abdom Imaging 2011;36:447-456.
22. Li T, Ji Y, Zhi XT, et al. A comparison of hepatic mucinous cystic neoplasms with biliary intraductal papillary neoplasms. Clin Gastroenterol Hepatol 2009;7:586-593.
23. Yeh TS, Tseng JH, Chiu CT, et al. Cholangiographic spectrum of intraductal papillary mucinous neoplasm of the bile ducts. Ann Surg 2006;244:248-253.
23a. Yokode M, Yamashita Y, Zen Y. Biliary intraductal papillary neoplasm with metachronous multiple tumors—true multicentric tumors or intrabiliary dissemination: a case report and review of the literature. Mol Clin Oncol 2017;6:315-320.
24. Nakanishi Y, Zen Y, Hirano S, et al. Intraductal oncocytic papillary neoplasm of the bile duct: the first case of peribiliary gland origin. J Hepatobiliary Pancreat Surg 2009;16:869-873.
25. Nakanishi Y, Nakanuma Y, Ohara M, et al. Intraductal papillary neoplasm arising from peribiliary glands connecting with the inferior branch of the bile duct of the anterior segment of the liver. Pathol Int 2011;61:773-777.
26. Adsay NV, Fukushima N, Furukawa T, et al. Intraductal neoplasms of the pancreas. In: Bosman FT, Carneiro F, Hruban RH, Theise ND, eds. WHO classification of tumours of the digestive system. Lyon: IARC; 2010:304-313.
27. Rocha FG, Lee H, Katabi N, et al. Intraductal papillary neoplasm of the bile duct: a biliary equivalent to intraductal papillary mucinous neoplasm of the pancreas? Hepatology 2012;56:1352-1360.

28. Sasaki M, Matsubara T, Nitta T, Sato Y, Nakanuma Y. GNAS and KRAS mutations are common in intraductal papillary neoplasms of the bile duct. PLoS One 2013;8:e81706.
29. Matthaei H, Wu J, Dal Molin M, et al. GNAS codon 201 mutations are uncommon in intraductal papillary neoplasms of the bile duct. HPB (Oxford) 2012;14:677-783.
30. Tsai JH, Yuan RH, Chen YL, Liau JY, Jeng YM. GNAS Is frequently mutated in a specific subgroup of intraductal papillary neoplasms of the bile duct. Am J Surg Pathol 2013;37:1862-1870.
31. Wu J, Matthaei H, Maitra A, et al. Recurrent GNAS mutations define an unexpected pathway for pancreatic cyst development. Sci Transl Med 2011;3:92ra66.
32. Furukawa T, Kuboki Y, Tanji E, et al. Whole-exome sequencing uncovers frequent GNAS mutations in intraductal papillary mucinous neoplasms of the pancreas. Sci Rep 2011;1:161.
33. Nakanishi Y, Zen Y, Kondo S, Itoh T, Itatsu K, Nakanuma Y. Expression of cell cycle-related molecules in biliary premalignant lesions: biliary intraepithelial neoplasia and biliary intraductal papillary neoplasm. Hum Pathol 2008;39:1153-1161.
34. Abraham SC, Lee JH, Boitnott JK, Argani P, Furth EE, Wu TT. Microsatellite instability in intraductal papillary neoplasms of the biliary tract. Mod Pathol 2002;15:1309-1317.
35. Aishima S, Nishihara Y, Tsujita E, et al. Biliary neoplasia with extensive intraductal spread associated with liver cirrhosis: a hitherto unreported variant of biliary intraepithelial neoplasia. Hum Pathol 2008;39:939-947.
36. Zen Y, Amarapurkar AD, Portmann BC. Intraductal tubulopapillary neoplasm of the bile duct: potential origin from peribiliary cysts. Hum Pathol 2012;43:440-445.
37. Schlitter AM, Jang KT, Kloppel G, et al. Intraductal tubulopapillary neoplasms of the bile ducts: clinicopathologic, immunohistochemical, and molecular analysis of 20 cases. Mod Pathol 2015;28:1249-1264.
38. Zen Y, Pedica F, Patcha VR, et al. Mucinous cystic neoplasms of the liver: a clinicopathological study and comparison with intraductal papillary neoplasms of the bile duct. Mod Pathol 2011;24:1079-1089.
39. Yamaguchi H, Shimizu M, et al. Intraductal tubulopapillary neoplasms of the pancreas distinct from pancreatic intraepithelial neoplasia and intraductal papillary mucinous neoplasms. Am J Surg Pathol 2009;33(8):1164-1172.
40. Katabi N, Torres J, Klimstra DS. Intraductal tubular neoplasms of the bile ducts. Am J Surg Pathol 2012;36:1647-1655.
41. Park HJ, Jang KT, Heo JS, Choi YL, Han J, Kim SH. A potential case of intraductal tubulopapillary neoplasms of the bile duct. Pathol Int 2010;60:630-635.
42. Jang KT, Saka B, Zen Y, Pambuccian S, Bacchi C, Adsay V. Tubulocystic carcinoma of bile ducts: A hitherto unrecognized and diagnostically challenging entity often mistaken as a benign lesion; clinicopathologic analysis of 6 cases. Mod Pathol 2013;26:404A.
43. Yamaguchi H, Kuboki Y, Hatori T, et al. Somatic mutations in PIK3CA and activation of AKT in intraductal tubulopapillary neoplasms of the pancreas. Am J Surg Pathol 2011;35:1812-1817.
44. Tsui WM, Adsay NV, Crawford JM, Hruban R, Kloppel G, Wee A. Mucinous cystic neoplasms of the liver. In: Bosman FT, Carneiro F, Hruban RH, Theise ND, eds. WHO classification of tumours of the digestive system. Lyon: IARC; 2010:236-238.
45. Shima Y, Horimi T, Shibuya Y, Sakurama K, Nishie M, Morita S. Resected cystadenoma of the common bile duct. J Hepatobiliary Pancreat Surg 2004;11:438-440.
46. Ishak KG, Willis GW, Cummins SD, Bullock AA. Biliary cystadenoma and cystadenocarcinoma: report of 14 cases and review of the literature. Cancer 1977;39:322-338.
47. Devaney K, Goodman ZD, Ishak KG. Hepatobiliary cystadenoma and cystadenocarcinoma. A light microscopic and immunohistochemical study of 70 patients. Am J Surg Pathol 1994;18:1078-1091.
48. Arnaoutakis DJ, Kim Y, Pulitano C, et al. Management of biliary cystic tumors: a multi-institutional analysis of a rare liver tumor. Ann Surg 2015;261:361-367.
49. Crippa S, Salvia R, Warshaw AL, et al. Mucinous cystic neoplasm of the pancreas is not an aggressive entity: lessons from 163 resected patients. Ann Surg 2008;247:571-579.
50. Zamboni G, Scarpa A, Bogina G, et al. Mucinous cystic tumors of the pancreas: clinicopathological features, prognosis, and relationship to other mucinous cystic tumors. Am J Surg Pathol 1999;23:410-422.
51. Albores-Saavedra J, Cordova-Ramon JC, Chable-Montero F, Dorantes-Heredia R, Henson DE. Cystadenomas of the liver and extrahepatic bile ducts: morphologic and immunohistochemical characterization of the biliary and intestinal variants. Ann Diagn Pathol 2015;19:124-129.
52. Wheeler DA, Edmondson HA. Cystadenoma with mesenchymal stroma (CMS) in the liver and bile ducts. A clinicopathologic study of 17 cases, 4 with malignant change. Cancer 1985;56:1434-1445.

53. Lempinen M, Halme L, Numminen K, Arola J, Nordin A, Makisalo H. Spontaneous rupture of a hepatic cystadenoma and cystadenocarcinoma: report of two cases. J Hepatobiliary Pancreat Surg 2005;12:409-414.
54. Takayasu K, Mizuguchi Y, Muramatsu Y, et al. Late complication of a large simple cyst of the liver mimicking cystadenocarcinoma after sclerotherapy. AJR Am J Roentgenol 2003;181:464-466.
55. Kitajima Y, Okayama Y, Hirai M, et al. Intracystic hemorrhage of a simple liver cyst mimicking a biliary cystadenocarcinoma. J Gastroenterol 2003;38:190-193.
56. Jang KT, Park SM, Basturk O, et al. Clinicopathologic characteristics of 29 invasive carcinomas arising in 178 pancreatic mucinous cystic neoplasms with ovarian-type stroma: implications for management and prognosis. Am J Surg Pathol 2015;39:179-187.
57. Logrono R, Rampy BA, Adegboyega PA. Fine needle aspiration cytology of hepatobiliary cystadenoma with mesenchymal stroma. Cancer 2002;96:37-42.
58. Kim JY, Kim SH, Eun HW, et al. Differentiation between biliary cystic neoplasms and simple cysts of the liver: accuracy of CT. AJR Am J Roentgenol 2010;195:1142-1148.
59. Seo JK, Kim SH, Lee SH, et al. Appropriate diagnosis of biliary cystic tumors: comparison with atypical hepatic simple cysts. Eur J Gastroenterol Hepatol 2010;22:989-996.
60. Doussot A, Gluskin J, Groot-Koerkamp B, et al. The accuracy of pre-operative imaging in the management of hepatic cysts. HPB (Oxford) 2015;17:889-895.
61. Zen Y, Terahata S, Miyayama S, et al. Multicystic biliary hamartoma: a hitherto undescribed lesion. Hum Pathol 2006;37:339-344.
62. Ryu Y, Matsui O, Zen Y, et al. Multicystic biliary hamartoma: imaging findings in four cases. Abdom Imaging 2010;35:543-547.
63. Hsu M, Terris B, Wu TT, et al. Endometrial cysts within the liver: a rare entity and its differential diagnosis with mucinous cystic neoplasms of the liver. Hum Pathol 2014;45:761-767.
64. Czermak BV, Akhan O, Hiemetzberger R, et al. Echinococcosis of the liver. Abdom Imaging 2008;33:133-143.
65. Pedrosa I, Saiz A, Arrazola J, Ferreiros J, Pedrosa CS. Hydatid disease: radiologic and pathologic features and complications. Radiographics 2000;20:795-817.
66. McManus DP, Zhang W, Li J, Bartley PB. Echinococcosis. Lancet 2003;362:1295-1304.
67. Bhathal PS, Hughes NR, Goodman ZD. The so-called bile duct adenoma is a peribiliary gland hamartoma. Am J Surg Pathol 1996;20:858-864.
68. Allaire GS, Rabin L, Ishak KG, Sesterhenn IA. Bile duct adenoma. A study of 152 cases. Am J Surg Pathol 1988;12:708-715.
69. Wu WW, Gu M, Lu D. Cytopathologic, histopathologic, and immunohistochemical features of intrahepatic clear cell bile duct adenoma: a case report and review of the literature. Case Rep Pathol 2014;2014:874826.
70. Albores-Saavedra J, Hoang MP, Murakata LA, Sinkre P, Yaziji H. Atypical bile duct adenoma, clear cell type: a previously undescribed tumor of the liver. Am J Surg Pathol 2001;25:956-960.
71. Johannesen EJ, Wu Z, Holly JS. Bile duct adenoma with oncocytic features. Case Rep Pathol 2014;2014:282010.
72. Hastir D, Verset L, Demetter P. Intrahepatic bile duct adenoma with oncocytic features. Liver Int 2013;33:273.
73. Arena V, Arena E, Stigliano E, Capelli A. Bile duct adenoma with oncocytic features. Histopathology 2006;49:318-320.
74. Hornick JL, Lauwers GY, Odze RD. Immunohistochemistry can help distinguish metastatic pancreatic adenocarcinomas from bile duct adenomas and hamartomas of the liver. Am J Surg Pathol 2005;29:381-389.
75. Hughes NR, Goodman ZD, Bhathal PS. An immunohistochemical profile of the so-called bile duct adenoma: clues to pathogenesis. Am J Surg Pathol 2010;34:1312-1318.
76. Gutgemann I, Haas S, Berg JP, Zhou H, Buttner R, Fischer HP. CD56 expression aids in the differential diagnosis of cholangiocarcinomas and benign cholangiocellular lesions. Virchows Arch 2006;448:407-411.
77. Zen Y, Britton D, Mitra V, et al. Tubulin beta-III: a novel immunohistochemical marker for intrahepatic peripheral cholangiocarcinoma. Histopathology 2014;65:784-792.
78. Sasaki M, Matsubara T, Kakuda Y, Sato Y, Nakanuma Y. Immunostaining for polycomb group protein EZH2 and senescent marker p16INK4a may be useful to differentiate cholangiolocellular carcinoma from ductular reaction and bile duct adenoma. Am J Surg Pathol 2014;38:364-369.
79. Govindarajan S, Peters RL. The bile duct adenoma. A lesion distinct from Meyenburg complex. Arch Pathol Lab Med 1984;108:922-924.
80. Redston MS, Wanless IR. The hepatic von Meyenburg complex: prevalence and association with hepatic and renal cysts among 2843 autopsies [corrected]. Mod Pathol 1996;9:233-237.
81. Gouw AS, Clouston AD, Theise ND. Ductular reactions in human liver: diversity at the interface. Hepatology 2011;54:1853-1863.

82. Hasebe T, Sakamoto M, Mukai K, et al. Cholangiocarcinoma arising in bile duct adenoma with focal area of bile duct hamartoma. Virchows Arch 1995;426:209-213.
83. Pujals A, Amaddeo G, Castain C, et al. BRAF V600E mutations in bile duct adenomas. Hepatology 2015;61:403-405.
84. Goodman ZD, Luigi MT, Wee A. Tumours and tumour-like lesions of the liver. In: Burt A, Portmann B, Ferrell L, eds. MacSween's pathology of the liver, 6th ed. Edinburgh: Elsevier; 2012:761-851.
85. Desmet VJ. Congenital diseases of intrahepatic bile ducts: variations on the theme "ductal plate malformation." Hepatology 1992;16:1069-1083.
86. Singhal A, Kanagala R, Wright HI, Kohli V. Multiple bile duct hamartomas mimicking diffuse hepatic metastasis: GI image. J Gastrointest Surg 2010;14:1629-1631.
87. Wohlgemuth WA, Bottger J, Bohndorf K. MRI, CT, US and ERCP in the evaluation of bile duct hamartomas (von Meyenburg complex): a case report. Eur Radiol 1998;8:1623-1626.
88. Panaro F, Gauff G, Dong G, Testa G, Benedetti E. Images of interest. Hepatobiliary and pancreatic: multiple biliary hamartomas (von Meyenburg complex). J Gastroenterol Hepatol 2004;19:463.
89. Rocken C, Pross M, Brucks U, Ridwelski K, Roessner A. Cholangiocarcinoma occurring in a liver with multiple bile duct hamartomas (von Meyenburg complexes). Arch Pathol Lab Med 2000;124:1704-1706.
90. Ishak KG, Goodman ZD, Stocker JT. Tumors of the liver and intrahepatic bile ducts. AFIP Atlas of Tumor Pathology, 3rd Series, Fascicle 31. Washington, DC: American Registry of Pathology; 1999.
91. Nakanuma Y, Sato Y, Ikeda H, et al. Intrahepatic cholangiocarcinoma with predominant "ductal plate malformation" pattern: a new subtype. Am J Surg Pathol 2012;36:1629-1635.
92. Jain D, Sarode VR, Abdul-Karim FW, Homer R, Robert ME. Evidence for the neoplastic transformation of Von-Meyenburg complexes. Am J Surg Pathol 2000;24:1131-9.
93. Wheeler DA, Edmondson HA. Ciliated hepatic foregut cyst. Am J Surg Pathol 1984;8:467-470.
94. Kadoya M, Matsui O, Nakanuma Y, et al. Ciliated hepatic foregut cyst: radiologic features. Radiology 1990;175:475-477.
95. Bishop KC, Perrino CM, Ruzinova MB, Brunt EM. Ciliated hepatic foregut cyst: a report of 6 cases and a review of the English literature. Diagn Pathol 2015;10:81.
96. Sharma S, Corn A, Kohli V, Wright HI, Sebastian A, Jabbour N. Ciliated hepatic foregut cyst: an increasingly diagnosed condition. Dig Dis Sci 2008;53:2818-2821.
97. Ben Mena N, Zalinski S, Svrcek M, et al. Ciliated hepatic foregut cyst with extensive squamous metaplasia: report of a case. Virchows Arch 2006;449:730-733.
98. Zhang X, Wang Z, Dong Y. Squamous cell carcinoma arising in a ciliated hepatic foregut cyst: case report and literature review. Pathol Res Pract 2009;205:498-501.
99. Wilson JM, Groeschl R, George B, et al. Ciliated hepatic cyst leading to squamous cell carcinoma of the liver. A case report and review of the literature. Int J Surg Case Rep 2013;4:972-975.
100. Vick DJ, Goodman ZD, Ishak KG. Squamous cell carcinoma arising in a ciliated hepatic foregut cyst. Arch Pathol Lab Med 1999;123:1115-1117.
101. Furlanetto A, Dei Tos AP. Squamous cell carcinoma arising in a ciliated hepatic foregut cyst. Virchows Arch 2002;441:296-298.
102. de Lajarte-Thirouard AS, Rioux-Leclercq N, Boudjema K, Gandon Y, Ramee MP, Turlin B. Squamous cell carcinoma arising in a hepatic forgut cyst. Pathol Res Pract 2002;198:697-700.
103. Song JS, Noh SJ, Cho BH, Moon WS. Multicystic biliary hamartoma of the liver. Korean J Pathol 2013;47:275-278.
104. Kai K, Takahashi T, Miyoshi A, Yasui T, Tokunaga O, Miyazaki K. Intrahepatic multicystic biliary hamartoma: report of a case. Hepatol Res 2008;38:629-634.
105. Varnholt H, Vauthey JN, Dal Cin P, et al. Biliary adenofibroma: a rare neoplasm of bile duct origin with an indolent behavior. Am J Surg Pathol 2003;27:693-698.
106. Tsui WM, Loo KT, Chow LT, Tse CC. Biliary adenofibroma. A heretofore unrecognized benign biliary tumor of the liver. Am J Surg Pathol 1993;17:186-192.
107. Nguyen NT, Harring TR, Holley L, Goss JA, O'Mahony CA. Biliary adenofibroma with carcinoma in situ: a rare case report. Case Reports Hepatol 2012;2012:793963.
108. Gurrera A, Alaggio R, Leone G, Aprile G, Magro G. Biliary adenofibroma of the liver: report of a case and review of the literature. Patholog Res Int 2010;2010:504584.
109. Aepli P, Vosbeck J, Metzger J. An unusual mass in a cirrhotic liver. Gastroenterology 2012;143:e12-13.
110. Parada LA, Bardi G, Hallen M, et al. Monosomy 22 in a case of biliary adenofibroma. Cancer Genet Cytogenet 1997;93:183-184.
111. Akin O, Coskun M. Biliary adenofibroma with malignant transformation and pulmonary metastases: CT findings. AJR Am J Roentgenol 2002;179:280-281.

7 INTRAHEPATIC CHOLANGIOCARCINOMA AND PRECURSOR LESIONS

INTRAHEPATIC CHOLANGIOCARCINOMA

Intrahepatic cholangiocarcinoma is a primary liver cancer with cholangiocyte differentiation but no hepatocellular components. Cholangiocarcinoma can emerge at any portion of the biliary tree, from the smallest ductules to the periampullary bile duct. It is classified into *intrahepatic* and *extrahepatic cancers*, with the latter further divided into *perihilar* and *distal carcinomas* based on the predominant location. The boundary between the intrahepatic and extrahepatic ducts is the proximal end of the right and left hepatic ducts, with both hepatic ducts grouped into the perihilar bile ducts (1,2). Although this definition is currently most widely used, another international group of surgeons and physicians recently proposed an even larger perihilar region, up to and including the second branches of the right and left hepatic ducts (3). Even using a single standard, the separation of intrahepatic from perihilar cholangiocarcinoma is sometimes difficult and can be arbitrary, particularly at advanced stages.

Synonyms of intrahepatic cholangiocarcinoma include *cholangiocellular carcinoma, peripheral cholangiocarcinoma,* and *intrahepatic bile duct cancer*. Intraductal papillary neoplasm of the bile duct (IPNB) and mucinous cystic neoplasm (MCN) can progress to invasive adenocarcinoma, but they are classified separately, and should be diagnosed as such (i.e., IPNB with an associated invasive carcinoma) (4) (see chapter 6).

General Features

There are two major subtypes of intrahepatic cholangiocarcinoma, each with distinct clinical, pathologic, and molecular features. One group consists of carcinomas arising from the intrahepatic large bile ducts (*large duct cholangiocarcinoma*), while the other consists of adenocarcinomas with an origin in the smaller bile ducts (*small duct cholangiocarcinoma*) (Table 7-1) (5).

Intrahepatic cholangiocarcinoma accounts for 5 to 10 percent of all bile duct cancers and 15 to 20 percent of primary liver cancers (6–10). Its prevalence shows wide geographic variation. The highest incidence is reported in northeast Thailand, where the age-standard incidence is 88/100,000 in men and 37/100,000 in women (11). It is also common in other Asian countries such as China and Korea (1 to 3/100,000 in men) (12). It occurs at lower incidence rates in all Western countries, where the age-standardized incidence in men is less than 1/100,000 (12,13). The incidence and mortality rates of intrahepatic cholangiocarcinoma are rising, while those of extrahepatic biliary malignancy are declining worldwide (14–17).

Several forms of cholangiopathy are known to increase the risk of bile duct cancers, but many patients with intrahepatic cholangiocarcinoma do not have any of the risk conditions. Primary sclerosing cholangitis (PSC) is one of the most widely recognized preceding cholangiopathies (18–21). Patients with PSC have a 1.5 percent cumulative annual risk of developing cholangiocarcinoma, and 10 to 20 percent of patients eventually have a biliary malignancy (21,22). Congenital abnormalities of the biliary tree, such as Caroli disease, congenital hepatic fibrosis, choledochal cyst, and pancreaticobiliary maljunction, carry a 15 percent risk of bile duct cancer including extrahepatic cholangiocarcinoma, unless preventative procedures such as excision of the choledochal cyst are used (23–28). Malignant complication usually occurs after the second decade of life, at an average age of 34 years (27).

Liver flukes contribute to the high incidence of cholangiocarcinoma in Asia. *Opisthorchis viverrini,* found primarily in Thailand, and *Clonorchis sinensis,* endemic in Taiwan, Korea, and southern China, are both strong risk factors (29). Almost all cases of intrahepatic cholangiocarcinoma in Khon Kaen, a city in northeastern

Table 7-1

CLASSIFICATION OF INTRAHEPATIC CHOLANGIOCARCINOMA

	Large Duct Cholangiocarcinoma[a]		Small Duct Cholangiocarcinoma
	Intraductal-Growth Type	Periductal-Infiltrating Type	Mass-Forming Type
Incidence	10%	30-40%	50-60%
Postulated ducts of origin	Intrahepatic large bile ducts	Intrahepatic large bile ducts	Bile ductules, interlobular bile ducts, septal bile ducts
Clinical presentation	Painless jaundice, dark urine, abdominal pain	Painless jaundice, dark urine, abdominal pain	Nonspecific abdominal symptoms, incidentally found liver tumor
Associated conditions	PSC[b], hepatolithiasis, liver flukes	PSC, hepatolithiasis, liver flukes	Chronic viral hepatitis, liver cirrhosis of any cause
Premalignant lesions	BilIN	BilIN	Unknown
Histologic features	Papillary or papillotubular adenocarcinoma	Infiltrative ductal adenocarcinoma with fibrotic stroma	Tubular adenocarcinoma with or without trabecular foci, ductal adenocarcinoma
Tumor cell phenotype	Pancreatobiliary or intestinal type	Pancreatobiliary type	Pancreatobiliary type, hepatoid foci
KRAS mutations	20-30%	20-30%	Probably <10%
IDH mutations	Rare	Rare	20-30%
Differential diagnosis	IPNB, metastatic colorectal cancer with intrabiliary growth	IgG4-related sclerosing cholangitis, follicular cholangitis	HCC, combined hepatocellular cholangiocarcinoma

[a]Large duct cholangiocarcinoma forms nodular tumors when it invades the liver parenchyma.
[b]PSC = primary sclerosing cholangitis; BilIN = biliary intraepithelial neoplasia; IPNB = intraductal papillary neoplasm; HCC = hepatocellular carcinoma; IDH = isocitrate dehydrogenase.

Thailand, are related to chronic infection by *Opisthorchis viverrini*. Humans are infected by eating undercooked fish, with adult worms inhabiting and laying eggs in the biliary system.

Hepatolithiasis is another risk factor contributing to the higher incidence of intrahepatic cholangiocarcinoma in Asia (30–33). Up to 10 percent of patients with intrahepatic stones develop cholangiocarcinoma at some time in their life (31–33). Bilirubin calcium stones are more strongly associated with cholangiocarcinoma than cholesterol stones.

Recent studies of a large population database have identified multiple new risk factors including cholangitis, cholelithiasis, choledocholithiasis, diabetes mellitus, inflammatory bowel disease, smoking, human immunodeficiency virus (HIV), duodenal ulcer, and chronic pancreatitis (9,34,35). Growing evidence has also suggested that cirrhosis of any cause increases the risk of small duct cholangiocarcinoma (34,36). A cohort study of more than 11,000 patients with cirrhosis, followed up over 6 years, showed a 10-fold risk of cholangiocarcinoma compared with the general population (36). Infection with hepatitis B or C virus (HBV or HCV) increases the risk of intrahepatic cholangiocarcinoma up to 5-fold (37). Sixteen percent of intrahepatic cholangiocarcinomas are diagnosed in patients with cirrhosis (38).

Some chemical toxins are associated with the development of cholangiocarcinoma. Thorotrast, a radiologic contrast agent banned in the 1960s for its carcinogenic properties, has been strongly associated with bile duct carcinogenesis (27,30,39). It increases the risk to 300 times that of the general population. Associations have also been suggested with exposure to by-products from rubber and nitrosamines, but these have not yet been definitively proved (39). More recently, dichloromethane and 1,2-dichloropropane were found to have carcinogenic effects in the bile ducts (40). Prolonged exposure to these chemical toxins caused cholangiocarcinoma in young men (25 to 45 years of age) who had been working in printing companies in Japan (40).

Clinical Features

Patients are usually over 40 years of age, with the peak in the seventh decade (27,41,42). The cancer develops earlier in patients who have chronic cholangiopathy, which increases the risk of biliary malignancy. Men have a slightly higher incidence of intrahepatic cholangiocarcinoma and mortality from the cancer than women (27,41,42). Nonspecific symptoms, such as abdominal pain, malaise, and weight loss, are common, while tumors involving the large bile ducts may present with the sequelae of biliary obstruction such as painless jaundice, pale stools, dark urine, and pruritus (27,43). Cholangitis is an uncommon presentation. For patients with chronic cholangiopathy, deteriorating unexplained cholestasis can be an initial clinical sign of cancer development (44). Extrahepatic metastasis is noted in approximately 40 percent of patients at the time of diagnosis (45).

Although histologic diagnosis is the gold standard, a multidisciplinary approach is required for the differentiation from benign biliary strictures, other primary liver tumors, and metastatic malignancies (46). CA19-9 is the most widely used biomarker for cholangiocarcinoma diagnosis. This assay, however, detects intrahepatic cholangiocarcinoma with only 62 percent sensitivity and 63 percent specificity (47). Using a higher cut-off value (100 U/mL) rather than the usual cut-off value (37 U/mL) increases the specificity to 80 to 90 percent, while sensitivity becomes around 50 percent (48). CA19-9 concentrations higher than 1,000 U/mL indicate advanced disease, usually with extrahepatic metastasis (49–51). The most reliable cut-off value of CA19-9 for patients with PSC is 129 U/mL, which yields sensitivity of 79 percent, specificity of 98 percent, but adjusted positive predictive value of only 57 percent (50,51). Serum CA19-9 is undetectable in patients who are negative for Lewis antigen (7 percent of the general population) (48). This possibility should be considered if the serum CA19-9 level is extremely low, but there is a high index of clinical suspicion of cholangiocarcinoma.

Imaging is essential for the diagnosis and staging of intrahepatic cholangiocarcinoma. Transabdominal ultrasound is probably the first radiologic investigation for patients with suspected cholangiocarcinoma (52,53). This approach is highly sensitive for confirming bile duct dilatation as well as for detecting intrahepatic masses. Computerized tomography (CT) and magnetic resonance imaging (MRI) with contrast enhancement have greater diagnostic value for liver tumors (fig. 7-1) (54–57). A classic feature of cholangiocarcinoma is progressive uptake of contrast during the venous phase (57–60). In contrast, hepatocellular carcinoma (HCC) is characterized by rapid contrast uptake during the arterial phase (hypervascular tumors), followed by contrast washout in the venous phase (58,59,61,62). Positron emission tomography with ^{18}F-fluorodeoxyglucose (FDG-PET) helps detect extrahepatic lesions, leading to the alteration of a surgical management plan in up to 20 percent of cases (63–66). Its role in the diagnosis of primary liver tumor is limited, however, as cholangiocarcinoma, particularly periductal infiltrating cancer, is often FDG-PET negative (64).

The diagnostic approach depends on the tumor location. The main entity in the differential diagnosis of peripheral nodular cholangiocarcinoma is HCC. A general approach is to perform a liver biopsy from the intrahepatic tumor, if patients do not have a history of chronic liver disease or the typical imaging features of HCC. For patients with a more centrally located tumor, surgical intervention without histologic confirmation of the malignancy is sometimes justified because of the technical difficulty in obtaining sufficient tissue samples.

Gross Findings

On the basis of the gross appearance, the tumors are classified into three types: mass-forming (50 to 60 percent), periductal-infiltrating (30 to 40 percent), and intraductal-growth (10 percent) types (67–69). Cholangiocarcinomas arising from small bile ducts are usually mass-forming tumors, while large duct cholangiocarcinomas more commonly are periductal-infiltrative tumors, the same as perihilar cholangiocarcinoma. The gross type is closely linked to the histologic findings, biologic behavior, and molecular characteristics (Table 7-1) (70,71).

The *mass-forming type* is a well-circumscribed nodular lesion located within the liver parenchyma (fig. 7-2, left) (72,73). It is homogeneously gray, firm, and usually solid on cut section, but cystic degeneration of variable size

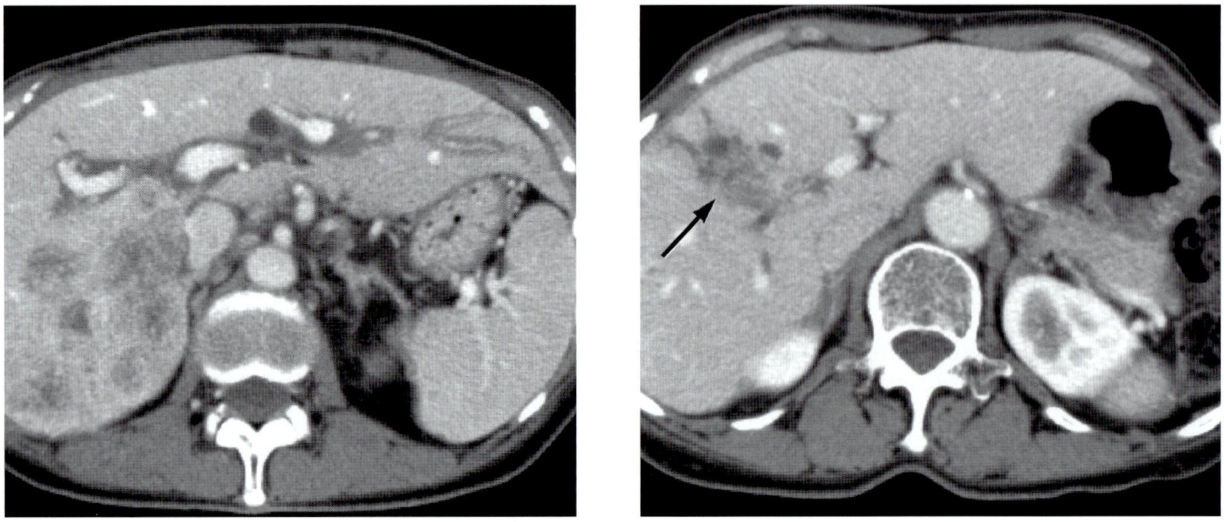

Figure 7-1

INTRAHEPATIC CHOLANGIOCARCINOMA

Left: Computerized tomography (CT) shows a mass-forming tumor in the right lobe.

Right: On CT, localized bile duct dilatation with a periductal low-density area indicates a periductal infiltrating cholangiocarcinoma.

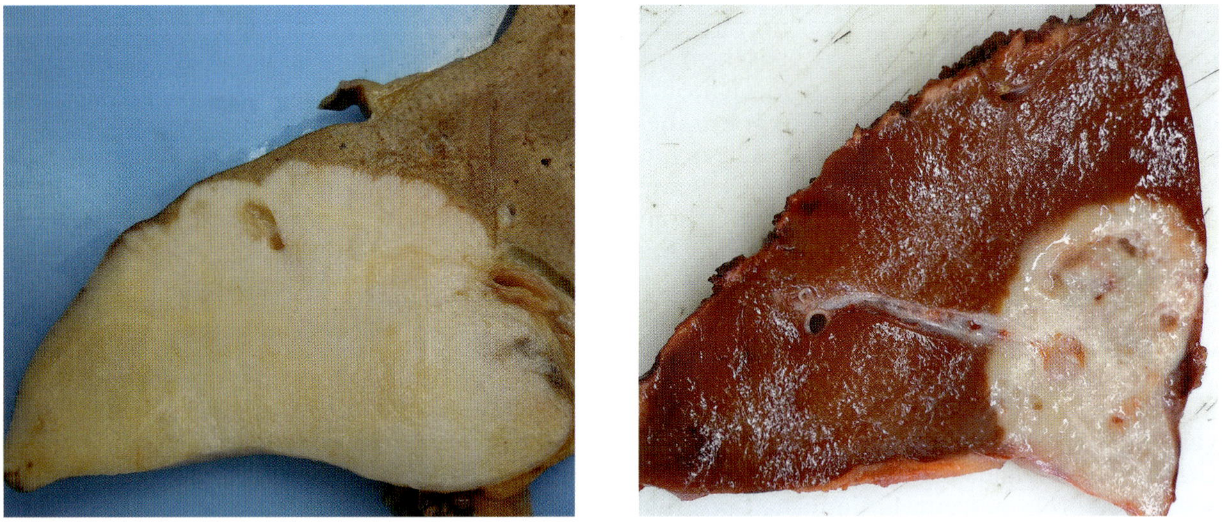

Figure 7-2

MASS-FORMING INTRAHEPATIC CHOLANGIOCARCINOMA

Left: The tumor is well defined and homogeneous on cut section.

Right: Small foci of cystic degeneration are present.

sometimes occurs, particularly in large tumors (fig. 7-2, right). The intracystic content is serous fluid or necrotic debris. The tumor is well demarcated, but with no surrounding fibrous capsule. Satellite nodules are common and remote intrahepatic metastases may be present in the same or contralateral lobe (fig. 7-3). The tumor may be associated with periductal infiltration when it invades large portal tracts (fig. 7-4). Unlike the other two types, which most often develop in noncirrhotic livers, mass-forming cholangiocarcinoma has been increasingly

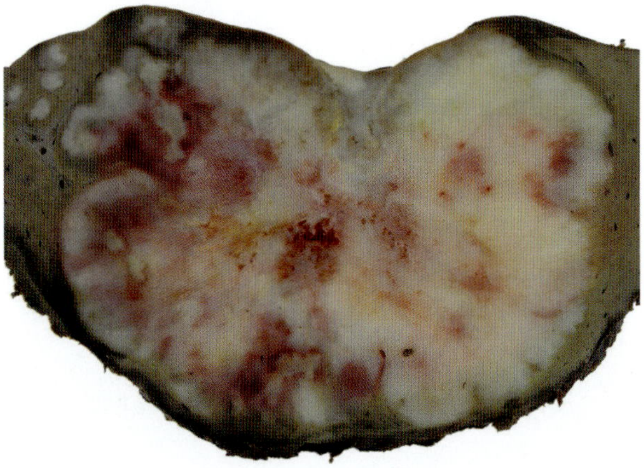

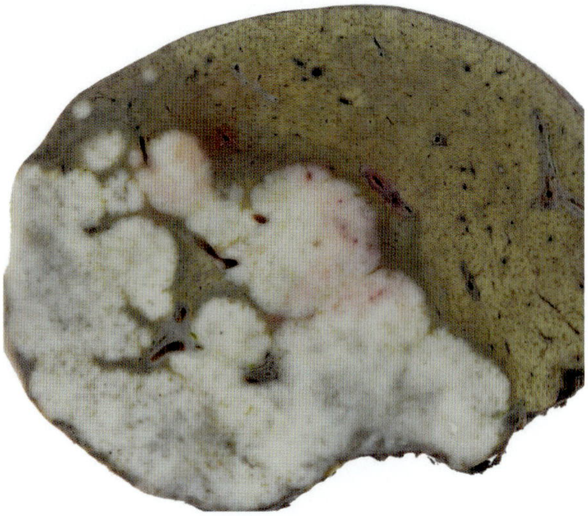

Figure 7-3

LARGE MASS-FORMING INTRAHEPATIC CHOLANGIOCARCINOMA

Left: This tumor is associated with satellite nodules.
Right: There is a multinodular appearance.

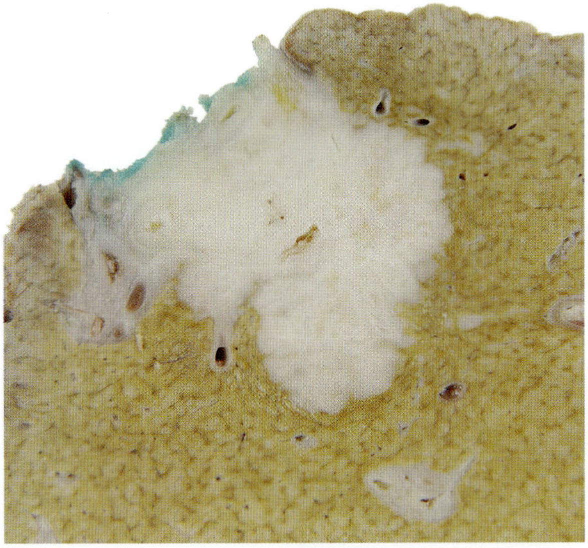

Figure 7-4

MASS-FORMING INTRAHEPATIC CHOLANGIOCARCINOMA

The tumor invades the portal tract. Large blood vessels are identifiable within the mass.

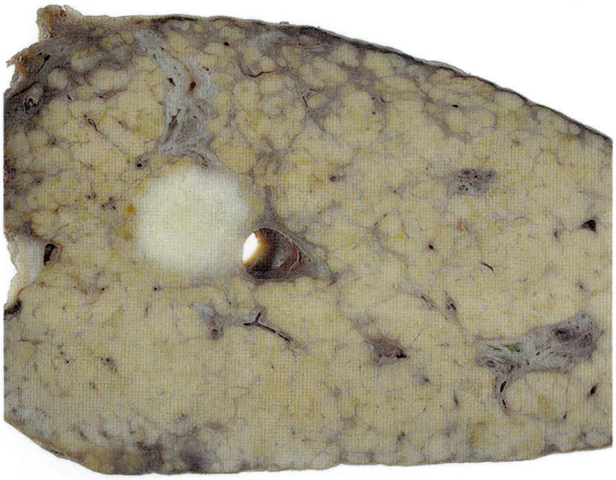

Figure 7-5

MASS-FORMING INTRAHEPATIC CHOLANGIOCARCINOMA

Chronic hepatitis is seen in the background.

diagnosed in patients with chronic liver disease or liver cirrhosis (fig. 7-5) (73–76).

The *periductal-infiltrating type* of cholangiocarcinoma presents with localized, zonal, or widespread biliary obstruction (fig. 7-6) (77,78). On cut section, it appears as a fibrotic tumor extending along periductal connective tissue (fig. 7-7). It is generally difficult to determine the extent of tumor spread grossly. When the tumor invades the adjacent liver parenchyma, it shows

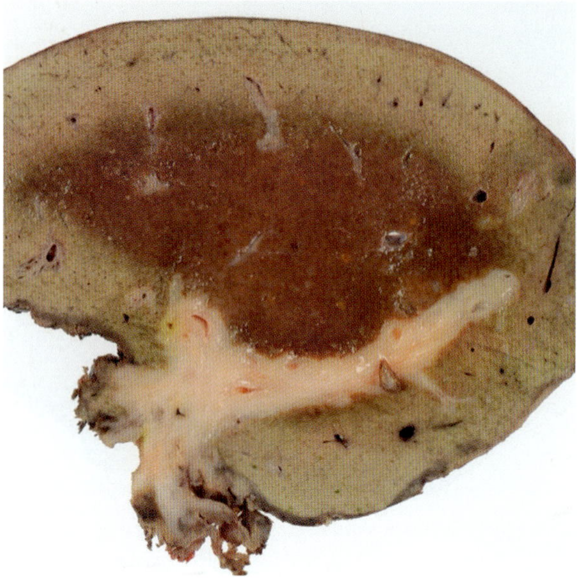

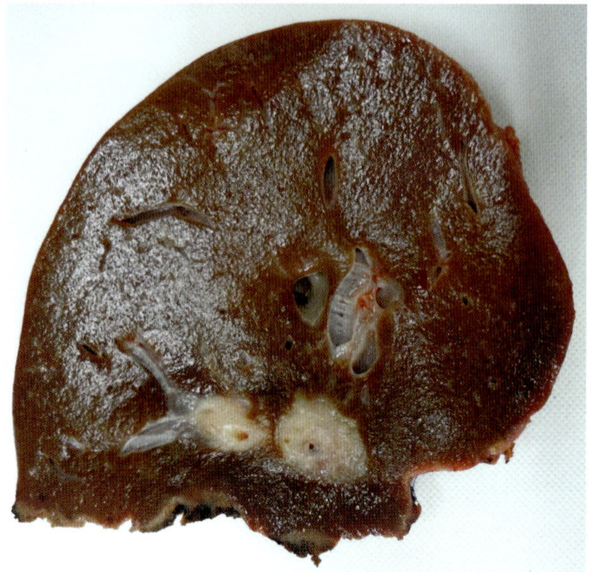

Figure 7-6

PERIDUCTAL-INFILTRATING CHOLANGIOCARCINOMA

Left: The bile ducts are broadly affected by the tumor.
Right: The cholangiocarcinoma is localized.

Figure 7-7

PERIDUCTAL-INFILTRATING CHOLANGIOCARCINOMA

This cholangiocarcinoma developed in a patient with primary sclerosing cholangitis.

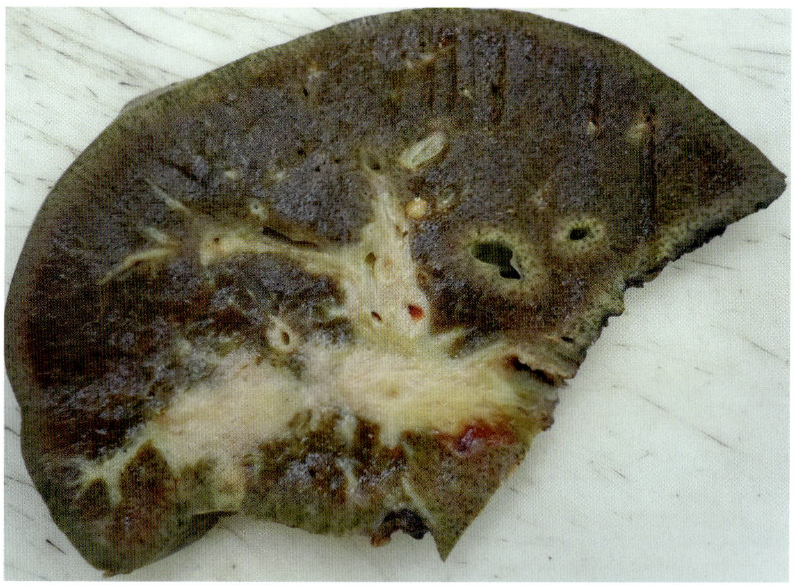

a well-defined nodule or mass (mixed periductal-infiltrating and mass-forming tumors) (fig. 7-8) (79). It causes dilatation of the upper bile ducts, which contain watery bile or mucinous pus. Accompanying branches of the artery and vein may also be obliterated. The affected hepatic lobe sometimes becomes atrophic.

The *intraductal-growth type* is a papillary or nodular tumor in the dilated bile duct (fig. 7-9) (80). It typically develops in the large ducts up to the second branch of the right or left hepatic duct. The intraductal-growth type of cholangiocarcinoma often resembles IPNB, however, in contrast to IPNB, where the bile ducts are

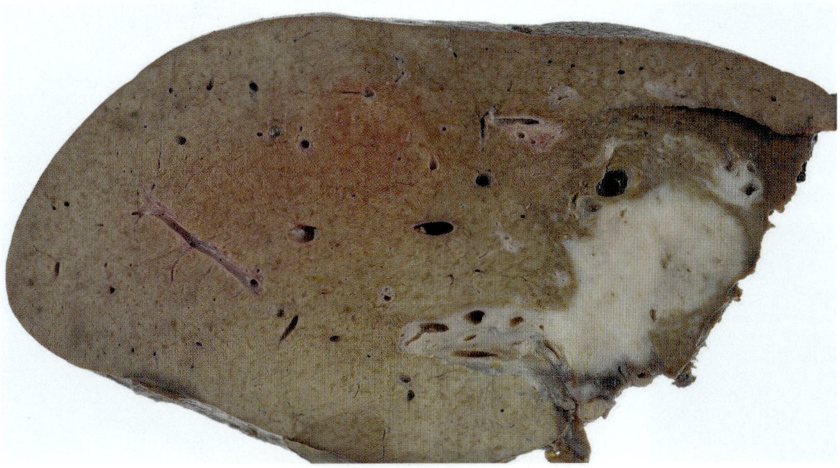

Figure 7-8

MIXED PERIDUCTAL-INFILTRATING AND MASS-FORMING CHOLANGIOCARCINOMA

The tumor appears as a well-defined mass.

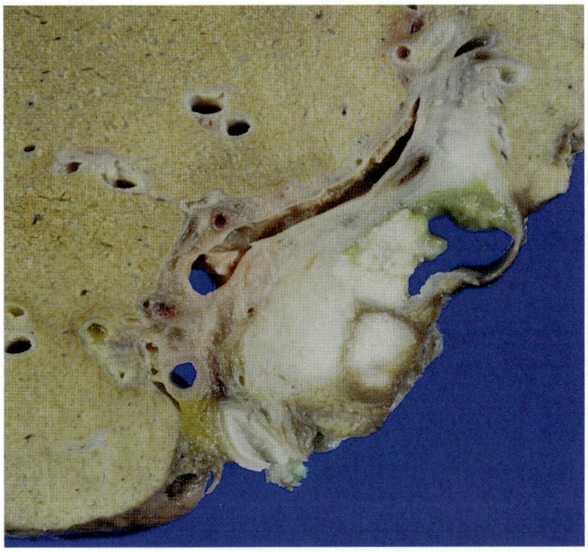

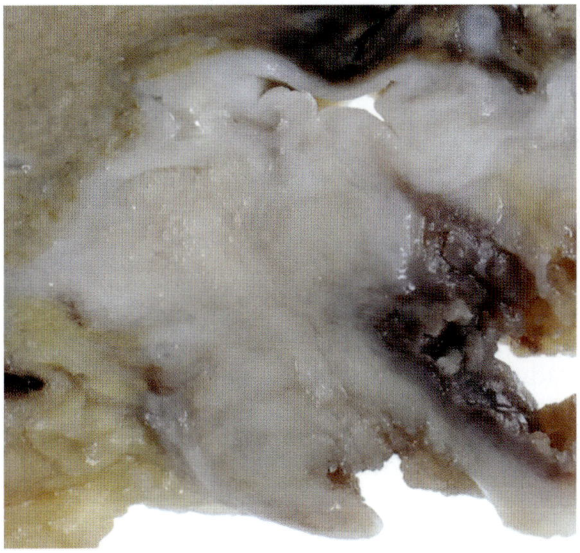

Figure 7-9

INTRADUCTAL-GROWTH CHOLANGIOCARCINOMA

Left: A papillary tumor is noted in the dilated bile duct.
Right: The large bile duct is filled with a papillary cholangiocarcinoma.

typically broadly involved, tumors of the intraductal-growth type are grossly more localized (81–83). The presence or absence of mucin overproduction helps in the discrimination of these two entities, as it is more common in IPNB (72 versus 7 percent). Although the proximal bile ducts are dilated, large cystic dilatation reminiscent of a cystic tumor is uncommon in this type. The intraductal mass may lead to cholestasis and atrophy of the liver parenchyma.

The size of the tumor varies considerably among cases, ranging from microscopic lesions to large bulky masses over 10 cm. The mass-forming cancer is the largest of the three gross types, since it is generally diagnosed at a more advanced stage (67,70). Direct invasion into extrahepatic tissue, such as the stomach, gallbladder, diaphragm, and abdominal wall, is common (fig. 7-10). The periductal-infiltrating cancer may show extensive lateral spread

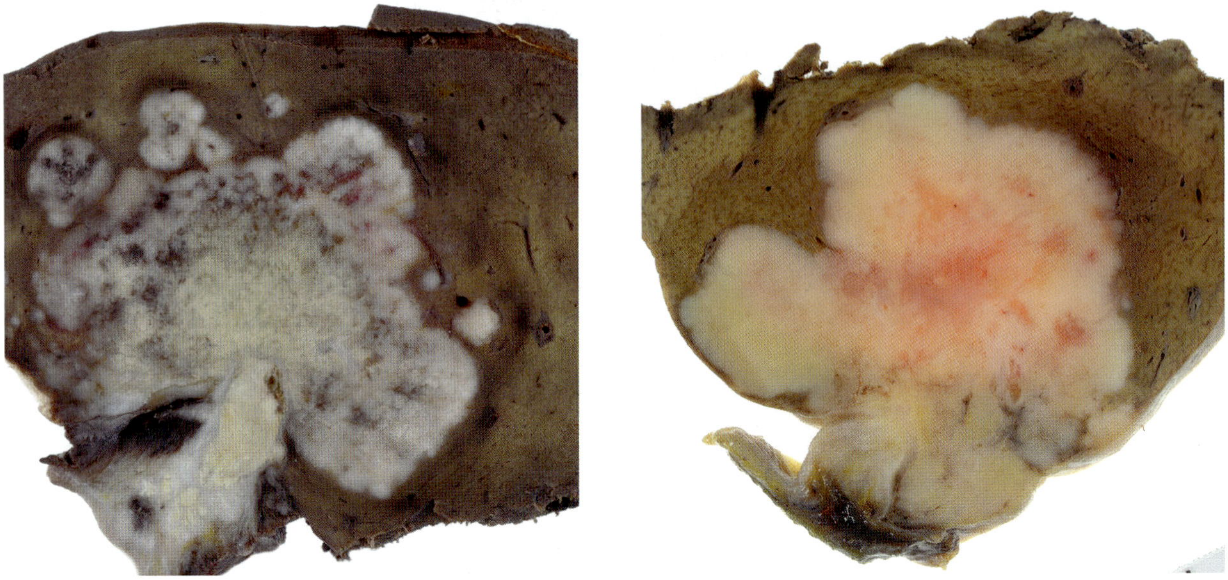

Figure 7-10

MASS-FORMING CHOLANGIOCARCINOMA

Left: This tumor invades the diaphragm (lower left).
Right: Cholangiocarcinoma directly infiltrates into extrahepatic fibroadipose tissue (lower left).

down to the perihilar or even distal bile ducts (see fig. 7-6, left) (67,70). It sometimes reaches over 5 cm in longitudinal diameter without forming a dominant mass. Tumors of the intraductal-growth type generally appear small upon gross examination, but this may be an underestimate as microscopic intraepithelial spread frequently occurs. In this rarest subtype, separate papillary tumors may be present in the bile ducts, but they are microscopically continuous with widespread intraepithelial carcinoma (84). True multifocal intrahepatic cholangiocarcinoma is rare even in patients who have a condition putting them at risk for biliary malignancy (i.e., PSC).

Microscopic Findings

Tumor cells are arranged in glands, tubules, papillae, solid nests, trabeculae, and small clusters against a background of fibrotic stroma (fig. 7-11) (4). Multiple growth patterns can coexist in a single tumor or even in a single microscopic field (85). Mucin production is easily found on hematoxylin and eosin (H&E)-stained sections in gland-forming or papillary adenocarcinomas, but is less conspicuous in other types. Neoplastic glands are typically equivalent in size to interlobular or septal bile ducts, but some cases form larger ducts. Carcinomas of tubular structure consist of anastomosing twisted tubules with narrow lumens (fig. 7-11D) (85). This growth pattern, somewhat reminiscent of ductular reaction, is more characteristic of intrahepatic cholangiocarcinoma than gland-forming adenocarcinomas. Tubular adenocarcinoma sometimes shows a cellular or fibrotic lobular architecture at low magnification (fig. 7-12).

The histologic features differ between small duct and large duct cholangiocarcinomas. Small duct cholangiocarcinoma commonly shows the tubular or small-glandular growth pattern. Trabecular growth can also be present, particularly at the interface between the tumor and liver parenchyma (fig. 7-13). Unlike HCC, in which neoplastic liver cell plates are surrounded by sinusoids, cholangiocarcinoma grows in trabeculae embedded in fibrotic stroma, and may contain entrapped hepatocytes (fig. 7-14). For equivocal cases, immunohistochemistry is required to rule out combined hepatocellular-cholangiocarcinoma. Minor histologic features of small duct cholangiocarcinoma include solid-nested growth reminiscent of the fetal liver (fig. 7-15A), intraglandular micropapillary architecture (fig.

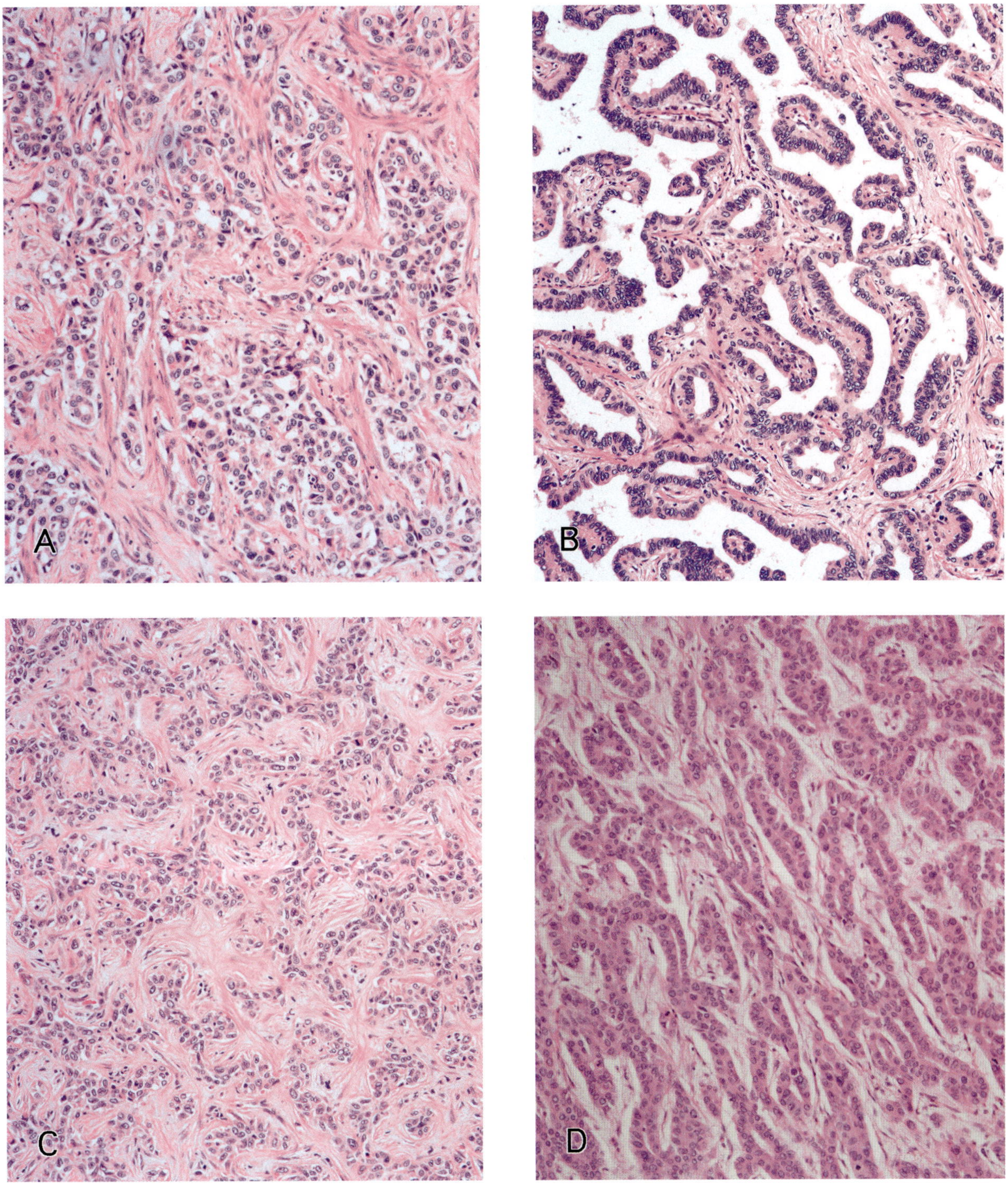

Figure 7-11

CHOLANGIOCARCINOMA

A: The tumor cells are arranged in small glandular nests.
B: Papillotubular growth.
C: Branching and anastomosing trabecular growth.
D: The carcinoma forms anastomosing twisted tubules with narrow lumens.

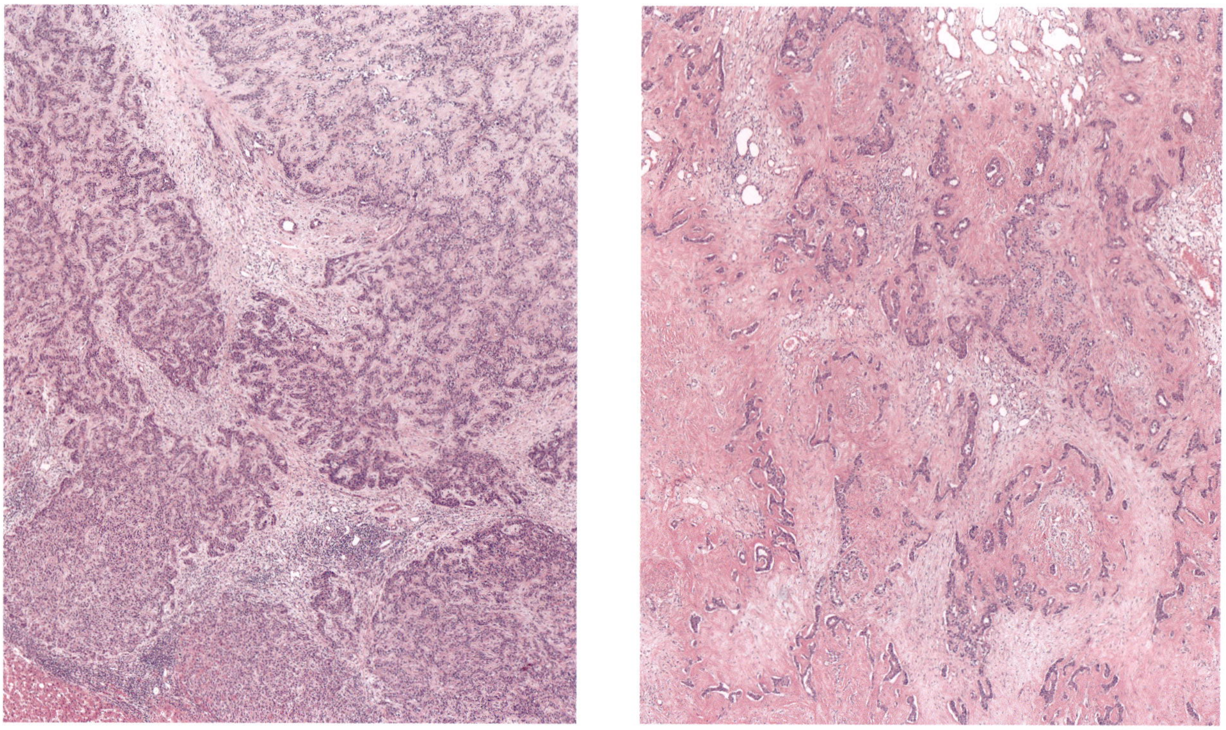

Figure 7-12

CHOLANGIOCARCINOMA

Left: This tumor shows a lobular architecture at low magnification.
Right: The lobular architecture appears to be fibrotic.

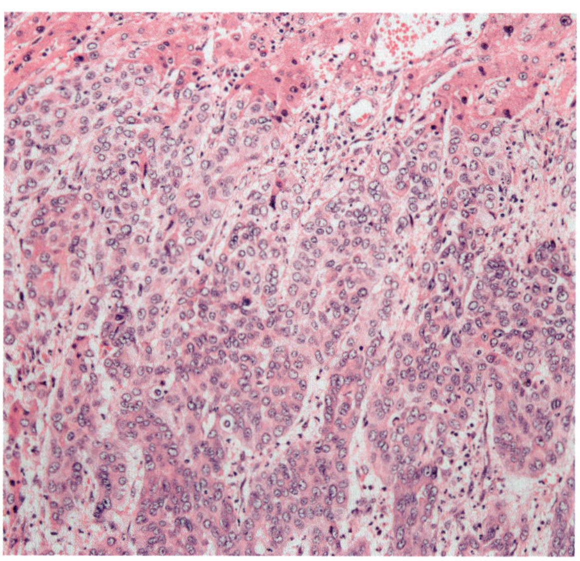

Figure 7-13

CHOLANGIOCARCINOMA

A trabecular pattern is seen at the interface between the tumor and liver parenchyma.

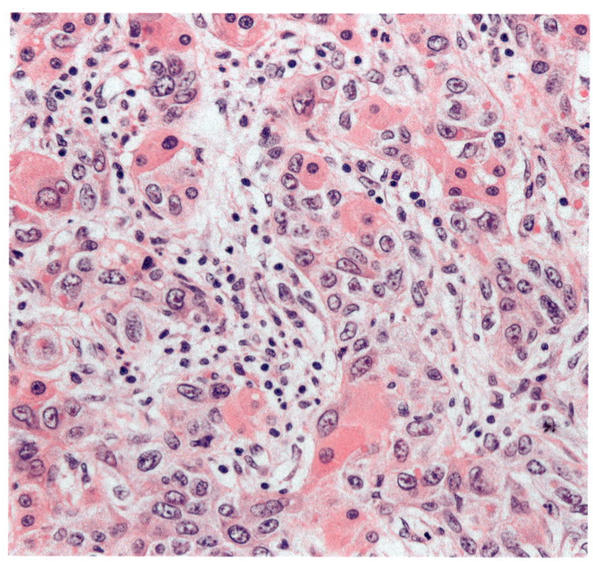

Figure 7-14

CHOLANGIOCARCINOMA

Non-neoplastic hepatocytes are entrapped in tumor cell nests. Nuclear features differ between the hepatocytes and cancer cells.

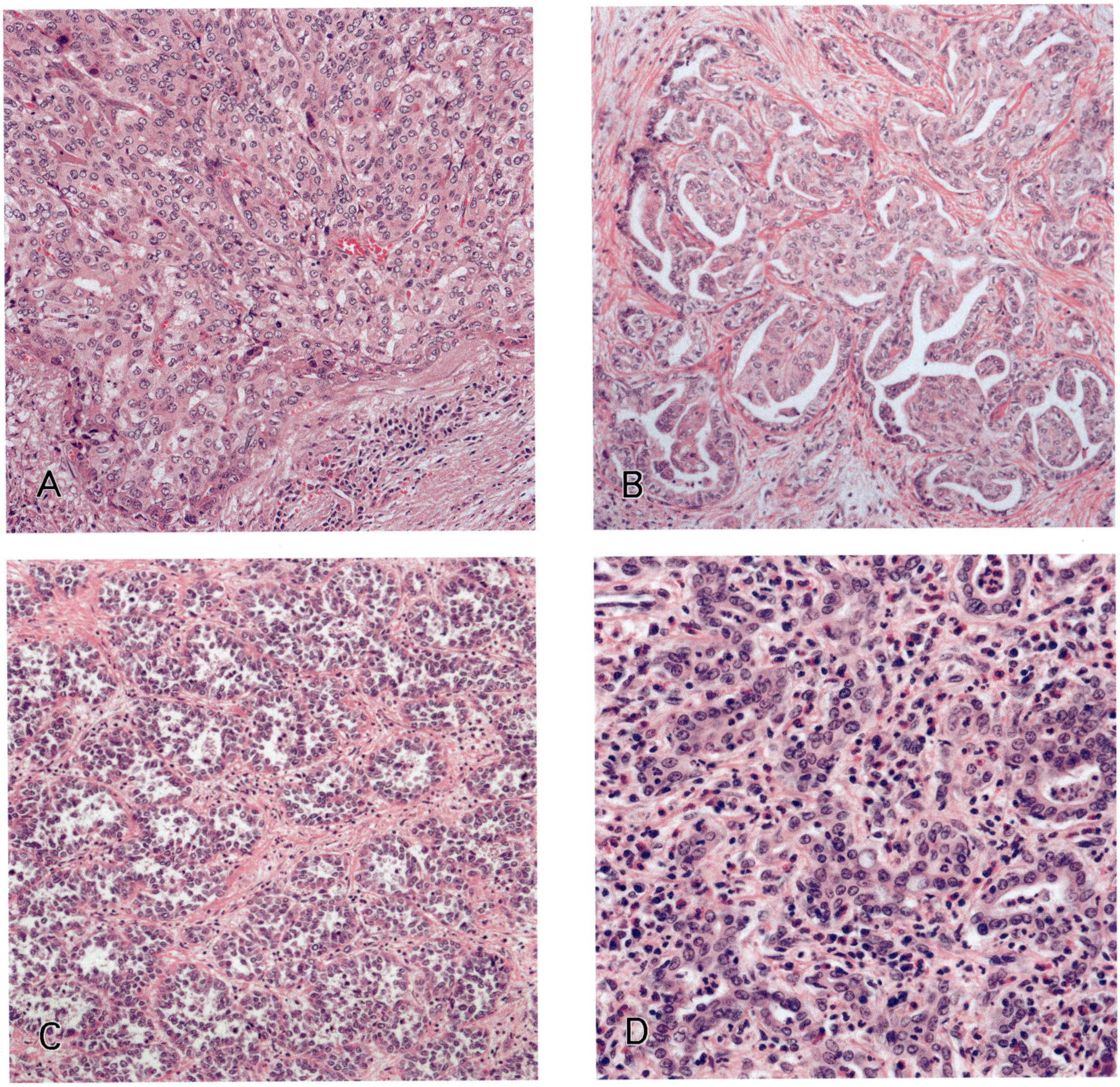

Figure 7-15

CHOLANGIOCARCINOMA

A: A solid nested growth pattern reminiscent of the fetal liver.
B: Intraglandular papillary growth.
C: Pseudopapillary pattern.
D: Extensive granulocytic infiltrate.

7-15B), pseudopapillary pattern (fig. 7-15C), and massive granulocytic infiltrates of unknown cause (fig. 7-15D) (86).

In large duct cholangiocarcinoma, periductal infiltrating-type tumors are typically gland-forming adenocarcinomas that are highly fibrotic and infiltrative. Minor tubular components, if present, are restricted to the tumor-liver interface (5). In the intraductal growth-type tumors, the cells are arranged with a papillary or papillotubular architecture (fig. 7-16). Compared with IPNB, the papillary architecture is more complex and often associated with tubular components and necrotic foci (fig. 7-17) (87).

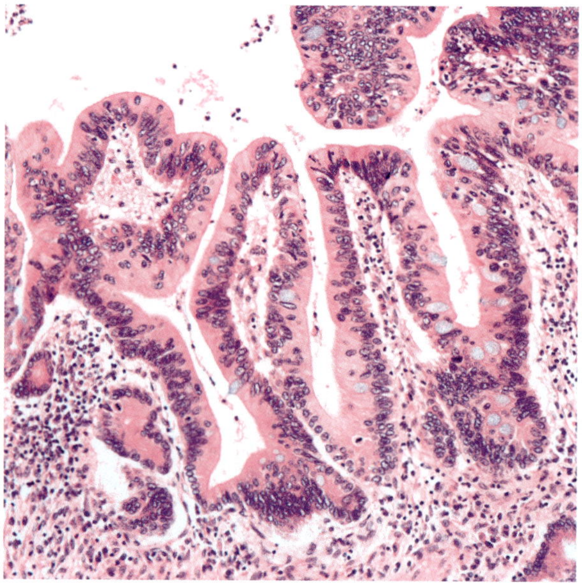

Figure 7-16

CHOLANGIOCARCINOMA WITH PAPILLARY ARCHITECTURE

Tumor cells show intestinal-type features.

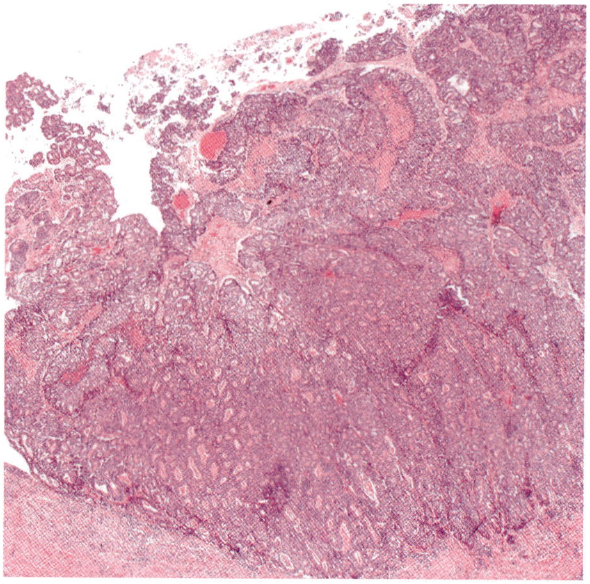

Figure 7-17

CHOLANGIOCARCINOMA

The intraductal tumor has a papillotubular growth pattern.

Intraepithelial cancers are frequently seen in the bile ducts adjacent to invasive foci in large duct cholangiocarcinoma, but are rare in small duct cholangiocarcinoma (88). They extend more than 2 cm beyond the main mass in 15 percent of large duct cancers, and tend to be widespread in the grossly intraductal growth-type tumors (84,89,90). Intraepithelial components are histologically completely flat or micropapillary (fig. 7-18). The latter is generally less dysplastic and more frequently associated with subepithelial inflammation (84), and it is difficult to histologically determine the extent of intraepithelial spread in those cases. The interpretation becomes much more challenging on frozen section diagnosis if the surgical margin contains micropapillary dysplastic cells.

The cancer cells have eosinophilic cytoplasm with occasional intracytoplasmic mucin. Clear cells may coexist, and cases with extensive clear cell change are often referred to as *clear cell cholangiocarcinoma* (fig. 7-19) (91). Other cytoplasmic alterations include oxyphilic change and mucin-negative vacuolation (figs. 7-20, 7-21). Nuclei are hyperchromatic and irregular in shape. The cellular polarity is distorted, with nuclei piled up to the luminal surface. Bizarre cells or spindle cell transformation may be seen in poorly differentiated adenocarcinomas (fig. 7-22).

Most intrahepatic cholangiocarcinomas are morphologically of the pancreatobiliary type, but intestinal differentiation such as goblet cells, nuclear stratification, and brush borders can be seen in large duct cholangiocarcinoma (fig. 7-23) (92,93). Intestinal-type adenocarcinomas sometimes have components of invasive mucinous carcinoma with abundant extracellular mucin (92). Intracytoplasmic globules mimicking Mallory-Denk bodies may be present, particularly in cholangiocarcinoma associated with chronic liver disease (fig. 7-24) (94). As intrahepatic cholangiocarcinoma resembles adenocarcinomas in other organs, such as the pancreas and gallbladder, clinical exclusion of other primary sites is required, particularly for biopsy cases.

Special stains help in the identification of mucin production. Normal cholangiocytes are positive for mucicarmine, high-iron diamine (HID), and periodic acid-Schiff (PAS) after digestion with diastase stains. As the proportion of sialomucin increases in the neoplastic biliary epithelium, the Alcian blue (pH 2.5) stain, in addition to the above three, becomes positive (95,96). The lack of identifiable mucin does not

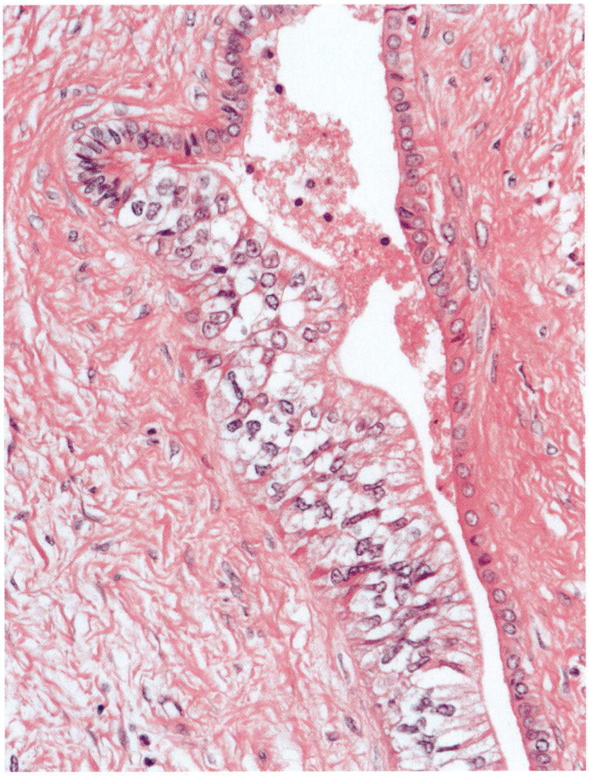

Figure 7-18

CHOLANGIOCARCINOMA

Flat intraepithelial carcinoma is seen.

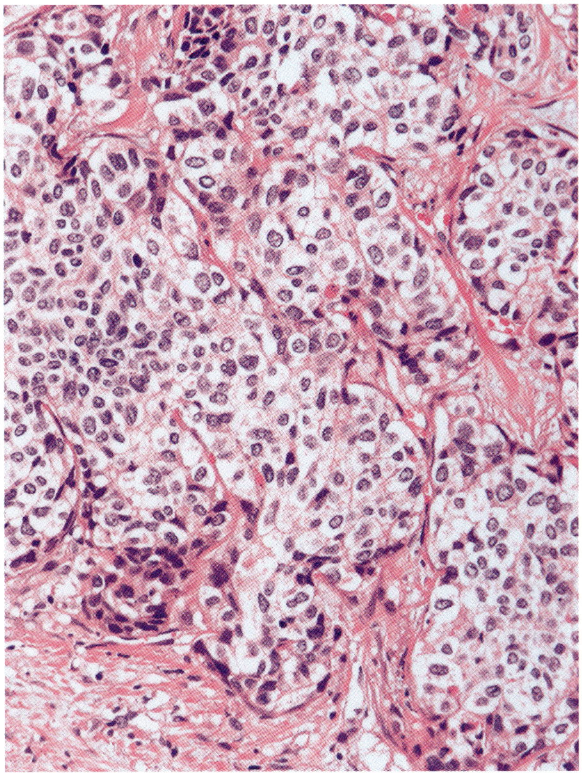

Figure 7-19

CHOLANGIOCARCINOMA WITH CLEAR CELL CHANGE

Extensive clear cell change is seen.

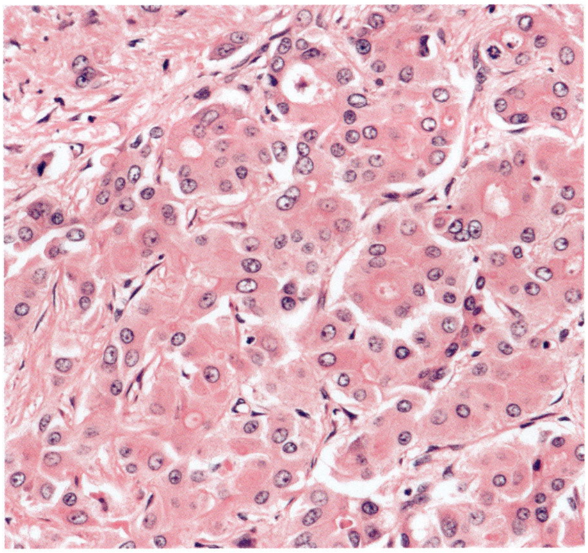

Figure 7-20

CHOLANGIOCARCINOMA WITH OXYPHILIC CHANGE

Oxyphilic appearance of the cytoplasm of the tumor cells is seen.

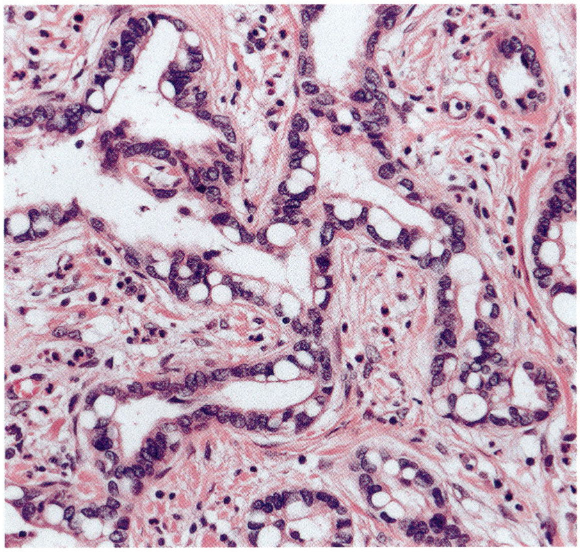

Figure 7-21

CHOLANGIOCARCINOMA

Cytoplasmic vacuoles are present.

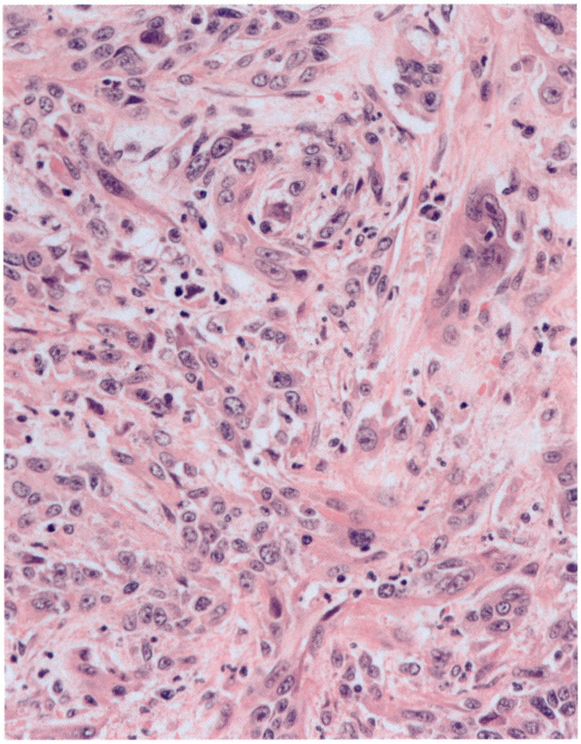

Figure 7-22

CHOLANGIOCARCINOMA

Spindle and pleomorphic cancer cells are seen.

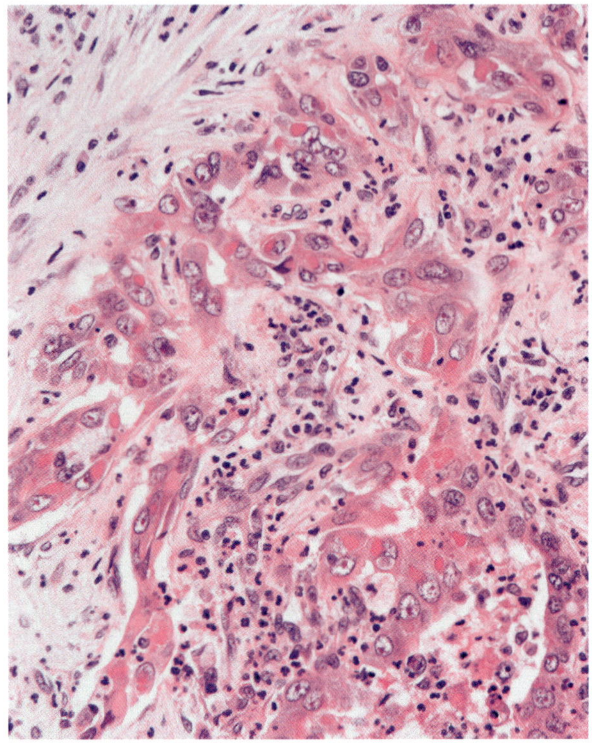

Figure 7-24

INTRACYTOPLASMIC EOSINOPHLILIC GLOBULES IN CHOLANGIOCARCINOMA

These mimic Mallory-Denk bodies.

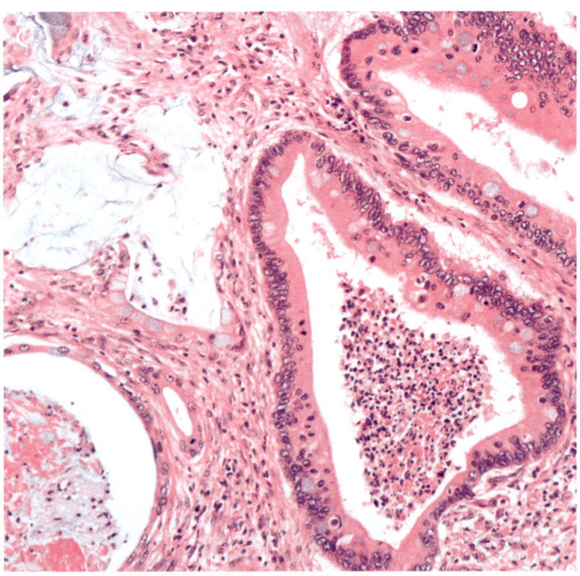

Figure 7-23

INTESTINAL-TYPE CHOLANGIOCARCINOMA

The presence of occasional goblet cells is associated with mucin overproduction.

rule out the possibility of cholangiocarcinoma, as it is not uncommon, particularly in poorly differentiated cholangiocarcinoma.

Liver needle biopsy is the most common approach for the tissue diagnosis of intrahepatic cholangiocarcinoma. As this procedure is often considered for mass-forming cases, tubular-appearing adenocarcinomas with or without trabecular components are commonly encountered in biopsy samples (fig. 7-25, left). Tumor cells in the biopsy may be few in number because of extensive fibrosis (fig. 7-25, right).

Another method of tissue sampling is bile duct biopsies, which are generally considered for large duct cholangiocarcinoma. In cases with suspected intraepithelial lateral extension, bile duct biopsies may be preoperatively taken from the contralateral hepatic duct to make sure that complete resection is possible. The small sample size and associated inflammatory changes in bile duct biopsies restrict the histologic examination. In small biopsy samples, interpretation depends

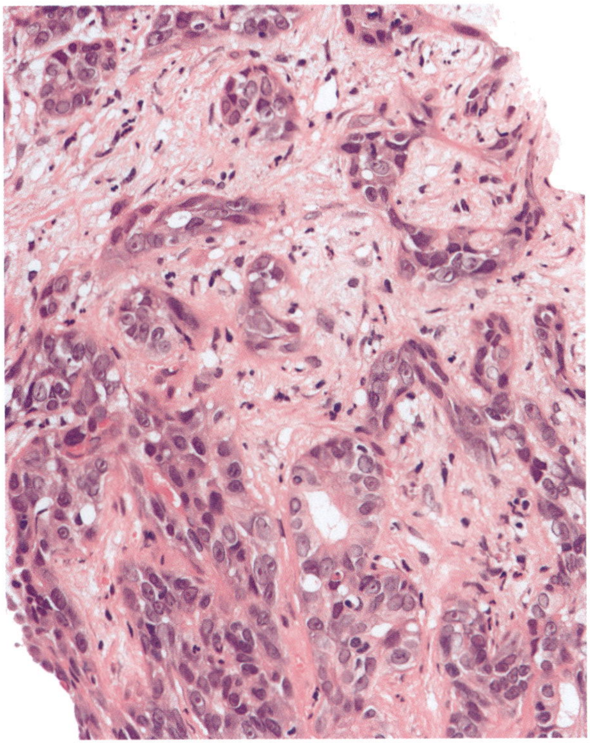

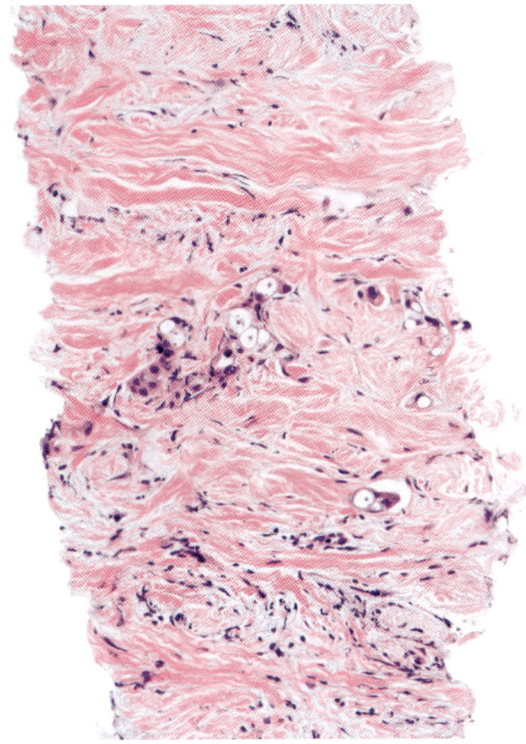

Figure 7-25

CHOLANGIOCARCINOMA IN NEEDLE BIOPSY

Left: Tubular adenocarcinoma in a liver needle biopsy.
Right: A small number of cancer cells is seen against the background of highly fibrotic stroma.

more on the cytologic features. Even if dysplastic changes are not obvious, intestinal metaplasia may suggest a neoplastic lesion nearby (fig. 7-26), as it is unlikely to occur in the non-neoplastic biliary epithelium unless patients have a history of chronic cholangiopathy (97).

Cholangiocarcinoma rarely shows extensive intrahepatic spread along portal tracts without forming a large dominant mass. The cancer cells in small portal tracts may resemble non-neoplastic bile ducts or ductules (fig. 7-27). The interpretation becomes challenging, particularly in liver biopsies that contain a few neoplastic ducts in small portal tracts. This type of tumor extension may give rise to imaging features mimicking sclerosing cholangitis, which may lead to a low clinical suspicion of malignancy.

Microscopic vascular invasion and perineural infiltration are common (38 and 29 percent, respectively, in surgical cases) (38). Many small lymphatic vessels are present in periductal connective tissue of the bile ducts, irrespective

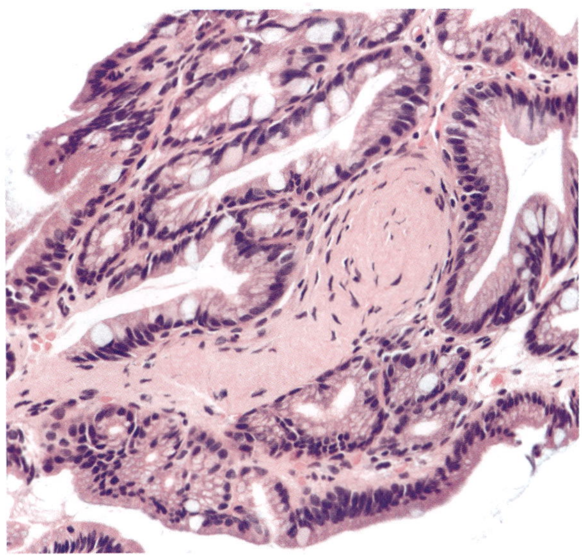

Figure 7-26

INTESTINAL METAPLASIA IN BILE DUCT BIOPSY

Although no significant atypia is noted in this sample, overt malignancy was confirmed nearby in the resected specimen.

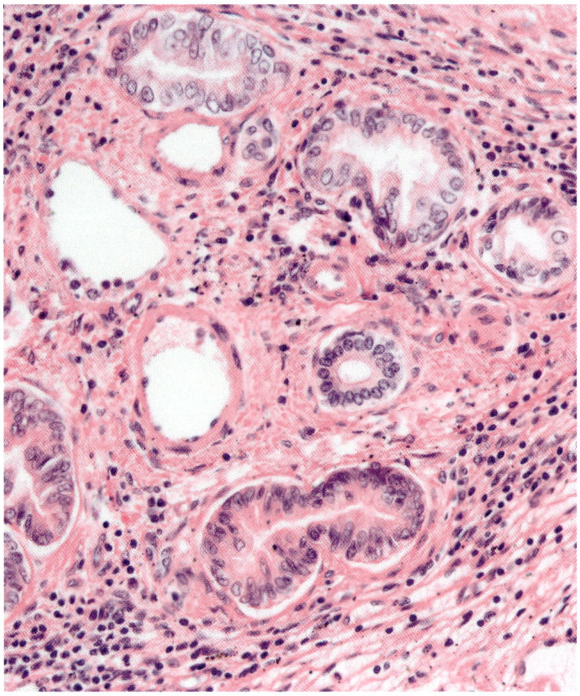

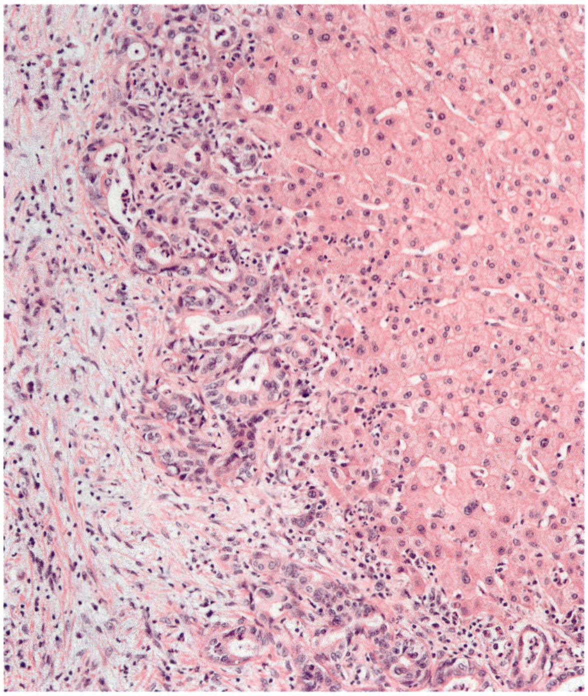

Figure 7-27

CHOLANGIOCARCINOMA MIMICKING BILE DUCTS

Left: Tumor infiltrating the small portal tract mimics non-neoplastic small bile ducts. The principal bile duct is present at the center of this figure.

Right: Cholangiocarcinoma is invading the interface between the portal tracts and liver parenchyma mimicking ductular reaction.

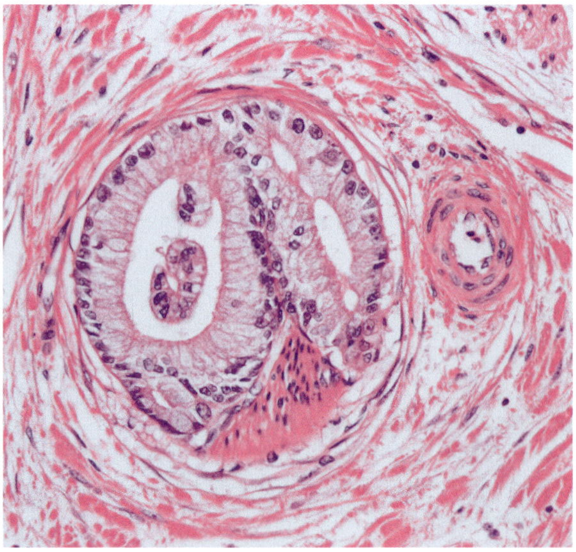

Figure 7-28

CHOLANGIOCARCINOMA

Perineural infiltration.

of their size. Lymphatic invasion can be noted away from the invasive foci. In addition to small veins, large branches of the portal or hepatic vein may be infiltrated by cancer cells. Perineural infiltration is particularly common in large duct cholangiocarcinoma of the periductal-infiltrating type (fig. 7-28).

Cholangiocarcinoma is graded by a three-tiered system. *Well-differentiated adenocarcinomas* form well-defined ducts consisting of columnar or cuboidal cells with eosinophilic cytoplasm and occasional intracytoplasmic mucin (fig. 7-29). Nuclei are basally oriented, round to oval in shape, with evenly distributed fine chromatin. Nuclear pleomorphism is not conspicuous. Compared with the non-neoplastic biliary epithelium, the nuclei of the cancer cells are larger and more hyperchromatic, but the changes may be subtle. Therefore, it is crucial to confirm the invasive nature.

Moderately differentiated adenocarcinomas show a more disorganized growth pattern (fig.

7-30). Neoplastic glands and tubules are irregular in shape, some associated with isolated "budding" cancer cells in the adjacent stroma. The cells have pleomorphic nuclei with occasional mitotic figures. The fibromyxoid tumor stroma contains enlarged myofibroblasts. The diagnosis of malignancy is generally easy based on the histologic appearance.

Poorly differentiated adenocarcinomas are characterized by poorly formed glands and tubules, and individual isolated cells (fig. 7-31, left). The cells have enlarged nuclei with an irregular nuclear membrane. Although mucin production may be difficult to prove, glandular differentiation is suggested by the vaguely tubular arrangement of the cells and the cytologic appearance of peripherally located nuclei (fig. 7-31, right). Brisk mitotic figures, including atypical ones, are noted. Necrosis is common. The tumor cell nests are surrounded by the cellular stroma containing plump myofibroblasts, which should not be interpreted as the pseudosarcomatous change of the cancer.

Histologic Types

Several histologic variants of intrahepatic cholangiocarcinoma are recognized. Although a majority of intrahepatic biliary malignancies are adenocarcinomas with conventional ductal

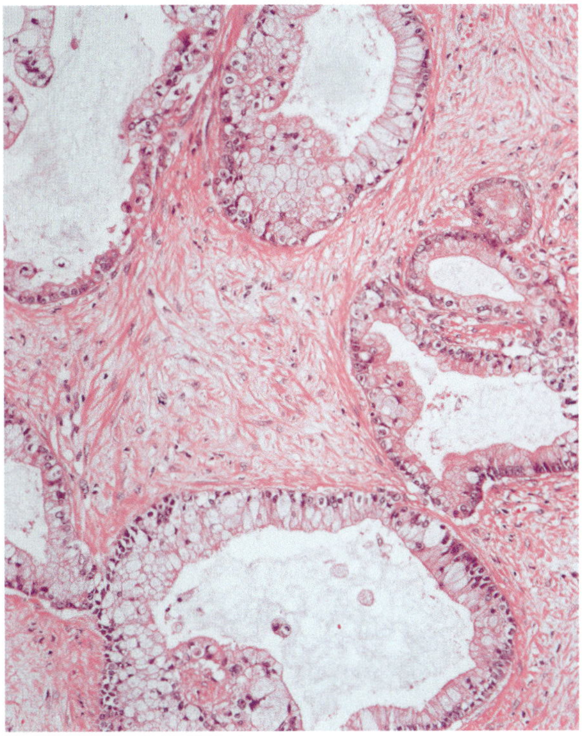

Figure 7-29

WELL-DIFFERENTIATED DUCTAL ADENOCARCINOMA (LARGE DUCT CHOLANGIOCARCINOMA)

The carcinoma forms well-defined glandular structures with inconspicuous pleomorphism.

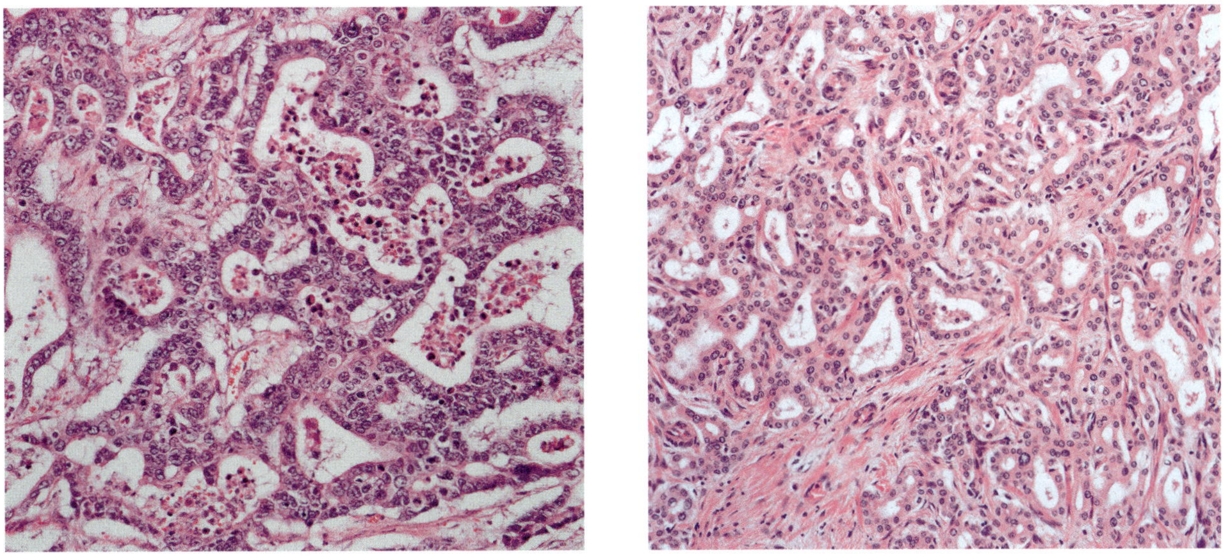

Figure 7-30

MODERATELY DIFFERENTIATED ADENOCARCINOMA

Left: The neoplastic glands are irregular, with pleomorphic nuclei and occasional mitotic figures (large duct cholangiocarcinoma). Right: Cancer cells form fused small tubules (small duct cholangiocarcinoma).

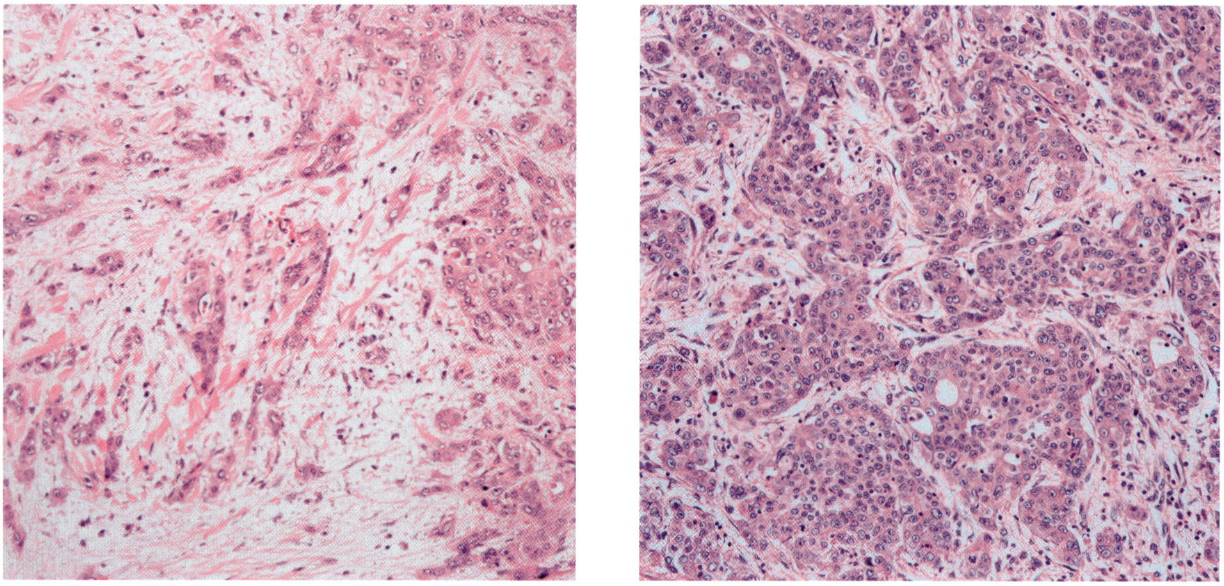

Figure 7-31

POORLY DIFFERENTIATED ADENOCARCINOMA (LARGE DUCT CHOLANGIOCARCINOMA)

Left: The tumor glands are poorly formed, with individual cancer cells in the stroma.
Right: A vaguely formed glandular appearance is appreciated.

or tubular morphology, the variants can develop purely or in conjunction with conventional cholangiocarcinoma. These subtypes are rare, each accounting for less than 5 percent of intrahepatic cholangiocarcinomas. It is important to recognize the histologic subtypes, as they confer a better or worse prognosis than conventional cholangiocarcinoma.

Adenosquamous Carcinoma. Adenosquamous carcinoma accounts for 2 to 3 percent of intrahepatic cholangiocarcinomas (98). This variant is defined as a primary liver cancer containing significant proportions of both adenocarcinoma and squamous cell carcinoma (99). Squamous differentiation should be evidenced by morphologic features such as keratinization or intercellular bridges (fig. 7-32). Immunoreactivity to the markers that are commonly expressed in squamous cell carcinoma (i.e., p63) is insufficient for the diagnosis.

The tumors can develop in both lobes, with no specific preference in location. They are large, being greater than 5 cm in 60 percent of cases (99). Necrosis and cystic degeneration are common.

Histologically, squamous cell carcinoma components are irregularly intermixed with adenocarcinoma. The degree of squamous cell differentiation ranges from well-formed keratin pearls to faint single-cell keratinization (fig. 7-33). Some reported cases were associated with preceding conditions such as hepatolithiasis and liver cysts lined by stratified epithelium (98,99).

Lymph node metastasis is present in 50 percent of patients at the time of diagnosis. The prognosis is poor: the 3-year survival rate is 8 percent, with no reported patients surviving over 5 years (99).

There are two theories about the tumorigenesis of intrahepatic adenosquamous carcinoma. One hypothesis is that the tumor develops from the metaplastic squamous epithelium lining the bile ducts, while the other possibility is squamous differentiation of conventional adenocarcinoma. Given that most tumors do not have identifiable non-neoplastic squamous epithelium nearby, the latter possibility may be more likely for the majority of cases. Pure squamous cell carcinoma can develop, but is extremely rare in the liver (100).

Mucoepidermoid Carcinoma. Mucoepidermoid carcinoma is rare, with only around 20 cases reported in the literature (101–104). The same as for the prototype in the salivary glands, mucoepidermoid carcinoma of the liver

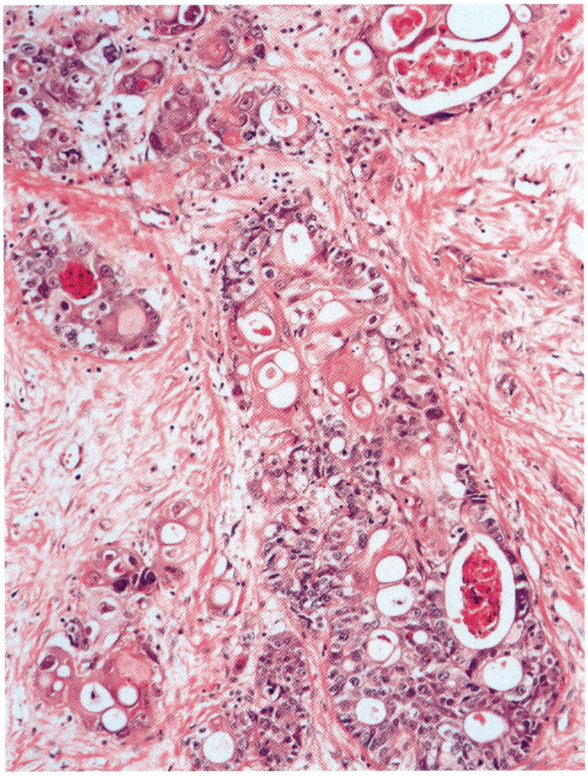

Figure 7-32

ADENOSQUAMOUS CARCINOMA VARIANT OF CHOLANGIOCARCINOMA

Both keratinization and tubule formation are observed.

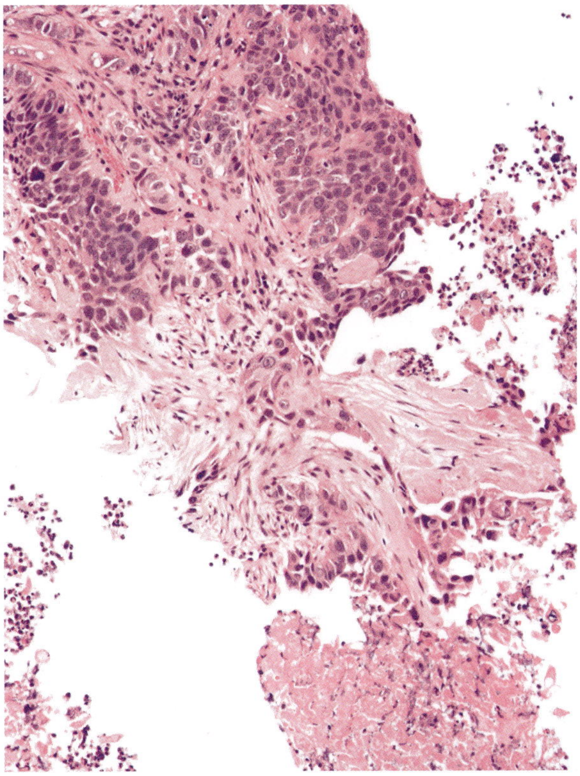

Figure 7-33

ADENOSQUAMOUS CARCINOMA VARIANT OF CHOLANGIOCARCINOMA

Vague squamous differentiation is seen in a biopsy sample.

is defined as a malignant epithelial neoplasm consisting of mucous, intermediate, and epidermoid cells. The tumors grossly do not differ from conventional intrahepatic cholangiocarcinoma, particularly of the mass-forming type (fig. 7-34). In 60 percent of cases tumors are larger than 10 cm (101).

Histologically, the three cellular components are easily identifiable, but their proportions vary among cases (fig. 7-35). The tumors are solid in most parts, but small cystic spaces lined by the neoplastic cells may be present. Intermediate and epidermoid cells may have clear cytoplasm. Special stains help in the identification of mucous cells, while p63 is positive particularly in epidermoid cells (102).

The grading scheme for mucoepidermoid carcinoma of the salivary glands is not useful for intrahepatic tumors, as the liver equivalent is always high grade. According to the reported cases, the prognosis seems to be extremely poor (101). A single patient survived more than 1 year after surgery. There is no known association with preceding hepatobiliary conditions, but we saw a case of mucoepidermoid carcinoma that developed against a background of PSC.

Mucinous Carcinoma (Colloid Carcinoma). Intrahepatic mucinous carcinoma is an invasive adenocarcinoma characterized by mucin-producing neoplastic cells floating in large amounts of extracellular mucus (fig. 7-36) (105–108). Focal mucinous features are sometimes seen in conventional cholangiocarcinoma, but mucinous components should be predominant (usually over 80 percent of the tumor) for this variant. Most tumors have intestinal features such as scattered goblet cells and immunoreactivity to CDX2 and MUC2. The expression of a gastric mucin, MUC5AC, is also common, as in conventional cholangiocarcinoma.

Nonmucinous components are sometimes papillary adenocarcinomas. Intestinal-type

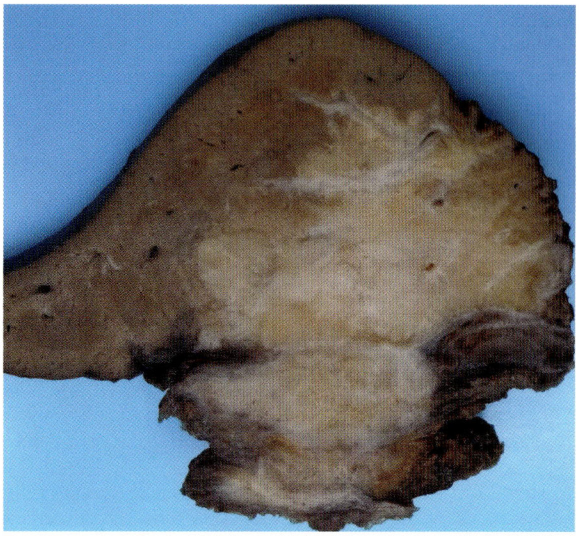

Figure 7-34

MUCOEPIDERMOID CARCINOMA VARIANT OF CHOLANGIOCARCINOMA

The tumor is large, with a mass-forming appearance.

biliary intraepithelial neoplasia (BilIN) can be present in the adjacent bile duct, particularly in patients with PSC, suggesting a dysplasia-carcinoma sequence (92). IPNB can also progress to mucinous carcinoma when it becomes invasive, but it is currently separately categorized (IPNB with an associated mucinous carcinoma) (4,109). Mucinous carcinoma should be discriminated from mucous lake with no floating cancer cells. Patients with mucinous carcinoma are known to have better prognosis than those with conventional cholangiocarcinoma.

Cholangiolocellular Carcinoma. Cholangiolocellular carcinoma is characterized by tumor cells arranged in regularly anastomosing and branching tubules, an appearance mimicking reactive bile ductules (110,111). A histologic and molecular link to hepatic progenitor cells has been suggested. As similar microscopic features are sometimes seen focally in conventional intrahepatic cholangiocarcinoma, this

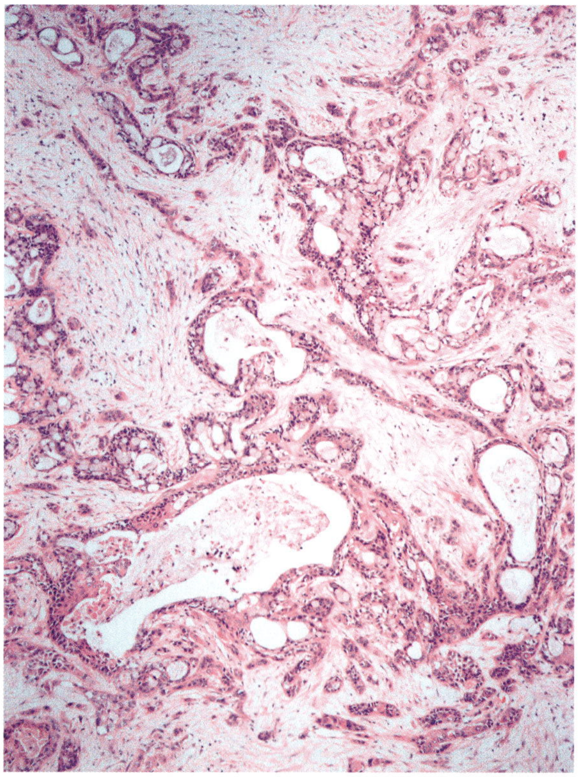

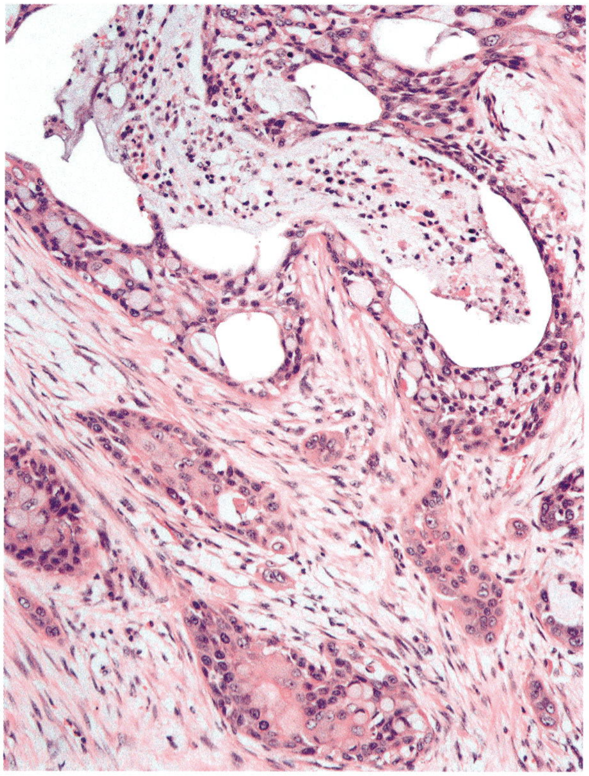

Figure 7-35

MUCOEPIDERMOID CARCINOMA VARIANT OF CHOLANGIOCARCINOMA

Left: Small cystic changes are noted.
Right: The tumor consists of epidermoid, intermediate, and mucous cells.

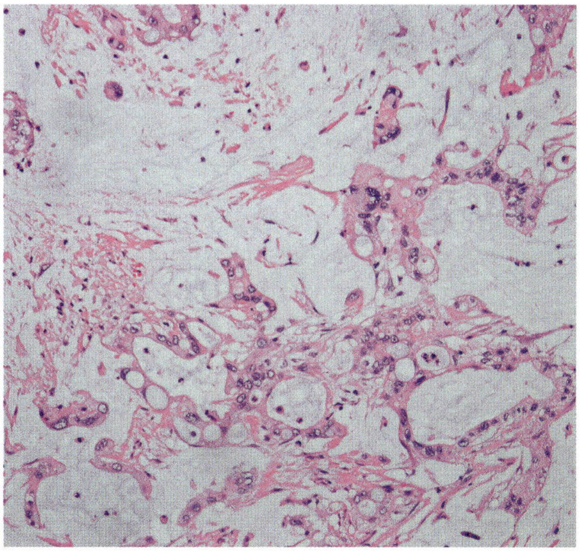

Figure 7-36

MUCINOUS CARCINOMA
VARIANT OF CHOLANGIOCARCINOMA

The neoplastic cells float in abundant extracellular mucin.

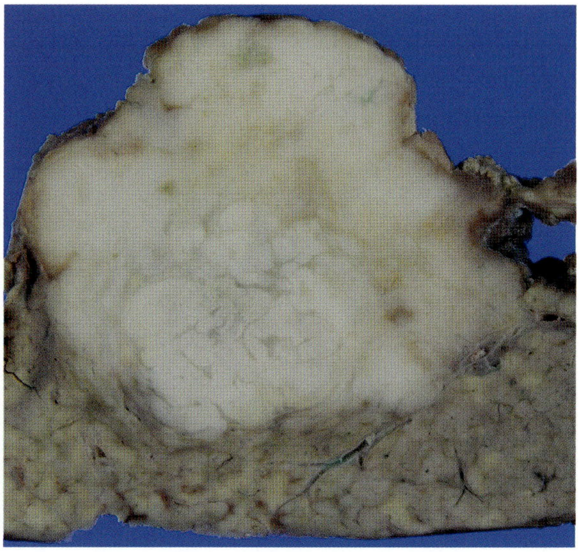

Figure 7-37

CHOLANGIOLOCELLUAR CARCINOMA

The tumor appears as a solid mass, without capsule.

diagnostic term should be given to neoplasms consisting predominantly of this growth pattern. The World Health Organization (WHO) classification describes this tumor group under the category of combined hepatocellular cholangiocarcinoma (112). However, we prefer to consider this neoplasm as a variant of intrahepatic cholangiocarcinoma unless there is a histology-proven hepatocellular component.

Cholangiolocellular carcinoma shares clinical and imaging features with both HCC and cholangiocarcinoma. At least 50 percent of patients have a history of chronic liver disease, such as viral hepatitis and hemochromatosis (110). Like HCC, it may show global or peripheral enhancement at the early phase of the contrast-enhanced image (113). Similar to cholangiocarcinoma, the enhancement typically remains until the delayed phase. The hypervascular tumors on the background of chronic liver disease are often clinically misdiagnosed as HCC. The tumor forms a solid mass with no surrounding fibrous capsule (fig. 7-37).

Histologically, the tubular growth pattern is fairly homogeneous throughout the tumor, and may be associated with minor trabecular components (fig. 7-38). Necrosis is not common even in large tumors. At the interface with the liver parenchyma, the tumor cells are

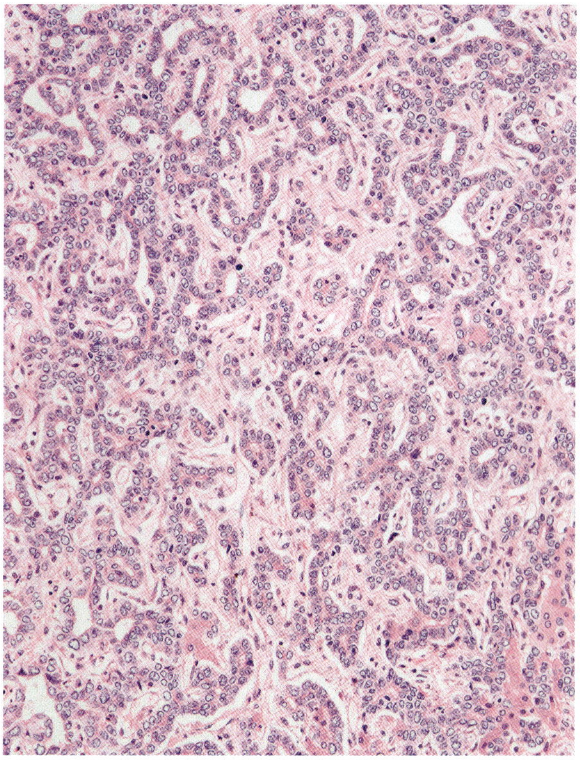

Figure 7-38

CHOLANGIOLOCELLULAR CARCINOMA

The tumor cells are arranged in an anastomosing tubular architecture mimicking reactive bile ductules.

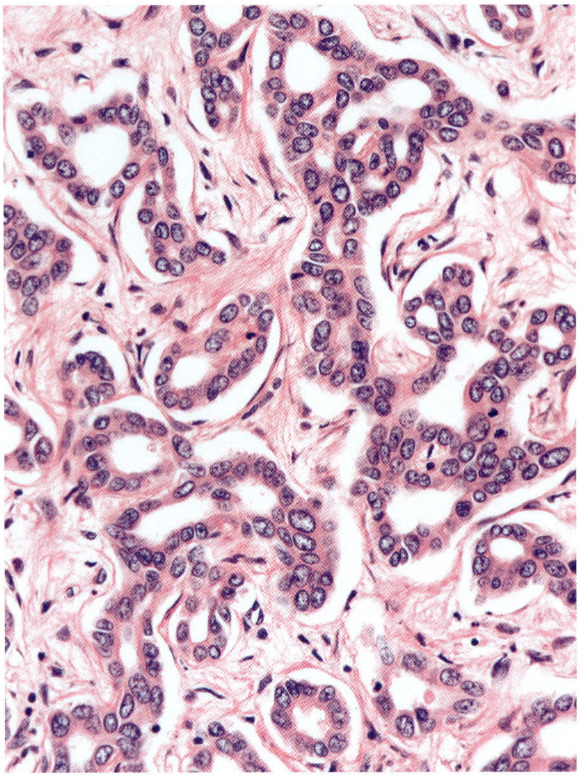

Figure 7-39

CHOLANGIOLOCELLULAR CARCINOMA

The tumor cells are less dysplastic than those in conventional cholangiocarcinoma.

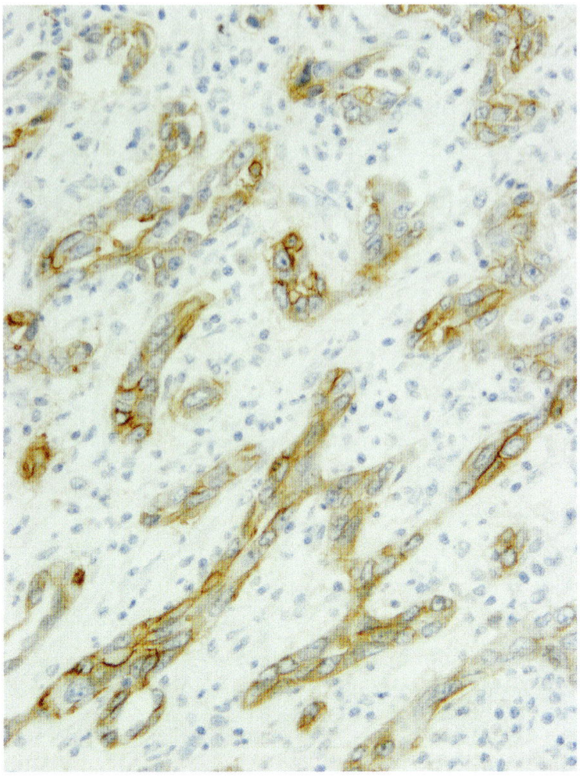

Figure 7-40

CHOLANGIOLOCELLULAR CARCINOMA

CD56 expression.

continuous with the liver cell plates, suggesting a replacing growth pattern. The cells are small, with less pleomorphic oval nuclei (fig. 7-39). The neoplastic cords are embedded in fibrotic stroma. Mucin production is usually absent.

On immunostaining, the cells are positive for cholangiocyte markers (CK7 and CK19). CD56 (NCAM), which is known to be positive in bile ductules but negative in bile ducts in non-neoplastic liver, is useful for determining the cholangiolocellular phenotype (fig. 7-40). It is not always expressed in cholangiolocellular carcinoma (positive in 70 to 80 percent), however, and could be positive in conventional cholangiocarcinoma (10 to 20 percent) (114). The 5-year survival rate is 75 percent, which is significantly better than that for patients with conventional intrahepatic cholangiocarcinoma (115).

Ductal Plate Malformation Type. This recently reported variant has tumor cells arranged in irregularly dilated ducts with peculiar projections and bridges, the microscopic features reminiscent of ductal plate malformation seen in congenital hepatic fibrosis, Caroli disease, and polycystic liver (116). According to a 10-case series, 60 percent of patients have a history of chronic liver disease (116). The tumor is usually less than 5 cm (fig. 7-41). Some patients have HCC or conventional cholangiocarcinoma elsewhere in the liver.

Histologically, the tumor shows a vague multinodular architecture with intervening fibrous bands. The tumor cells are small, oval, and not pleomorphic. Portal tracts and central veins are regularly distributed within the mass, suggesting a replacing growth pattern. Mitotic figures are rare, and the MIB-1 index is usually less than 5 percent. Similar to ductal plate malformation, bile plugs are present in dilated neoplastic lumens (fig. 7-42).

This variant is always intermixed with components of cholangiolocellular carcinoma.

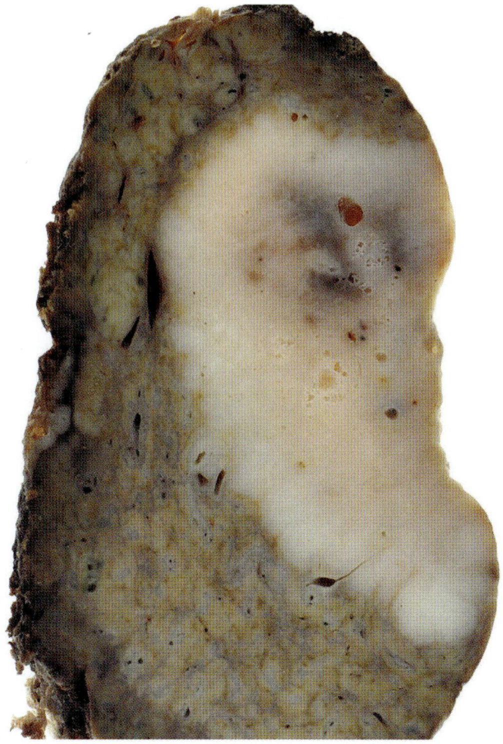

Figure 7-41

DUCTAL PLATE MALFORMATION TYPE CHOLANGIOCARCINOMA

A small cystic change representing dilated neoplastic glands is seen.

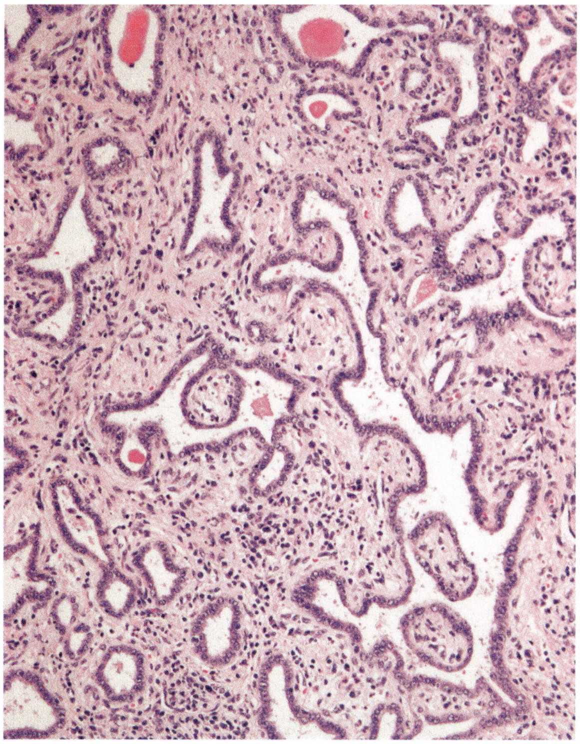

Figure 7-42

DUCTAL PLATE MALFORMATION TYPE CHOLANGIOCARCINOMA

Irregularly dilated ducts contain eosinophilic bile plugs.

Given the considerable overlap in histologic features between the two, this subtype is probably best regarded as a morphologic variant of cholangiolocellular carcinoma. The immunophenotype is also similar, since CD56 is positive.

Lymphoepithelioma-Like Carcinoma. Lymphoepithelioma-like carcinoma, which is histologically similar to nasopharyngeal carcinoma, is extremely rare in the liver, with less than 30 cases reported in the literature (117, 118). Most patients are diagnosed in East Asia.

Histologically, the tumor is an undifferentiated carcinoma or poorly differentiated adenocarcinoma with an abundant lymphoid stroma (fig. 7-43A–C). Components of more differentiated adenocarcinoma may focally coexist. The tumor cells are large and polygonal, with vesicular nuclei and distinct nucleoli. The cells are arranged in solid nests, cords, or tubules with indistinct intercellular borders. The lymphoid stroma consists of mixed T cells, B cells, and mature plasma cells. Neutrophils and eosinophils are rare, while a granulomatous reaction may be present. In situ hybridization for Epstein-Barr encoded RNA (EBER) is positive in the cancer cells (fig. 7-43D) (119). Conventional intrahepatic cholangiocarcinoma may have lymphoplasmacytic infiltration, while the lymphoid stroma may be less prominent in lymphoepithelioma-like carcinoma. Thus, confirmation by EBER positivity is required for the diagnosis. The presence of many intraepithelial lymphocytes may be a diagnostic clue in equivocal cases (fig. 7-44).

The tumor is usually positive for CK7 and CK19, and negative for HepPar1. Immunostaining for cytokeratins highlights the cancer cells, which are ambiguous on H&E-stained sections. This variant has a favorable prognosis, with one study on seven patients indicating a 100 percent 5-year overall survival rate (120).

Spindle Cell Carcinoma and Carcinosarcoma. The same as carcinomas in other organs,

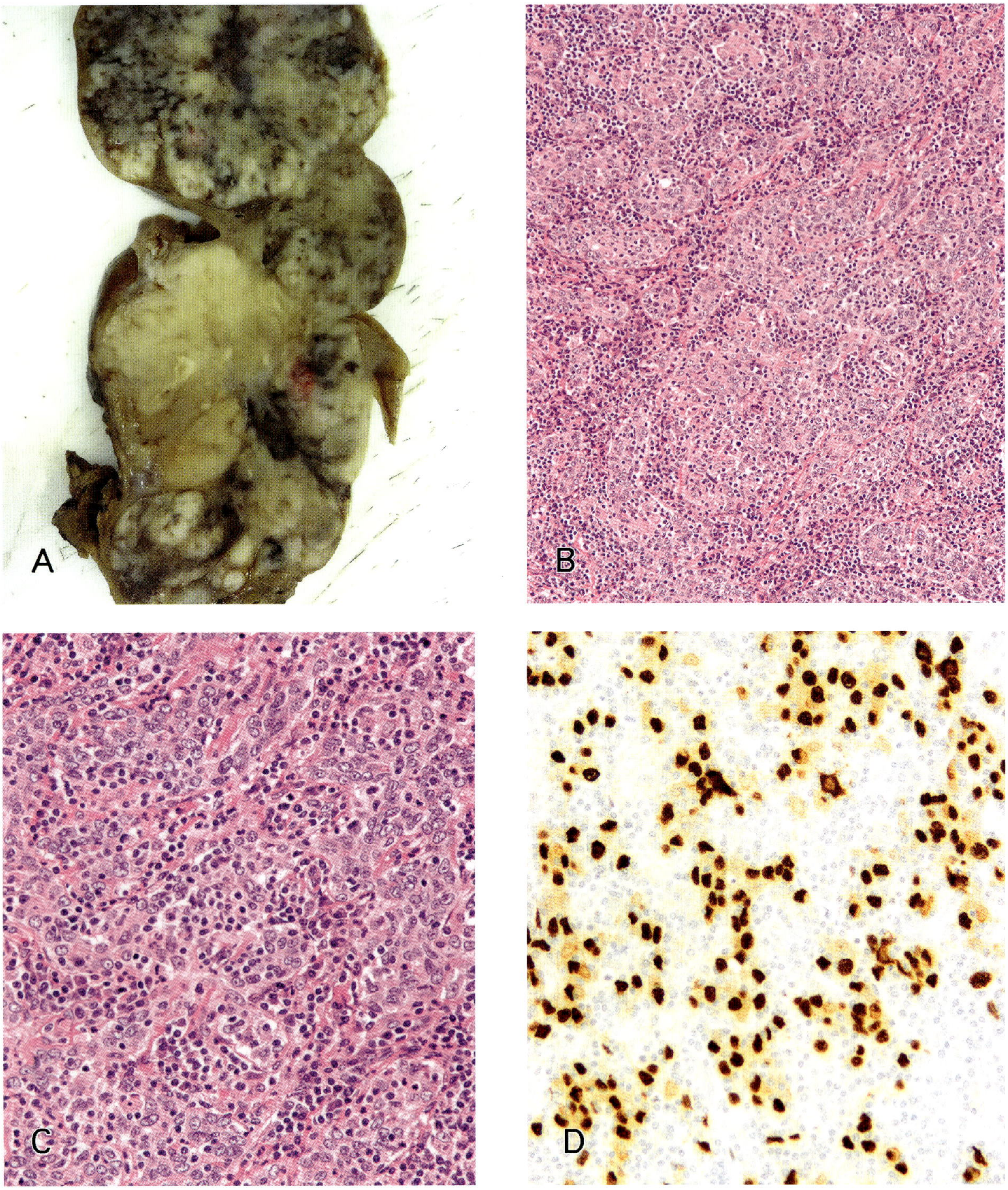

Figure 7-43

LYMPHOEPITHELIOMA-LIKE CARCINOMA

A: The lobulated tumor mass contains darkly brown areas.
B: The tumor is associated with an extensive lymphoplasmacytic infiltrate.
C: Tumor cells have plump large nuclei.
D: Tumor cells are positive for EBER staining.

cholangiocarcinoma can show pseudosarcomatous transformation (121,122). The spindle-shaped neoplastic cells have pleomorphic nuclei and occasional mitotic figures (fig. 7-45, left). They are arranged in a cellular fascicular pattern (fig. 7-45, right). Necrosis is common. On immunostaining, the sarcomatous components at least focally express epithelial markers such as cytokeratins and epithelial membrane antigen (EMA), confirming the epithelial nature. Mesenchymal markers that are frequently positive in sarcomatoid carcinomas include vimentin, HHF35, and alpha-smooth muscle actin (SMA) (123).

The diagnostic term carcinosarcoma should be restricted to the tumors with proven heterologous sarcomatous elements such as osteosarcoma, chondrosarcoma, and rhabdomyosarcoma (fig. 7-46). As carcinosarcoma of the liver typically contains HCC components, pure intrahepatic cholangiocarcinoma with heterologous sarcomatous elements is extremely rare. These

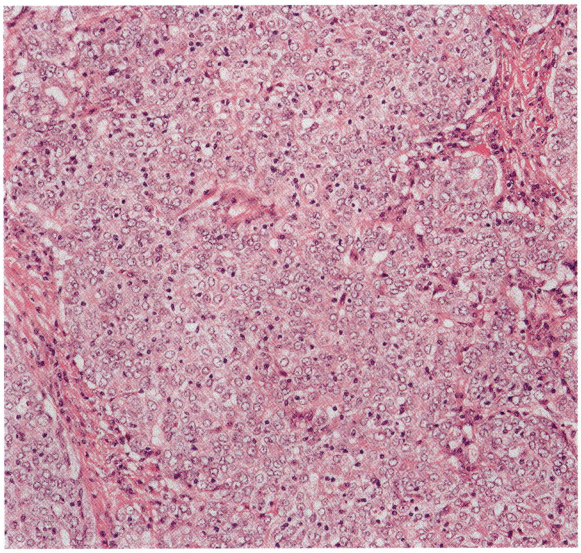

Figure 7-44

LYMPHOEPITHELIOMA-LIKE CARCINOMA

Although lymphoplasmacytic infiltration is not conspicuous, many intraepithelial lymphocytes are noted. This case was positive for EBER.

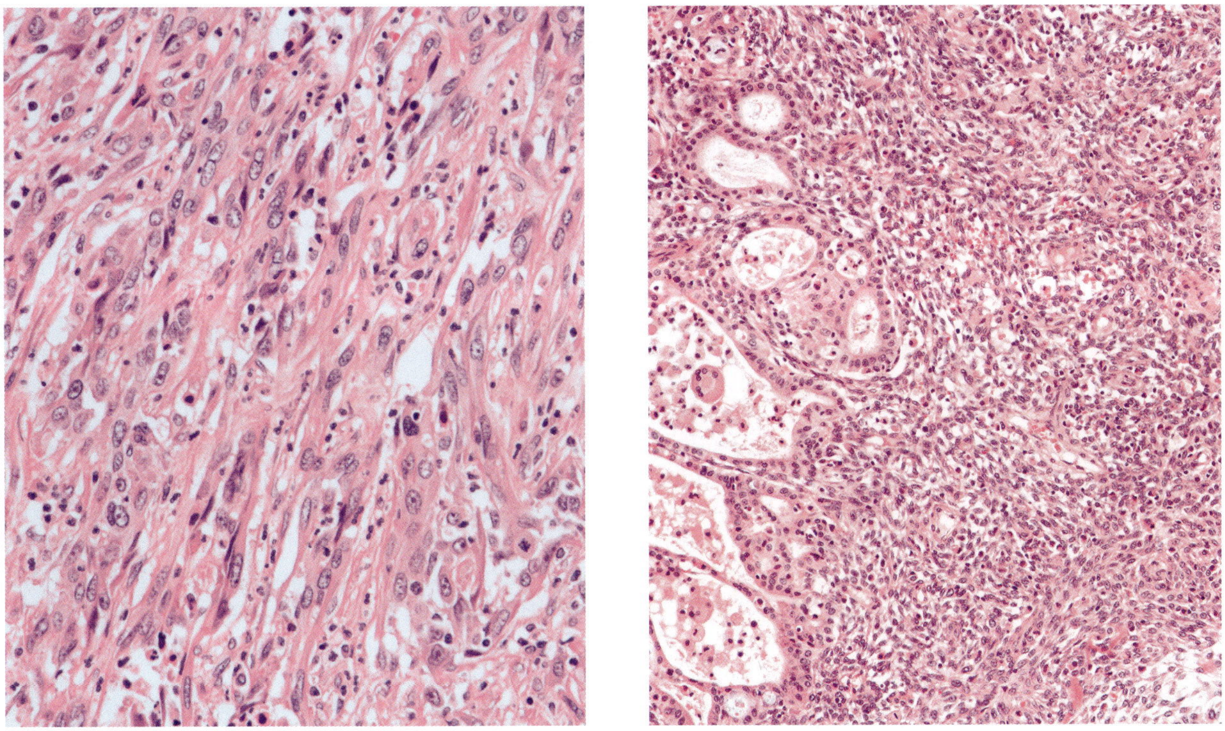

Figure 7-45

SPINDLE CELL CARCINOMA VARIANT OF CHOLANGIOCARCINOMA

Left: Spindle tumor cells are arranged in a diffuse fashion.
Right: Glandular and sarcomatous areas are intermixed.

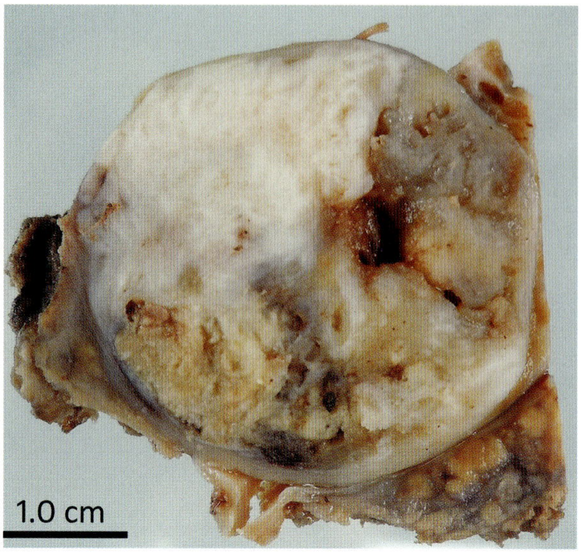

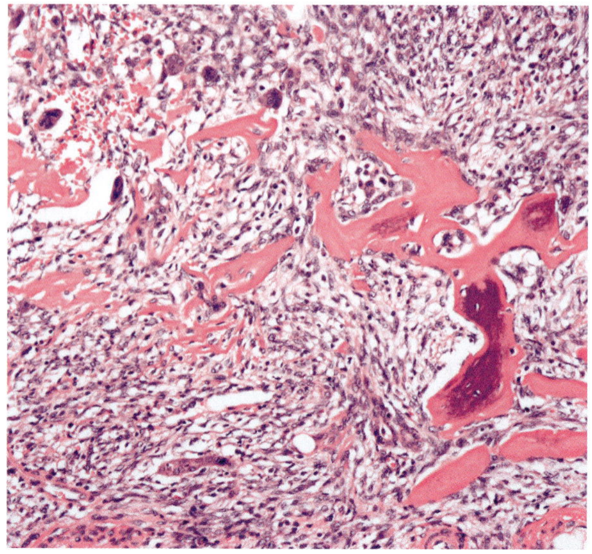

Figure 7-46

CARCINOSARCOMA

Left: Grossly, fibrotic and calcified foci are noted.
Right: The sarcomatous component creates osteoid, indicating osteosarcoma differentiation.

variants generally show aggressive clinical behavior and confer a poorer prognosis than ordinary cholangiocarcinoma (122).

Tubulocystic Carcinoma. This peculiar form of cholangiocarcinoma was recently proposed (124). Of five cases in the original series, two were intrahepatic and three developed at the perihilar region. The tumors share morphologic features with tubulocystic carcinomas of the kidney. Numerous variably sized cysts form a fairly circumscribed mass (3 to 7 cm in diameter) with an overall "honeycomb" appearance (fig. 7-47, left) (125). Most of the tubules are small, up to 1 cm, and have eosinophilic secretory contents. The lining epithelium consists of atypical cuboidal to flat cells with no intracytoplasmic mucin. Foci of intracystic papillary proliferation are present. Because of attenuation, cellular atypia may not be obvious, but dysplastic features, such as nuclear enlargement and hyperchromasia, and distinct nucleoli, are seen at least focally (fig. 7-47, right). The apical cytoplasm often contains projections resembling snouts.

Well-defined tubules, bland-looking cells, and little desmoplastic reaction may give an impression of a noninvasive lesion, but the tumor seems to be invasive since the numerous tubules cannot be explained by non-neoplastic processes. Unlike mucinous cystic neoplasm of the liver, there is no ovarian-like stroma. An indolent clinical course was suggested in the original report (124), but we recently observed a case of high-grade sarcomatoid transformation.

Acinar Cell Carcinoma. Whether the rare acinar cell carcinoma is a variant of intrahepatic cholangiocarcinoma or HCC remains unclear, however, it is probably best described here as another form of primary liver cancer with glandular differentiation. Only five cases have been described in the literature (126,127). The tumor forms a solid mass ranging from 7 to 19 cm.

Histologically, the tumor cells are arranged predominantly in well-organized glands with small lumen, reminiscent of pancreatic acini. Occasional foci show small cystic dilatation of glands, and solid or trabecular architecture. The cells have round, basally located nuclei and eosinophilic cytoplasm. There is no identifiable additional component of conventional cholangiocarcinoma or HCC.

The tumor is positive for at least one of the three acinar markers: trypsin, amylase, and lipase. Synaptophysin may be focally positive. The tumor is negative for HepPar1, CK7, CK19, CK20, CD56, alpha-fetoprotein (AFP), and CDX2 (126).

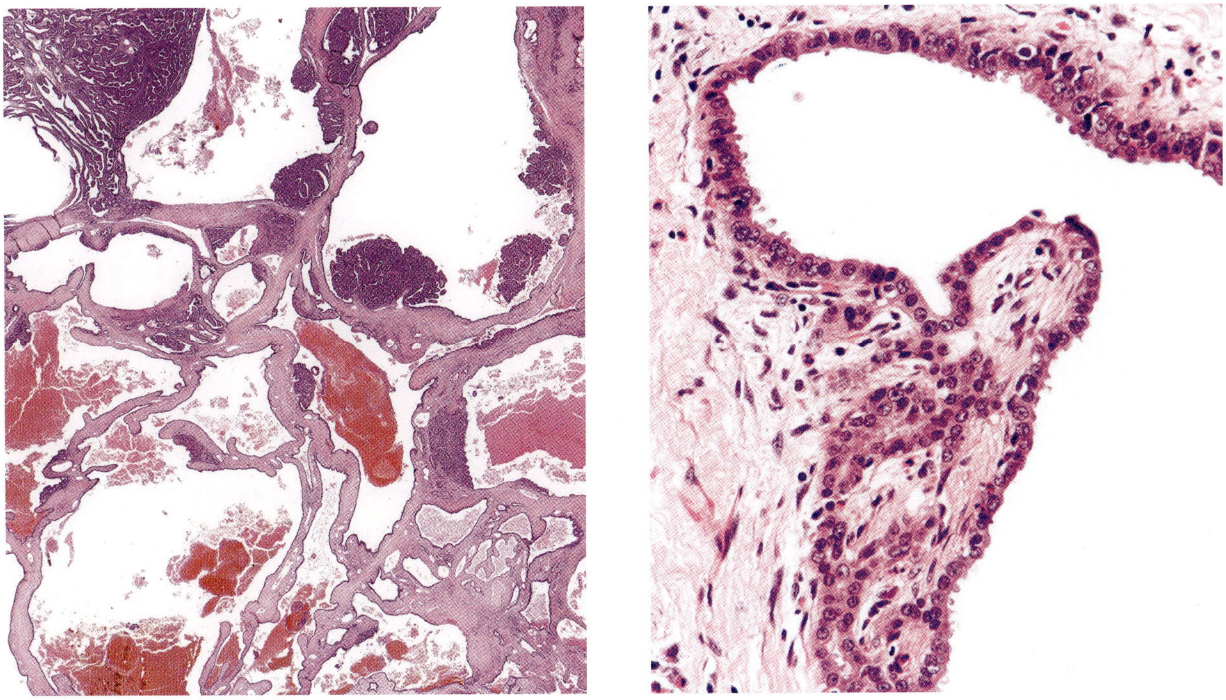

Figure 7-47

TUBULOCYSTIC CARCINOMA

Left: The tumor is characterized by large cystic spaces and intracystic tumor growth.
Right: The epithelium lining the cystic space shows atypical features and cytoplasmic projections like apocrine snouts.

The prognosis seems to be favorable, with no recurrence noted at a mean follow-up of 22 months, except for one patient who had recurrent disease in the liver at 18 months (126,127). Although peribiliary glands sometimes show acinar metaplasia, they are less likely to be a precursor since the tumors are more peripherally located. It is important to exclude metastasis from clinically occult acinar cell carcinoma of the pancreas and salivary glands.

Frozen Sections

For patients with intrahepatic cholangiocarcinoma, intraoperative frozen section diagnosis is considered for making the diagnosis of the main tumor or suspected metastatic lesions and for assessing the surgical margin. A common scenario is that a small nodular lesion just beneath the hepatic capsule is submitted to rule out metastatic adenocarcinoma. The size of the nodule is important because benign lesions such as bile duct adenoma (peribiliary gland hamartoma) and von Meyenburg complex (bile duct hamartoma) are generally less than 1.5 cm. In bile duct adenoma, the tubules are regular in size and shape. Bile plugs in the dilated tubules usually suggest a benign hamartomatous nature. The presence of unremarkable portal tracts within the lesion also supports benignity (fig. 7-48). Unlike cholangiocarcinoma, where neoplastic glands invade the adjacent liver cell plates, the tissue-destructive nature is not identified in peribiliary gland and bile duct hamartomas. As it is generally difficult to assess the degree of cytologic atypia on frozen sections, the overall architecture may be more informative. Another entity in the differential diagnosis is a suppurative or xanthogranulomatous inflammatory nodule secondary to bile duct obstruction. Small bile ducts involved in the inflammation may show an irregular architecture (fig. 7-49).

Frozen section diagnosis of the bile duct margin is challenging, particularly if the duct is inflamed or a biliary stent is placed (fig. 7-50). The reactive lining epithelial cells may be slightly cellular, with enlarged nuclei, but the nuclear

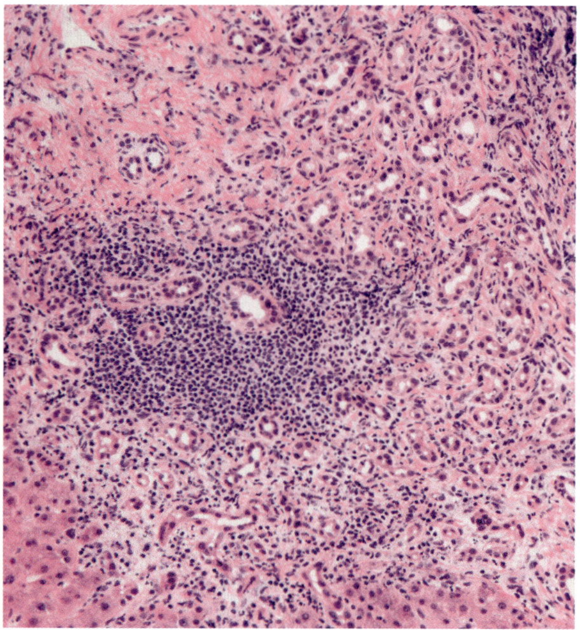

Figure 7-48

BILE DUCT ADENOMA

Glandular structures are embedded in the stroma with or without inflammatory infiltrates (frozen section).

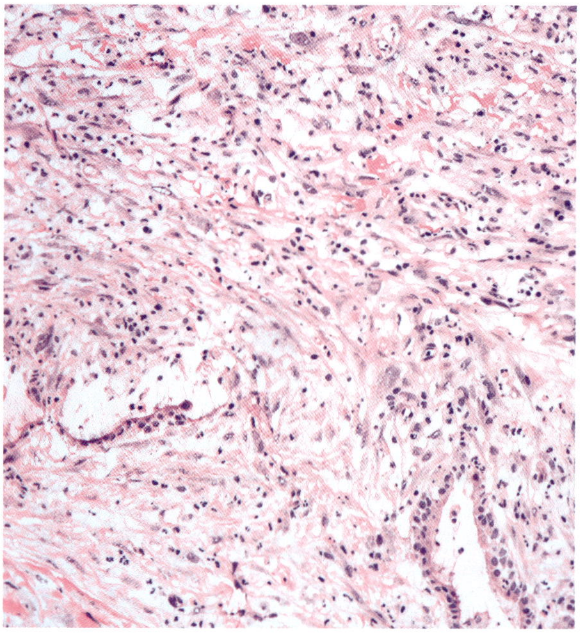

Figure 7-49

INFLAMMATORY NODULE DUE TO BILIARY OBSTRUCTION

Small bile ducts involved in the process become irregular in shape (frozen section).

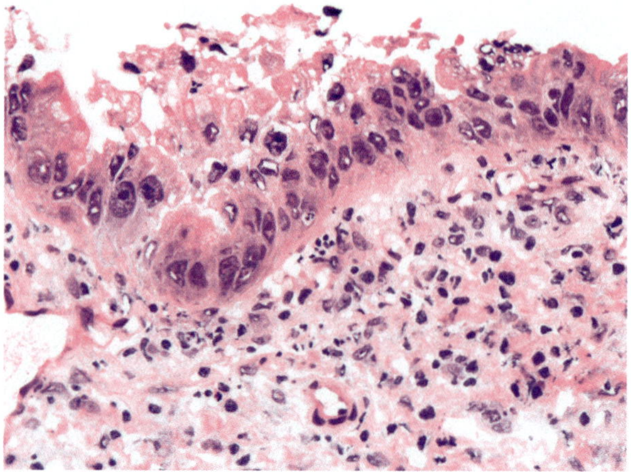

Figure 7-50

CARCINOMA IN SITU AT BILE DUCT SURGICAL MARGIN

The epithelium shows pleomorphic nuclei and prominent nucleoli that reach to the top of the surface. No invasion is seen (frozen section).

membrane generally remains round, and chromatin is fine and homogeneously distributed (fig. 7-51). The presence of many intraepithelial neutrophils suggests a reactive process rather than BilIN or intraepithelial carcinoma. Well-differentiated adenocarcinomas infiltrating the bile duct wall are sometimes misinterpreted as benign, as they can form well-defined ducts with minimal desmoplastic reaction. The large bile ducts lack ductal structures in their wall, except for conduits of peribiliary glands. Therefore, ductal structures with no peribiliary glands nearby are most likely infiltrating carcinomas (fig. 7-52).

Immunohistochemical Findings

Several immunohistochemical markers for intrahepatic cholangiocarcinoma that are useful for the histologic diagnosis have been identified in the last two decades. They are classified into biliary markers that are expressed in both non-neoplastic and neoplastic cholangiocytes, and "neoplastic" markers that are positive in cholangiocarcinoma but negative in the non-neoplastic biliary epithelium (Table 7-2).

The cytokeratin profile of intrahepatic cholangiocarcinoma is basically similar to that of non-neoplastic biliary epithelium, but expression becomes weaker or patchier in poorly differentiated adenocarcinomas. As in normal

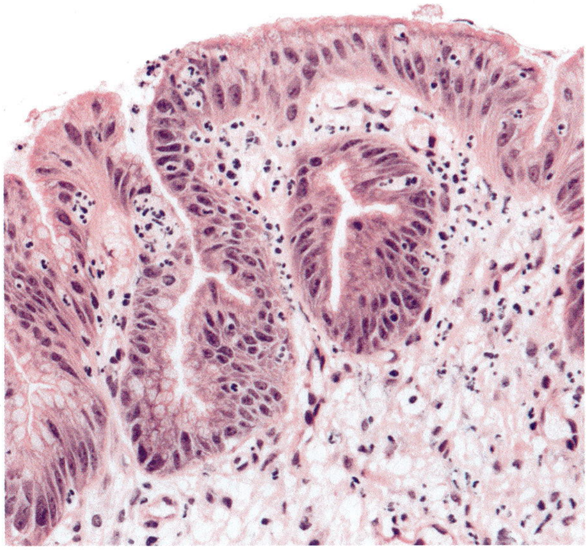

Figure 7-51

REGENERATIVE EPITHELIUM AT BILE DUCT SURGICAL MARGIN

A slight papillary architecture and many intraepithelial neutrophils are seen in a frozen section specimen.

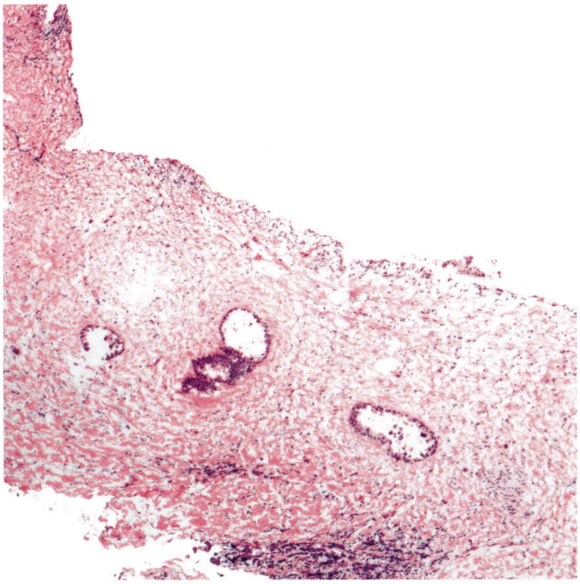

Figure 7-52

INFILTRATING WELL-DIFFERENTIATED ADENOCARCINOMA AT BILE DUCT SURGICAL MARGIN

Ducts with no associated glands in the bile duct wall indicate malignancy (frozen section).

bile ducts and peribiliary glands, intrahepatic cholangiocarcinoma expresses CK7 (91 percent), CK8 (82 percent), CK18 (51 percent), and CK19 (70 percent) (96). Of these four, CK7 and CK19 are more valuable for the diagnosis, as CK8 and CK18 are also positive in hepatocytes and HCC (fig. 7-53). Keratin 903 (34βE12), a high molecular weight cytokeratin, is expressed in 74 percent of intrahepatic cholangiocarcinomas and only 10 percent of HCCs (128). The loss of keratin 903 expression is an unfavorable prognostic factor for patients with intrahepatic cholangiocarcinoma (128). CK20 expression may be focally present in intrahepatic cholangiocarcinomas, particularly those arising from large bile ducts.

The expression patterns of mucin core proteins (MUCs) change during the malignant transformation of biliary epithelial cells (129). MUC1 is used for the pathologic diagnosis, as it is believed to be aberrantly expressed in malignant neoplasms. In fact, its expression is noted in 80 percent of intrahepatic cholangiocarcinomas (fig. 7-54) (130,131). A caveat is that staining patterns of MUC1 in normal bile ducts depend on the clones of monoclonal antibodies used (132). MUC1 (clone DF3) is negative

Table 7-2

IMMUNOHISTOCHEMICAL MARKERS FOR INTRAHEPATIC CHOLANGIOCARCINOMA

Cholangiocyte Markers[a]	"Neoplastic" Markers
CK7 (91%)	p53 (80%)
Keratin 903 (34βE12) (74%)	MUC1 (80%)
CK19 (70%)	Maspin (73%)
CA19-9 (60%)	S-100 protein P (53%)
	Tubulin beta-3 (50%)
	Fascin (40%)
	MUC4 (37%)
	Mesothelin (21%)

[a]Cholangiocyte markers are expressed in both non-neoplastic and neoplastic biliary epithelium, while "neoplastic" markers are more specific for cholangiocarcinoma. Percentages in parentheses are expression rates in intrahepatic cholangiocarcinoma.

in normal bile ducts, but can be positive with other monoclonal antibodies (132). Nevertheless, MUC1 expression is associated with poor outcome, irrespective of the type of antibody used (133). Although MUC2 expression is rare in the bile duct, it may be focally expressed in intrahepatic large duct cholangiocarcinoma (28

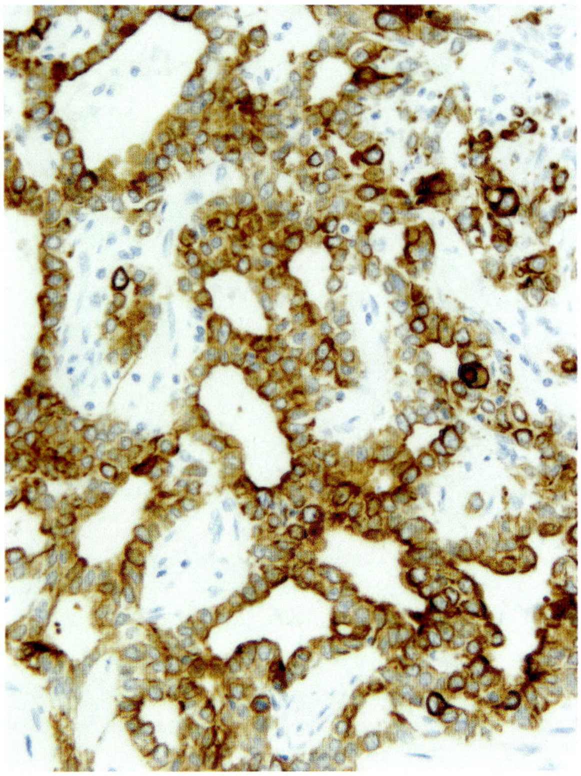

Figure 7-53

CHOLANGIOCARCINOMA: IMMUNOHISTOCHEMISTRY

CK19 expression in cholangiocarcinoma.

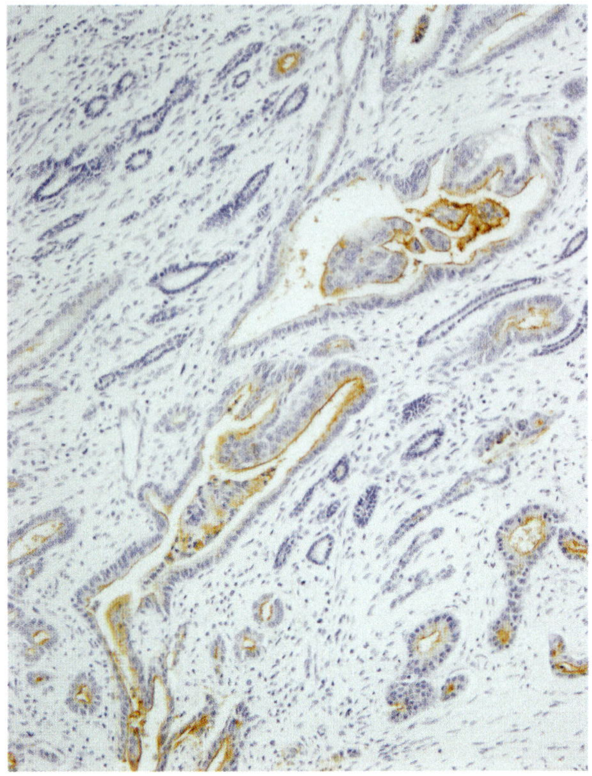

Figure 7-54

CHOLANGIOCARCINOMA: IMMUNOHISTOCHEMISTRY

MUC1 (clone DF3) expression. Cancer cells express MUC1 on the luminal surface, while non-neoplastic ducts are negative.

percent) (134). MUC4 is negative in non-neoplastic liver tissue, but is aberrantly expressed in cholangiocarcinoma (37 percent) (130). As MUC4 is an intramembrane ligand for receptor tyrosine kinase ErbB2, the expression of these two molecules is correlated in intrahepatic cholangiocarcinoma (130). Gastric-type mucins, MUC5AC and MUC6, are expressed in 40 percent and 20 percent of intrahepatic cholangiocarcinomas, respectively (134).

Immunohistochemical "neoplastic" markers for intrahepatic cholangiocarcinoma include p53, maspin, fascin, mesothelin, and S-100 protein P. Overexpression of p53 is found in approximately 50 percent of intrahepatic cholangiocarcinomas (135). As diffuse and strong expression of p53 is unlikely to occur in reactive processes, it indicates the neoplastic nature of the biliary epithelium. p53 is also positive in less than 10 percent of BilIN-3 cases, while its expression is exceptional in lower-grade lesions (136). Maspin is overexpressed in 73 percent of intrahepatic cholangiocarcinomas and 40 to 60 percent of BilINs (fig. 7-55) (137). Fascin is also positive in 35 to 50 percent of intrahepatic cholangiocarcinoma (138,139). Its expression is more commonly seen in poorly differentiated carcinomas and larger tumors, and at the invasive front. Fascin expression is correlated with the overexpression of MMP-9 and cyclin D1, and could be an unfavorable prognostic factor (138,139). Mesothelin is a mesothelial marker aberrantly expressed in 21 percent of cases (140). These neoplastic markers are fairly specific for cholangiocarcinoma and are useful for small biopsy samples and cytologic specimens.

The cancer cell phenotype differs based on the size of the originating bile ducts. Immunohistochemical markers that are more commonly expressed in large duct or small duct cholangiocarcinoma are shown in Table 7-3 (141–146). Intrahepatic cholangiocarcinoma arising from

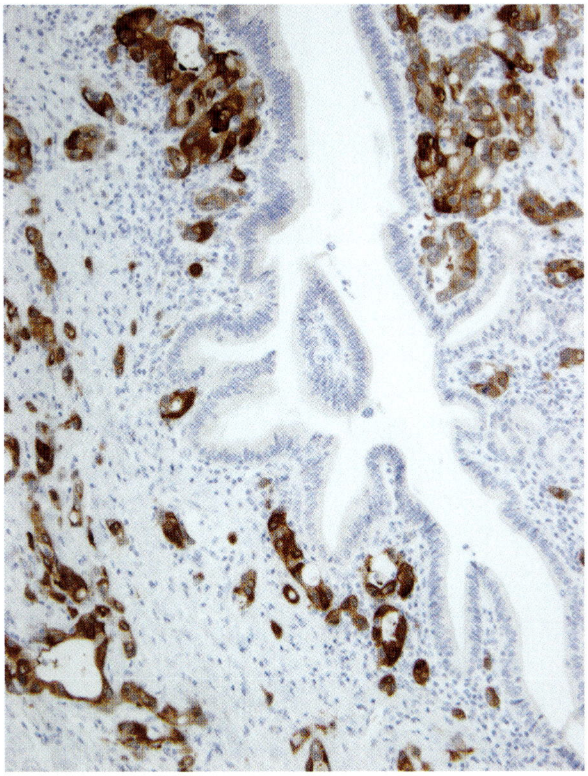

Figure 7-55

CHOLANGIOCARCINOMA: IMMUNOHISTOCHEMISTRY

Maspin is negative in the non-neoplastic biliary epithelium, but is strongly expressed in infiltrating cholangiocarcinoma.

the large bile ducts shares some immunohistochemical phenotypes with perihilar cholangiocarcinoma (145). However, given that the expression of most markers overlaps between large duct and small duct cholangiocarcinoma, the origin of tumors cannot be determined based on a single molecule. Panels of immunohistochemical markers may be developed to identify subgroups of intrahepatic cholangiocarcinoma that have distinct clinicopathologic and molecular features (146).

Immunostaining for serum tumor markers may be positive in cholangiocarcinoma. CA19-9 is diffusely expressed in the non-neoplastic epithelium of the pancreas and bile ducts. It is detectable in 60 percent of cholangiocarcinomas (147). CEA and CA125 are only rarely expressed in the non-neoplastic biliary epithelium, while CEA is positive in 46 percent of cholangiocarcinomas, particularly in large duct cancers (143).

Table 7-3

IMMUNOHISTOCHEMICAL MARKERS THAT ARE MORE FREQUENTLY EXPRESSED IN EITHER LARGE-DUCT OR SMALL-DUCT INTRAHEPATIC CHOLANGIOCARCINOMA

Markers More Commonly Expressed in Large Duct Cholangiocarcinoma	Markers More Commonly Expressed in Small Duct Cholangiocarcinoma
CK20	CK18
MUC2	VEGF-A
MUC5AC	Filamin-A
Akt2	CD56 (NCAM)
Annexin II	Tubulin beta-3
S-100 protein P	N-cadherin
Anterior gradient 2 (AGR2)	
Trefoil factor 1 (TFF1)	

CA125, also named MUC16, is expressed in 48 percent of cases, and its expression is known to be a poor prognostic factor (140).

Nuclear proteins involved in the cell cycle are upregulated or downregulated in carcinomas and premalignant lesions, leading to the proliferation of tumor cells. Essential modulators of the G1-S phase, including p16, p21, and cyclin D1, are dysregulated in cholangiocarcinoma (136). Cyclin D1 is overexpressed in 64 percent of cases, and p21 in 73 percent (136). p16 is stable in non-neoplastic biliary epithelium or low-grade BilIN, but significantly downregulated in cholangiocarcinoma, where the expression is detectable in only 20 percent (148). SMAD4/DPC4 is encoded by *DPC4* located on chromosome 18q, and its inactivation occurs in some malignant neoplasms (149). In cholangiocarcinoma, 73 percent of cases show the loss of SMAD4 immunolabeling (fig. 7-56) (136).

Cadherins play a major role in cell adhesion, and are known to be disrupted in malignant neoplasms, which facilitates invasive growth (150). In intrahepatic cholangiocarcinoma, E-cadherin expression on the cell membrane remains in only 20 percent of cases (151). The loss of E-cadherin is correlated with the overexpression of MMP7 and MT1-MMP (151). N-cadherin is another cell adhesion molecule more commonly expressed in mesenchymal cells than in epithelial cells. In non-neoplastic

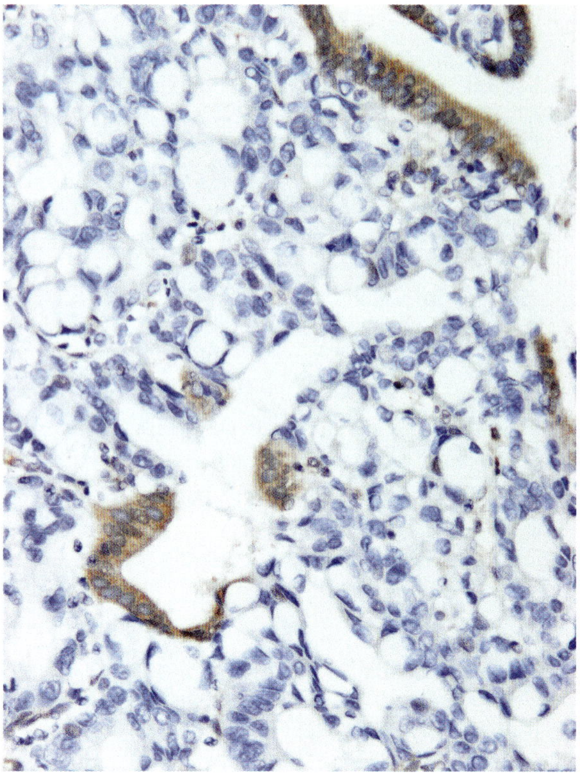

Figure 7-56

CHOLANGIOCARCINOMA: IMMUNOHISTOCHEMISTRY

SMAD4 expression is preserved in entrapped nonneoplastic cholangiocytes but lost in the cholangiocarcinoma.

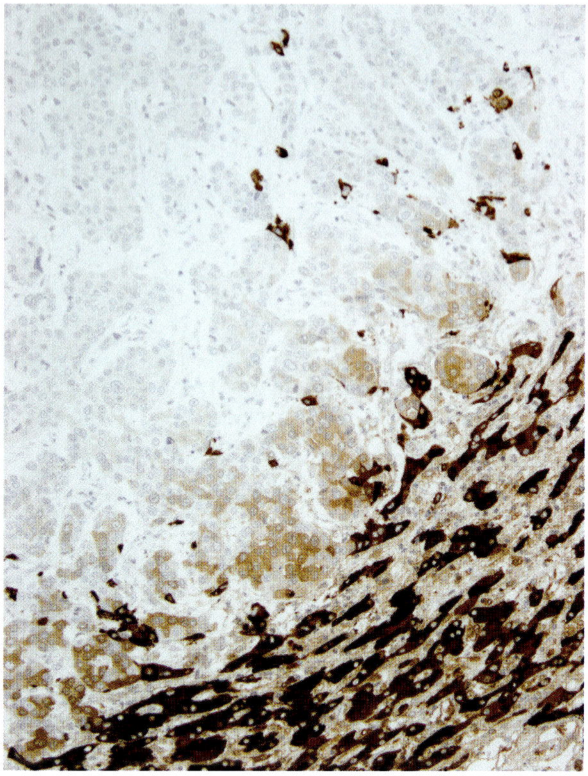

Figure 7-57

CHOLANGIOCARCINOMA: IMMUNOHISTOCHEMISTRY

HepPar1 highlights entrapped hepatocytes at the invasive front. Weak staining in tumor cells probably represents enzymes released from dying hepatocytes.

human tissue, this form of cadherin is constantly expressed in hepatocytes and intrahepatic biliary epithelium, but not in extrahepatic bile ducts (152). N-cadherin is positive in 79 percent of intrahepatic, 48 percent of perihilar, and none of extrahepatic cholangiocarcinomas (145,152). N-cadherin positivity is strongly associated with cholangiolar morphology and a history of chronic viral hepatitis (153). Its expression is rare in other carcinomas except for HCC and gallbladder cancers, suggesting its diagnostic value in discriminating intrahepatic cholangiocarcinoma from metastatic adenocarcinomas (152).

Hepatocellular markers are generally negative in intrahepatic cholangiocarcinoma. Oncofetal proteins such as AFP and glypican-3 are not expressed. Immunostaining for HepPar1 may exhibit weak cytoplasmic staining in cholangiocarcinoma, but coarse granular staining is not a feature and indicates a concomitant hepatocellular component if present. Entrapped hepatocytes positive for HepPar1 should not be interpreted as an HCC component. This finding is commonly seen at the invasive front. Arginase-1 is also generally negative in cholangiocarcinoma. However, a caveat is that staining for HepPar1 or arginase-1 may yield moderate nonspecific signals at the interface between the cholangiocarcinoma and liver parenchyma, probably representing the antigens released from dying hepatocytes (fig. 7-57).

The stroma of intrahepatic cholangiocarcinoma has a unique immunophenotype. Laminin gamma 2 chain is an extracellular matrix protein that plays a role in cell migration and tumor invasion. It is overexpressed in the stroma around the malignant cholangiocytes at the invasive front, and the expression is correlated with a poor prognosis (154). Stromal expression of tenascin, decorin, osteopontin, and heparan

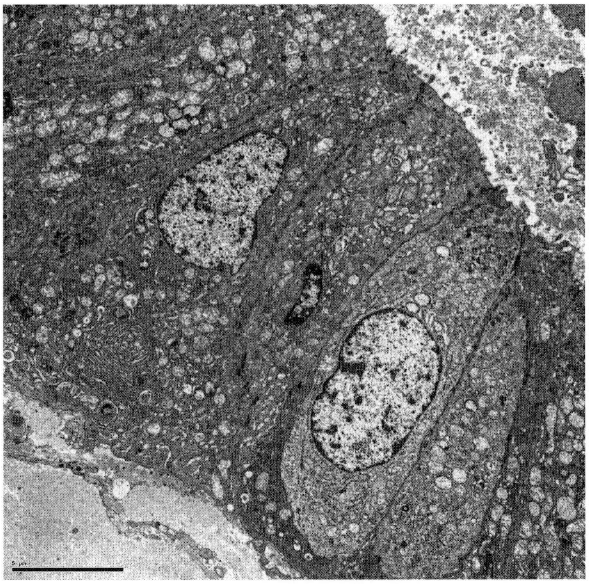

Figure 7-58

CHOLANGIOCARCINOMA: ELECTRON MICROSCOPIC FEATURES

Cellular polarity is preserved with intracytoplasmic mucin.

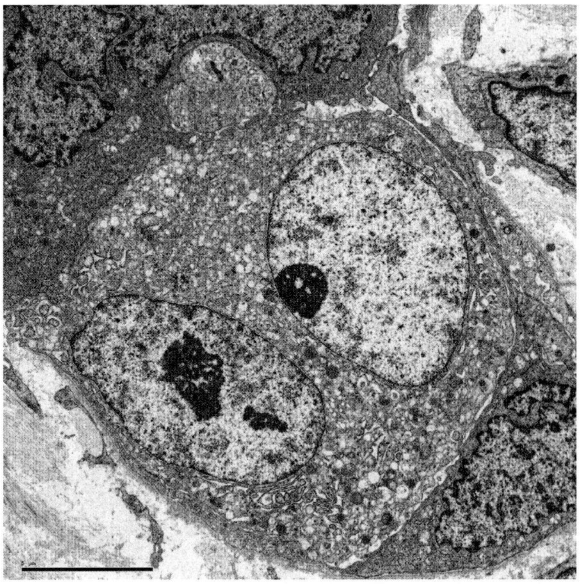

Figure 7-59

CHOLANGIOCARCINOMA: ELECTRON MICROSCOPIC FEATURES

The cells are connected by tight junctions and desmosomes.

sulfate proteoglycan also contributes to the development of the unique tumor stroma in cholangiocarcinoma (155–157). The stromal expression of osteopontin is an independent prognostic marker for overall and disease-free survival (156).

A recent gene profiling analysis of stroma identified a signature of 1,073 genes that can discriminate the tumor stroma from nontumor fibrous tissue. Functional analysis of differentially expressed genes demonstrated that upregulated genes are related to the cell cycle, extracellular matrix, and transforming growth factor beta (TGF-β) pathways (156). TGF-β1 expressed in cancer cells and myofibroblasts in cholangiocarcinoma seems to be one of the profibrogenic factors underlying the dynamic stromal remodeling (158).

Ultrastructural Findings

Electron microscopy examination is rarely considered for the diagnosis of intrahepatic cholangiocarcinoma. The cancer cells form lumens consisting of apical membranes with microvilli (fig. 7-58). The nuclei are medium in size, with large or finely dispersed heterochromatin. In the cytoplasm, there are small mucin granules at the subapical area, round to oval mitochondria, and numerous rough endoplasmic reticuli. The cells are connected by tight junctions and desmosomes (fig. 7-59).

Some tumor cells in the histologically trabecular area may have abnormal canalicular lumens sealed by junctional complexes and containing a few irregular or sometimes numerous microvilli, suggesting early hepatocellular differentiation (110). Intracytoplasmic electron-dense granular bodies can also be present (94).

Cytologic Findings

Cytology samples are obtained from patients with suspected intrahepatic cholangiocarcinoma by percutaneous fine-needle aspiration, biliary brushing, and bile cytology (fig. 7-60). Percutaneous aspiration cytology has been replaced by core needle biopsies, and is less commonly used in clinical practice than before. The abundant fibrotic stroma in cholangiocarcinoma may result in hypocellular aspirates (159). For biliary brushing and bile samples, a general rule is that the further the tumor is from the site at which the specimen is taken, the less sensitive the cytologic diagnosis (159,160).

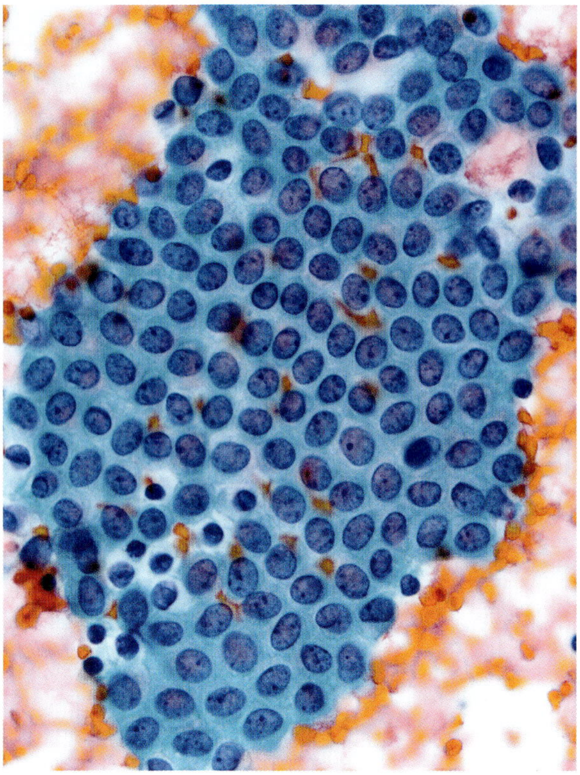

Figure 7-60

NORMAL BILIARY EPITHELIUM

Brush cytology (Papanicolaou stain).

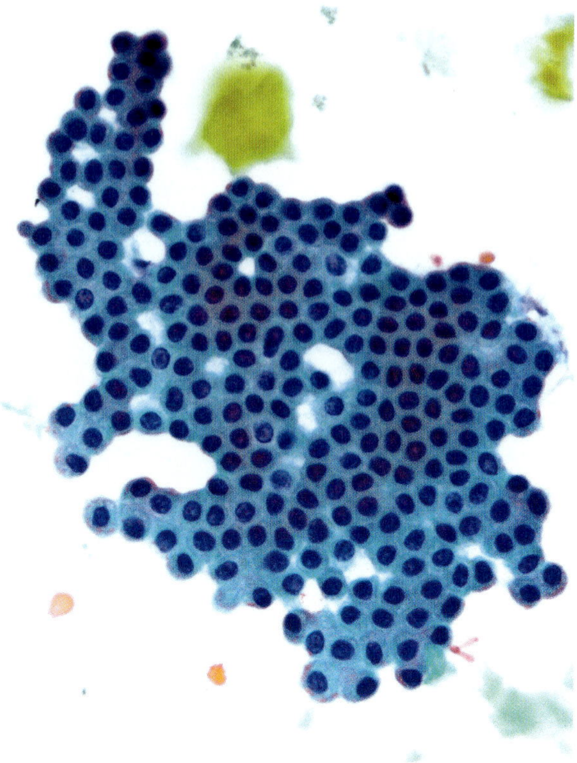

Figure 7-61

NORMAL BILIARY EPITHELIUM

Bile cytology (Papanicolaou stain).

Table 7-4

SIX KEY FEATURES FOR BILE CYTOLOGY INTERPRETATION OF CHOLANGIOCARCINOMA[a,b]

Loss of honeycomb arrangement
Enlarged nuclei
Loss of polarity
Bloody background
Flat nuclei
Cell-in-cell arrangement

[a]The presence of three or more of these findings indicates malignancy with 86% sensitivity and 77% specificity.
[b]Modified from data in reference 163.

In addition, the tumor must infiltrate into the ductal system to be diagnosed. False negative results are associated with poor sampling, concomitant cholangitis, and cellular degeneration due to bile (161,162).

It is important to recognize variations of degenerative atypia in biliary epithelial cells. As bile is toxic to the cells, bile samples usually yield considerable degenerative changes, such as nuclear pyknosis, karyorrhexis, and increased nuclear to cytoplasmic ratios (fig. 7-61). The cells are arranged in isolation, and occasionally in sheets. Cytoplasmic degeneration is also common. Intracytoplasmic vacuoles may be reminiscent of signet ring cell carcinomas. Six key features of bile cytology are summarized in Table 7-4 (163).

In moderately to poorly differentiated cholangiocarcinoma, the cellular features of malignancy are generally obvious (164). The malignant cells are poorly cohesive with scattered isolated atypical cells. The cells are generally large, with a wide size variation. The nuclei are enlarged, with increased coarse chromatin, and covered by irregular membranes (fig. 7-62) (164,165). Malignant giant cells or spindle cells may be present (fig. 7-63). Other features include cell-in-cell patterns, nuclear molding, and necrosis, either single cell or coagulation type

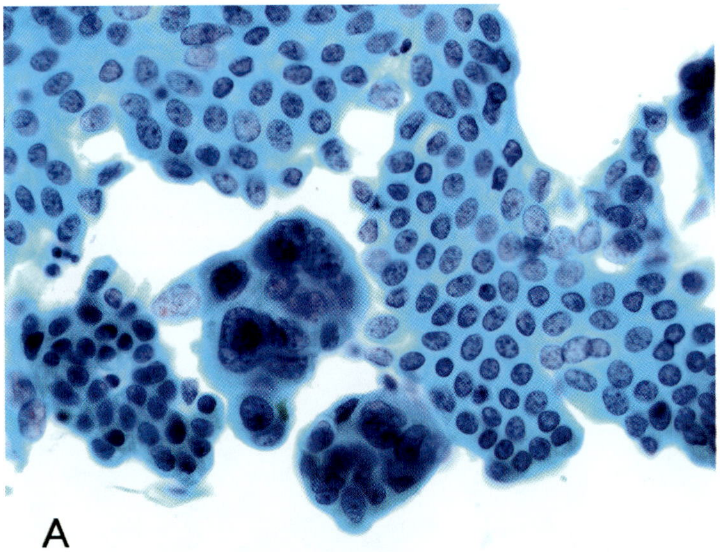

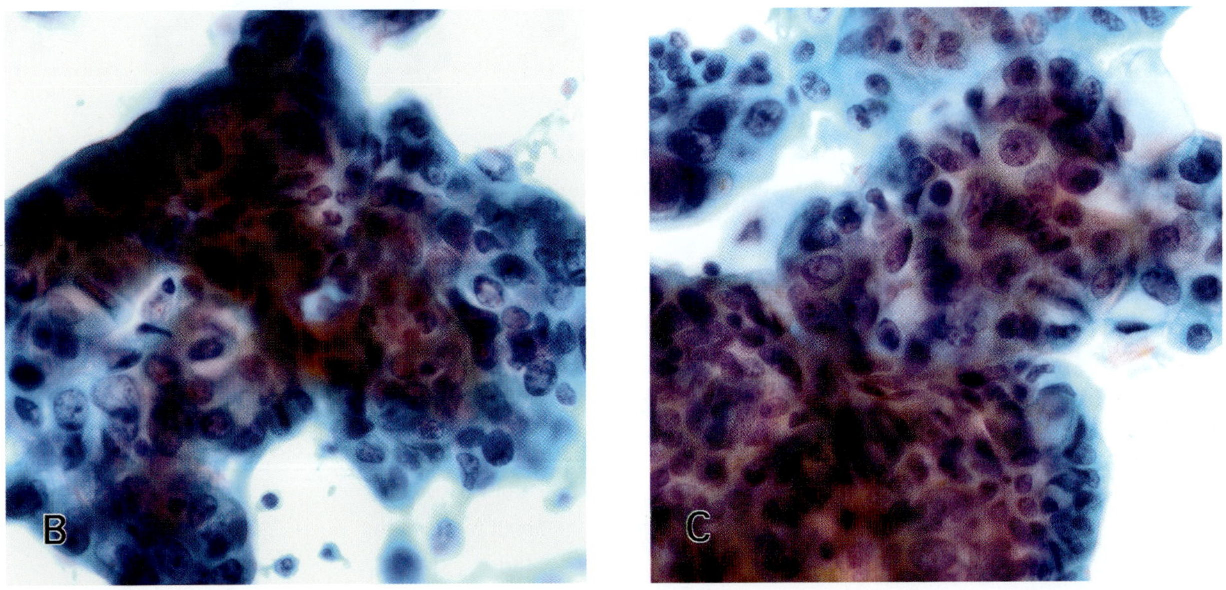

Figure 7-62

CHOLANGIOCARCINOMA CYTOLOGY

A: Poorly differentiated adenocarcinoma. B: Moderately differentiated adenocarcinoma. C: Moderately differentiated adenocarcinoma (all: Papanicolaou stain).

(163). Mitotic figures are common, and atypical mitotic figures may also be present (Table 7-5).

In well-differentiated cholangiocarcinoma, the cells have more abundant cytoplasm and are arranged in a larger sheet. The variation in cell size leads to the appearance termed "drunken honeycomb," where the cells are unevenly distributed with variable nucleus-nucleus distances (fig. 7-64A). Irregularly crowded and piled up foci may be present (fig. 7-64B–D). These features contrast well to the uniform distribution of benign cholangiocytes. For the diagnosis of well-differentiated adenocarcinoma, it helps to compare the atypical cells and clearly benign cholangiocytes present on the same slide. Both cells can have fine, evenly distributed chromatin, but the nuclei are darker in the malignant cells. An abrupt transition from the normal to atypical cells in a cluster also suggests a neoplastic nature.

In response to inflammation, stones, and biliary stents, the biliary epithelium may undergo significant reactive changes (fig. 7-65) (165,166). Benign atypical cells can show marked variation

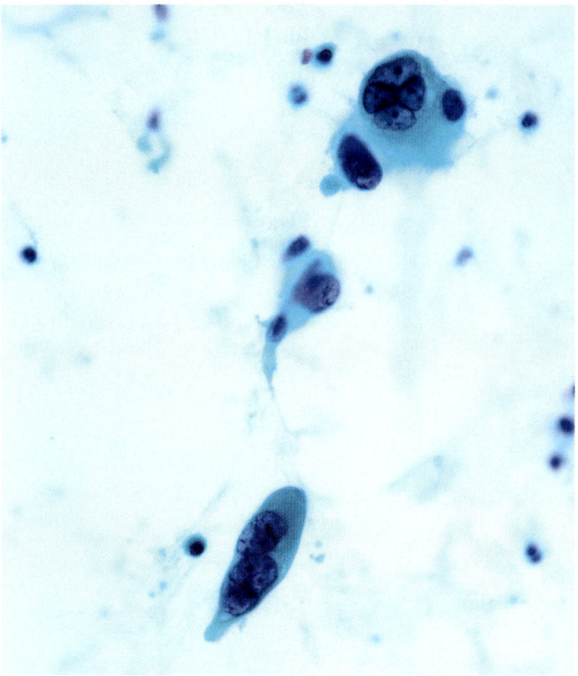

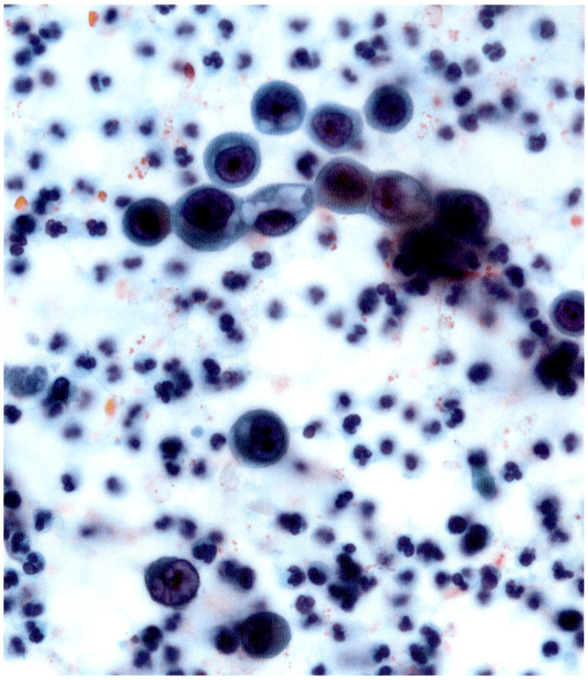

Figure 7-63

CHOLANGIOCARCINOMA CYTOLOGY

Left: Poorly differentiated adenocarcinoma.
Right: Poorly differentiated adenocarcinoma (both: Papanicolaou stain).

Table 7-5

CYTOLOGIC FEATURES OF NORMAL, REACTIVE, AND MALIGNANT BILIARY EPITHELIAL CELLS

	Normal Cholangiocytes	Reactive Changes	Well-Differentiated Adenocarcinoma	Poorly Differentiated Adenocarcinoma
Architecture	Flat sheets with honeycomb appearance	Sheets or nests slightly irregular in shape	Sheets or nests with piled up foci (drunken honeycomb)	Variably sized clusters with individual cells
Cell size	Small	Small to large	Small to medium	Small to large
Pleomorphism	None	Minimal	Mild	Extensive
Nuclear features	Round nuclei with fine, homogeneously distributed chromatin	Variably sized round nuclei with coarse, but not significantly increased chromatin	Dark nuclei with evenly distributed chromatin; partly irregular nuclear membrane; rare mitotic figures	Large, hyperchromatic nuclei with coarse chromatin and distinct nucleoli; occasional mitotic figures
Other findings	Degenerative changes are common in bile cytology	Intraepithelial neutrophils and metaplastic changes are common	Three-dimensional architecture can be present	Bizarre or spindle-shaped cells may be present; necrosis is common

in nuclear size, and enlargement of up to four times the normal size may occur (166). In contrast with carcinomas, reactive cells are arranged in well-ordered, cohesive clusters or sheets with only focal nuclear crowding or overlap (164,167). The cells have abundant clear cytoplasm, smooth nuclear membranes, and less abundant chromatin (fig. 7-66). Intraepithelial

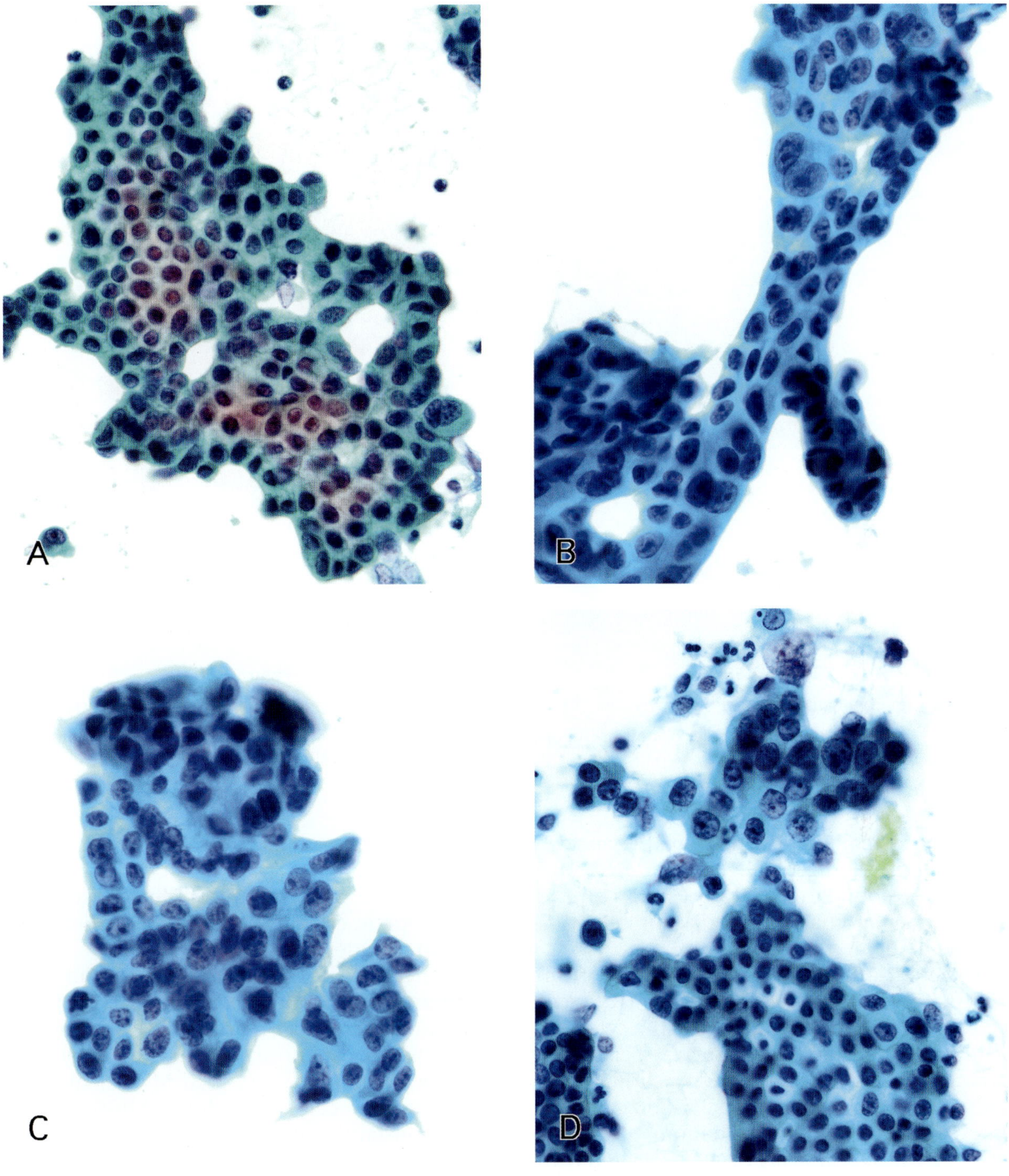

Figure 7-64

WELL-DIFFERENTIATED CHOLANGIOCARCINOMA CYTOLOGY

A: The adenocarcinoma has a "drunken honeycomb" appearance.

B: The carcinoma cells are irregular in nuclear size, and show hyperchromatic nuclei and an increased nuclear to cytoplasmic ratio.

C: The carcinoma shows coarse chromatin and distorted cellular polarity.

D: The carcinoma shows irregularity in nuclear size and distorted nuclear membranes (all: Papanicolaou stain).

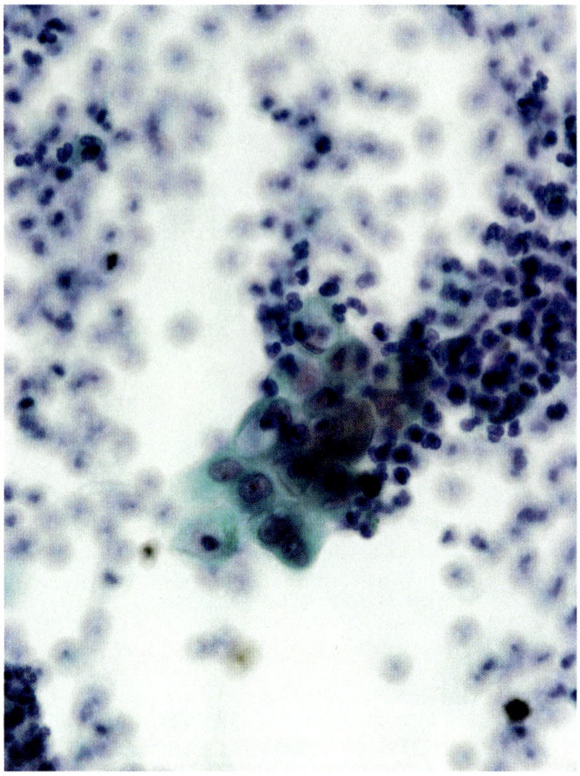

Figure 7-65

BILIARY EPITHELIUM CYTOLOGY

Reactive changes are seen in a background of inflammation (Papanicolaou stain).

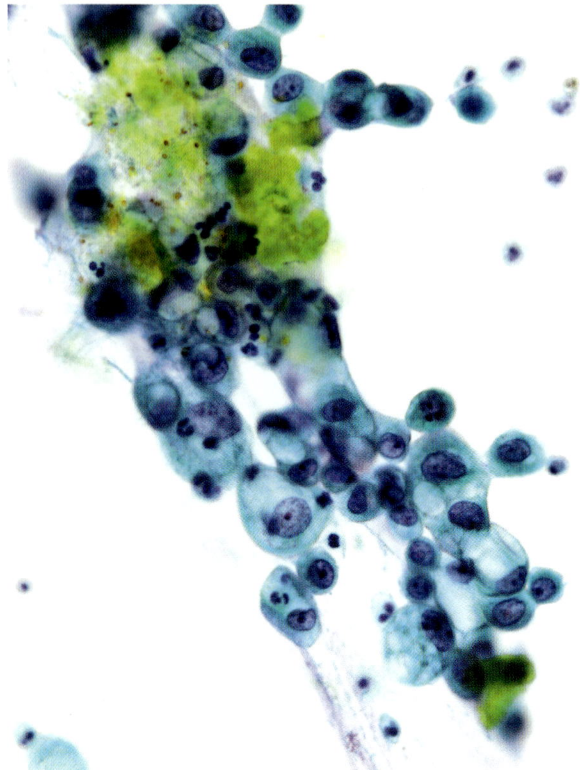

Figure 7-66

BILIARY EPITHELIUM WITH REACTIVE CHANGES

Abundant clear cytoplasm, smooth nuclear membrane, and less abundant chromatin are present. The background has mixed inflammation (Papanicolaou stain).

neutrophils may be present in malignant cell clusters, but they generally suggest a reactive process, if abundant. It always helps to find similar cellular changes in adjacent cells that are clearly benign (168).

Differentiating cholangiocarcinoma from HCC is easy in most cases. Unlike HCC, the cells in cholangiocarcinoma have the cytologic features of adenocarcinoma, such as a glandular arrangement with lumens, preserved cellular polarity with basally located nuclei, and cytoplasmic vacuoles. Cholangiocarcinoma cells lack glycogen and fat, and are never associated with bile production. It is more challenging to discriminate cholangiocarcinoma from metastatic adenocarcinomas that originate from other organs (169). It is almost impossible to differentiate from metastatic pancreatic or gallbladder cancer based on purely cytologic grounds. Intestinal features such as elongated stratified nuclei and goblet cells are more common in metastatic adenocarcinoma of gastrointestinal origin. The presence of many ductular clusters suggests intrahepatic cholangiocarcinoma rather than metastatic adenocarcinoma (170).

Cell block cytology is useful for an additional immunocytochemical examination (171). Immunohistochemical markers that are positive in cholangiocarcinoma but negative in normal biliary epithelium (i.e., p53, MUC1, maspin) work on the cell block slides. Multi-epitope immunostaining using multiple antibodies can decrease the risk of false positive results (fig. 7-67). This approach is also useful for ruling out the possibility of metastatic adenocarcinomas using site-specific markers.

Molecular Genetic Findings

Growing molecular data on intrahepatic cholangiocarcinoma have promoted understanding

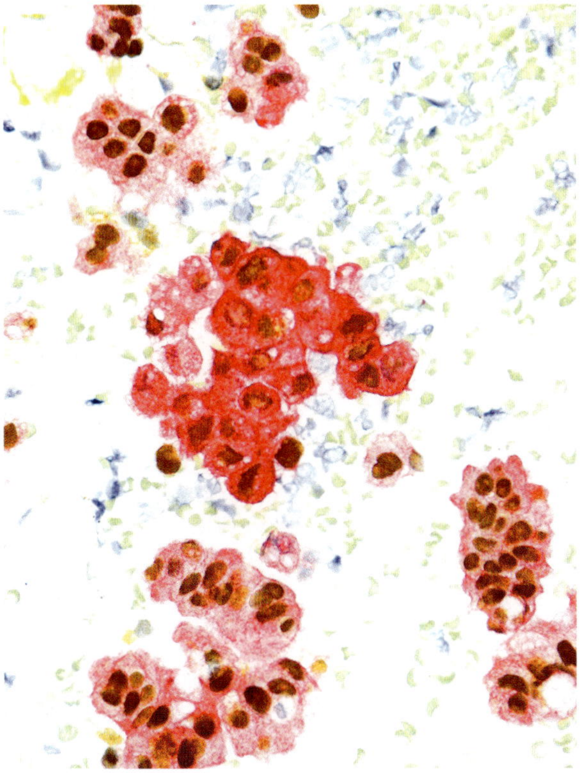

Figure 7-67

CHOLANGIOCARCINOMA CYTOLOGY

Double immunostaining for maspin (red) and p53 (brown) in cholangiocarcinoma (cell block).

of the tumorigenetic process and potential drug targets in this liver tumor. Although genetic examination is not routinely used in most institutes, the increasing knowledge of the molecular pathology will be used to develop new diagnostic tests and to select suitable chemotherapeutic drugs on a patient-by-patient basis. Some genetic alterations that differ in incidence between intrahepatic and extrahepatic cholangiocarcinoma suggest the distinct carcinogenetic process of the intrahepatic bile ducts.

Chromosomal aberrations of intrahepatic cholangiocarcinoma were examined in five studies using comparative genomic hybridization (172–176). A meta-analysis on 98 cases that were investigated in these five studies identified copy number losses at 1p, 4q, 8p, 9p, 17p, and 18q, and gains at 1q, 5p, 7p, 8q, 17q, and 20q (177). Considerable variations between Asian and European patients are postulated to be due to differences in ethnicity and etiologic background (42). The fluorescence in situ hybridization (FISH) technique helps in the detection of quantitative genetic chromosomal changes indicating aneusomy (chromosome pair imbalance) in clinical samples. The FISH method applied to biliary brushing cytology increases the diagnostic sensitivity of conventional cytology from 15 percent to 40 to 50 percent (178–181). PSC patients who are repeatedly positive for polysomy by FISH have an increased risk of developing cholangiocarcinoma (179). The FISH analysis may be positive up to 2.7 years before a tumor becomes detectable on imaging (179).

Microsatellite instability is seen in 23 percent of cases. Its frequency is considerably higher in thorotrast-induced cholangiocarcinoma (63 percent) (182). Hypermethylation of the promoter region of *MLH1* supposedly leads to this genetic trait in thorotrast-related cancers. The reported incidence of microsatellite instability in liver fluke-associated cholangiocarcinoma varies widely among studies, probably because of the different microsatellite markers used (183,184). On the basis of the largest study, where 12 highly polymorphic loci, including 5 microsatellite markers for evaluating microsatellite status with the Bethesda panel, were examined, cholangiocarcinoma associated with liver flukes seems to be a microsatellite-stable neoplasm (184).

Various oncogenes and tumor suppressor genes have been examined in intrahepatic cholangiocarcinoma, but, unfortunately, mutations in each gene are not common. *KRAS* is the oncogene most intensively analyzed. This oncogene is less commonly mutated in intrahepatic cholangiocarcinoma (15 to 25 percent) than in perihilar and distal cholangiocarcinoma (40 percent), and pancreatic ductal carcinoma (90 percent) (145,185,186). In intrahepatic cholangiocarcinoma, *KRAS* mutations are found in up to 23 percent of the tumors that supposedly have the large bile ducts as their origin, while they are less common in cancers arising from the small bile ducts or cholangiocarcinoma in chronic advanced liver disease (i.e., viral hepatitis, alcoholic liver disease; 1 to 8 percent) (145,185). One study suggested that *KRAS* mutations are an unfavorable prognostic factor for patients with intrahepatic cholangiocarcinoma, but another study failed to validate this finding (145,185).

EGFR mutations occur in up to 15 percent of cases (185,187). These genetic alterations are more common in patients who have a history of chronic nonbiliary liver disease (i.e., viral hepatitis, alcoholic liver disease), while *EGFR* is known to be the wild type in cholangiocarcinoma associated with *Opisthorchis viverrini* infection (185,188). Similar to lung cancers, the deletion of exon 19 of *EGFR* can result in an enhanced sensitivity to the effect of EGF in cholangiocarcinoma. Therefore, patients with these mutations may be good candidates for targeted therapy with EGFR inhibitors.

Somatic mutations in genes encoding isocitrate dehydrogenases (IDH) 1 and 2 have attracted attention, as these genetic events seem to be fairly specific to intrahepatic cholangiocarcinoma among various gastrointestinal and biliary malignancies (41). *IDH1* and *IDH2* mutations have been intensively investigated in gliomas, and are believed to occur only rarely in solid neoplasms. *IDH1* and *IDH2* mutations are found in 10 to 28 percent of intrahepatic cholangiocarcinomas and 0 to 7 percent of extrahepatic and gallbladder cancers (189–191). Mutated *IDH* leads to the aberrant production and accumulation of an oncometabolite, 2-hydroxyglutarate, which may play a crucial oncogenic role in cholangiocarcinoma. It is also interesting that serum concentrations of 2-hydroxyglutarate are elevated in these patients (192). This metabolite may thus serve as a diagnostic and therapeutic biomarker.

Experimental models of cholangiocarcinoma have suggested the crucial role of *p53* in the development of intrahepatic cholangiocarcinoma (193,194). The exact incidence of *p53* mutations in human intrahepatic cholangiocarcinoma remains unclear, however, and vary widely (14 percent to over 50 percent), probably representing differences in ethnicity and etiologic factors among regions (195–198). Another reason for this variation is that some of the previous studies examined both intrahepatic and extrahepatic cholangiocarcinomas in a single study group. Combining all available data, *p53* is supposedly mutated in about 20 percent of cholangiocarcinomas, including both intrahepatic and extrahepatic types (135). However, this genetic event may be much less common in the intrahepatic type, since two recent studies that examined only intrahepatic cholangiocarcinomas identified the mutation in only 1 to 2 percent of cases (185,199). Immunohistochemical expression of p53 does not necessarily indicate *p53* mutations. For example, nuclear overexpression of p53 is common in *IDH*-mutated cholangiocarcinoma, but the *p53* mutation is rare in this subtype (190).

Other mutated but less investigated genes include *BRAF, GNAS, NRAS, MCL1, CTNNB1,* and *PIK3CA*. *BRAF* is mutated in 3 to 5 percent of cases (199–201). Interestingly, this mutation is restricted to intrahepatic cholangiocarcinoma among biliary tract malignancies (200). The fact that 53 percent of bile duct adenomas have the *BRAF* mutation may suggest a possible link in tumorigenesis between bile duct adenoma and intrahepatic cholangiocarcinoma (202). Immunostaining with the BRAF V600E protein-specific antibody (clone VE1) has been proven to be a highly specific and sensitive method to identify *BRAF*-mutated cholangiocarcinoma (200). Another 5 percent of intrahepatic cholangiocarcinoma cases harbor *PIK3CA* mutations (201). Mutations in *BRAF* and *PIK3CA* are not common but may be worth investigating in clinical samples (199), as intrahepatic cholangiocarcinoma harboring these mutations is expected to respond well to specific kinase inhibitors (203).

Gene fusions are driver mutations in malignant tumors, as has been well studied in chronic myeloid leukemia (*BCR-ABL* gene) and lung adenocarcinomas (*ALK1* fusions). Recent studies identified fusions involving *FGFR2* and *ROS1* in bile duct cancers (204,205). *FGFR2* fusions can be found in 13 percent of intrahepatic cholangiocarcinomas particularly of the small duct type, but are exceptional in extrahepatic bile duct cancers (206,207,207a). Conversely, *ROS1* translocations seem to be fairly restricted to extrahepatic cholangiocarcinoma (208). Patients harboring these gene fusions may be good candidates for therapy with FGFR or ROS1 kinase inhibitors. A recent study also identified *MDM2* amplification in 12 percent of large duct intrahepatic cholangiocarcinomas but none of small duct cancers (207b).

Differential Diagnosis

HCC. Intrahepatic cholangiocarcinoma should be differentiated from HCC. Although most HCC cases develop in patients with chronic liver disease, they also occur in normal liver. Conversely, intrahepatic cholangiocarcinoma typically occurs in normal liver, but bile duct cancers in chronic liver disease are increasingly recognized (111). Therefore, the presence or absence of chronic liver disease does not differentiate these two tumors. Imaging studies are also not always conclusive, as cholangiocarcinoma that develops against a background of chronic liver disease can be a hypervascular tumor on imaging, reminiscent of HCC (58,209,210). From the pathologic point of view, mucin production and a glandular architecture support the diagnosis of intrahepatic cholangiocarcinoma, while bile production and a trabecular pattern are diagnostic of HCC. Immunohistochemistry is required for morphologically equivocal cases.

The expression of hepatocyte-specific markers such as HepPar1, glypican-3, and arginase-1 suggests HCC rather than cholangiocarcinoma (211). Scirrhous HCC is sometimes HepPar1 negative, but is usually positive for glypican-3 or arginase-1 (212). CD10 and polyclonal CEA can be positive in either neoplasm, but their expression in a canalicular pattern indicates that HCC is more likely. Diffuse expression of CK7 and CK19 supports the diagnosis of bile duct cancer, but these biliary markers are focally expressed in 10 to 20 percent of HCCs. MUC1 is known to be more specific for cholangiocarcinoma.

Intrahepatic cholangiocarcinoma sometimes has hepatoid histologic foci. To establish the diagnosis of combined hepatocellular cholangiocarcinoma, histologic evidence of both hepatocellular and biliary differentiation is required. Whether immunoreactivity to lineage-specific markers is sufficient evidence remains controversial. However, the expression of hepatocyte markers (HepPar1, glypican-3, and arginase-1) in an otherwise typical adenocarcinoma is insufficient to confirm it as an HCC component. In combined hepatocellular cholangiocarcinoma, these hepatocyte markers are usually expressed in a trabecular or solid area with no glandular differentiation.

Benign Biliary Lesions. Benign biliary lesions that mimic intrahepatic cholangiocarcinoma are bile duct adenoma (peribiliary gland hamartoma), von Meyenburg complex (bile duct hamartoma), and extensive ductular reaction. Although these lesions share some histologic findings with cholangiocarcinoma, their clinical presentation is different. The former two are small in size, and are more commonly found incidentally during surgery by surgeons or in resected specimens by pathologists. Both benign lesions can be multifocal. Extensive ductular reaction occurs following parenchymal extinction due to severe hepatitis or ischemia (fig. 7-68). The lesion zonally replaces the liver parenchyma, but the affected area becomes atrophic rather than bulging. Immunohistochemistry for p16, EZH2, and tubulin beta-3 may help: p16 expression is common in benign biliary lesions (more than 80 percent), but rare in cholangiocarcinoma (12 percent) (213). The expression of EZH2 and tubulin beta-3 suggests that cholangiocarcinoma is more likely (144,213).

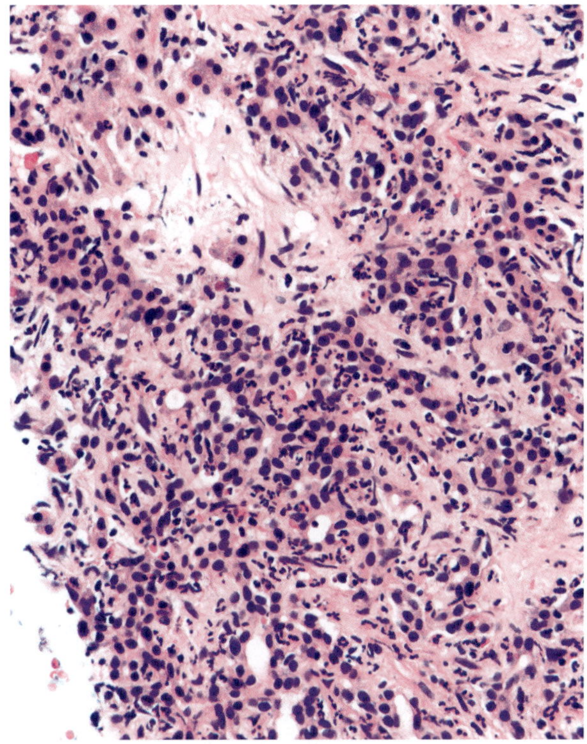

Figure 7-68

EXTENSIVE DUCTULAR REACTION

Typically associated with a neutrophilic infiltrate.

Metastatic Adenocarcinoma. Intrahepatic cholangiocarcinoma needs to be differentiated from metastatic adenocarcinomas. Metastatic cancers present typically as liver masses and rarely as intraductal tumors. Periductal-infiltrating tumors are an uncommon manifestation of metastatic liver cancers. Histologically, ductal adenocarcinomas are most frequently seen in both

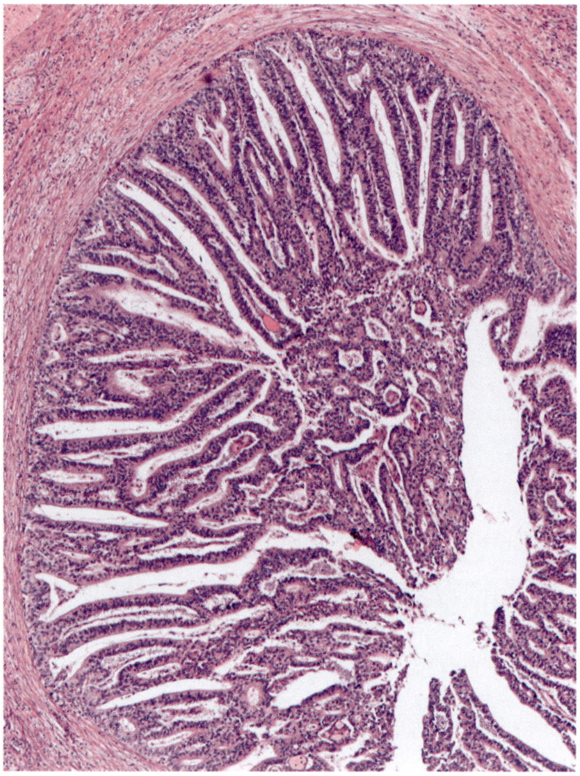

Figure 7-69

METASTATIC COLORECTAL CARCINOMA

Intrabiliary growth is seen.

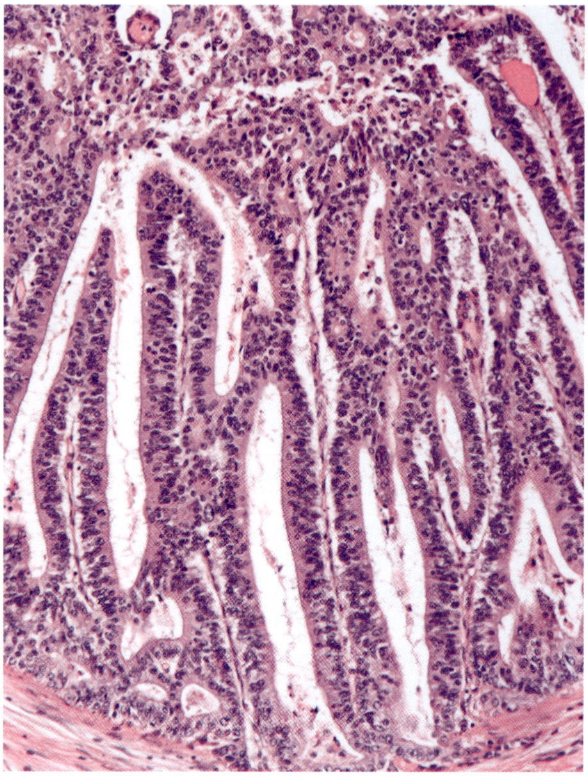

Figure 7-70

METASTATIC COLORECTAL CARCINOMA

The growth pattern is intrabiliary. Intestinal-type cancer cells are arranged in a papillotubular architecture.

primary and secondary neoplasms, while anastomosing tubular adenocarcinomas are more common in cholangiocarcinoma. If patients have a history of cancer in other organs, it always helps to compare the histologic features and immunophenotypes between the liver tumor and the extrahepatic primary carcinoma. In intrahepatic cholangiocarcinoma, the immunophenotype CK7(+)/CK20(-) is most common (70 percent), followed by CK7(+)/CK20(+) (20 to 30 percent), CK7(-)/CK20(+) (less than 5 percent), and CK7(-)/CK20(-) (less than 5 percent) (96,214,215). Immunohistochemical markers that are relatively specific to other organ systems and less likely to be positive in intrahepatic cholangiocarcinoma include ER, PR, TTF-1, and PAX8.

Metastatic colorectal cancers can show intrabiliary growth that mimics intraductal papillary cholangiocarcinoma (216). In some patients, the intrabiliary components are continuous with intraparenchymal metastatic nodules, while in other patients the tumor is entirely within the ducts (fig. 7-69) (217). Intrabiliary growth is seen in 3 to 6 percent of liver metastases with a primary colorectal site, but is extremely uncommon in liver metastases from other primary sites (less than 1 percent) (217,218). The intraductal tumor histologically consists of classic intestinal-type adenocarcinoma showing intraductal papillotubular growth (fig. 7-70). The mass is associated with intraepithelial cancer, which shows an abrupt transition from the benign biliary epithelium (218). Therefore, the presence of intraepithelial carcinoma does not necessarily indicate a primary biliary neoplasm. Intestinal morphologic features, the immunophenotype of CK7(-)/CK20(+), and a history of colorectal cancer suggest metastatic tumor rather than cholangiocarcinoma. A caveat is that papillary cholangiocarcinoma with intestinal features (i.e., goblet cells) can develop in the large bile ducts (92). CK20 and CDX2 can also be expressed

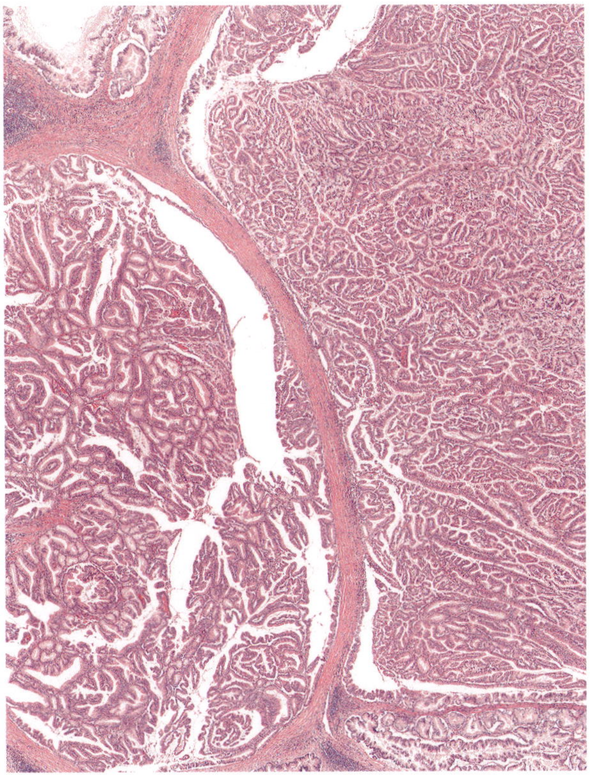

Figure 7-71

INTRADUCTAL PAPILLARY NEOPLASM OF BILE DUCT

Papillary architecture is well organized with delicate fibrovascular stalks.

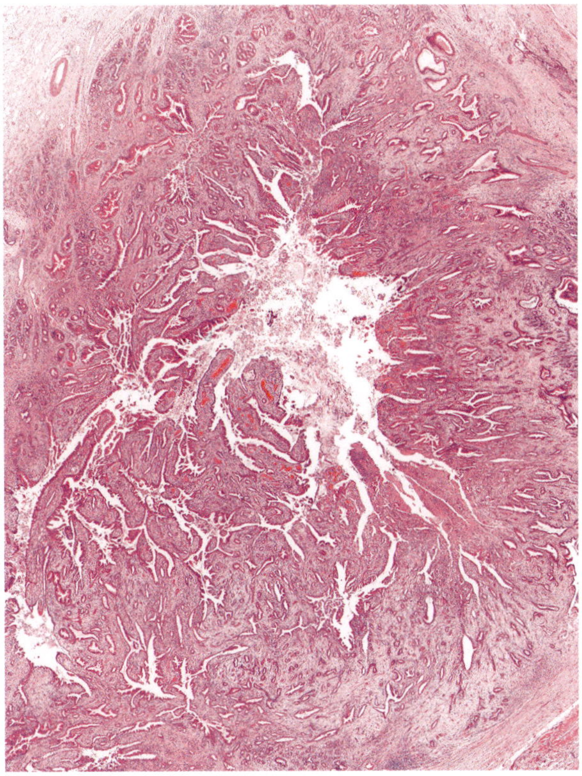

Figure 7-72

PAPILLARY CHOLANGIOCARCINOMA

The papillary architecture is more complex than that in IPNB.

in those neoplasms, but CK7 typically remains positive (92). Papillary cholangiocarcinoma is generally less dysplastic and less necrotic than intrabiliary colorectal cancer metastases.

IPNB. Another mimic of papillary cholangiocarcinoma is IPNB (109,219). IPNB is more common in the intrahepatic bile ducts, while papillary cholangiocarcinoma more frequently develops in the extrahepatic bile ducts (fig. 7-71). Mucin overproduction is less common in papillary cholangiocarcinoma than in IPNB (7 versus 72 percent). Unlike IPNB, where neoplastic cells are arranged in a delicate papillary fashion, papillary cholangiocarcinoma shows a more complex papillary or papillotubular architecture with small necrotic foci (fig. 7-72) (220). Intestinal features can be seen in either, but oncocytic- or gastric-type tumors are restricted to IPNB. The pathologic features of papillary cholangiocarcinoma, intrabiliary colorectal metastasis, and IPNB are summarized in Table 7-6.

Gallbladder Cancers Invading the Liver. These often form a nodular tumor beneath the gallbladder bed, a liver mass often reminiscent of intrahepatic cholangiocarcinoma on imaging. Even histologically, it is sometimes difficult to determine whether it is a gallbladder cancer invading the liver or intrahepatic cancer involving the gallbladder. Given that both tumors originate from the biliary epithelium, there are considerable overlapping morphologic and immunophenotypic features.

The general rule that the location of an intraepithelial cancer is the primary site cannot be applied in this context, as intrahepatic cholangiocarcinoma invading the gallbladder can replace the lining epithelium of the gallbladder mucosa, a finding called cancerization. A potential diagnostic clue is the presence or absence of non-neoplastic cholangiocytes entrapped in the intraepithelial cancer in the gallbladder (fig. 7-73). In primary gallbladder cancers, the intraepithelial

Table 7-6

CLINICOPATHOLOGIC FEATURES OF PAPILLARY CHOLANGIOCARCINOMA, INTRABILIARY METASTASIS OF COLORECTAL CANCER, AND IPNB

	Papillary Cholangiocarcinoma	Intrabiliary Colorectal Metastasis	IPNB
Medical history	None	Advanced colorectal cancer	May have intrahepatic stones
Location	More common in extrahepatic bile ducts	Intrahepatic bile ducts	More common in intrahepatic bile ducts
Gross features	Grossly localized tumor (intraepithelial lateral spread is histologically common)	Intraductal tumor with or without intraparenchymal mass	Papillary tumor in the dilated bile duct; sometimes cystic
Mucus overproduction	Rare	Sometimes	Common
Histologic features	Complex papillary or papillotubular architecture with small necrotic foci	Intestinal-type adenocarcinoma with papillotubular or cribriform architecture; necrosis is common	Delicate papillary architecture; no necrosis
Cellular types	Pancreatobiliary or intestinal	Intestinal	Pancreatobiliary, intestinal, gastric, or oncocytic

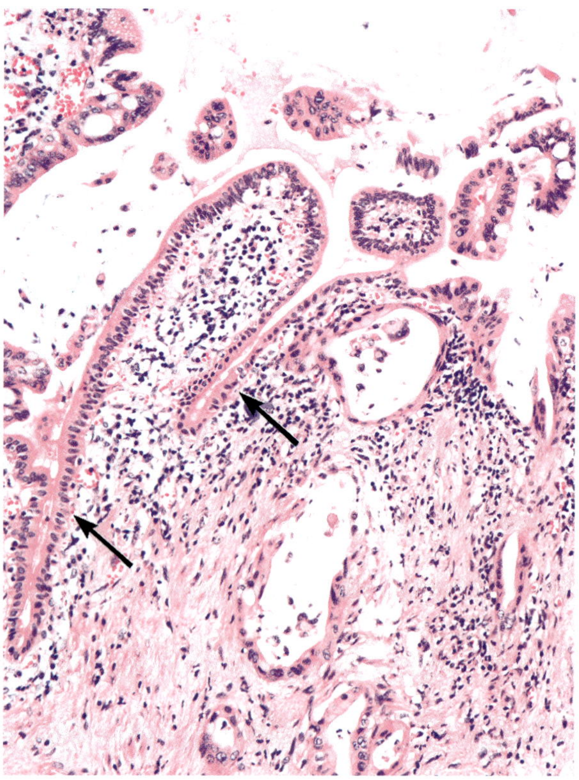

Figure 7-73

INTRAHEPATIC CHOLANGIOCARCINOMA INVADING GALLBLADDER MUCOSA

The non-neoplastic epithelium is entrapped in the intraepithelial carcinoma (arrows).

cancer cells are zonally present, with no residual benign cholangiocytes between. In contrast, the residual non-neoplastic cholangiocytes can be entrapped in epithelium secondarily infiltrated by carcinoma.

Epithelioid Hemangioendothelioma. Another primary liver tumor that histologically mimics intrahepatic cholangiocarcinoma is epithelioid hemangioendothelioma, a sometimes difficult differential diagnosis in liver biopsies. In both conditions, neoplastic cells can be arranged in single cells or clusters against the background of an abundant fibrotic stroma. CK7 and CK19 highlight entrapped biliary epithelium and reactive bile ductules scattered within the mass, which may be misinterpreted as neoplastic cells. Compared with intrahepatic cholangiocarcinoma, the tumor stroma is more myxoid in this vascular neoplasm, and the intravascular architecture is polypoid. Immunostaining for endothelial markers helps in differentiation. Epithelioid hemangioendothelioma needs to be ruled out when intrahepatic cholangiocarcinoma is suspected in young patients.

Chronic Cholangiopathies. Hepatolithiasis and PSC can have peribiliary gland hyperplasia (221,222). Peribiliary glands that are increased in size and number should be differentiated from cholangiocarcinoma, particularly if they are associated with dysplastic features. It is important to recognize the overall lobular architecture in keeping with the benign process. IgG4-related sclerosing cholangitis, follicular cholangitis, and pseudolymphoma often mimic intrahepatic cholangiocarcinoma on imaging, but their discrimination is not difficult histologically (223–225).

Spread and Metastases

Intrahepatic cholangiocarcinoma progresses by local invasion, lymph node involvement, and remote metastasis including peritoneal dissemination. At initial presentation, primary intrahepatic cholangiocarcinoma forms a solitary mass (37 percent), a dominant mass with satellite lesions in the same affected segments (21 percent), or multiple liver lesions beyond the segment of the primary mass (42 percent) (45). The last group has a higher risk of distant metastasis. As described above, the primary tumors sometimes invade adjacent organs such as stomach and transverse colon. The tumors involve the liver hilum, including the portal vein, hepatic artery, and biliary confluence, in 26 percent of cases (226).

Lymph node metastases are seen in 30 to 35 percent of patients on imaging (46,227); half of them have three or more positive nodes (228). The most commonly affected lymph nodes are in the hepatoduodenal ligament or along the common hepatic artery (over 90 percent), followed by retroperitoneal nodes (50 percent), epiphrenic nodes (18 percent), mediastinal nodes (16 percent), and supraclavicular nodes (13 percent) (45). In left lobe cholangiocarcinoma, the tumor sometimes spreads to the lymph nodes around the cardia, along the lesser curvature of the stomach, or along the left gastric artery. The size of the primary tumor does not correlate with the presence or absence of nodal involvement (228).

Up to 40 percent of patients have distant metastases at initial presentation. An additional 20 percent subsequently develop metastatic disease within the first 2 years. The common sites of distant metastases are the lungs (45 percent), peritoneum (35 percent), and bones (27 percent) (45). Metastatic cancer has been reported in almost every organ and tissue, including the adrenal gland, brain, dura mater, heart, intestines, soft tissue, oral mucosa, and testis (229,230).

Table 7-7

AMERICAN JOINT COMMITTEE ON CANCER (AJCC) STAGING OF INTRAHEPATIC CHOLANGIOCARCINIOMA[a]

T Category	T Criteria
TX	Primary tumor cannot be assessed
T0	No evidence of primary tumor
Tis	Carcinoma in situ (intraductal tumor)
T1	Solitary tumor without vascular invasion, ≤5 cm or >5 cm
T1a	Solitary tumor ≤5 cm without vascular invasion
T1b	Solitary tumor >5 cm without vascular invasion
T2	Solitary tumor with intrahepatic vascular invasion, or multiple tumors with or without vascular invasion
T3	Tumor perforating the visceral peritoneum
T4	Tumor involving local extrahepatic structures by direct invasion
N Category	**N Criteria**
NX	Regional lymph nodes cannot be assessed
N0	No regional lymph node metastasis
N1	Regional lymph node metastasis present
M Category	**M Criteria**
M0	No distant metastasis
M1	Distant metastasis present

[a]AJCC 8th edition, 2017.

Staging

The same TNM staging system is endorsed by the American Joint Committee on Cancer (AJCC) and Union International Contra Cancer (UICC) (Tables 7-7, 7-8) (1,2). In the most current (8th) AJCC edition, intrahepatic cholangiocarcinoma continues to be categorized separately from extrahepatic cholangiocarcinoma. This system also includes combined hepatocellular cholangiocarcinoma.

The T classification is based on the number of tumors (solitary or multiple), the presence of vascular invasion, the presence of visceral peritoneal perforation, and direct invasion into local extrahepatic tissue. The definition of the term "multiple tumors" described in T2 includes satellitosis, intrahepatic metastasis, and multifocal tumors (231). Both macroscopic and microscopic vascular infiltration is qualified as "vascular invasion" for T2. Tumor size was previously not considered for the T classification (232), but is now accounted for by using 5 cm as the cutoff to subdivide T1 into T1a and T1b (1). This is one of the most significant revisions

Table 7-8

STAGE GROUPING FOR INTRAHEPATIC CHOLANGIOCARCINOMA[a]

Stage 0	Tis	N0	M0
Stage IA	T1a	N0	M0
Stage IB	T1b	N0	M0
Stage II	T2	N0	M0
Stage IIIA	T3	N0	M0
Stage IIIB	T4	N0	M0
Stage IIIB	Any T	N1	M0
Stage IV	Any T	Any N	M1

[a]AJCC 8th edition, 2017.

from the previous edition. Interestingly, a study using the Surveillance, Epidemiology and End Results (SEER) database found that tumor size is not associated with survival when taking into account the tumor number and the presence of vascular invasion (231). The most current T2 category combines solitary tumors with intrahepatic vascular invasion and multiple tumors with or without vascular invasion since vascular invasion and multifocality of tumors share equivalent prognostic parameters (1).

T4 disease is currently defined as tumor involving local extrahepatic structures by direct invasion (1). The 8th edition eliminates the periductal tumor growth pattern as a criterion for T4 staging, as data have shown there is no prognostic difference between cholangiocarcinoma with and without periductal infiltration (233).

The current N category (8th edition) is classified into positive (N1) and negative (N0) regional nodal involvement. Although multiple positive nodes (three or more) indicate a worse prognosis, this is not considered for the current classification (228). One limitation is that lymph nodes have not been well examined in patients with intrahepatic cholangiocarcinoma. Lymphadenectomy is performed in 67 percent of the patients, with three or fewer lymph nodes histologically examined (38,234). Extraregional nodal involvement and other distant metastatic sites are classified as M1 disease.

Treatment

Surgical resection is the single, potentially curable treatment for intrahepatic cholangiocarcinoma. Surgery should be considered if the patient has a potentially resectable tumor and is an appropriate surgical candidate (8). Unfortunately, 54 percent of patients with intrahepatic cholangiocarcinoma are not candidates for resection at initial presentation. After surgical exploration, an additional 14 percent of patients are found to have unresectable disease. The extent of the intrahepatic tumors (i.e., locally advanced or multiple nodules) is the most common reason for irresectability, followed by metastatic diseases (226). Only 32 percent of patients can undergo surgical resection (226,235). Three-quarters of them require a major liver resection, and negative surgical margins can be achieved in 81 percent (234). Additional extrahepatic bile duct resection is required in up to one quarter (38).

Most patients with intrahepatic cholangiocarcinoma present with or eventually develop advanced disease and need systemic therapy. Chemotherapy with a gemcitabine and cisplatin combination is currently the first-line treatment for advanced disease (236). There is no consensus in terms of effective regimens for patients who have failed first-line chemotherapy (46).

As intrahepatic cholangiocarcinoma is typically confined to the liver and systemic chemotherapy has limited efficacy, there has been increasing interest in locoregional therapy. Potential approaches include transarterial chemoembolization, radiofrequency ablation, and hepatic artery infusion therapy, but none of these has yet been accepted as a standard treatment for locally advanced cholangiocarcinoma (237).

Prognosis

The resectability of tumors significantly affects patient prognosis. Survival rates for patients who undergo surgery and those who have unresectable disease are summarized in Table 7-9. The median disease-specific survival period for the entire cohort is around 19 months: 30 to 36 months for patients who undergo surgery, and 9 to 11 months for those with unresectable disease (46,226,235).

The pT classification is also linked to survival. Many patients with cholangiocarcinoma who have surgical resection have disease recurrence in the first 5 years, and the majority of these occur within the liver, either alone or in combination with one or more extrahepatic sites. Only 20 to

Table 7-9

OVERALL AND DISEASE-FREE SURVIVAL OF PATIENTS WHO UNDERGO SURGERY AND PATIENTS WITH UNRESECTABLE DISEASE

	Overall Survival		Disease-Free Survival	
	3 years	5 years	3 years	5 years
Patients with surgical resection	45-50%	25-30%	22%	15%
Patients with unresectable disease	20%	<5%	0%	0%

Table 7-10

POOR PROGNOSTIC FACTORS FOR INTRAHEPATIC CHOLANGIOCARCINOMA

Large tumor size
Presence of multiple tumors
Satellite nodules
Major vascular invasion
Microvascular invasion
Perineural invasion
Lymph node metastases
Poor tumor differentiation
Positive surgical margin
Older age
No postoperative adjuvant therapy given

30 percent of patients develop recurrences solely outside the liver (226).

In patients who have surgical resection, several potential prognostic factors have been determined by univariate analysis (Table 7-10) (38). Gender and a history of viral hepatitis are not associated with prognosis. On multivariate analysis, independent prognostic factors include the presence of multiple tumors and lymph node metastases (238–242). Of the patients with solitary primary tumor and no lymph node metastases, the recurrence rate is 47 percent compared with 93 percent in those with multiple tumors or nodal metastases (226). A surgical margin positive for cancer (R1 resection) is an independent poor prognostic factor for patients with no lymph node metastases, but does not significantly affect prognosis in those with N1 disease (239).

In patients with unresectable disease, the outcome is largely dictated by the tumor extent at presentation. Patients with disease confined to the liver have an overall better outcome than those with extrahepatic metastases.

Among three gross types of intrahepatic cholangiocarcinoma, patients with intraductal tumors have the best prognosis (69). The second most favorable prognosis is expected in mass-forming cholangiocarcinomas. S-100 protein P, expressed in up to 15 percent of mass-forming intrahepatic cholangiocarcinomas indicates poorer survival in this group (141). In PSC patients, intrahepatic cholangiocarcinoma with intestinal features shows longer recurrence-free survival than classic cholangiocarcinoma (92). This is at least partly because intestinal-type cholangiocarcinoma often has intraductal growth, leading to early detection.

PRECURSOR LESIONS

Biliary Intraepithelial Neoplasia

Definition. *Biliary intraepithelial neoplasia* (BilIN) is defined as noninvasive dysplastic epithelium lining the bile ducts and peribiliary glands. This is generally a microscopic lesion showing flat or micropapillary architecture. Noninvasive high-papillary neoplasms such as IPNB and cystic tumors such as MCN are outside this category. BilIN includes the previous diagnostic terms of *biliary dysplasia* and *carcinoma in situ*. The same classification scheme is used for the extrahepatic bile duct.

Clinical Features. BilIN usually develops in the large bile ducts. As the microscopic precursor lesions cannot be identified by current imaging modalities, it is most often incidentally found in surgically resected or explanted livers. On the basis of data from an autopsy series (243), dysplastic changes are supposedly present in less than 1 percent of the general population. This incidence increases up to 2 percent in patients with non-biliary-type liver

Table 7-11

HISTOLOGIC FEATURES OF REACTIVE BILIARY EPITHELIUM AND BilIN[a]

Hyperplasia or regenerative change:
These lesions are most commonly flat. Low-papillary or micropapillary architecture, when observed, is often associated with hepatolithiasis or choledochal cyst, but tall papillary structures are rare. Cellularity is only slightly increased compared to normal biliary epithelium. Nuclei are round or oval, and slightly enlarged with smooth nuclear membranes. Chromatin is fine and homogeneously distributed. Intraepithelial neutrophil infiltration can be seen. Mitoses can be observed in some lesions.

BilIN-1 (biliary intraepithelial neoplasia-1):
These lesions show flat or micropapillary architecture. Nuclei are basally located. Some lesions show focal nuclear pseudostratification; however, the nuclei remain within the lower two thirds of the epithelium. Cytologically, mild nuclear abnormalities, such as subtle irregularities of nuclear membrane, high nuclear/cytoplasmic ratios, and nuclear elongation are seen. Nuclear size and shape are relatively uniform, and the presence of large nuclei suggest a diagnosis of BilIN-2 or BilIN-3.

BilIN-2 (biliary intraepithelial neoplasia-2):
These lesions show flat, pseudopapillary or micropapillary architecture. Loss of cellular polarity is easily found, but it is not a diffuse feature. Nuclear pseudostratification reaching the luminal surface is common. Cytologically, dysplastic nuclear changes, which include enlargement, hyperchromasia and irregular nuclear membranes, are evident. Some variations in nuclear size and shape are seen. Peribiliary glands are sometimes involved (glandular involvement). Mitoses are rare.

BilIN-3 (biliary intraepithelial neoplasia-3):
These lesions usually show pseudopapillary or micropapillary architecture, and are only rarely flat. They cytologically resemble carcinoma, but invasion through the basement membrane is absent. Cellular polarity is diffusely and severely distorted with nuclei reaching and piling up on the luminal surface. "Budding off" of small clusters of epithelial cells into the lumen and cribriforming can be seen. Cytologically malignant features with severe nuclear membrane irregularities, hyperchromasia, or abnormally large nuclei are typically noted. Mitoses can be observed. Peribiliary gland involvement is sometimes found.

[a]Table/data from Zen Y, Adsay NV, Bardadin K, et al. Biliary intraepithelial neoplasia: an international interobserver agreement study and proposal for diagnostic criteria. Mod Pathol 2007;20:701-9.

cirrhosis, particularly hepatitis C (HCV)-related or alcoholic cirrhosis (244). BilIN is considerably more common in patients with biliary diseases (i.e., PSC, hepatolithiasis), which also increase the risk of cholangiocarcinoma. It is incidentally found in up to 15 percent of patients who have surgical resection for intrahepatic stones or liver transplantation for end-stage PSC (97,245).

Microscopic Findings. BilIN shows variable cytologic and architectural changes (246). Based on the degree of dysplasia, BilIN is classified into three grades (Table 7-11) (247). BilIN-1 is the lowest grade, characterized by increased cellularity and irregularity of the nuclear membrane, but preserved cellular polarity (fig. 7-74). BilIN-2 has more obvious dysplastic changes, such as focally piled-up nuclei and more variations in nuclear size and shape. Intermediate-grade lesions sometimes replace the lining epithelium of peribiliary glands, which should not be interpreted as an associated invasive malignancy (fig. 7-75). BilIN-3 has overt dysplastic features, including enlarged nuclei, nuclear pleomorphism, and extensive loss of cellular polarity. Mitosis is frequently seen in BilIN-3 (fig. 7-76).

The abrupt transition from nondysplastic epithelium, which is commonly seen in BilIN-2 to BilIN-3 helps to determine the neoplastic nature. It is also common that variable grades are intermixed in a single lesion, for which the highest grade should be reported. Although BilIN is typically a focal lesion, widespread BilIN has been described (248,249). In such cases, extensive sampling is required to exclude an associated invasive malignancy. Multiple BilIN lesions also occur, particularly in patients with an underlying risk condition. BilIN most commonly develops on the surface lining epithelium, but similar changes occur in the peribiliary glands (fig. 7-77) (243).

BilIN most commonly has the pancreatobiliary-type morphology, but also shows rare intestinal differentiation, such as stratified nuclei, brush borders, and occasional goblet cells, an appearance mimicking intestinal dysplasia in inflammatory bowel disease (fig. 7-78, left) (92). At least one of the three intestinal markers (CK20, MUC2, and CDX2) is positive on immunostaining (fig. 7-78, right). The intestinal variant is more common in patients with biliary

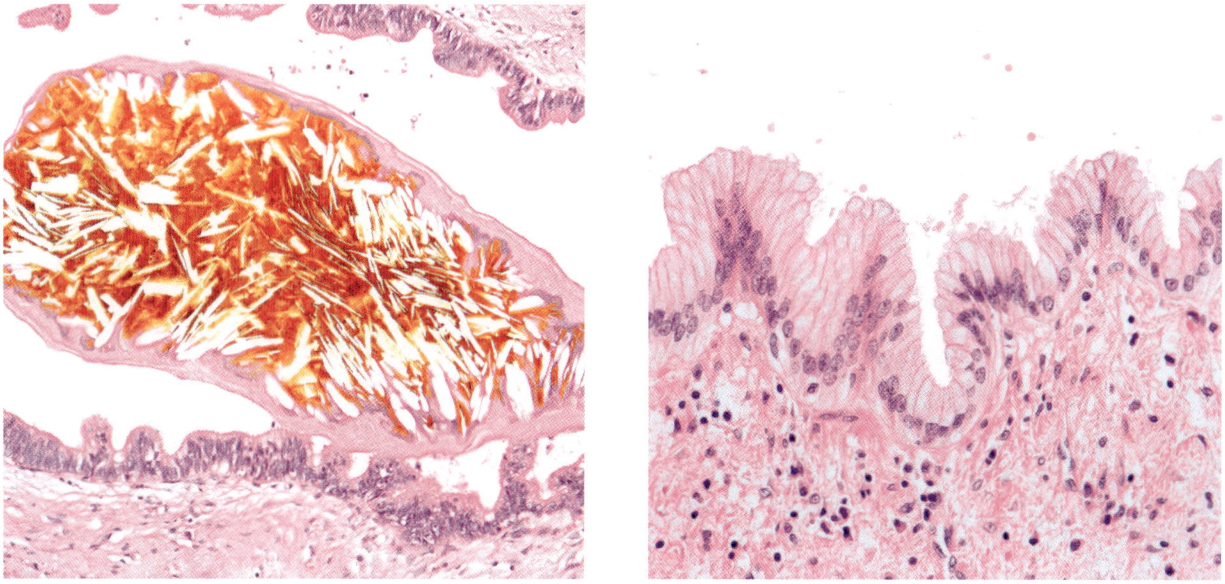

Figure 7-74

BILIARY INTRAEPITHELIAL NEOPLASIA (BilIN)-1

Left: This BilIN-1 lesion shows a micropapillary architecture. The nuclei are basally located, remaining within the lower two thirds of the epithelium, with preserved polarity. There is focal nuclear pseudostratification. Mild irregularities in the nuclear membrane, high nuclear to cytoplasmic ratios, and nuclear elongation are seen.

Right: The nuclear size and shape in the lesion are fairly uniform. The nuclear polarity is preserved.

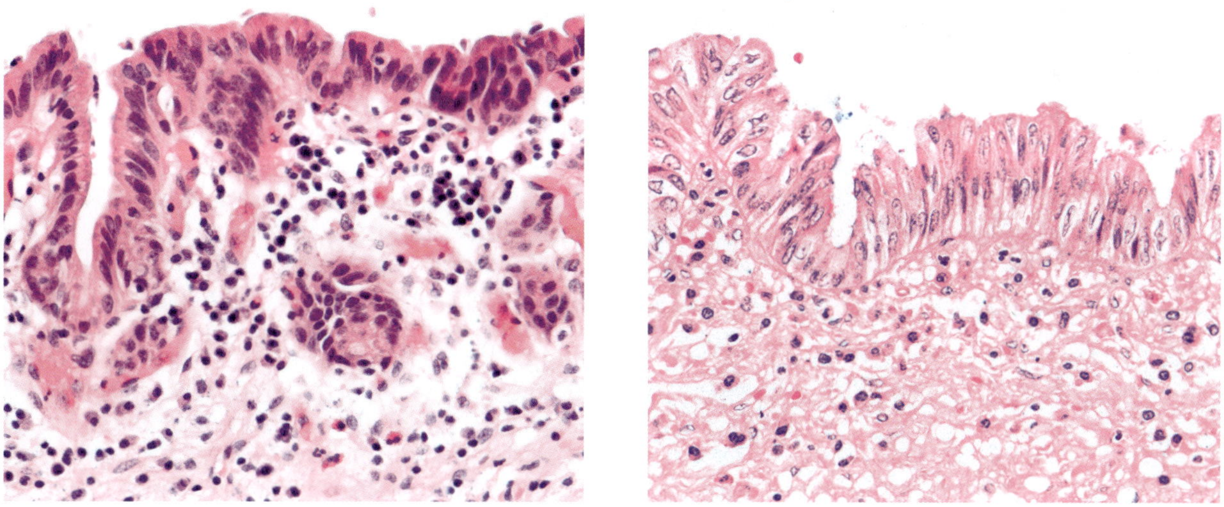

Figure 7-75

BILIARY INTRAEPITHELIAL NEOPLASIA (BilIN)-2

Left: There is focal loss of cellular polarity, but it is not diffuse. Nuclear pseudostratification reaches the luminal surface. The nuclei show pronounced enlargement, hyperchromasia, and an irregular nuclear membrane. Some variations in nuclear size and shape are seen.

Right: The nuclear pseudostratification reaches the luminal surface. Irregular size and shape of the nuclear membrane are present.

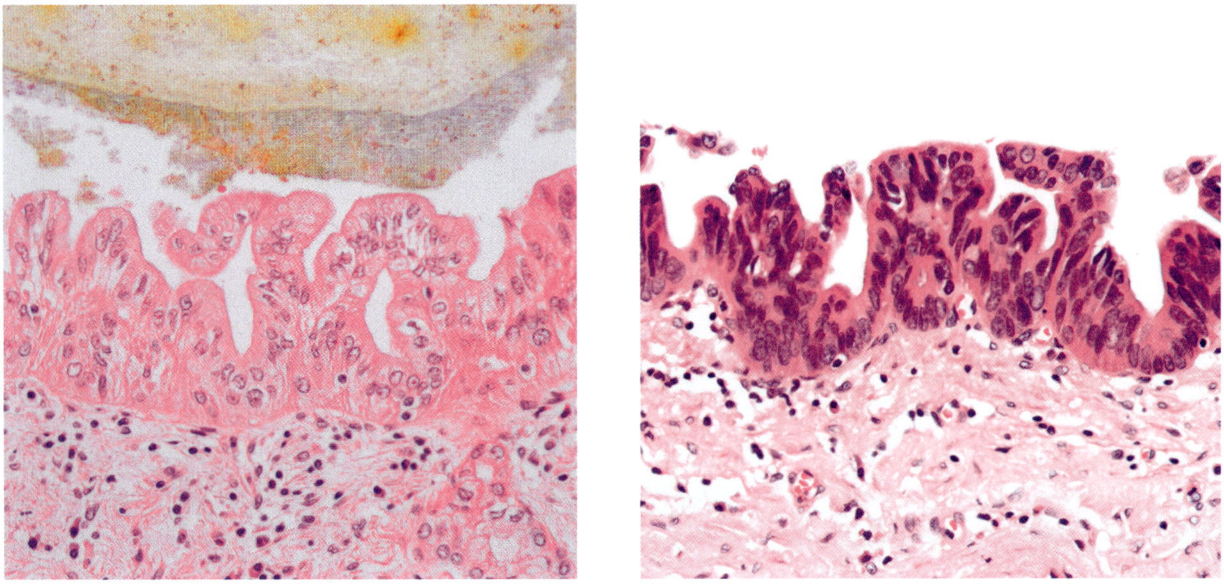

Figure 7-76

BILIARY INTRAEPITHELIAL NEOPLASIA (BilIN)-3

Left: The lesion has a micropapillary architecture. The cellular polarity is diffusely and severely distorted, with nuclei reaching and piling up on the luminal surface. There is cribriforming.

Right: Another lesion cytologically resembles carcinoma, but invasion through the basement membrane is absent. The cellular polarity is diffusely and severely lost. "Budding off" of small clusters of epithelial cells into the lumen is seen. The nuclei show hyperchromasia and enlargement. Mitoses are present.

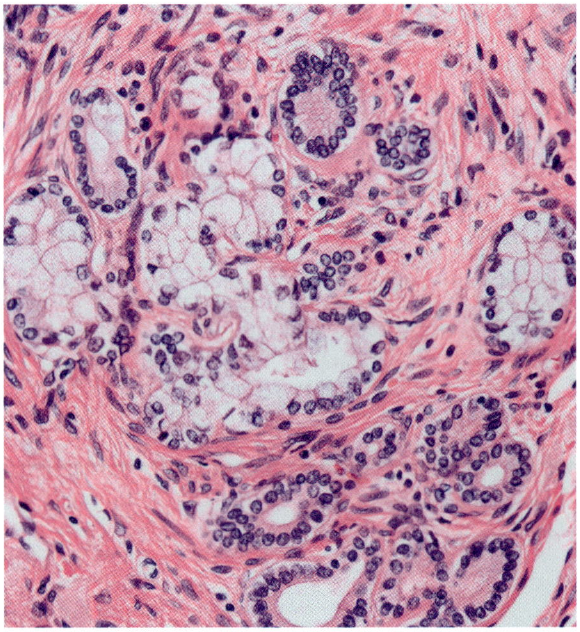

Figure 7-77

BILIARY INTRAEPITHELIAL NEOPLASIA (BilIN) IN PERIBILIARY GLANDS

Atypical large cells with clear cytoplasm are present.

disease, accounting for 10 percent of BilINs in hepatolithiasis and 50 to 60 percent in PSC (92,219). This variant is frequently associated with intestinal metaplasia nearby or elsewhere in the bile ducts, suggesting the metaplasia-dysplasia sequence. This less common variant of BilIN has been determined to be a precursor of papillary cholangiocarcinoma, with or without mucinous carcinoma components (92).

Not surprisingly, most of the immunohistochemical markers for intrahepatic cholangiocarcinoma are also positive in BilIN at lower frequencies and intensities. Markers related to the cell cycle (i.e., p16, p21, and DPC4) are stepwisely upregulated or downregulated in the three-tiered grading scheme (136). Although immunohistochemistry is not required for the diagnosis of BilIN, potentially useful markers are S-100 protein P and maspin, which are generally negative in nondysplastic epithelium and often positive in BilIN (141). p53 is less useful since its expression is rare even in BilIN-3.

Cytologic Findings. BilIN-1 is extremely difficult to diagnose by cytology samples, as

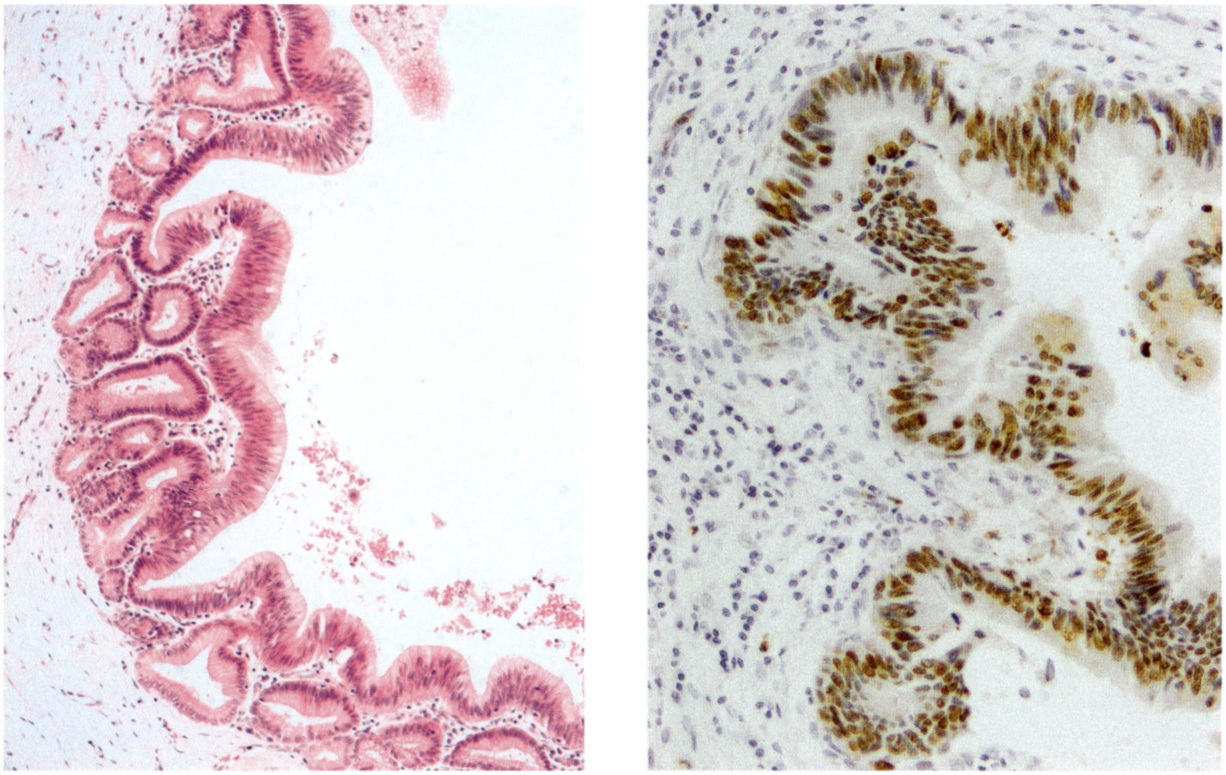

Figure 7-78

INTESTINAL-TYPE BILIARY INTRAEPITHELIAL NEOPLASIA (BilIN)-1

Left: The histologic appearance resembles intestinal dysplasia in inflammatory bowel disease. Right: CDX2 expression (immunohistochemical stain).

there is considerable overlap in cytologic features between BilIN-1 and regenerative atypia of the biliary epithelium. Because of the focal nature of BilIN-1, it is also unlikely to yield sufficient numbers of dysplastic cells in cytology specimens. BilIN-2 is still challenging to diagnose based on purely cytologic grounds, but occasional dysplastic cells with enlarged hyperchromatic nuclei may be present. BilIN-3 can show cytologic features that are diagnostic of adenocarcinoma, particularly if it is widespread on the biliary epithelium (fig. 7-79).

The cytologic features of BilIN are basically similar to those of invasive cholangiocarcinoma, but the changes are less conspicuous and necrosis is uncommon. As significant regenerative changes are seen in the biliary epithelium in patients with PSC and hepatolithiasis, attention should be paid if no tumor mass is detected on imaging. Repeat cytologic examinations may be in order for those cases.

Molecular Genetic Findings. Around 40 percent of BilIN cases associated with PSC harbor polysomy and 10 to 20 percent display homozygous 9p21 loss (250). Patients with prior or current cholangiocarcinoma are more likely to display polysomy in dysplasia. Similar chromosomal abnormalities are detectable in cholangiocarcinoma in PSC patients, suggesting a dysplasia-carcinoma sequence (250).

Genetic alterations are supposedly accumulated during the carcinogenetic process from BilIN to cholangiocarcinoma. Some genes are involved in the early events, while others play important roles at the late phases. Around 30 percent of BilIN cases harbor *KRAS* mutations (251). Given that the incidence is similar to that in intrahepatic large duct cholangiocarcinoma, *KRAS* mutation seems to be an early molecular event in the process of biliary carcinogenesis. Although *p53* mutations have not been well examined in BilIN, molecular alterations of

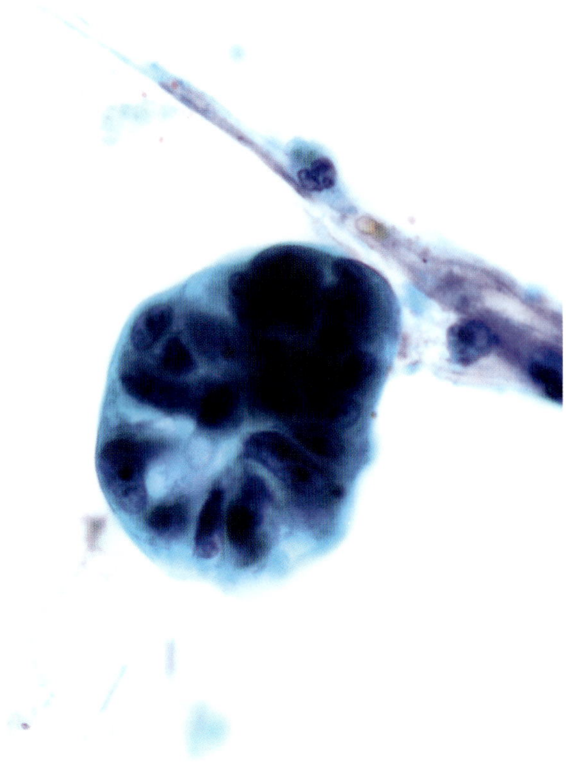

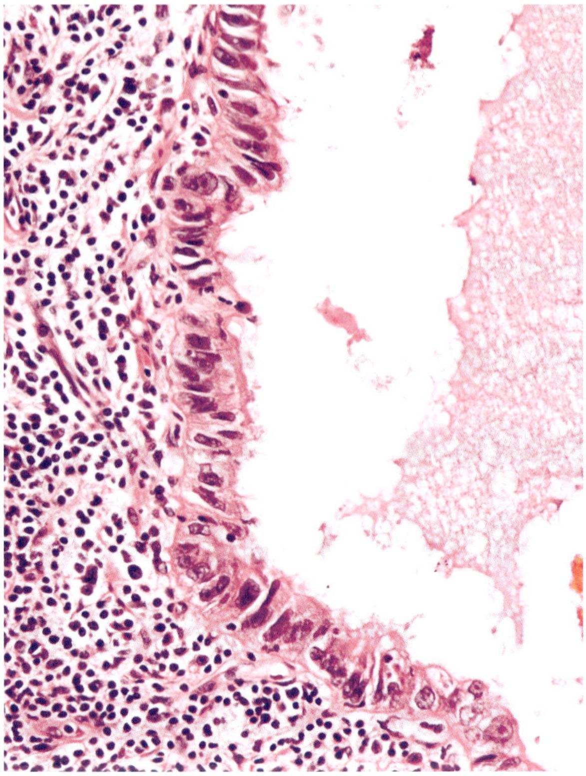

Figure 7-79

BILIARY INTRAEPITHELIAL NEOPLASIA (BilIN)-3 IN PATIENT WITH HEPATOLITHIASIS

Left: Nuclear changes in the cytology sample are consistent with carcinoma.
Right: The resected specimen confirmed the diagnosis of BilIN-3 with no invasive cancer.

this tumor suppressor gene seem to occur at the late phase (136,251). Little is known about molecular alterations of other genes in BilIN.

Differential Diagnosis. *Reactive Changes.* As described above, the biliary epithelium often displays considerable reactive changes, particularly in patients with PSC or hepatolithiasis, and this needs to be differentiated from BilIN (figs. 7-80, 7-81). Zonal distribution of dysplastic cells with abrupt transition from the benign epithelium supports a neoplastic nature. The presence of mitotic figures does not indicate a diagnosis of BilIN; mitotic figures are seen in reactive epithelium. Similarly, MIB-1 indices can be significantly elevated in the regenerative epithelium. The lining biliary epithelium often shows metaplastic changes, such as foveolar, pseudopyloric, and intestinal metaplasia, which should be discriminated from BilIN based on the lack of nuclear atypia. Squamous metaplasia also rarely occurs in the bile duct (fig. 7-82).

IPNB. BilIN is distinguished from IPNB on the basis of the tumor size and histologic features (109,219). BilIN is a microscopic lesion, while IPNB forms a macroscopically visible tumor. Unlike IPNB, high-papillary architecture with delicate fibrovascular stalks is not a feature in BilIN. A caveat is that IPNB may have flat or micropapillary dysplastic epithelium at the laterally spreading area. Mucin overproduction is unusual in BilIN.

Treatment and Prognosis. There is no consensus in terms of suitable treatment of BilIN, but in general, surgical resection is considered for high-grade lesions such as BilIN-3 based on the risk of malignant transformation. How long it takes for BilIN-3 to become an invasive malignancy is another controversial issue. Some investigators have looked into how rapidly residual BilIN-3 progresses to an invasive cancer in patients with cholangiocarcinoma, for whom surgical resection was performed but BilIN-3

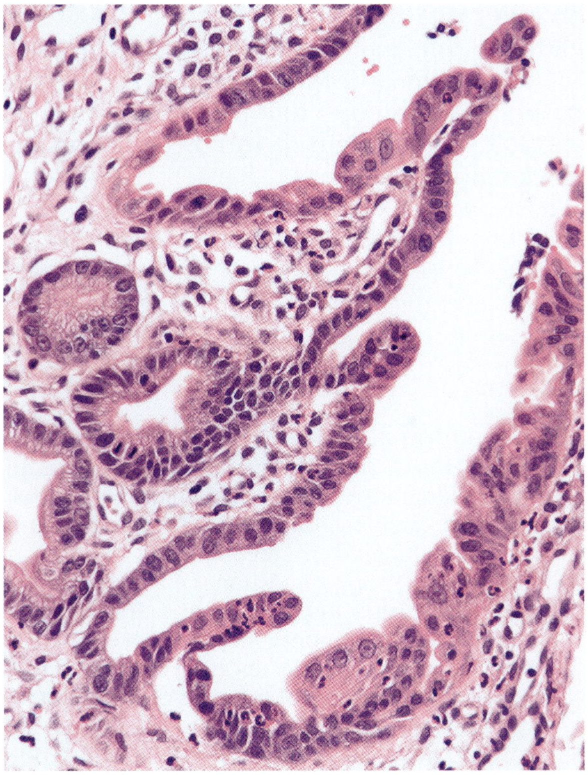

Figure 7-80

REACTIVE CHANGES OF BILIARY EPITHELIUM

The cells show nuclear enlargement and piled-up nuclei on a background of many intraepithelial neutrophils.

remained at the surgical margin (84,89,90). Anastomotic recurrence has been shown to occur at 3 years or later postsurgery, suggesting that the malignant transformation of BilIN-3 may take longer than previously thought (84).

Other Precursor Lesions

BilIN is supposedly a major premalignant lesion for large duct cholangiocarcinoma, but it is debatable which conditions can progress to small duct cholangiocarcinoma. Potential precursor lesions include *peribiliary gland hamartoma (bile duct adenoma)* and *bile duct hamartoma (von Meyenburg complex)* (202,252). It is rare, however, to identify these lesions within or adjacent to peripheral nodular cholangiocarcinoma. These conditions are described in chapter 6.

The lining epithelium of the small bile ducts is another possible origin of cholangiocarcinoma, but it is also uncommon to see dysplastic

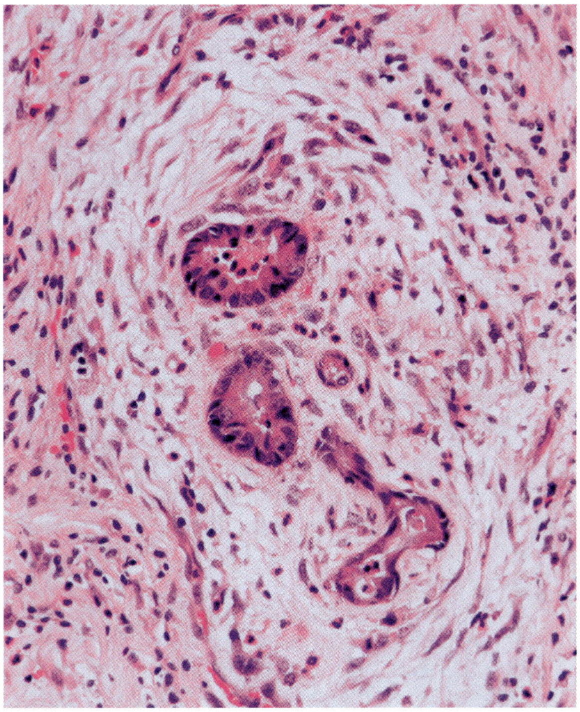

Figure 7-81

DEGENERATIVE CHANGES OF PERIBILIARY GLAND

These changes, reminiscent of BilIN, can be incidentally seen in livers explanted for acute liver failure due to paracetamol (acetaminophen) overdose.

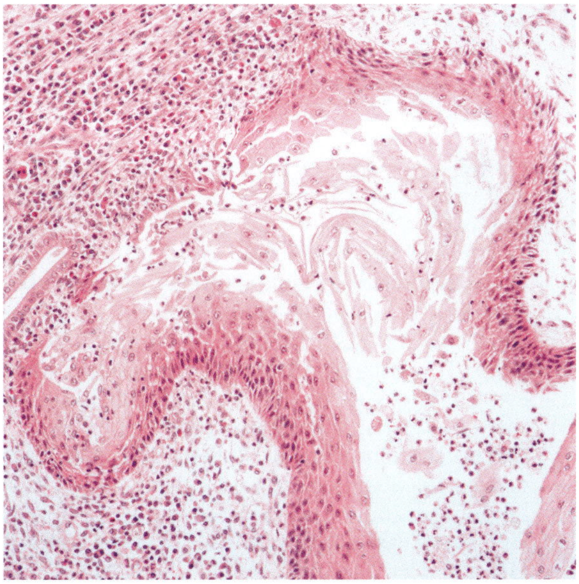

Figure 7-82

SQUAMOUS METAPLASIA OF THE BILIARY EPITHELIUM

The patient had PSC.

changes in septal or smaller bile ducts. Given the fact that both HCC and small duct cholangiocarcinoma can develop in cirrhotic livers, bipotent or intermediate cells, such as bile ductules or even stem cells, may be involved in the carcinogenesis (253). A recent study also observed that activation of Notch and AKT signaling within mature hepatocytes can induce the formation of intrahepatic biliary cancers, raising the possibility that hepatocytes may be another cell of origin of intrahepatic cholangiocarcinoma (254).

REFERENCES

1. Aloia T, Pawlik TM, Taouli B, Rubbia-Brandt L, Vauthey JN. Intrahepatic bile ducts. In: Amin MB, Edge SB, Greene FL, et al., eds. AJCC cancer staging manual, 8th ed. Switzerland: Springer; 2017:295-302.
2. Sobin LH, Gospodarowicz MK, Wittekind C, International Union against Cancer. TNM classification of malignant tumours, 7th ed. Chichester, West Sussex, UK; Hoboken, NJ: Wiley-Blackwell; 2010.
3. Deoliveira ML, Schulick RD, Nimura Y, et al. New staging system and a registry for perihilar cholangiocarcinoma. Hepatology 2011;53:1363-1371.
4. Nakanuma Y, Curado MP, Franceschi S, et al. Intrahepatic cholangiocarcinoma. In: Bosman FT, Carneiro F, Hruban RH, Theise ND, eds. World Health Organization classification of tumours of the digestive system. Lyon: IARC; 2010:217-224.
5. Akita M, Fujikura K, Ajiki T, et al. Dichotomy in intrahepatic cholangiocarcinomas based on histologic similarities to hilar cholangiocarcinomas. Mod Pathol 2017;30:986-997.
6. Nakeeb A, Pitt HA, Sohn TA, et al. Cholangiocarcinoma. A spectrum of intrahepatic, perihilar, and distal tumors. Ann Surg 1996;224:463-73; discussion 73-75.
7. DeOliveira ML, Cunningham SC, Cameron JL, et al. Cholangiocarcinoma: thirty-one-year experience with 564 patients at a single institution. Ann Surg 2007;245:755-762.
8. Malhi H, Gores GJ. Cholangiocarcinoma: modern advances in understanding a deadly old disease. J Hepatol 2006;45:856-867.
9. Welzel TM, Graubard BI, El-Serag HB, et al. Risk factors for intrahepatic and extrahepatic cholangiocarcinoma in the United States: a population-based case-control study. Clin Gastroenterol Hepatol 2007;5:1221-1228.
10. Yamanaka N, Okamoto E, Ando T, et al. Clinicopathologic spectrum of resected extraductal mass-forming intrahepatic cholangiocarcinoma. Cancer 1995;76:2449-2256.
11. Parkin DM, Ohshima H, Srivatanakul P, Vatanasapt V. Cholangiocarcinoma: epidemiology, mechanisms of carcinogenesis and prevention. Cancer Epidemiol Biomarkers Prev 1993;2:537-544.
12. Nakanuma Y, Sripa B, Vatanasapt V, Leong AS, Ponchon T, Ishak KG. Intrahepatic cholangiocarcinoma. In: Hamilton SR, Aaltonen LA, eds. World Health Organization classification of tumours, pathology and genetics of tumours of the digestive system. Lyon: IARC Press; 2000:173-180.
13. Bragazzi MC, Cardinale V, Carpino G, et al. Cholangiocarcinoma: epidemiology and risk factors. Transl Gastrointest Cancer 2012;1:21-32.
14. Khan SA, Taylor-Robinson SD, Toledano MB, Beck A, Elliott P, Thomas HC. Changing international trends in mortality rates for liver, biliary and pancreatic tumours. J Hepatol 2002;37:806-813.
15. Patel T. Increasing incidence and mortality of primary intrahepatic cholangiocarcinoma in the United States. Hepatology 2001;33:1353-1357.
16. Patel T. Worldwide trends in mortality from biliary tract malignancies. BMC Cancer 2002;2:10.
17. Taylor-Robinson SD, Toledano MB, Arora S, et al. Increase in mortality rates from intrahepatic cholangiocarcinoma in England and Wales 1968-1998. Gut 2001;48:816-8120.
18. Eaton JE, Talwalkar JA, Lazaridis KN, Gores GJ, Lindor KD. Pathogenesis of primary sclerosing cholangitis and advances in diagnosis and management. Gastroenterology 2013;145:521-536.
19. Hirschfield GM, Karlsen TH, Lindor KD, Adams DH. Primary sclerosing cholangitis. Lancet 2013;382:1587-1599.
20. Karlsen TH, Boberg KM. Update on primary sclerosing cholangitis. J Hepatol 2013;59:571-582.
21. Chapman RW. Risk factors for biliary tract carcinogenesis. Ann Oncol 1999;10(Suppl 4):308-311.
22. Bergquist A, Ekbom A, Olsson R, et al. Hepatic and extrahepatic malignancies in primary sclerosing cholangitis. J Hepatol 2002;36:321-327.

23. Dayton MT, Longmire WP Jr, Tompkins RK. Caroli's Disease: a premalignant condition? Am J Surg 1983;145:41-48.
24. Yamato T, Sasaki M, Hoso M, et al. Intrahepatic cholangiocarcinoma arising in congenital hepatic fibrosis: report of an autopsy case. J Hepatol 1998;28:717-22.
25. Voyles CR, Smadja C, Shands WC, Blumgart LH. Carcinoma in choledochal cysts. Age-related incidence. Arch Surg 1983;118:986-988.
26. Scott J, Shousha S, Thomas HC, Sherlock S. Bile duct carcinoma: a late complication of congenital hepatic fibrosis. Case report and review of literature. Am J Gastroenterol 1980;73:113-119.
27. Khan SA, Thomas HC, Davidson BR, Taylor-Robinson SD. Cholangiocarcinoma. Lancet 2005;366:1303-1314.
28. Lipsett PA, Pitt HA, Colombani PM, Boitnott JK, Cameron JL. Choledochal cyst disease. A changing pattern of presentation. Ann Surg 1994;220:644-652.
29. Parkin DM, Srivatanakul P, Khlat M, et al. Liver cancer in Thailand. I. A case-control study of cholangiocarcinoma. Int J Cancer 1991;48:323-328.
30. Shaib Y, El-Serag HB. The epidemiology of cholangiocarcinoma. Semin Liver Dis 2004;24:115-25.
31. Kubo S, Kinoshita H, Hirohashi K, Hamba H. Hepatolithiasis associated with cholangiocarcinoma. World J Surg 1995;19:637-641.
32. Chen MF. Peripheral cholangiocarcinoma (cholangiocellular carcinoma): clinical features, diagnosis and treatment. J Gastroenterol Hepatol 1999;14:1144-1149.
33. Okuda K, Nakanuma Y, Miyazaki M. Cholangiocarcinoma: recent progress. Part 1: epidemiology and etiology. J Gastroenterol Hepatol 2002;17:1049-1055.
34. Shaib YH, El-Serag HB, Davila JA, Morgan R, McGlynn KA. Risk factors of intrahepatic cholangiocarcinoma in the United States: a case-control study. Gastroenterology 2005;128:620-626.
35. Welzel TM, Mellemkjaer L, Gloria G, et al. Risk factors for intrahepatic cholangiocarcinoma in a low-risk population: a nationwide case-control study. Int J Cancer 2007;120:638-6341.
36. Sorensen HT, Friis S, Olsen JH, et al. Risk of liver and other types of cancer in patients with cirrhosis: a nationwide cohort study in Denmark. Hepatology 1998;28:921-925.
37. Palmer WC, Patel T. Are common factors involved in the pathogenesis of primary liver cancers? A meta-analysis of risk factors for intrahepatic cholangiocarcinoma. J Hepatol 2012;57:69-76.
38. Mavros MN, Economopoulos KP, Alexiou VG, Pawlik TM. Treatment and prognosis for patients with intrahepatic cholangiocarcinoma: systematic review and meta-analysis. JAMA Surg 2014;149:565-574.
39. Sahani D, Prasad SR, Tannabe KK, Hahn PF, Mueller PR, Saini S. Thorotrast-induced cholangiocarcinoma: case report. Abdom Imaging 2003;28:72-74.
40. Kubo S, Nakanuma Y, Takemura S, et al. Case series of 17 patients with cholangiocarcinoma among young adult workers of a printing company in Japan. J Hepatobiliary Pancreat Sci 2014;21:479-488.
41. Razumilava N, Gores GJ. Cholangiocarcinoma. Lancet 2014;383:2168-2179.
42. Rizvi S, Gores GJ. Pathogenesis, diagnosis, and management of cholangiocarcinoma. Gastroenterology 2013;145:1215-1229.
43. Khan SA, Davidson BR, Goldin RD, et al. Guidelines for the diagnosis and treatment of cholangiocarcinoma: an update. Gut 2012;61:1657-1669.
44. van Leeuwen DJ, Reeders JW. Primary sclerosing cholangitis and cholangiocarcinoma as a diagnostic and therapeutic dilemma. Ann Oncol 1999;10(Suppl 4):89-93.
45. Baheti AD, Tirumani SH, Shinagare AB, et al. Correlation of CT patterns of primary intrahepatic cholangiocarcinoma at the time of presentation with the metastatic spread and clinical outcomes: retrospective study of 92 patients. Abdom Imaging 2014;39:1193-1201.
46. Maithel SK, Gamblin TC, Kamel I, Corona-Villalobos CP, Thomas M, Pawlik TM. Multidisciplinary approaches to intrahepatic cholangiocarcinoma. Cancer 2013;119:3929-3942.
47. Blechacz B, Gores GJ. Cholangiocarcinoma: advances in pathogenesis, diagnosis, and treatment. Hepatology 2008;48:308-321.
48. Nehls O, Gregor M, Klump B. Serum and bile markers for cholangiocarcinoma. Semin Liver Dis 2004;24:139-154.
49. Venkatesh PG, Navaneethan U, Shen B, McCullough AJ. Increased serum levels of carbohydrate antigen 19-9 and outcomes in primary sclerosing cholangitis patients without cholangiocarcinoma. Dig Dis Sci 2013;58:850-857.
50. Sinakos E, Saenger AK, Keach J, Kim WR, Lindor KD. Many patients with primary sclerosing cholangitis and increased serum levels of carbohydrate antigen 19-9 do not have cholangiocarcinoma. Clin Gastroenterol Hepatol 2011;9:434-439.e1.
51. Patel AH, Harnois DM, Klee GG, LaRusso NF, Gores GJ. The utility of CA 19-9 in the diagnoses of cholangiocarcinoma in patients without primary sclerosing cholangitis. Am J Gastroenterol 2000;95:204-207.
52. Saini S. Imaging of the hepatobiliary tract. N Engl J Med 1997;336:1889-1894.

53. Chung YE, Kim MJ, Park YN, et al. Varying appearances of cholangiocarcinoma: radiologic-pathologic correlation. Radiographics 2009;29:683-700.
54. Fukukura Y, Hamanoue M, Fujiyoshi F, et al. Cholangiolocellular carcinoma of the liver: CT and MR findings. J Comput Assist Tomogr 2000;24:809-812.
55. Han JK, Choi BI, Kim AY, et al. Cholangiocarcinoma: pictorial essay of CT and cholangiographic findings. Radiographics 2002;22:173-187.
56. Manfredi R, Barbaro B, Masselli G, Vecchioli A, Marano P. Magnetic resonance imaging of cholangiocarcinoma. Semin Liver Dis 2004;24:155-164.
57. Kang Y, Lee JM, Kim SH, Han JK, Choi BI. Intrahepatic mass-forming cholangiocarcinoma: enhancement patterns on gadoxetic acid-enhanced MR images. Radiology 2012;264:751-760.
58. Iavarone M, Piscaglia F, Vavassori S, et al. Contrast enhanced CT-scan to diagnose intrahepatic cholangiocarcinoma in patients with cirrhosis. J Hepatol 2013;58:1188-1193.
59. Rimola J, Forner A, Reig M, et al. Cholangiocarcinoma in cirrhosis: absence of contrast washout in delayed phases by magnetic resonance imaging avoids misdiagnosis of hepatocellular carcinoma. Hepatology 2009;50:791-798.
60. Kim SH, Lee CH, Kim BH, et al. Typical and atypical imaging findings of intrahepatic cholangiocarcinoma using gadolinium ethoxybenzyl diethylenetriamine pentaacetic acid-enhanced magnetic resonance imaging. J Comput Assist Tomogr 2012;36:704-709.
61. Matsui O, Kadoya M, Kameyama T, et al. Benign and malignant nodules in cirrhotic livers: distinction based on blood supply. Radiology 1991; 178:493-497.
62. Matsui O. Imaging of multistep human hepatocarcinogenesis by CT during intra-arterial contrast injection. Intervirology 2004;47:271-276.
63. Lan BY, Kwee SA, Wong LL. Positron emission tomography in hepatobiliary and pancreatic malignancies: a review. Am J Surg 2012;204:232-241.
64. Anderson CD, Rice MH, Pinson CW, Chapman WC, Chari RS, Delbeke D. Fluorodeoxyglucose PET imaging in the evaluation of gallbladder carcinoma and cholangiocarcinoma. J Gastrointest Surg 2004;8:90-97.
65. Kim YJ, Yun M, Lee WJ, Kim KS, Lee JD. Usefulness of 18F-FDG PET in intrahepatic cholangiocarcinoma. Eur J Nucl Med Mol Imaging 2003;30:1467-1472.
66. Fritscher-Ravens A, Bohuslavizki KH, Broering DC, et al. FDG PET in the diagnosis of hilar cholangiocarcinoma. Nucl Med Commun 2001;22:1277-1285.
67. Sano T, Kamiya J, Nagino M, et al. Macroscopic classification and preoperative diagnosis of intrahepatic cholangiocarcinoma in Japan. J Hepatobiliary Pancreat Surg 1999;6:101-107.
68. Yamamoto M, Takasaki K, Yoshikawa T, Ueno K, Nakano M. Does gross appearance indicate prognosis in intrahepatic cholangiocarcinoma? J Surg Oncol 1998;69:162-167.
69. Ohtsuka M, Ito H, Kimura F, et al. Results of surgical treatment for intrahepatic cholangiocarcinoma and clinicopathological factors influencing survival. Br J Surg 2002;89:1525-1531.
70. Yamasaki S. Intrahepatic cholangiocarcinoma: macroscopic type and stage classification. J Hepatobiliary Pancreat Surg 2003;10:288-291.
71. Suh KS, Chang SH, Lee HJ, Roh HR, Kim SH, Lee KU. Clinical outcomes and apomucin expression of intrahepatic cholangiocarcinoma according to gross morphology. J Am Coll Surg 2002;195:782-789.
72. Uenishi T, Hirohashi K, Kubo S, Yamamoto T, Yamazaki O, Kinoshita H. Clinicopathological factors predicting outcome after resection of mass-forming intrahepatic cholangiocarcinoma. Br J Surg. 2001;88:969-974.
73. Kubo S, Uenishi T, Yamamoto S, et al. Clinicopathologic characteristics of small intrahepatic cholangiocarcinomas of mass-forming type. Hepatol Res 2004;29:223-227.
74. Ariizumi SI, Yamamoto M. Intrahepatic cholangiocarcinoma and cholangiolocellular carcinoma in cirrhosis and chronic viral hepatitis. Surg Today 2015;45:682-687.
75. Kim SJ, Lee JM, Han JK, Kim KH, Lee JY, Choi BI. Peripheral mass-forming cholangiocarcinoma in cirrhotic liver. AJR Am J Roentgenol 2007;189:1428-1434.
76. Wu ZF, Yang N, Li DY, Zhang HB, Yang GS. Characteristics of intrahepatic cholangiocarcinoma in patients with hepatitis B virus infection: clinicopathologic study of resected tumours. J Viral Hepat 2013;20:306-310.
77. Imai K, Yamamoto M, Ariizumi S. Surgery for periductal infiltrating type intrahepatic cholangiocarcinoma without hilar invasion provides a better outcome than for mass-forming type intrahepatic cholangiocarcinoma without hilar invasion. Hepatogastroenterology 2010;57:1333-1336.
78. Uno M, Shimada K, Yamamoto Y, et al. Periductal infiltrating type of intrahepatic cholangiocarcinoma: a rare macroscopic type without any apparent mass. Surg Today 2012;42:1189-1194.
79. Shimada K, Sano T, Sakamoto Y, Esaki M, Kosuge T, Ojima H. Surgical outcomes of the mass-forming plus periductal infiltrating types of intrahepatic cholangiocarcinoma: a comparative study with the typical mass-forming type of intrahepatic cholangiocarcinoma. World J Surg 2007;31:2016-2022.

80. Yeh CN, Jan YY, Yeh TS, Hwang TL, Chen MF. Hepatic resection of the intraductal papillary type of peripheral cholangiocarcinoma. Ann Surg Oncol 2004;11:606-611.
81. Kim YI, Yu ES, Kim ST. Intraductal variant of peripheral cholangiocarcinoma of the liver with Clonorchis sinensis infection. Cancer 1989;63:1562-1566.
82. Suh KS, Roh HR, Koh YT, Lee KU, Park YH, Kim SW. Clinicopathologic features of the intraductal growth type of peripheral cholangiocarcinoma. Hepatology 2000;31:12-17.
83. Yeh TS, Tseng JH, Chen TC, et al. Characterization of intrahepatic cholangiocarcinoma of the intraductal growth-type and its precursor lesions. Hepatology 2005;42:657-664.
84. Nakanishi Y, Zen Y, Kawakami H, et al. Extrahepatic bile duct carcinoma with extensive intraepithelial spread: a clinicopathological study of 21 cases. Mod Pathol 2008;21:807-816.
85. Komuta M, Govaere O, Vandecaveye V, et al. Histological diversity in cholangiocellular carcinoma reflects the different cholangiocyte phenotypes. Hepatology 2012;55:1876-1888.
86. Sasaki M, Tsuneyama K, Ishikawa A, Nakanuma Y. Intrahepatic cholangiocarcinoma in cirrhosis presents granulocyte and granulocyte-macrophage colony-stimulating factor. Hum Pathol 2003;34:1337-1344.
87. Fujikura K, Fukumoto T, Ajiki T, et al. Comparative clinicopathological study of biliary intraductal papillary neoplasms and papillary cholangiocarcinomas. Histopathology 2016;69:950-961.
88. Aishima S, Kuroda Y, Nishihara Y, et al. Proposal of progression model for intrahepatic cholangiocarcinoma: clinicopathologic differences between hilar type and peripheral type. Am J Surg Pathol 2007;31:1059-1067.
89. Wakai T, Shirai Y, Moroda T, Yokoyama N, Hatakeyama K. Impact of ductal resection margin status on long-term survival in patients undergoing resection for extrahepatic cholangiocarcinoma. Cancer 2005;103:1210-1216.
90. Igami T, Nagino M, Oda K, et al. Clinicopathologic study of cholangiocarcinoma with superficial spread. Ann Surg 2009;249:296-302.
91. Haas S, Gutgemann I, Wolff M, Fischer HP. Intrahepatic clear cell cholangiocarcinoma: immunohistochemical aspects in a very rare type of cholangiocarcinoma. Am J Surg Pathol 2007;31:902-906.
92. Zen Y, Quaglia A, Heaton N, Rela M, Portmann B. Two distinct pathways of carcinogenesis in primary sclerosing cholangitis. Histopathology 2011;59:1100-1110.
93. Choi JE, Noh SJ, Lee JH, et al. Expression of keratin 20 and its clinicopathological significance in intrahepatic cholangiocarcinoma. Oncol Lett 2012;4:534-540.
94. Aishima S, Fujita N, Mano Y, et al. p62+ Hyaline inclusions in intrahepatic cholangiocarcinoma associated with viral hepatitis or alcoholic liver disease. Am J Clin Pathol 2010;134:457-465.
95. Inagaki Y, Xu H, Nakata M, et al. Clinicopathology of sialomucin: MUC1, particularly KL-6 mucin, in gastrointestinal, hepatic and pancreatic cancers. Biosci Trends 2009;3:220-232.
96. Shimonishi T, Miyazaki K, Nakanuma Y. Cytokeratin profile relates to histological subtypes and intrahepatic location of intrahepatic cholangiocarcinoma and primary sites of metastatic adenocarcinoma of liver. Histopathology 2000;37:55-63.
97. Lewis JT, Talwalkar JA, Rosen CB, Smyrk TC, Abraham SC. Precancerous bile duct pathology in end-stage primary sclerosing cholangitis, with and without cholangiocarcinoma. Am J Surg Pathol 2010;34:27-34.
98. Yeh CN, Jan YY, Chen MF. Adenosquamous carcinoma of the liver: clinicopathologic features in 12 patients and review of the literature. Int Surg 2002;87:125-129.
99. Kobayashi M, Okabayashi T, Okamoto K, Namikawa T, Araki K. A clinicopathologic study of primary adenosquamous carcinoma of the liver. J Clin Gastroenterol 2005;39:544-548.
100. Nakajima T, Kondo Y, Miyazaki M, Okui K. A histopathologic study of 102 cases of intrahepatic cholangiocarcinoma: histologic classification and modes of spreading. Hum Pathol 1988;19:1228-1234.
101. Arakawa Y, Shimada M, Ikegami T, et al. Mucoepidermoid carcinoma of the liver: report of a rare case and review of the literature. Hepatol Res 2008;38:736-742.
102. Choi D, Kim H, Lee KS, Lee KG, Park CK. Mucoepidermoid carcinoma of the liver diagnosed as a liver abscess: report of a case. Surg Today 2004;34:968-972.
103. Katsuda S, Nakanishi I, Kajikawa K, Takabatake S. Mucoepidermoid carcinoma of the liver. Acta Pathol Jpn 1984;34:153-157.
104. Pianzola LE, Drut R. Mucoepidermoid carcinoma of the liver. Am J Clin Pathol 1971;56:758-61.
105. Chen MF, Jan YY, Chen TC. Clinical studies of mucin-producing cholangiocellular carcinoma: a study of 22 histopathology-proven cases. Ann Surg 1998;227:63-69.
106. Chow LT, Ahuja AT, Kwong KH, Fung KS, Lai CK, Lau JW. Mucinous cholangiocarcinoma: an unusual complication of hepatolithiasis and recurrent pyogenic cholangitis. Histopathology 1997;30:491-494.

107. Hayashi M, Matsui O, Ueda K, et al. Imaging findings of mucinous type of cholangiocellular carcinoma. J Comput Assist Tomogr 1996; 20:386-389.
108. Mizukami Y, Ohta H, Arisato S, et al. Case report: mucinous cholangiocarcinoma featuring a multicystic appearance and periportal collar in imaging. J Gastroenterol Hepatol 1999;14: 1223-1226.
109. Zen Y, Fujii T, Itatsu K, et al. Biliary papillary tumors share pathological features with intraductal papillary mucinous neoplasm of the pancreas. Hepatology 2006;44:1333-1343.
110. Komuta M, Spee B, Vander Borght S, et al. Clinicopathological study on cholangiolocellular carcinoma suggesting hepatic progenitor cell origin. Hepatology 2008;47:1544-1556.
111. Sempoux C, Jibara G, Ward SC, et al. Intrahepatic cholangiocarcinoma: new insights in pathology. Semin Liver Dis 2011;31:49-60.
112. Theise ND, Nakashima O, Park YN, Nakanuma Y. Combined hepatocellular-cholangiocarcinoma. In: Bosman FT, Carneiro F, Hruban RH, Theise ND, eds. World Health Organization classification of tumours of the digestive system. Lyon: IARC; 2010:225-227.
113. Motosugi U, Ichikawa T, Nakajima H, et al. Cholangiolocellular carcinoma of the liver: imaging findings. J Comput Assist Tomogr 2009;33:682-688.
114. Kozaka K, Sasaki M, Fujii T, et al. A subgroup of intrahepatic cholangiocarcinoma with an infiltrating replacement growth pattern and a resemblance to reactive proliferating bile ductules: 'bile ductular carcinoma'. Histopathology 2007;51:390-400.
115. Ariizumi S, Kotera Y, Katagiri S, et al. Long-term survival of patients with cholangiolocellular carcinoma after curative hepatectomy. Ann Surg Oncol 2014;21(Suppl 3):S451-458.
116. Nakanuma Y, Sato Y, Ikeda H, et al. Intrahepatic cholangiocarcinoma with predominant "ductal plate malformation" pattern: a new subtype. Am J Surg Pathol 2012;36:1629-1635.
117. Chen TC, Ng KF, Kuo T. Intrahepatic cholangiocarcinoma with lymphoepithelioma-like component. Mod Pathol 2001;14:527-532.
118. Hsu HC, Chen CC, Huang GT, Lee PH. Clonal Epstein-Barr virus associated cholangiocarcinoma with lymphoepithelioma-like component. Hum Pathol 1996;27:848-850.
119. Jeng YM, Chen CL, Hsu HC. Lymphoepithelioma-like cholangiocarcinoma: an Epstein-Barr virus-associated tumor. Am J Surg Pathol 2001;25:516-520.
120. Chan AW, Tong JH, Sung MY, Lai PB, To KF. Epstein-Barr virus-associated lymphoepithelioma-like cholangiocarcinoma: a rare variant of intrahepatic cholangiocarcinoma with favourable outcome. Histopathology 2014;65:674-683.
121. Kaibori M, Kawaguchi Y, Yokoigawa N, et al. Intrahepatic sarcomatoid cholangiocarcinoma. J Gastroenterol 2003;38:1097-1101.
122. Nakajima T, Tajima Y, Sugano I, Nagao K, Kondo Y, Wada K. Intrahepatic cholangiocarcinoma with sarcomatous change. Clinicopathologic and immunohistochemical evaluation of seven cases. Cancer 1993;72:1872-1877.
123. Tsou YK, Wu RC, Hung CF, Lee CS. Intrahepatic sarcomatoid cholangiocarcinoma: clinical analysis of seven cases during a 15-year period. Chang Gung Med J 2008;31:599-605.
124. Jang KT, Saka B, Zen Y, Pambuccian S, Bacchi C, Adsay V. Tubulocystic carcinoma of bile ducts: A hitherto unrecognized and diagnostically challenging entity often mistaken as a benign lesion; clinicopathologic analysis of 6 cases. Mod Pathol 2013;26:404A.
125. Amin MB, MacLennan GT, Gupta R, et al. Tubulocystic carcinoma of the kidney: clinicopathologic analysis of 31 cases of a distinctive rare subtype of renal cell carcinoma. Am J Surg Pathol 2009;33:384-392.
126. Agaimy A, Kaiser A, Becker K, et al. Pancreatic-type acinar cell carcinoma of the liver: a clinicopathologic study of four patients. Mod Pathol 2011;24:1620-1626.
127. Hervieu V, Lombard-Bohas C, Dumortier J, Boillot O, Scoazec JY. Primary acinar cell carcinoma of the liver. Virchows Arch 2008;452:337-341.
128. Aishima S, Asayama Y, Taguchi K, et al. The utility of keratin 903 as a new prognostic marker in mass-forming-type intrahepatic cholangiocarcinoma. Mod Pathol 2002;15:1181-1190.
129. Yonezawa S, Higashi M, Yamada N, Yokoyama S, Goto M. Significance of mucin expression in pancreatobiliary neoplasms. J Hepatobiliary Pancreat Sci 2010;17:108-124.
130. Shibahara H, Tamada S, Higashi M, et al. MUC4 is a novel prognostic factor of intrahepatic cholangiocarcinoma-mass forming type. Hepatology 2004;39:220-229.
131. Matsumura N, Yamamoto M, Aruga A, Takasaki K, Nakano M. Correlation between expression of MUC1 core protein and outcome after surgery in mass-forming intrahepatic cholangiocarcinoma. Cancer 2002;94:1770-1706.
132. Yamashita K, Yonezawa S, Tanaka S, et al. Immunohistochemical study of mucin carbohydrates and core proteins in hepatolithiasis and cholangiocarcinoma. Int J Cancer 1993;55:82-91.

133. Higashi M, Yonezawa S, Ho JJ, et al. Expression of MUC1 and MUC2 mucin antigens in intrahepatic bile duct tumors: its relationship with a new morphological classification of cholangiocarcinoma. Hepatology 1999;30:1347-1355.
134. Aishima S, Kuroda Y, Nishihara Y, et al. Gastric mucin phenotype defines tumour progression and prognosis of intrahepatic cholangiocarcinoma: gastric foveolar type is associated with aggressive tumour behaviour. Histopathology 2006;49:35-44.
135. Khan SA, Thomas HC, Toledano MB, Cox IJ, Taylor-Robinson SD. p53 mutations in human cholangiocarcinoma: a review. Liver Int 2005;25:704-716.
136. Nakanishi Y, Zen Y, Kondo S, Itoh T, Itatsu K, Nakanuma Y. Expression of cell cycle-related molecules in biliary premalignant lesions: biliary intraepithelial neoplasia and biliary intraductal papillary neoplasm. Hum Pathol 2008;39:1153-1161.
137. Lok T, Chen L, Lin F, Wang HL. Immunohistochemical distinction between intrahepatic cholangiocarcinoma and pancreatic ductal adenocarcinoma. Hum Pathol 2014;45:394-400.
138. Iguchi T, Aishima S, Taketomi A, et al. Fascin overexpression is involved in carcinogenesis and prognosis of human intrahepatic cholangiocarcinoma: immunohistochemical and molecular analysis. Hum Pathol 2009;40:174-180.
139. Onodera M, Zen Y, Harada K, et al. Fascin is involved in tumor necrosis factor-alpha-dependent production of MMP9 in cholangiocarcinoma. Lab Invest 2009;89:1261-1274.
140. Higashi M, Yamada N, Yokoyama S, et al. Pathobiological implications of MUC16/CA125 expression in intrahepatic cholangiocarcinoma-mass forming type. Pathobiology 2012;79:101-106.
141. Aishima S, Fujita N, Mano Y, et al. Different roles of S100P overexpression in intrahepatic cholangiocarcinoma: carcinogenesis of perihilar type and aggressive behavior of peripheral type. Am J Surg Pathol 2011;35:590-598.
142. Guedj N, Zhan Q, Perigny M, et al. Comparative protein expression profiles of hilar and peripheral hepatic cholangiocarcinomas. J Hepatol 2009;51:93-101.
143. Tsai JH, Huang WC, Kuo KT, Yuan RH, Chen YL, Jeng YM. S100P immunostaining identifies a subset of peripheral-type intrahepatic cholangiocarcinomas with morphological and molecular features similar to those of perihilar and extrahepatic cholangiocarcinomas. Histopathology 2012;61:1106-1116.
144. Zen Y, Britton D, Mitra V, et al. Tubulin beta-III: a novel immunohistochemical marker for intrahepatic peripheral cholangiocarcinoma. Histopathology 2014;65:784-792.
145. Liau JY, Tsai JH, Yuan RH, Chang CN, Lee HJ, Jeng YM. Morphological subclassification of intrahepatic cholangiocarcinoma: etiological, clinicopathological, and molecular features. Mod Pathol 2014;27:1163-1173.
146. Hayashi A, Misumi K, Shibahara J, et al. Distinct clinicopathologic and genetic features of 2 histologic subtypes of intrahepatic cholangiocarcinoma. Am J Surg Pathol 2016;40:1021-1030.
147. Tsuji M, Kashihara T, Terada N, Mori H. An immunohistochemical study of hepatic atypical adenomatous hyperplasia, hepatocellular carcinoma, and cholangiocarcinoma with alpha-fetoprotein, carcinoembryonic antigen, CA19-9, epithelial membrane antigen, and cytokeratins 18 and 19. Pathol Int 1999;49:310-317.
148. Sasaki M, Yamaguchi J, Itatsu K, Ikeda H, Nakanuma Y. Over-expression of polycomb group protein EZH2 relates to decreased expression of p16 INK4a in cholangiocarcinogenesis in hepatolithiasis. J Pathol 2008;215:175-183.
149. Hahn SA, Schutte M, Hoque AT, et al. DPC4, a candidate tumor suppressor gene at human chromosome 18q21.1. Science 1996;271:350-353.
150. Techasen A, Loilome W, Namwat N, et al. Loss of E-cadherin promotes migration and invasion of cholangiocarcinoma cells and serves as a potential marker of metastasis. Tumour Biol 2014;35:8645-8652.
151. Itatsu K, Zen Y, Ohira S, et al. Immunohistochemical analysis of the progression of flat and papillary preneoplastic lesions in intrahepatic cholangiocarcinogenesis in hepatolithiasis. Liver Int 2007;27:1174-1184.
152. Mosnier JF, Kandel C, Cazals-Hatem D, et al. N-cadherin serves as diagnostic biomarker in intrahepatic and perihilar cholangiocarcinomas. Mod Pathol 2009;22:182-190.
153. Yu TH, Yuan RH, Chen YL, Yang WC, Hsu HC, Jeng YM. Viral hepatitis is associated with intrahepatic cholangiocarcinoma with cholangiolar differentiation and N-cadherin expression. Mod Pathol 2011;24:810-819.
154. Aishima S, Matsuura S, Terashi T, et al. Aberrant expression of laminin gamma 2 chain and its prognostic significance in intrahepatic cholangiocarcinoma according to growth morphology. Mod Pathol 2004;17:938-945.
155. Sabit H, Tsuneyama K, Shimonishi T, et al. Enhanced expression of basement-membrane-type heparan sulfate proteoglycan in tumor fibro-myxoid stroma of intrahepatic cholangiocarcinoma. Pathol Int 2001;51:248-256.

156. Sulpice L, Rayar M, Desille M, et al. Molecular profiling of stroma identifies osteopontin as an independent predictor of poor prognosis in intrahepatic cholangiocarcinoma. Hepatology 2013;58:1992-2000.
157. Aishima S, Taguchi K, Terashi T, Matsuura S, Shimada M, Tsuneyoshi M. Tenascin expression at the invasive front is associated with poor prognosis in intrahepatic cholangiocarcinoma. Mod Pathol 2003;16:1019-1027.
158. Zen Y, Harada K, Sasaki M, et al. Intrahepatic cholangiocarcinoma escapes from growth inhibitory effect of transforming growth factor-beta1 by overexpression of cyclin D1. Lab Invest 2005;85:572-581.
159. DeMay RM. The art and science of cytopathology. Chicago: ASCP Press; 1996.
160. DiMagno EP, Malagelada JR, Taylor WF, Go VL. A prospective comparison of current diagnostic tests for pancreatic cancer. N Engl J Med 1977;297:737-742.
161. Ferrari Junior AP, Lichtenstein DR, Slivka A, Chang C, Carr-Locke DL. Brush cytology during ERCP for the diagnosis of biliary and pancreatic malignancies. Gastrointest Endosc 1994;40:140-145.
162. Mohandas KM, Swaroop VS, Gullar SU, Dave UR, Jagannath P, DeSouza LJ. Diagnosis of malignant obstructive jaundice by bile cytology: results improved by dilating the bile duct strictures. Gastrointest Endosc 1994;40:150-154.
163. Nakajima T, Tajima Y, Sugano I, et al. Multivariate statistical analysis of bile cytology. Acta Cytol 1994;38:51-55.
164. Layfield LJ, Wax TD, Lee JG, Cotton PB. Accuracy and morphologic aspects of pancreatic and biliary duct brushings. Acta Cytol 1995;39:11-18.
165. Kurzawinski T, Deery A, Davidson BR. Diagnostic value of cytology for biliary stricture. Br J Surg 1993;80:414-421.
166. Rupp M, Hawthorne CM, Ehya H. Brushing cytology in biliary tract obstruction. Acta Cytol 1990;34:221-226.
167. Kline TS, Joshi LP, Goldstein F. Preoperative diagnosis of pancreatic malignancy by the cytologic examination of duodenal secretions. Am J Clin Pathol 1978;70:851-4.
168. Kameya S, Kuno N, Kasugai T. The diagnosis of pancreatic cancer by pancreatic juice cytology. Acta Cytol 1981;25:354-360.
169. Suen KC. Diagnosis of primary hepatic neoplasms by fine-needle aspiration cytology. Diagn Cytopathol 1986;2:99-109.
170. Sampatanukul P, Leong AS, Kosolbhand P, Tangkijvanich P. Proliferating ductules are a diagnostic discriminator for intrahepatic cholangiocarcinoma in FNA biopsies. Diagn Cytopathol 2000;22:359-363.
171. Jain D, Mathur SR, Iyer VK. Cell blocks in cytopathology: a review of preparative methods, utility in diagnosis and role in ancillary studies. Cytopathology 2014;25:356-371.
172. Koo SH, Ihm CH, Kwon KC, Park JW, Kim JM, Kong G. Genetic alterations in hepatocellular carcinoma and intrahepatic cholangiocarcinoma. Cancer Genet Cytogenet 2001;130:22-28.
173. Uhm KO, Park YN, Lee JY, Yoon DS, Park SH. Chromosomal imbalances in Korean intrahepatic cholangiocarcinoma by comparative genomic hybridization. Cancer Genet Cytogenet 2005;157:37-41.
174. Lee JY, Park YN, Uhm KO, Park SY, Park SH. Genetic alterations in intrahepatic cholangiocarcinoma as revealed by degenerate oligonucleotide primed PCR-comparative genomic hybridization. J Korean Med Sci 2004;19:682-687.
175. Wong N, Li L, Tsang K, Lai PB, To KF, Johnson PJ. Frequent loss of chromosome 3p and hypermethylation of RASSF1A in cholangiocarcinoma. J Hepatol 2002;37:633-639.
176. Homayounfar K, Gunawan B, Cameron S, et al. Pattern of chromosomal aberrations in primary liver cancers identified by comparative genomic hybridization. Hum Pathol 2009;40:834-842.
177. Andersen JB, Thorgeirsson SS. Genetic profiling of intrahepatic cholangiocarcinoma. Curr Opin Gastroenterol 2012;28:266-272.
178. Razumilava N, Gores GJ. Classification, diagnosis, and management of cholangiocarcinoma. Clin Gastroenterol Hepatol 2013;11:13-21.e1; quiz e3-4.
179. Barr Fritcher EG, Kipp BR, Voss JS, et al. Primary sclerosing cholangitis patients with serial polysomy fluorescence in situ hybridization results are at increased risk of cholangiocarcinoma. Am J Gastroenterol 2011;106:2023-2028.
180. Kipp BR, Stadheim LM, Halling SA, et al. A comparison of routine cytology and fluorescence in situ hybridization for the detection of malignant bile duct strictures. Am J Gastroenterol 2004;99:1675-1681.
181. Gonda TA, Glick MP, Sethi A, et al. Polysomy and p16 deletion by fluorescence in situ hybridization in the diagnosis of indeterminate biliary strictures. Gastrointest Endosc 2012;75:74-79.
182. Liu D, Momoi H, Li L, Ishikawa Y, Fukumoto M. Microsatellite instability in thorotrast-induced human intrahepatic cholangiocarcinoma. Int J Cancer 2002;102:366-371.
183. Limpaiboon T, Krissadarak K, Sripa B, et al. Microsatellite alterations in liver fluke related cholangiocarcinoma are associated with poor prognosis. Cancer Lett 2002;181:215-222.

184. Liengswangwong U, Nitta T, Kashiwagi H, et al. Infrequent microsatellite instability in liver fluke infection-associated intrahepatic cholangiocarcinomas from Thailand. Int J Cancer 2003;107:375-380.
185. Jang S, Chun SM, Hong SM, et al. High throughput molecular profiling reveals differential mutation patterns in intrahepatic cholangiocarcinomas arising in chronic advanced liver diseases. Mod Pathol 2014;27:731-739.
186. Churi CR, Shroff R, Wang Y, et al. Mutation profiling in cholangiocarcinoma: prognostic and therapeutic implications. PLoS One 2014;9: e115383.
187. Gwak GY, Yoon JH, Shin CM, et al. Detection of response-predicting mutations in the kinase domain of the epidermal growth factor receptor gene in cholangiocarcinomas. J Cancer Res Clin Oncol 2005;131:649-652.
188. Ong CK, Subimerb C, Pairojkul C, et al. Exome sequencing of liver fluke-associated cholangiocarcinoma. Nat Genet 2012;44:690-693.
189. Borger DR, Tanabe KK, Fan KC, et al. Frequent mutation of isocitrate dehydrogenase (IDH)1 and IDH2 in cholangiocarcinoma identified through broad-based tumor genotyping. Oncologist 2012;17:72-79.
190. Wang P, Dong Q, Zhang C, et al. Mutations in isocitrate dehydrogenase 1 and 2 occur frequently in intrahepatic cholangiocarcinomas and share hypermethylation targets with glioblastomas. Oncogene 2013;32:3091-3100.
191. Kipp BR, Voss JS, Kerr SE, et al. Isocitrate dehydrogenase 1 and 2 mutations in cholangiocarcinoma. Hum Pathol 2012;43:1552-1558.
192. Fathi AT, Sadrzadeh H, Comander AH, et al. Isocitrate dehydrogenase 1 (IDH1) mutation in breast adenocarcinoma is associated with elevated levels of serum and urine 2-hydroxyglutarate. Oncologist 2014;19:602-607.
193. O'Dell MR, Huang JL, Whitney-Miller CL, et al. Kras(G12D) and p53 mutation cause primary intrahepatic cholangiocarcinoma. Cancer Res 2012;72:1557-1567.
194. Farazi PA, Zeisberg M, Glickman J, Zhang Y, Kalluri R, DePinho RA. Chronic bile duct injury associated with fibrotic matrix microenvironment provokes cholangiocarcinoma in p53-deficient mice. Cancer Res 2006;66:6622-6627.
195. Kang YK, Kim WH, Lee HW, Lee HK, Kim YI. Mutation of p53 and K-ras, and loss of heterozygosity of APC in intrahepatic cholangiocarcinoma. Lab Invest 1999;79:477-483.
196. Tullo A, Sbisa E. Mutation of p53 tumor suppressor gene in hepatocellular carcinoma. Methods Mol Med 2000;45:113-130.
197. Sturm PD, Baas IO, Clement MJ, et al. Alterations of the p53 tumor-suppressor gene and K-ras oncogene in perihilar cholangiocarcinomas from a high-incidence area. Int J Cancer 1998; 78:695-698.
198. Momoi H, Itoh T, Nozaki Y, et al. Microsatellite instability and alternative genetic pathway in intrahepatic cholangiocarcinoma. J Hepatol 2001;35:235-244.
199. Zhu AX, Borger DR, Kim Y, et al. Genomic profiling of intrahepatic cholangiocarcinoma: refining prognosis and identifying therapeutic targets. Ann Surg Oncol 2014;21:3827-3834.
200. Goeppert B, Frauenschuh L, Renner M, et al. BRAF V600E-specific immunohistochemistry reveals low mutation rates in biliary tract cancer and restriction to intrahepatic cholangiocarcinoma. Mod Pathol 2014;27:1028-1034.
201. Ross JS, Wang K, Gay L, et al. New routes to targeted therapy of intrahepatic cholangiocarcinomas revealed by next-generation sequencing. Oncologist 2014;19:235-242.
202. Pujals A, Amaddeo G, Castain C, et al. BRAF V600E mutations in bile duct adenomas. Hepatology 2015;61:403-405.
203. Loaiza-Bonilla A, Clayton E, Furth E, O'Hara M, Morrissette J. Dramatic response to dabrafenib and trametinib combination in a BRAF V600E-mutated cholangiocarcinoma: implementation of a molecular tumour board and next-generation sequencing for personalized medicine. Ecancermedicalscience 2014;8:479.
204. Wu YM, Su F, Kalyana-Sundaram S, et al. Identification of targetable FGFR gene fusions in diverse cancers. Cancer Discov 2013;3:636-647.
205. Borad MJ, Champion MD, Egan JB, et al. Integrated genomic characterization reveals novel, therapeutically relevant drug targets in FGFR and EGFR pathways in sporadic intrahepatic cholangiocarcinoma. PLoS Genet 2014;10:e1004135.
206. Arai Y, Totoki Y, Hosoda F, et al. Fibroblast growth factor receptor 2 tyrosine kinase fusions define a unique molecular subtype of cholangiocarcinoma. Hepatology 2014;59:1427-1434.
207. Graham RP, Barr Fritcher EG, Pestova E, et al. Fibroblast growth factor receptor 2 translocations in intrahepatic cholangiocarcinoma. Hum Pathol 2014;45:1630-1638.
207a. Hayashi A, Misumi K, Shibahara J, et al. Distinct clinicopathologic and genetic features of 2 histologic subtypes of intrahepatic cholangiocarcinoma. Am J Surg Pathol 2016;40:1021-1030.
207b. Kim SJ, Akita M, Sung YN, et al. MDM2 amplification in intrahepatic cholangiocarcinomas: its relationship with large-duct type morphology and uncommon KRAS mutations. Am J Surg Pathol 2018;42:512-21.

208. Peraldo Neia C, Cavalloni G, Balsamo A, et al. Screening for the FIG-ROS1 fusion in biliary tract carcinomas by nested PCR. Genes Chromosomes Cancer 2014;53:1033-1040.
209. Xu J, Igarashi S, Sasaki M, et al. Intrahepatic cholangiocarcinomas in cirrhosis are hypervascular in comparison with those in normal livers. Liver Int 2012;32:1156-1164.
210. Vilana R, Forner A, Bianchi L, et al. Intrahepatic peripheral cholangiocarcinoma in cirrhosis patients may display a vascular pattern similar to hepatocellular carcinoma on contrast-enhanced ultrasound. Hepatology 2010;51:2020-2029.
211. Radwan NA, Ahmed NS. The diagnostic value of arginase-1 immunostaining in differentiating hepatocellular carcinoma from metastatic carcinoma and cholangiocarcinoma as compared to HepPar-1. Diagn Pathol 2012;7:149.
212. Krings G, Ramachandran R, Jain D, et al. Immunohistochemical pitfalls and the importance of glypican 3 and arginase in the diagnosis of scirrhous hepatocellular carcinoma. Mod Pathol 2013;26:782-791.
213. Sasaki M, Matsubara T, Kakuda Y, Sato Y, Nakanuma Y. Immunostaining for polycomb group protein EZH2 and senescent marker p16INK4a may be useful to differentiate cholangiolocellular carcinoma from ductular reaction and bile duct adenoma. Am J Surg Pathol 2014;38:364-369.
214. Chu PG, Weiss LM. Keratin expression in human tissues and neoplasms. Histopathology 2002;40:403-439.
215. Rullier A, Le Bail B, Fawaz R, Blanc JF, Saric J, Bioulac-Sage P. Cytokeratin 7 and 20 expression in cholangiocarcinomas varies along the biliary tract but still differs from that in colorectal carcinoma metastasis. Am J Surg Pathol 2000;24:870-876.
216. Povoski SP, Klimstra DS, Brown KT, et al. Recognition of intrabiliary hepatic metastases from colorectal adenocarcinoma. HPB Surg 2000;11:383-90; discussion 90-91.
217. Sugiura T, Nagino M, Oda K, et al. Hepatectomy for colorectal liver metastases with macroscopic intrabiliary tumor growth. World J Surg 2006;30:1902-1908.
218. Estrella JS, Othman ML, Taggart MW, et al. Intrabiliary growth of liver metastases: clinicopathologic features, prevalence, and outcome. Am J Surg Pathol 2013;37:1571-1579.
219. Zen Y, Sasaki M, Fujii T, et al. Different expression patterns of mucin core proteins and cytokeratins during intrahepatic cholangiocarcinogenesis from biliary intraepithelial neoplasia and intraductal papillary neoplasm of the bile duct—an immunohistochemical study of 110 cases of hepatolithiasis. J Hepatol 2006;44:350-358.
220. Hoang MP, Murakata LA, Katabi N, Henson DE, Albores-Saavedra J. Invasive papillary carcinomas of the extrahepatic bile ducts: a clinicopathologic and immunohistochemical study of 13 cases. Mod Pathol 2002;15:1251-1258.
221. Hughes NR, Pairojkul C, Royce SG, Clouston A, Bhathal PS. Liver fluke-associated and sporadic cholangiocarcinoma: an immunohistochemical study of bile duct, peribiliary gland and tumour cell phenotypes. J Clin Pathol 2006;59:1073-1078.
222. Nakanuma Y, Terada T, Tanaka Y, Ohta G. Are hepatolithiasis and cholangiocarcinoma aetiologically related? A morphological study of 12 cases of hepatolithiasis associated with cholangiocarcinoma. Virchows Arch A Pathol Anat Histopathol 1985;406:45-58.
223. Zen Y, Harada K, Sasaki M, et al. IgG4-related sclerosing cholangitis with and without hepatic inflammatory pseudotumor, and sclerosing pancreatitis-associated sclerosing cholangitis: do they belong to a spectrum of sclerosing pancreatitis? Am J Surg Pathol 2004;28:1193-1203.
224. Zen Y, Ishikawa A, Ogiso S, Heaton N, Portmann B. Follicular cholangitis and pancreatitis—clinicopathological features and differential diagnosis of an under-recognized entity. Histopathology 2012;60:261-269.
225. Zen Y, Fujii T, Nakanuma Y. Hepatic pseudolymphoma: a clinicopathological study of five cases and review of the literature. Mod Pathol 2010;23:244-250.
226. Endo I, Gonen M, Yopp AC, et al. Intrahepatic cholangiocarcinoma: rising frequency, improved survival, and determinants of outcome after resection. Ann Surg 2008;248:84-96.
227. Guglielmi A, Ruzzenente A, Campagnaro T, et al. Intrahepatic cholangiocarcinoma: prognostic factors after surgical resection. World J Surg 2009;33:1247-1254.
228. Nakagawa T, Kamiyama T, Kurauchi N, et al. Number of lymph node metastases is a significant prognostic factor in intrahepatic cholangiocarcinoma. World J Surg 2005;29:728-733.
229. Nakanishi Y, Xu B, LeVea C. Oral floor and gingival metastasis of cholangiocarcinoma: a case report and review of the literature. Case Rep Pathol 2014;2014:712912.
230. Chang SA, Kim HK, Oh DY, Kim YJ, Sohn DW. Myocardial metastasis in patient with cholangiocarcinoma. Echocardiography 2009;26:295-296.
231. Nathan H, Aloia TA, Vauthey JN, et al. A proposed staging system for intrahepatic cholangiocarcinoma. Ann Surg Oncol 2009;16:14-22.
232. Edge SB, Byrd DR, Compton CC, Fritz AG, Greene FL, Trotti A, et al. AJCC cancer staging manual, 7th ed. New York: Springer; 2010.

233. Igami T, Ebata T, Yokoyama Y, Sugawara G, Takahashi Y, Nagino M. Staging of peripheral-type intrahepatic cholangiocarcinoma: appraisal of the new TNM classification and its modifications. World J Surg 2011;35:2501-2509.
234. Farges O, Fuks D, Le Treut YP, et al. AJCC 7th edition of TNM staging accurately discriminates outcomes of patients with resectable intrahepatic cholangiocarcinoma: By the AFC-IH-CC-2009 study group. Cancer 2011;117:2170-2177.
235. Weber SM, Jarnagin WR, Klimstra D, DeMatteo RP, Fong Y, Blumgart LH. Intrahepatic cholangiocarcinoma: resectability, recurrence pattern, and outcomes. J Am Coll Surg 2001;193:384-391.
236. Valle J, Wasan H, Palmer DH, et al. Cisplatin plus gemcitabine versus gemcitabine for biliary tract cancer. N Engl J Med 2010;362:1273-1281.
237. Tanguturi SK, Wo JY, Zhu AX, Dawson LA, Hong TS. Radiation therapy for liver tumors: ready for inclusion in guidelines? Oncologist 2014;19:868-879.
238. Wang Y, Li J, Xia Y, et al. Prognostic nomogram for intrahepatic cholangiocarcinoma after partial hepatectomy. J Clin Oncol 2013;31:1188-1195.
239. Farges O, Fuks D, Boleslawski E, et al. Influence of surgical margins on outcome in patients with intrahepatic cholangiocarcinoma: a multicenter study by the AFC-IHCC-2009 study group. Ann Surg 2011;254:824-829; discussion 30.
240. de Jong MC, Nathan H, Sotiropoulos GC, et al. Intrahepatic cholangiocarcinoma: an international multi-institutional analysis of prognostic factors and lymph node assessment. J Clin Oncol 2011;29:3140-3145.
241. Jiang W, Zeng ZC, Tang ZY, et al. A prognostic scoring system based on clinical features of intrahepatic cholangiocarcinoma: the Fudan score. Ann Oncol 2011;22:1644-1652.
242. Ribero D, Pinna AD, Guglielmi A, et al. Surgical approach for long-term survival of patients with intrahepatic cholangiocarcinoma: a multi-institutional analysis of 434 patients. Arch Surg 2012;147:1107-1113.
243. Terada T, Nakanuma Y. Pathological observations of intrahepatic peribiliary glands in 1,000 consecutive autopsy livers. II. A possible source of cholangiocarcinoma. Hepatology 1990;12:92-97.
244. Torbenson M, Yeh MM, Abraham SC. Bile duct dysplasia in the setting of chronic hepatitis C and alcohol cirrhosis. Am J Surg Pathol 2007;31:1410-1413.
245. Terada T, Nakanuma Y, Ohta T, Nagakawa T. Histological features and interphase nucleolar organizer regions in hyperplastic, dysplastic and neoplastic epithelium of intrahepatic bile ducts in hepatolithiasis. Histopathology 1992;21:233-240.
246. Zen Y, Aishima S, Ajioka Y, et al. Proposal of histological criteria for intraepithelial atypical/proliferative biliary epithelial lesions of the bile duct in hepatolithiasis with respect to cholangiocarcinoma: preliminary report based on interobserver agreement. Pathol Int 2005;55:180-188.
247. Zen Y, Adsay NV, Bardadin K, et al. Biliary intraepithelial neoplasia: an international interobserver agreement study and proposal for diagnostic criteria. Mod Pathol 2007;20:701-709.
248. Aishima S, Nishihara Y, Tsujita E, et al. Biliary neoplasia with extensive intraductal spread associated with liver cirrhosis: a hitherto unreported variant of biliary intraepithelial neoplasia. Hum Pathol 2008;39:939-947.
249. Rougemont AL, Genevay M, McKee TA, Gremaud M, Mentha G, Rubbia-Brandt L. Extensive biliary intraepithelial neoplasia (BilIN) and multifocal early intrahepatic cholangiocarcinoma in non-biliary cirrhosis. Virchows Arch 2010;456:711-717.
250. Kerr SE, Barr Fritcher EG, Campion MB, et al. Biliary dysplasia in primary sclerosing cholangitis harbors cytogenetic abnormalities similar to cholangiocarcinoma. Hum Pathol 2014;45:1797-1804.
251. Hsu M, Sasaki M, Igarashi S, Sato Y, Nakanuma Y. KRAS and GNAS mutations and p53 overexpression in biliary intraepithelial neoplasia and intrahepatic cholangiocarcinomas. Cancer 2013;119:1669-1674.
252. Song JS, Lee YJ, Kim KW, Huh J, Jang SJ, Yu E. Cholangiocarcinoma arising in von Meyenburg complexes: report of four cases. Pathol Int 2008;58:503-512.
253. Roskams T. Liver stem cells and their implication in hepatocellular and cholangiocarcinoma. Oncogene 2006;25:3818-3822.
254. Sekiya S, Suzuki A. Intrahepatic cholangiocarcinoma can arise from Notch-mediated conversion of hepatocytes. J Clin Invest 2012;122:3914-3918.

8 COMBINED HEPATOCELLULAR-CHOLANGIOCARCINOMA

Combined hepatocellular-cholangiocarcinoma is a primary malignant epithelial neoplasm of the liver that contains components of both classic hepatocellular carcinoma and intrahepatic cholangiocarcinoma. It has several synonyms, including *hepatocholangiocarcinoma, biphenotypic hepatocellular carcinoma-cholangiocarcinoma,* and *mixed hepatocellular carcinoma-cholangiocarcinoma*. The most recent World Health Organization (WHO) Classification of Tumours of the Digestive System (1) defines this entity as an intimately mixed neoplasm with unequivocal components of both hepatocellular carcinoma and cholangiocarcinoma in the same tumor, but not two separate tumors either in the same liver or simply adjacent to each other.

Combined hepatocellular-cholangiocarcinoma is further subclassified into classic combined hepatocellular-cholangiocarcinoma or combined hepatocellular-cholangiocarcinoma with stem cell features (three subtypes: typical, intermediate cell, and cholangiolocellular) (Table 8-1) (1). Currently it is unclear whether to separate combined hepatocellular-cholangiocarcinoma with stem cell features as a unique subtype, but it is included here for completeness. In addition to a distinct component of hepatocellular carcinoma and a separate distinct component of cholangiocarcinoma, cases with stem cell features have additional features that suggest stem "cellness" in either or both components, either by morphology or by immunohistochemical stains.

Table 8-1

WORLD HEALTH ORGANIZATION (WHO) DEFINITIONS FOR COMBINED HEPATOCELLULAR-CHOLANGIOCARCINOMA WITH STEM CELL FEATURES

Subtype	H&E[a] and Immunohistochemical Features
Typical	Core histology: nests of tumor cells resemble mature hepatocytes with mild to moderate cytologic atypia, besides components of hepatocellular carcinoma and cholangiocarcinoma. These nests have a peripheral rim of smaller cells with a high nuclear to cytoplasmic ratio and hyperchromatic nuclei. Stains: nests of mature cells are positive for usual markers of hepatocytic differentiation. The peripheral cells but not the nests of mature cells are positive for CK7, CK19, and often CD56/NCAM1, c-Kit, and EpCAM. Other features: intratumoral fibrosis can be striking
Intermediate cell	Core histology: on morphology it is difficult to distinguish whether the tumor cells are hepatocytic or biliary. They are small and oval with mild cytologic atypia. Moderate atypia can be focally present. The tumor growth patterns are variable and can show solid nests, trabeculae, or thin cords with elongated and equivocal gland like structures. Stains: coexpression of markers of hepatocytic and biliary differentiation, e.g., HepPar1, α-fetoprotein, CK19, and polyclonal CEA. c-Kit expression is common. Mucicarmine is negative. Other features: intratumoral fibrosis can be striking
Cholangiolocellular	Core histology: resembles cholangiocarcinoma. The tumor cells are small cells with a high nuclear to cytoplasmic ratio but mild cytologic atypia. The tumor grows with a branching, anastomosing cord and antler-like pattern. Small tubular structures can be seen. Stains: tumor cells are positive for CK19, CK7, CD56/NCAM1, c-Kit, and EpCAM but negative for makers of hepatocytic differentiation such as HepPar1 and arginase-1. Other features: intratumoral fibrosis can be striking.

[a]H&E = hematoxylin and eosin; CEA = carcinoembryonic antigen.

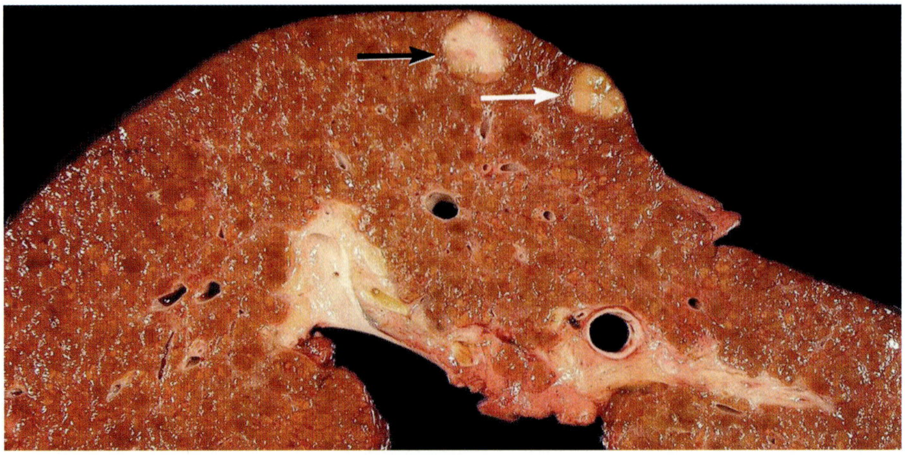

Figure 8-1

SEPARATE PRIMARY TUMORS

This cirrhotic liver contains two separate tumors: a yellowish, lobulated and soft hepatocellular carcinoma on the right (white arrow), and a white, infiltrative and firm cholangiocarcinoma on the left (black arrow). These are not considered as combined hepatocellular-cholangiocarcinoma.

GENERAL AND CLINICAL FEATURES

Combined hepatocellular-cholangiocarcinoma was first described and reviewed in detail by Allen and Lisa in 1949 (2). The first large series using immunohistochemistry was published by Goodman et al. (3), who examined 24 cases in the mid-1980s. Both studies attempted to classify these neoplasms into subtypes. Type 1 tumor by Allen and Lisa and type I tumor designated by Goodman et al. appear to be separate primary tumors (separate hepatocellular carcinoma and cholangiocarcinoma coincidentally found in the same liver) (fig. 8-1), currently excluded as combined hepatocellular-cholangiocarcinoma by the hepatopathology community including the WHO. The subtype with an intermingling of hepatocellular and cholangiocarcinoma elements, classified as type 3 tumor by Allen and Lisa and subsequently defined by Goodman et al. as type II (transitional) neoplasm, is the neoplasm of focus in this chapter.

Most of the intermingled type tumors in the above studies arose in cirrhotic livers. Subsequent studies also showed that combined hepatocellular-cholangiocarcinomas commonly arise in patients with underlying liver disease and advanced fibrosis (4,5). Cirrhosis, however, is not a prerequisite for combined hepatocellular-cholangiocarcinoma and it may also arise in the noncirrhotic liver. In fact, the prevalence of background cirrhosis in combined hepatocellular-cholangiocarcinoma varies among different studies, which may be the result of different patient populations as well as the diagnostic criteria (6,7). Likewise, the underlying cause of liver disease, such as chronic hepatitis B or hepatitis C infection, also varies among different studies and this may be at least partially explained by the different geographic regions and diagnostic criteria used in each study. Recently, cases of combined hepatocellular-cholangiocarcinoma in patients after tumor treatment, such as transarterial chemoembolization, have been increasingly observed (8,9).

Preoperative biopsies frequently misdiagnose these tumors as either hepatocellular carcinomas or cholangiocarcinomas (10). This is largely attributed to sampling error, when only one component is in the biopsy specimen. In a study by Lee et al. (11), patients with combined hepatocellular-cholangiocarcinoma had lower levels of serum bilirubin and alkaline phosphatase when compared with patients with cholangiocarcinoma alone.

Early studies estimated the frequency of combined hepatocellular-cholangiocarcinoma to be up to 5 percent of primary liver carcinomas, but more recent and larger studies show a frequency closer to 1 percent (12–15), possibly because of the stricter diagnostic criteria used in recent years. Lee et al. (11) showed a greater prevalence in male patients when compared with cholangiocarcinoma. In a review of 465 patients with combined hepatocellular-cholangiocarcinoma using the Surveillance, Epidemiology, and End Results (SEER) database, analyzed during the period between 1988 to 2009, the tumor was more common in patients who were white, male, and older than 65 years of age (12). Overall, the survival rates of patients with combined hepatocellular-cholangiocarcinoma are intermediate between those of patients with hepatocellular carcinoma and cholangiocarcinoma (12,16).

LABORATORY FINDINGS

Simultaneous elevation of both CA19-9 and alpha-fetoprotein (AFP) has been suggested as highly concerning for combined hepatocellular-cholangiocarcinoma (17). One study found serum AFP levels were greater than 200 ng/mL in 40 percent of cases and CA19-9 was elevated in 48 percent of cases (18). In another study, both tumor markers were elevated in about 50 percent of cases (19). Elevated CA19-9 levels indicate a worse prognosis (13,18), with a dose-effect curve seen in one study (13).

ETIOLOGY

Cumulated data suggest hepatobiliary stem cells as the cells of origin of combined hepatocellular-cholangiocarcinoma (20–23). This is based upon the combination of morphologic observation, showing cells have a range of differentiation, from stem-like cells through cells of intermediate morphology to cells of hepatocytic or cholangiocytic differentiation, and findings using immunohistochemical markers identifying progenitor cells within the tumor (24–30). Other theories have also been proposed, including collision tumors of hepatocellular carcinoma and cholangiocarcinoma that incidentally coexist in the same liver. Given that both carcinoma elements intermingle with each other in a transitional area in most combined hepatocellular-cholangiocarcinomas, this hypothesis is less likely (31). Another theory is subsequent differentiation of hepatocellular carcinoma or cholangiocarcinoma into the other component. This postulation cannot be completely excluded in all cases, but seems less likely to be the general mechanism for combined tumors.

An earlier investigation using a genome-wide allelotyping assay has shown that recurrent loss of heterozygosity at 3p and 14q is common in both cholangiocarcinoma and combined hepatocellular-cholangiocarcinoma, while β-*catenin* mutation, a common mutation in hepatocellular carcinoma, was not observed, suggesting common pathways shared by combined hepatocellular-cholangiocarcinoma and cholangiocarcinoma (32). The demographic and clinical characteristics of the patients with combined hepatocellular-cholangiocarcinoma in this study, however, were intermediate to those of patients with hepatocellular carcinoma and cholangiocarcinoma, with a disproportionate male predilection (M:F = 14:1), more similar to patients with hepatocellular carcinoma than cholangiocarcinoma.

In one study (33), a single clonal tumor with a homogeneous genetic background in both the hepatocellular carcinoma and cholangiocarcinoma components of combined hepatocellular-cholangiocarcinoma was identified. This finding suggests that histologic diversity reflects the divergent differentiation potential of a single clone, or single clonal process (31,33). It thus strongly supports the hypothesis that combined hepatocellular-cholangiocarcinoma is derived from a single clone.

Another study by Yano et al. (34) demonstrated a primary cell line derived from resected combined hepatocellular-cholangiocarcinoma differentiated to not only show the phenotypic features of hepatocellular carcinoma but also those of cholangiocarcinoma, corroborating that a single clonally expanded tumor cell can give rise to both hepatocytic and biliary phenotypes. Some subsequent investigations further highlighted the hypothesis that at least a subset of combined hepatocellular-cholangiocarcinomas derive from hepatic progenitor cells (24,27,35).

Theise et al. (24) showed that cells morphologically and immunohistochemically resembling hepatic progenitor cells merged with the hepatocellular carcinoma and cholangiocarcinoma components and with mature-appearing hepatocytes within combined hepatocellular-cholangiocarcinoma, supporting the concept that carcinogenesis of this unique neoplasm may be attributed to the malignant transformation of the hepatic progenitor cells.

Later investigations have revealed that genes associated with stem cells are enriched in combined hepatocellular-cholangiocarcinoma (36). This suggests an association of stem cellness in combined hepatocellular-cholangiocarcinoma (37).

GROSS FINDINGS

Grossly, combined hepatocellular-cholangiocarcinomas are in part similar to hepatocellular carcinomas, which are soft and bulge out from the cut surface of the liver, and in part similar

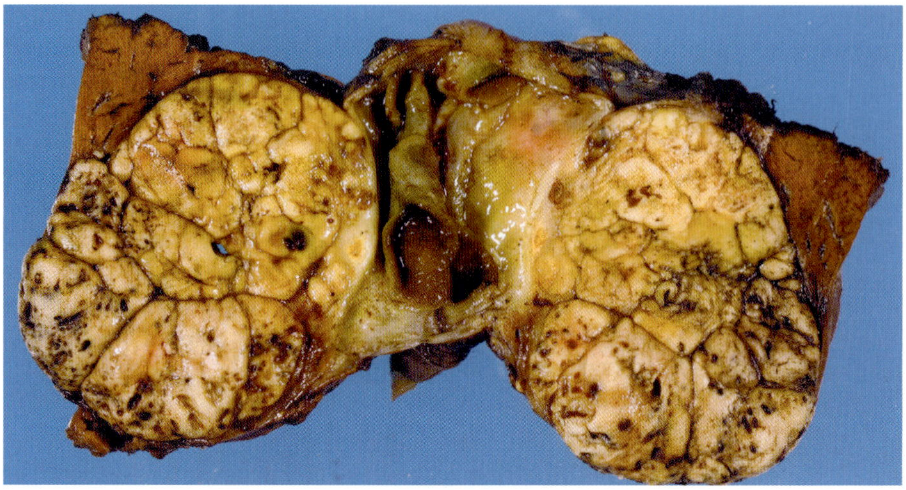

Figure 8-2

COMBINED HEPATOCELLULAR-CHOLANGIOCARCINOMA

A well-circumscribed, lobulated tumor with a soft, tan appearance is present in a background of noncirrhotic liver.

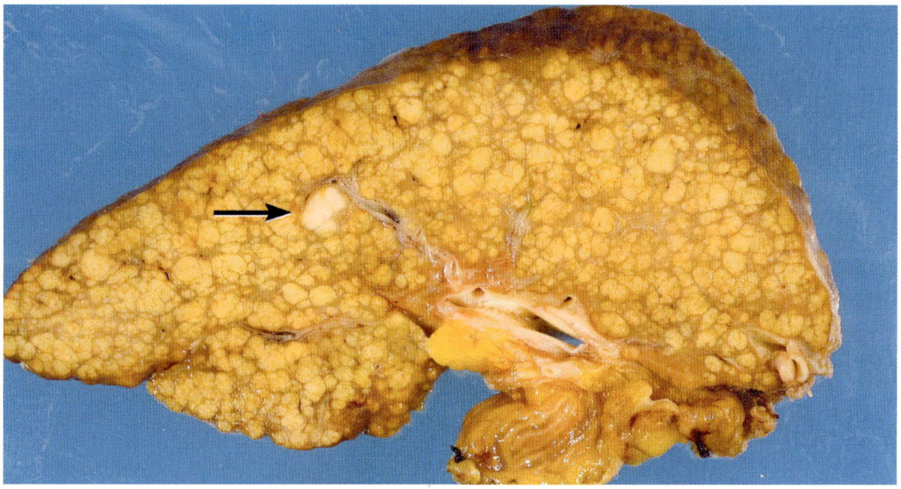

Figure 8-3

COMBINED HEPATOCELLULAR-CHOLANGIOCARCINOMA

A whitish firm tumor (arrow) containing both hepatocellular carcinoma and cholangiocarcinoma components is incidentally found in an explanted cirrhotic liver.

to cholangiocarcinomas, which are fibrotic and firm (figs. 8-2, 8-3).

MICROSCOPIC FINDINGS

Combined hepatocellular-cholangiocarcinoma arises in both cirrhotic and noncirrhotic livers (13). The definitive diagnosis can only be established by histopathology. By definition, classic combined hepatocellular-cholangiocarcinomas have two distinct and separate morphologies (fig. 8-4). The tumors can be multifocal (10 to 30 percent of cases) or unifocal (70 to 90 percent of cases) (14,38,39), but to qualify for the diagnosis of a combined hepatocellular-cholangiocarcinoma, the tumor should have both components in one nodule or in immediately adjacent nodules. The two morphologies should be in direct contact with each other, commonly with a thin transition zone, an interface in which these two components intermingle intimately with each other (fig. 8-5). Outside of the transition zone, the morphologies are histologically distinct, with one looking like hepatocellular carcinoma and the other like cholangiocarcinoma. The morphology should be distinctive enough to strongly suggest the diagnosis of combined hepatocellular-cholangiocarcinoma on hematoxylin and eosin (H&E)-stained slides, but immunostains are important to confirm the H&E impression (figs. 8-6, 8-7).

The WHO further subtypes combined hepatocellular-cholangiocarcinomas with stem cell features based on their morphology and immunostain results (Table 8-1; figs. 8-8–8-10) (1). All of the subtypes share some features in common, including frequent dense intratumoral fibrosis.

The first two subtypes (typical subtype and intermediate cell subtype) show evidence of hepatocyte differentiation based on either morphologic findings or immunohistochemical results, while the third subtype (cholangiolocellular subtype) is fundamentally a cholangiocarcinoma that stains with some markers suggestive of stem cell origin, although occasionally there can be foci at the periphery that appear more hepatoid.

These stem cell like patterns have been challenging to implement in studies (40) since they may coexist in different combination and their terminologies are cumbersome and will likely need to be refined to increase their usefulness. In some cases, this terminology has been applied to conventional hepatocellular carcinomas that had some features of stem cellness, as well as cholangiocarcinomas with some features of stem cellness, regardless of whether they were truly combined tumors with distinct components of hepatocellular carcinoma and cholangiocarcinoma. Thus, many of the cases reported in the literature under the rubric of combined hepatocellular-cholangiocarcinoma

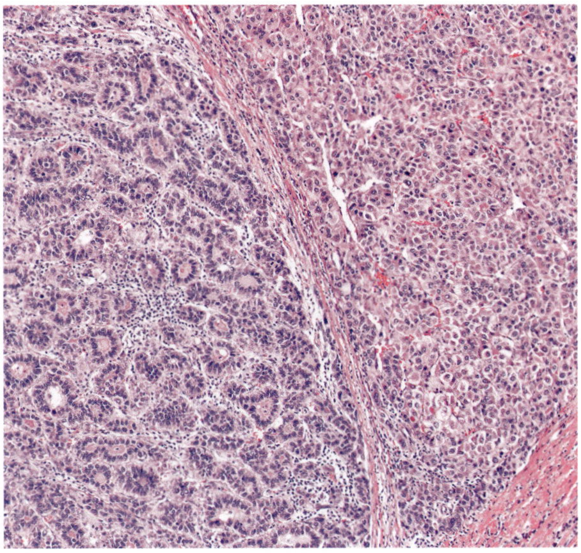

Figure 8-4

COMBINED HEPATOCELLULAR-CHOLANGIOCARCINOMA: CLASSIC TYPE

The cholangiocarcinoma component with neoplastic glands is evident on the left, while the hepatocellular carcinoma component is on the right of the image.

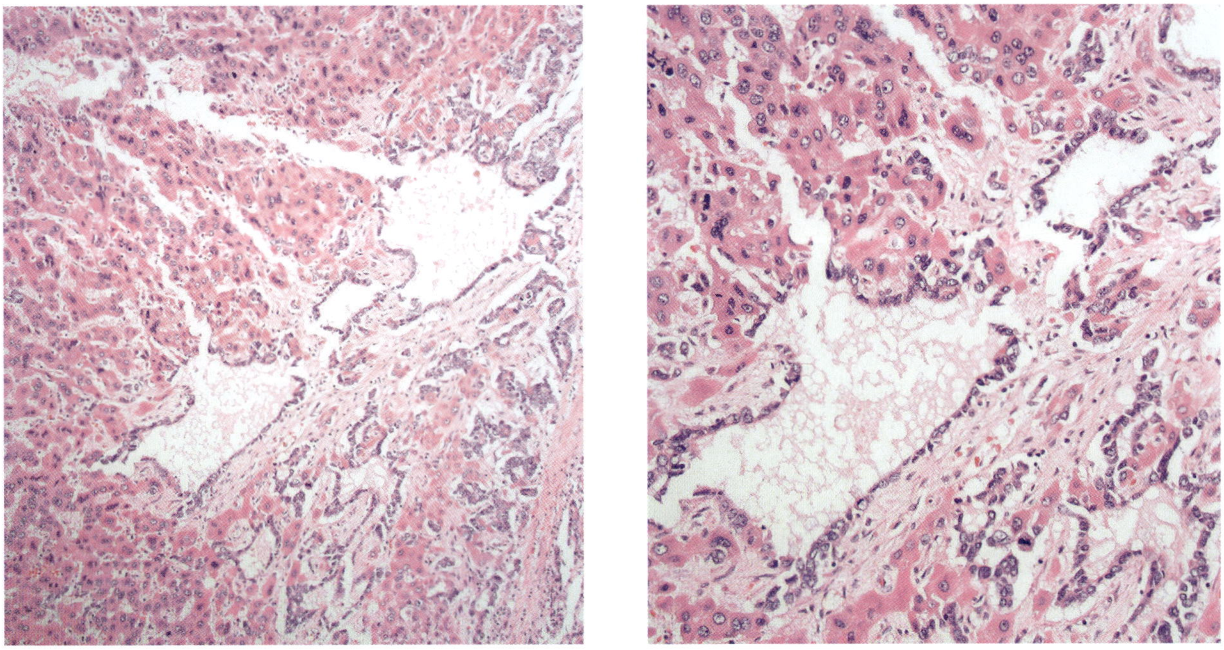

Figure 8-5

COMBINED HEPATOCELLULAR-CHOLANGIOCARCINOMA: CLASSIC TYPE

The hepatocellular carcinoma component with trabecular structures is on the upper left side, while the cholangiocarcinoma component with glandular structures is on the lower right (left), and they intermingle with each other intimately in the transitional area (right).

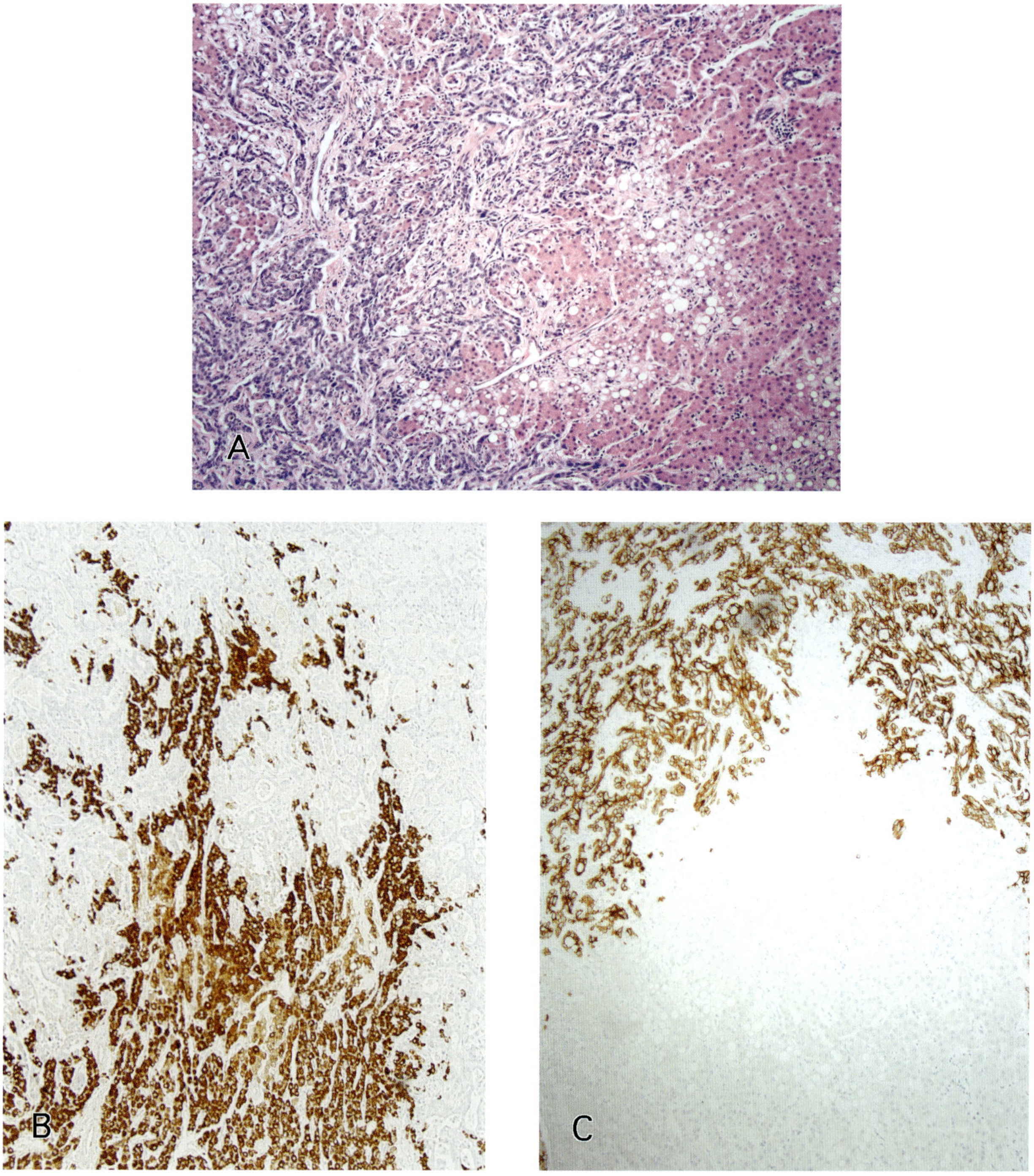

Figure 8-6

COMBINED HEPATOCELLULAR-CHOLANGIOCARCINOMA: CLASSIC TYPE

A: The hepatocellular carcinoma component (on the right side) and the cholangiocarcinoma component (on the left side) intermingle with each other in the transitional area.

B: Immunohistochemical staining for HepPar1 is positive in the hepatocellular carcinoma component on the bottom, and negative in the cholangiocarcinoma component on the top.

C: Immunohistochemical staining for CK19 is positive in the cholangiocarcinoma component at the top, and negative in the hepatocellular carcinoma component on the bottom.

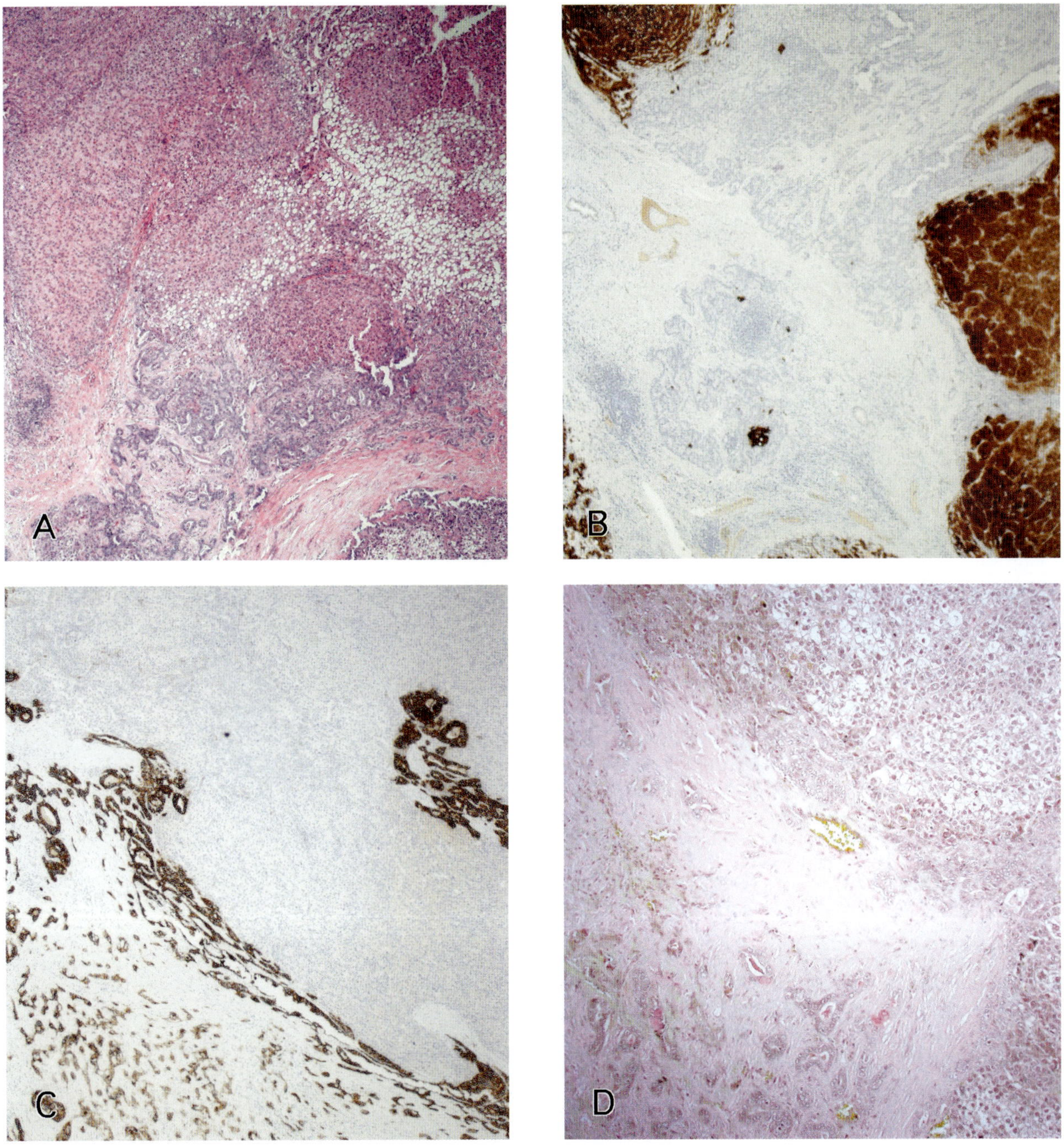

Figure 8-7

COMBINED HEPATOCELLULAR-CHOLANGIOCARCINOMA: CLASSIC TYPE

A: The hepatocellular carcinoma component and the cholangiocarcinoma component (lower right) intermingle in the transitional area. Fatty change is seen in the hepatocellular carcinoma component and desmoplastic stroma in the cholangiocarcinoma component.

B: Immunohistochemical staining for arginase 1 is positive in the hepatocellular carcinoma component, and negative in the cholangiocarcinoma component.

C: Immunohistochemical staining for MOC31 is positive in the cholangiocarcinoma component, but negative in the hepatocellular carcinoma component.

D: A mucin stain is positive in the cholangiocarcinoma component, but negative in the hepatocellular carcinoma component.

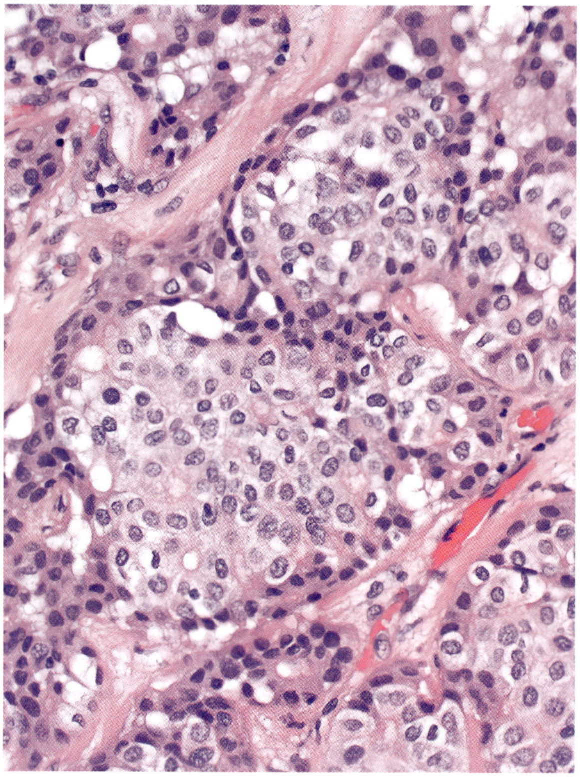

Figure 8-8

COMBINED HEPATOCELLULAR-CHOLANGIOCARCINOMA WITH STEM CELL FEATURES

Subtype 1 (typical subtype) shows nests of tumor cells surrounded by a thin rim of smaller and more basophilic cells. The cells in the center of the tumor nests stain with hepatocytic markers; those on the periphery less so, but they also stain with some putative stem cell markers.

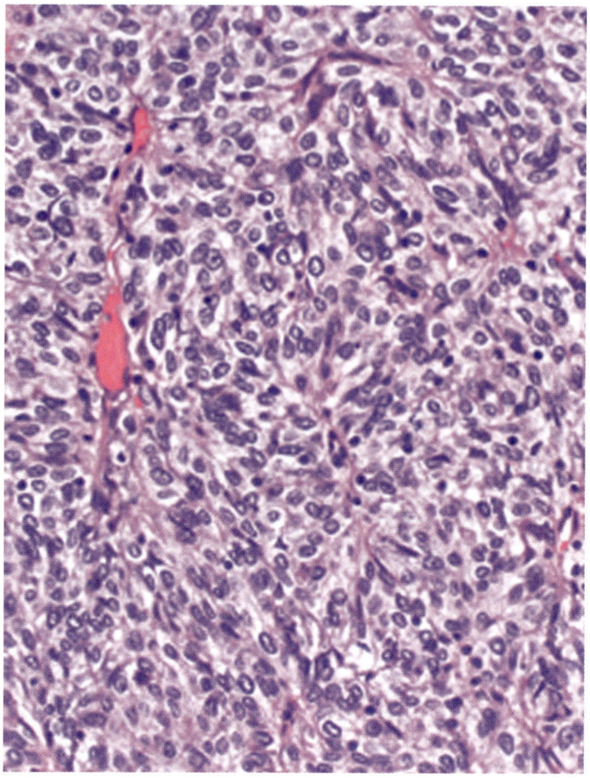

Figure 8-9

COMBINED HEPATOCELLULAR-CHOLANGIOCARCINOMA, WITH STEM CELL FEATURES

The subtype 2 (intermediate cell subtype) shows small basophilic cells that are difficult to classify, but the tumor stains primarily with hepatocytic markers.

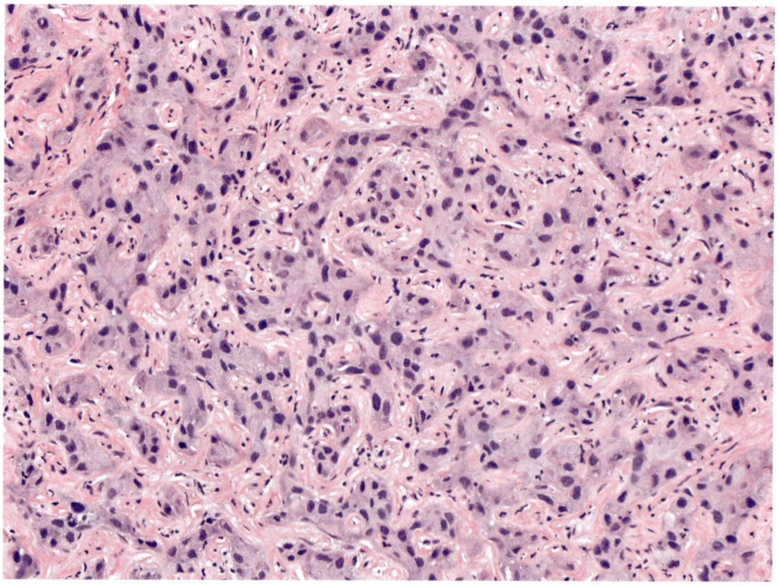

Figure 8-10

COMBINED HEPATOCELLULAR-CHOLANGIOCARCINOMA WITH STEM CELL FEATURES

Subtype 3 (cholangiolocellular subtype) is arranged in a tubular, "antler-like" pattern with dense fibrous stroma. It looks and stains like a cholangiocarcinoma. There can be some peripheral areas of tumor growth that look more like hepatocellular carcinoma.

with stem cell features do not have the classic combined hepatocellular-cholangiocarcinoma morphology: one component with hepatocellular carcinoma and one with cholangiocarcinoma. Instead, most are either all hepatocellular carcinomas or all cholangiocarcinomas, but have morphologic or immunostain findings that suggest stem cellness.

CYTOLOGIC FINDINGS

Combined hepatocellular-cholangiocarcinoma may be diagnosed in fine-needle aspiration specimens when correlated with clinical, imaging, and histologic findings. The cytology specimen shows distinct hepatocellular carcinoma cells, which are arranged in cohesive cords recapitulating anastomosing hepatocellular trabeculae, and cohesive columnar adenocarcinoma cells that show nuclear palisading arranged in papillary or glandular structures (fig. 8-11). Mucin production may be evident within the cytoplasm or glandular structures. Intermediate cells, when present, show mixed cytologic features bordering between hepatocellular carcinoma and cholangiocarcinoma cells. Immunohistochemical stains may be useful (41–43).

IMMUNOHISTOCHEMICAL FINDINGS

The immunohistochemical profiles of the different components of combined hepatocellular-cholangiocarcinomas should correlate with their morphology. The hepatocellular carcinoma component is positive for markers of hepatocytic differentiation such as HepPar1 (fig. 8-6B), arginase 1 (fig. 8-7B), glypican 3, and albumin by in situ hybridization. None of these stains is 100 percent specific and positivity has also been reported in cholangiocarcinoma (44–46). The use of multiple stains may be necessary, with prudent correlation with morphology, to arrive at an accurate diagnosis. The demonstration of a canalicular staining pattern using polyclonal carcinoembryonic antigen (CEA) or CD10 may be helpful in some instances, but the sensitivity is not optimal, and the interpretation needs experience. The cholangiocarcinoma component is typically negative for hepatocytic markers and positive for biliary type keratins, such as CK19 (fig. 8-6C). A positive mucicarmine stain in the neoplastic glands supports an adenocarcinoma component (fig. 8-7D).

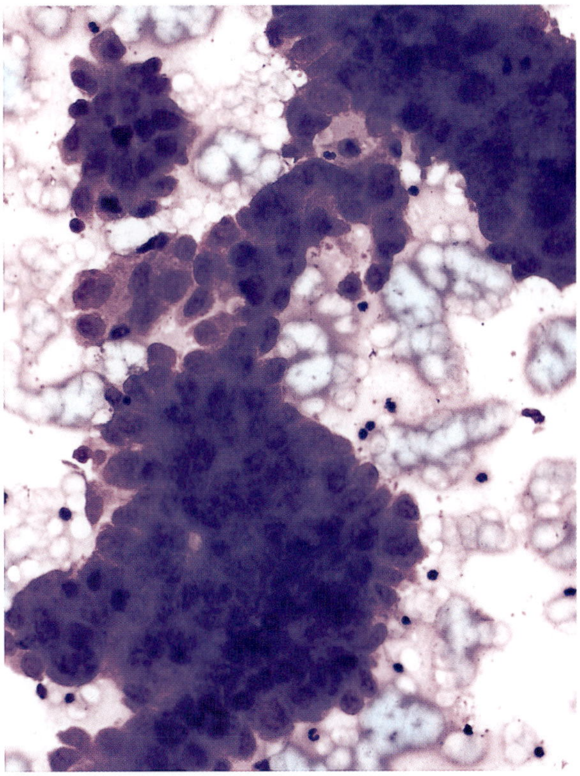

Figure 8-11

COMBINED HEPATOCELLULAR CHOLANGIOCARCINOMA

Fine-needle aspiration of combined hepatocellular-cholangiocarcinoma shows cohesive pleomorphic tumor cells that are arranged in broad tongues with a vague suggestion of an acinus. The tumor cells are generally polygonal and display round central nuclei with nuclear contour irregularities, high nuclear to cytoplasmic ratio, and a small to moderate amount of cytoplasm. No peripheral endothelium or nuclear palisading is discernible. The cells are from a transitional area of a combined hepatocellular-cholangiocarcinoma and they exhibit cytologic features hybrid between classic malignant hepatocytes and adenocarcinoma cells (May-Grunwald Giemsa stain). (Courtesy of Professor Aileen Wee, Singapore.)

There are several important diagnostic pitfalls when making a diagnosis of combined hepatocellular-cholangiocarcinoma, the most important of which is making this diagnosis based on immunohistochemical findings alone, without having separate and distinctive morphologies on the H&E stain. In this regard, an otherwise conventional hepatocellular carcinoma should not be diagnosed as combined hepatocellular-cholangiocarcinoma solely because there is positive staining for keratins that are normally

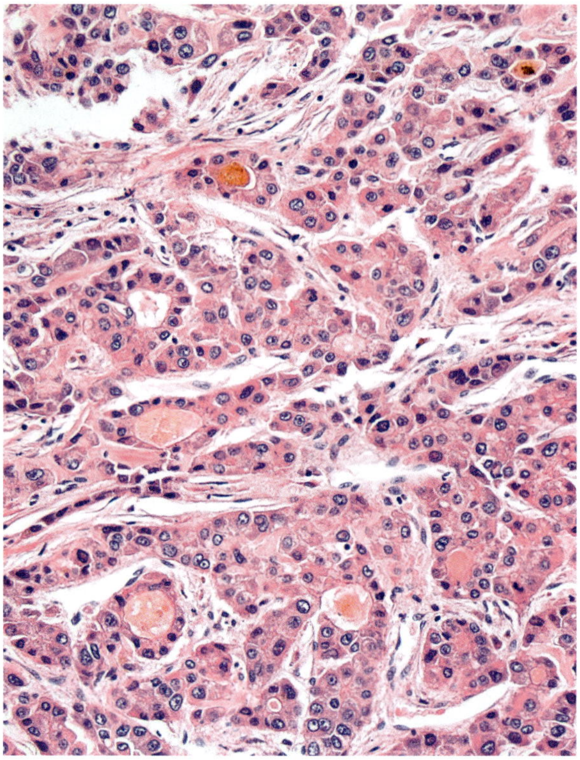

Figure 8-12

PSEUDOGLANDS IN HEPATOCELLULAR CARCINOMA

Prominent pseudoglands or pseudoacini in hepatocellular carcinoma may mimic the cholangiocarcinoma component and be misdiagnosed as a combined hepatocellular-cholangiocarcinoma. The presence of bile or proteinaceous material within the pseudoglands helps to distinguish them from the mucin within true neoplastic glands in cholangiocarcinoma.

expressed in the biliary tree, such as CK19 or CK7, as a significant number of hepatocellular carcinomas stain for these markers (28,47,48).

ULTRASTRUCTURAL FINDINGS

Electron microscopy is rarely or almost never used for the diagnosis of combined hepatocellular-cholangiocarcinoma. It may show dual differentiation in different neoplastic cells within the same acini, such as bile canaliculi and abundant organelles (lipid droplets, rough endoplasmic reticulum, mitochondria, and abundant glycogen—characteristic of hepatocytic differentiation), and microvillus projections at the luminal surface or junctional complexes between the neoplastic cells (features of biliary differentiation) (49).

MOLECULAR GENETIC FINDINGS

Mutational analysis has shown that combined hepatocellular-cholangiocarcinomas have various types of mutations, which may be attributed to different etiologies, underlying liver diseases, and diagnostic criteria adopted (33,36,50). Currently, molecular studies are not useful in making the diagnosis of combined hepatocellular-cholangiocarcinoma or predicting its prognosis.

DIFFERENTIAL DIAGNOSIS

Combined hepatocellular-cholangiocarcinomas need to be distinguished from conventional hepatocellular carcinomas and cholangiocarcinomas. Prominent pseudoglands or pseudoacini (fig. 8-12) are commonly seen in conventional hepatocellular carcinoma. They should not be mistaken for the true glandular structures in cholangiocarcinomas and hence misclassified as combined hepatocellular-cholangiocarcinoma. The proteinaceous material within the pseudoglandular structures may also be confused with mucin and thus mistaken as the cholangiocarcinoma component in combined hepatocellular-cholangiocarcinoma. Recognizing that pseudoglands can be prominent will prevent most of these diagnostic errors, but positive immunostains for HepPar1 or arginase 1 are helpful.

The expression of biliary markers such as CK7 and CK19 in conventional hepatocellular carcinoma is common and therefore a diagnosis solely based on immunohistochemistry alone should not be made. Morphologic diagnosis remains the key, with careful interpretation of the immunohistochemical stains (28,47,48). A marked bile ductular reaction (fig. 8-13) adjacent to hepatocellular carcinoma owing to mass effect, is common, and caution should be taken not to interpret these ductules as the cholangiocarcinoma component in combined hepatocellular-cholangiocarcinoma. Unfortunately, immunohistochemistry is not routinely helpful in distinguishing malignant biliary epithelium from reacting ductules. In general, a ductular reaction is commonly accompanied by an inflammatory cell infiltrate and is not mass forming, while the cholangiocarcinoma component in combined hepatocellular-cholangiocarcinoma is usually surrounded by a desmoplastic stroma that lacks inflammatory cells and is mass forming (fig. 8-7A) (31).

SPREAD AND METASTASES

The rate of regional lymph node disease at presentation varies from 5 to 30 percent in various studies (10,12). The overall frequency of lymph node metastases is between that of hepatocellular carcinoma and cholangiocarcinoma (12). One study found regional lymph node metastases in 2 percent of hepatocellular carcinomas, 13 percent of combined hepatocellular-cholangiocarcinomas, and 21 percent of cholangiocarcinomas (38). Combined hepatocellular-cholangiocarcinomas also more often present with distant spread than hepatocellular carcinoma (51).

STAGING AND TREATMENT

Combined hepatocellular-cholangiocarcinomas are staged in the current American Joint Committee on Cancer (AJCC) system using the cholangiocarcinoma protocol (52). However, these tumors are sufficiently biologically distinct from both hepatocellular carcinoma and cholangiocarcinoma that a unique staging system should be considered in the future.

Surgical resection remains the sole treatment choice to potentially cure localized combined hepatocellular-cholangiocarcinoma, particularly in patients with cirrhosis. The risk of recurrence may be greater than that for hepatocellular carcinoma (7,53–55). Recent studies showed that the prognosis of patients with combined hepatocellular-cholangiocarcinomas undergoing liver transplantation was comparable to the prognosis of patients undergoing hepatic resection (56–58), although the outcome may be worse if there is a major component of cholangiocarcinoma (58).

Due to its rarity and lack of uniformed diagnostic criteria, there are no standard systemic or loco-regional treatment modalities for recurrent or metastatic combined hepatocellular-cholangiocarcinoma (55). There are yet unmet needs to develop targeted therapies for this unique tumor.

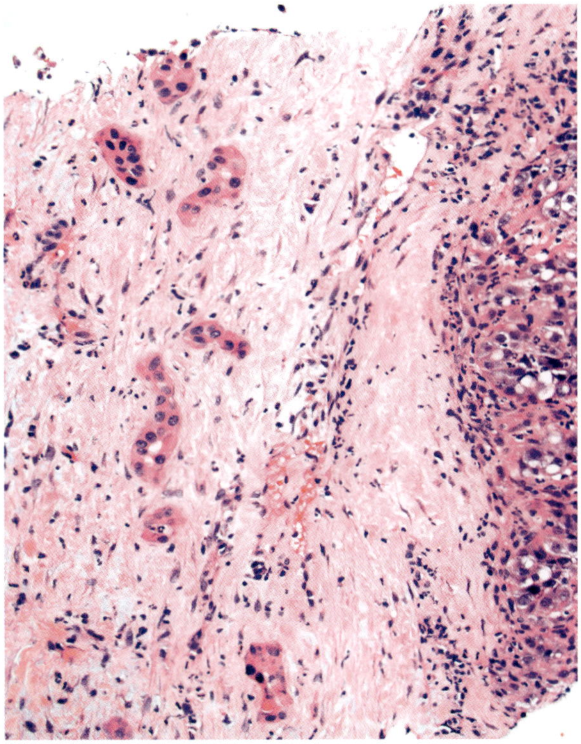

Figure 8-13

BILE DUCTULAR REACTION

A bile ductular reaction with mild cytological reactive atypia owing to mass effect (left side) adjacent to hepatocellular carcinoma (right side). This finding may mimic the cholangiocarcinoma component in combined hepatocellular-cholangiocarcinoma.

PROGNOSIS

The prognosis for patients with combined hepatocellular-cholangiocarcinoma is better than that for those with cholangiocarcinoma and worse than that for those with hepatocellular carcinoma (31,51,54). Combined hepatocellular-cholangiocarcinomas have a high risk for recurrence after resection (10) and a high risk for early tumor recurrence after liver transplantation, particularly in the first year (59). They are also more likely than hepatocellular carcinomas to metastasize to lymph nodes (38). Lymph node disease primarily shows the cholangiocarcinoma component.

REFERENCES

1. Theise ND, Park Y, Nakanuma Y. Combined hepatocellular-cholangiocarcinoma. In: Bosman FT, F. C, Hruban RH, Theise ND, eds. WHO classification of tumours of the digestive System, 4th ed. Lyon: IARC Press; 2010:225-227.
2. Allen RA, Lisa JR. Combined liver cell and bile duct carcinoma. Am J Pathol 1949;25:647-655.
3. Goodman ZD, Ishak KG, Langloss JM, Sesterhenn IA, Rabin L. Combined hepatocellular-cholangiocarcinoma. A histologic and immunohistochemical study. Cancer 1985;55:124-135.
4. Aoki K, Takayasu K, Kawano T, et al. Combined hepatocellular carcinoma and cholangiocarcinoma: clinical features and computed tomographic findings. Hepatology 1993;18:1090-1095.
5. Sempoux C, Fan C, Singh P, et al. Cholangiolocellular carcinoma: an innocent-looking malignant liver tumor mimicking ductular reaction. Semin Liver Dis 2011;31:104-110.
6. Maeda T, Adachi E, Kajiyama K, Sugimachi K, Tsuneyoshi M. Combined hepatocellular and cholangiocarcinoma: proposed criteria according to cytokeratin expression and analysis of clinicopathologic features. Hum Pathol 1995;26:956-964.
7. Jarnagin WR, Weber S, Tickoo SK, et al. Combined hepatocellular and cholangiocarcinoma: demographic, clinical, and prognostic factors. Cancer 2002;94:2040-2046.
8. Nishihara Y, Aishima S, Kuroda Y, et al. Biliary phenotype of hepatocellular carcinoma after preoperative transcatheter arterial chemoembolization. J Gastroenterol Hepatol 2008;23:1860-1868.
9. Zen C, Zen Y, Mitry RR, et al. Mixed phenotype hepatocellular carcinoma after transarterial chemoembolization and liver transplantation. Liver Transpl 2011;17:943-954.
10. Yap AQ, Chen CL, Yong CC, et al. Clinicopathological factors impact the survival outcome following the resection of combined hepatocellular carcinoma and cholangiocarcinoma. Surg Oncol 2013;22:55-60.
11. Lee CC, Wu CY, Chen JT, Chen GH. Comparing combined hepatocellular-cholangiocarcinoma and cholangiocarcinoma: a clinicopathological study. Hepatogastroenterology 2002;49:1487-1490.
12. Garancini M, Goffredo P, Pagni F, et al. Combined hepatocellular-cholangiocarcinoma: a population-level analysis of an uncommon primary liver tumor. Liver Transpl 2014;20:952-959.
13. Chu KJ, Lu CD, Dong H, Fu XH, Zhang HW, Yao XP. Hepatitis B virus-related combined hepatocellular-cholangiocarcinoma: clinicopathological and prognostic analysis of 390 cases. Eur J Gastroenterol Hepatol 2014;26:192-199.
14. Groeschl RT, Turaga KK, Gamblin TC. Transplantation versus resection for patients with combined hepatocellular carcinoma-cholangiocarcinoma. J Surg Oncol 2013;107:608-612.
15. Wang J, Wang F, Kessinger A. Outcome of combined hepatocellular and cholangiocarcinoma of the liver. J Oncol 2010;2010.
16. Lee WS, Lee KW, Heo JS, et al. Comparison of combined hepatocellular and cholangiocarcinoma with hepatocellular carcinoma and intrahepatic cholangiocarcinoma. Surg Today 2006;36:892-897.
17. Tang D, Nagano H, Nakamura M, et al. Clinical and pathological features of Allen's type C classification of resected combined hepatocellular and cholangiocarcinoma: a comparative study with hepatocellular carcinoma and cholangiocellular carcinoma. J Gastrointest Surg 2006;10:987-998.
18. Kim KH, Lee SG, Park EH, et al. Surgical treatments and prognoses of patients with combined hepatocellular carcinoma and cholangiocarcinoma. Ann Surg Oncol 2009;16:623-629.
19. Li R, Yang D, Tang CL, et al. Combined hepatocellular carcinoma and cholangiocarcinoma (biphenotypic) tumors: clinical characteristics, imaging features of contrast-enhanced ultrasound and computed tomography. BMC Cancer 2016;16:158.
20. Theise ND, Saxena R, Portmann BC, et al. The canals of Hering and hepatic stem cells in humans. Hepatology 1999;30:1425-1433.
21. Falkowski O, An HJ, Ianus IA, et al. Regeneration of hepatocyte 'buds' in cirrhosis from intrabiliary stem cells. J Hepatol 2003;39:357-364.
22. Kofman AV, Morgan G, Kirschenbaum A, et al. Dose- and time-dependent oval cell reaction in acetaminophen-induced murine liver injury. Hepatology 2005;41:1252-1261.
23. Kuwahara R, Kofman AV, Landis CS, Swenson ES, Barendswaard E, Theise ND. The hepatic stem cell niche: identification by label-retaining cell assay. Hepatology 2008;47:1994-2002.
24. Theise ND, Yao JL, Harada K, et al. Hepatic 'stem cell' malignancies in adults: four cases. Histopathology 2003;43:263-271.
25. Wu PC, Lai VC, Fang JW, Gerber MA, Lai CL, Lau JY. Hepatocellular carcinoma expressing both hepatocellular and biliary markers also expresses cytokeratin 14, a marker of bipotential progenitor cells. J Hepatol 1999;31:965-966.

26. Kim H, Choi GH, Na DC, et al. Human hepatocellular carcinomas with "Stemness"-related marker expression: keratin 19 expression and a poor prognosis. Hepatology 2011;54:1707-1717.
27. Kim H, Park C, Han KH, et al. Primary liver carcinoma of intermediate (hepatocyte-cholangiocyte) phenotype. J Hepatol 2004;40:298-304.
28. Durnez A, Verslype C, Nevens F, et al. The clinicopathological and prognostic relevance of cytokeratin 7 and 19 expression in hepatocellular carcinoma. A possible progenitor cell origin. Histopathology 2006;49:138-151.
29. Zhang F, Chen XP, Zhang W, et al. Combined hepatocellular cholangiocarcinoma originating from hepatic progenitor cells: immunohistochemical and double-fluorescence immunostaining evidence. Histopathology 2008;52:224-232.
30. Yamashita T, Ji J, Budhu A, et al. EpCAM-positive hepatocellular carcinoma cells are tumor-initiating cells with stem/progenitor cell features. Gastroenterology 2009;136:1012-1024.
31. Yeh MM. Pathology of combined hepatocellular-cholangiocarcinoma. J Gastroenterol Hepatol 2010;25:1485-1492.
32. Cazals-Hatem D, Rebouissou S, Bioulac-Sage P, et al. Clinical and molecular analysis of combined hepatocellular-cholangiocarcinomas. J Hepatol 2004;41:292-298.
33. Fujii H, Zhu XG, Matsumoto T, et al. Genetic classification of combined hepatocellular-cholangiocarcinoma. Hum Pathol 2000;31:1011-1017.
34. Yano H, Iemura A, Haramaki M, et al. A human combined hepatocellular and cholangiocarcinoma cell line (KMCH-2) that shows the features of hepatocellular carcinoma or cholangiocarcinoma under different growth conditions. J Hepatol 1996;24:413-422.
35. Tanaka S, Yamamoto T, Tanaka H, et al. Potentiality of combined hepatocellular and intrahepatic cholangiocellular carcinoma originating from a hepatic precursor cell: Immunohistochemical evidence. Hepatol Res 2005;32:52-57.
36. Coulouarn C, Cavard C, Rubbia-Brandt L, et al. Combined hepatocellular-cholangiocarcinomas exhibit progenitor features and activation of Wnt and TGFbeta signaling pathways. Carcinogenesis 2012;33:1791-1796.
37. Kim GJ, Kim H, Park YN. Increased expression of Yes-associated protein 1 in hepatocellular carcinoma with stemness and combined hepatocellular-cholangiocarcinoma. PLoS One 2013;8:e75449.
38. Yin X, Zhang BH, Qiu SJ, et al. Combined hepatocellular carcinoma and cholangiocarcinoma: clinical features, treatment modalities, and prognosis. Ann Surg Oncol 2012;19:2869-2876.
39. Kim SH, Park YN, Lim JH, Choi GH, Choi JS, Kim KS. Characteristics of combined hepatocelluar-cholangiocarcinoma and comparison with intrahepatic cholangiocarcinoma. Eur J Surg Oncol 2014;40:976-981.
40. Yoon YI, Hwang S, Lee YJ, et al. Postresection outcomes of combined hepatocellular carcinoma-cholangiocarcinoma, hepatocellular carcinoma and intrahepatic cholangiocarcinoma. J Gastrointest Surg 2016;20:411-420.
41. Kilpatrick SE, Geisinger KR, Loggie BW, Hopkins MB 3rd. Cytomorphology of combined hepatocellular-cholangiocarcinoma in fine needle aspirates of the liver. A report of two cases. Acta Cytol 1993;37:943-947.
42. Dusenbery D. Combined hepatocellular-cholangiocarcinoma. Cytologic findings in four cases. Acta Cytol 1997;41:903-909.
43. Wee A, Nilsson B. Combined hepatocellular-cholangiocarcinoma. Diagnostic challenge in hepatic fine needle aspiration biopsy. Acta Cytol 1999;43:131-138.
44. Radwan NA, Ahmed NS. The diagnostic value of arginase-1 immunostaining in differentiating hepatocellular carcinoma from metastatic carcinoma and cholangiocarcinoma as compared to HepPar-1. Diagn Pathol 2012;7:149.
45. Krings G, Ramachandran R, Jain D, et al. Immunohistochemical pitfalls and the importance of glypican 3 and arginase in the diagnosis of scirrhous hepatocellular carcinoma. Mod Pathol 2013;26:782-791.
46. Ferrone CR, Ting DT, Shahid M, et al. The ability to diagnose intrahepatic cholangiocarcinoma definitively using novel branched DNA-enhanced albumin RNA in situ hybridization technology. Ann Surg Oncol 2016;23:290-296.
47. Klein WM, Molmenti EP, Colombani PM, et al. Primary liver carcinoma arising in people younger than 30 years. Am J Clin Pathol 2005;124:512-518.
48. Wu PC, Fang JW, Lau VK, Lai CL, Lo CK, Lau JY. Classification of hepatocellular carcinoma according to hepatocellular and biliary differentiation markers. Clinical and biological implications. Am J Pathol 1996;149:1167-1175.
49. Ng IO, Shek TW, Nicholls J, Ma LT. Combined hepatocellular-cholangiocarcinoma: a clinicopathological study. J Gastroenterol Hepatol 1998;13:34-40.
50. Sasaki M, Sato Y, Nakanuma Y. Mutational landscape of combined hepatocellular carcinoma and cholangiocarcinoma, and its clinicopathological significance. Histopathology 2017;70:423-434.
51. Wachtel MS, Zhang Y, Xu T, Chiriva-Internati M, Frezza EE. Combined hepatocellular cholangiocarcinomas; analysis of a large database. Clin Med Pathol 2008;1:43-47.

52. Aloia T, Pawlik T, Taouli B, Rubbia-Brandt L, Vauthey JN. AJCC Cancer Staging Manual. In: Amin M, Edge S, Greene F, et al., 8th ed. Switzerland: Springer; 2017:295-302.
53. Park H, Choi KH, Choi SB, et al. Clinicopathological characteristics in combined hepatocellular-cholangiocarcinoma: a single center study in Korea. Yonsei Med J 2011;52:753-760.
54. Lee JH, Chung GE, Yu SJ, et al. Long-term prognosis of combined hepatocellular and cholangiocarcinoma after curative resection comparison with hepatocellular carcinoma and cholangiocarcinoma. J Clin Gastroenterol 2011;45:69-75.
55. Chi M, Mikhitarian K, Shi C, Goff LW. Management of combined hepatocellular-cholangiocarcinoma: a case report and literature review. Gastrointest Cancer Res 2012;5:199-202.
56. Song S, Moon HH, Lee S, et al. Comparison between resection and transplantation in combined hepatocellular and cholangiocarcinoma. Transplant Proc 2013;45:3041-3046.
57. Jung DH, Hwang S, Song GW, et al. Longterm prognosis of combined hepatocellular carcinoma-cholangiocarcinoma following liver transplantation and resection. Liver Transpl 2017;23:330-341.
58. Wu CH, Yong CC, Liew EH, et al. Combined hepatocellular carcinoma and cholangiocarcinoma: diagnosis and prognosis after resection or transplantation. Transplant Proc 2016;48:1100-1104.
59. Park YH, Hwang S, Ahn CS, et al. Long-term outcome of liver transplantation for combined hepatocellular carcinoma and cholangiocarcinoma. Transplant Proc 2013;45:3038-3040.

9 MESENCHYMAL TUMORS AND TUMOR-LIKE LESIONS

Among the various mesenchymal neoplasms that develop in the liver, some are unique to this anatomic site (e.g., embryonal sarcoma), while others, including angiosarcoma and rhabdomyosarcoma, are almost identical to those neoplasms in other organs. One of the factors complicating the classification of hepatic mesenchymal tumors is the use of many similar names and synonyms. Despite the similarity in their names, infantile hemangioendothelioma completely differs from epithelioid hemangioendothelioma in its histologic appearance and degree of malignancy. Also, susceptible ages differ widely among neoplasms. Although there are exceptional cases, some conditions occur within particular age groups (fig. 9-1).

The first group of tumors described in this chapter is endothelial and perivascular neoplasms, followed by pediatric mesenchymal tumors, which preferentially affect children or teenagers. The last section mainly summarizes the liver manifestations of soft tissue neoplasms that develop in almost every organ system. A comprehensive review of the entities in the last group is beyond the scope of this chapter. Readers interested in these neoplasms may refer to the Armed Forces Institute of Pathology (AFIP) Fascicle, Tumors of the Soft Tissues or the World Health Organization (WHO) Classification of Tumours of Soft Tissue and Bone for their general morphologic, immunohistochemical, and ultrastructural features (1,2). Inflammatory pseudotumors are also incorporated in the last section.

VASCULAR AND PERIVASCULAR NEOPLASMS

Cavernous Hemangioma

Definition. *Cavernous hemangioma* is a benign endothelial neoplasm that forms dilated thin-walled blood vessels. Other diagnostic

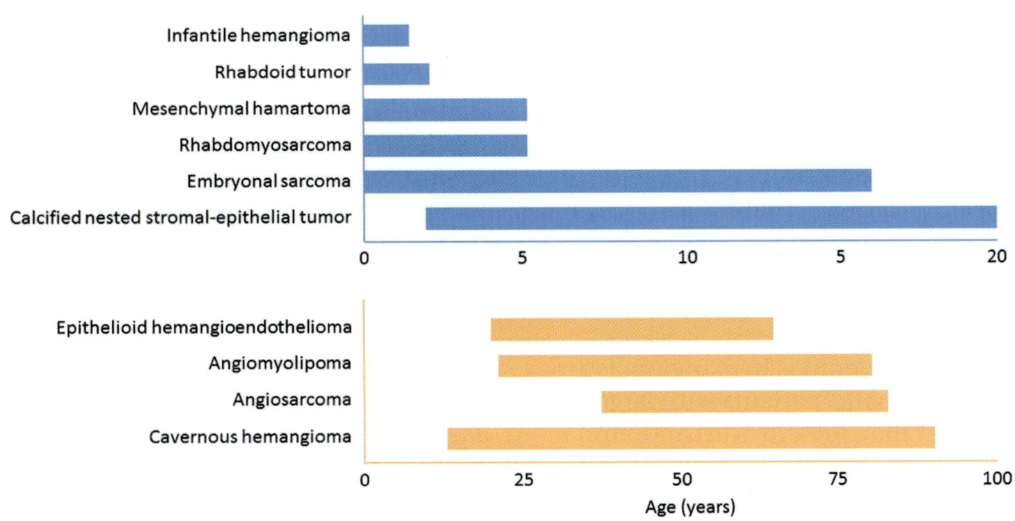

Figure 9-1

PRIMARY MESENCHYMAL TUMOR OF LIVER: PATIENT AGE

The upper chart indicates predilection ages of pediatric tumors, while the lower shows those of neoplasms that preferentially affect adults.

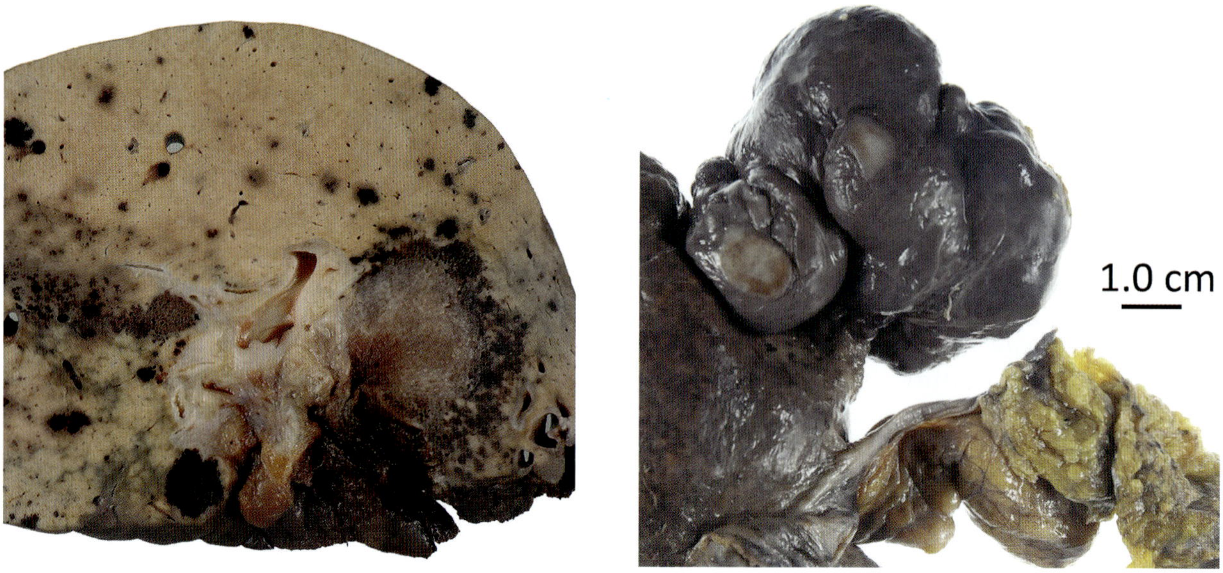

Figure 9-2

CAVERNOUS HEMANGIOMA

Left: Dark brown spots represent multiple foci of hemangioma.
Right: A polypoid tumor mass protrudes from the liver.

terms, including *sclerosing cavernous hemangioma, sclerosed hemangioma, giant hemangioma,* and *diffuse hemangiomatosis*, are used to characterize the various gross and microscopic appearances (3,4).

General and Clinical Features. This is the most common benign tumor of the liver (5). Its incidence ranges from less than 1 to 20 percent in autopsy series depending on how extensively the examination was performed (6). It occurs at all ages (mean age, 46 years), but is more common in young women. In a series of 114 cases of surgically resected hemangiomas, 76 percent occurred in women (7). However, this may be because hemangiomas tend to be larger in women and, thus, are more frequently diagnosed (4).

Although small cavernous hemangiomas are generally asymptomatic, patients with large tumors (over 4 cm) may present with abdominal pain. Other exceptional, but critical presentations are spontaneous rupture, acute thrombosis, and Kasabach-Merritt syndrome (8–10).

Cavernous hemangioma is typically solitary, but may be multiple in up to 10 percent of cases. Tumors may increase in size during pregnancy or in association with the use of estrogen. There is no known risk of malignant transformation. Surgical resection is only considered for large symptomatic tumors.

Gross Findings. The size of cavernous hemangioma varies widely from incidental microscopic lesions to huge tumors occupying most of the unilateral or bilateral liver lobes. Tumors greater than 10 cm in diameter are often called *giant hemangiomas* (3). They may form multiple lesions or a polypoid mass that protrudes from the hepatic capsule (fig. 9-2). The tumors contain large amounts of blood. In cut section, there is a spongy appearance, which is sometimes associated with mural thrombi and calcification (fig. 9-3).

Fibrosis of varying degrees often occurs, particularly at the center of the tumor, and may represent a regressive process. These cases are often referred to as *sclerosing cavernous hemangioma* (11). Another similar, but supposedly distinct group is *sclerosed hemangioma*, which exhibits fully fibrotic nodules with no identifiable cavernous area (11). Patients with sclerosed hemangioma are typically diagnosed with a solid liver mass on imaging, and the vascular origin may not be obvious based on the radiologic appearance (12–14). It has not yet been

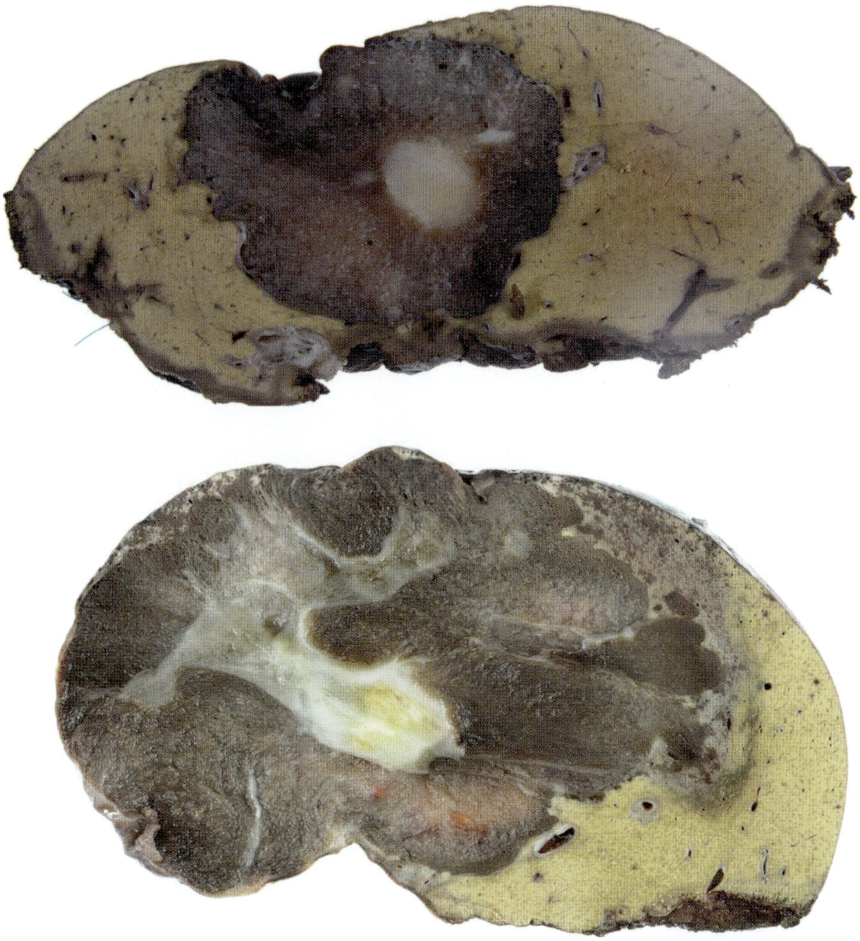

Figure 9-3

CAVERNOUS HEMANGIOMA

Top: A well-circumscribed sponge-like tumor is seen on cut section. The white solid nodule at the tumor center represents fibrosis.

Bottom: A large tumor mass is associated with a stellate central scar. There is focal irregular extension into the adjacent liver parenchyma (upper right).

established whether sclerosed and sclerosing hemangiomas are fundamentally similar or distinct lesions. The lack of typical cavernous areas and the focal presence of capillary vessels in sclerosed hemangioma suggest its origin from other vascular neoplasms, such as infantile hemangioma (11).

Although cavernous hemangioma is typically well demarcated, some cases extend irregularly into the adjoining parenchyma. Extreme examples extensively infiltrate the liver parenchyma and are referred to as *diffuse hemangiomatosis* (fig. 9-4) (15–17).

Microscopic Findings. Cavernous hemangioma consists of blood-filled dilated vascular channels with a flat endothelial lining (fig. 9-5). The intervening fibrous septa of variable thickness contain small blood vessels (fig. 9-6). Hemorrhage, fresh or organized thrombi, and calcification are often observed. Central solid

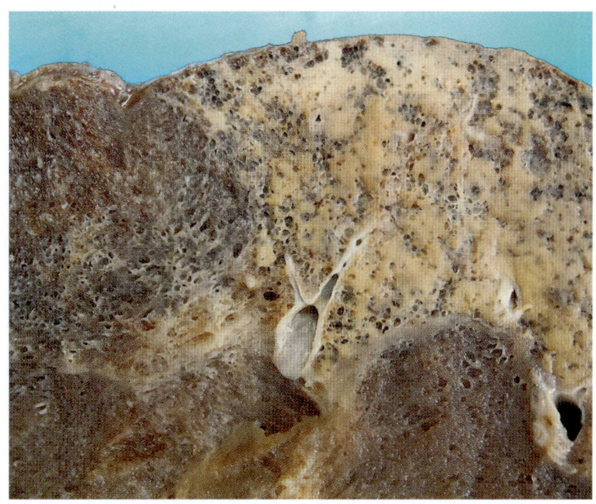

Figure 9-4

DIFFUSE HEMANGIOMATOSIS

The neoplastic process irregularly infiltrates the liver parenchyma and shows minute cystic changes, reflecting dilated vascular structures.

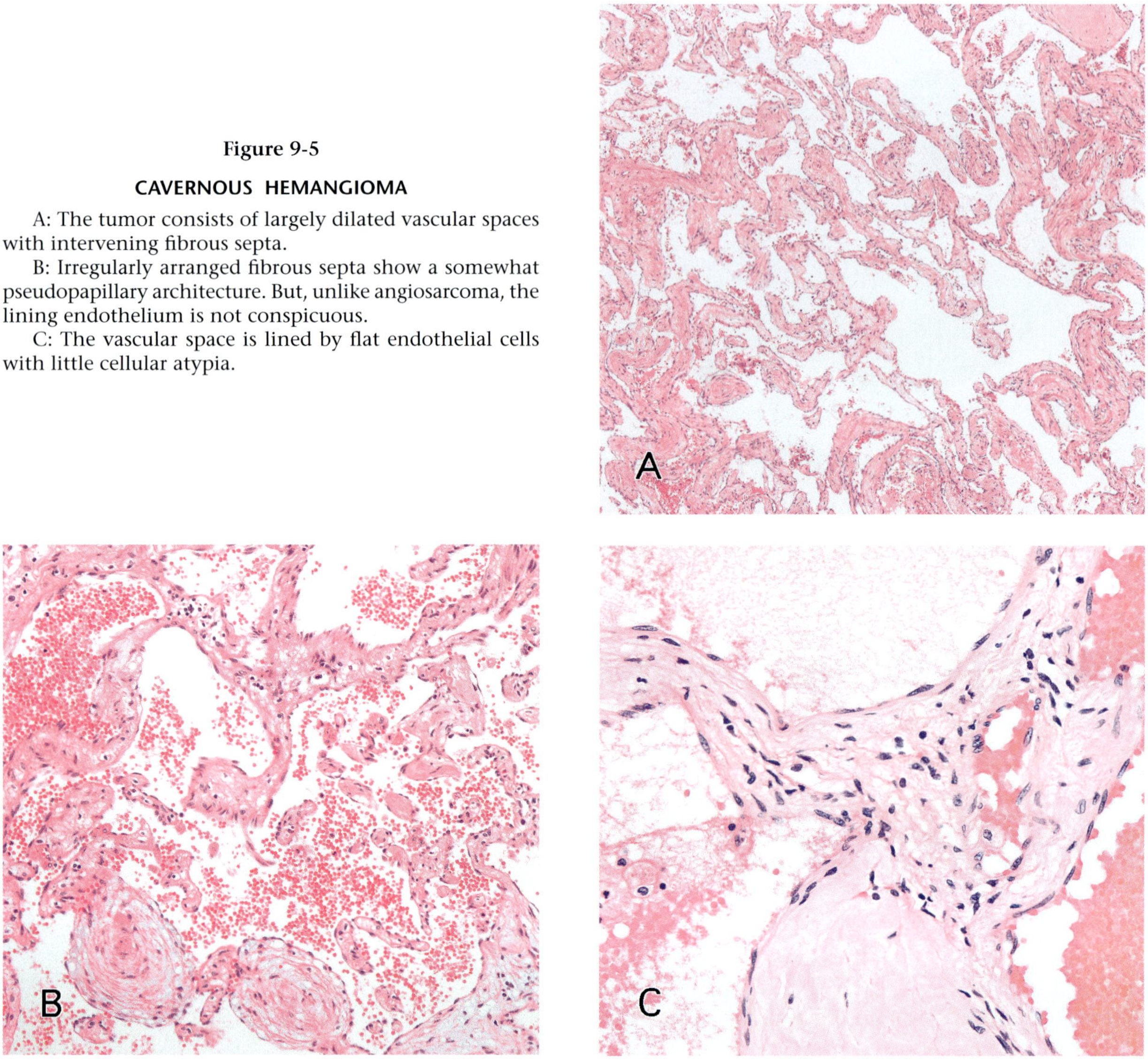

Figure 9-5

CAVERNOUS HEMANGIOMA

A: The tumor consists of largely dilated vascular spaces with intervening fibrous septa.

B: Irregularly arranged fibrous septa show a somewhat pseudopapillary architecture. But, unlike angiosarcoma, the lining endothelium is not conspicuous.

C: The vascular space is lined by flat endothelial cells with little cellular atypia.

foci consist of variably collagenized fibrosis (fig. 9-7). The liver parenchyma or bile ducts are entrapped in the tumor mass, particularly at peripheral areas. Similar dilated blood vessels may be present in the adjacent liver parenchyma (18).

Sclerosed hemangioma is characterized by extensive fibrosis with subsequent hyalinization and the marked narrowing or obliteration of vascular spaces; however, cavernous vascular structures are not identified (fig. 9-8) (11). The fibrotic stroma contains abundant amounts of collagen and elastic fibers (11). In diffuse hemangiomatosis, the tumor extends into the liver parenchyma irregularly and extensively (fig. 9-9). On immunostaining, the lining endothelial cells of the dilated vascular channels are positive for endothelial markers such as CD34, CD31, and factor VIII.

Differential Diagnosis. The diagnosis of cavernous hemangioma is straightforward in most cases. Sclerosed hemangioma needs to be discriminated from other fibrotic liver lesions, such as bile duct adenoma, hamartoma, and intrahepatic cholangiocarcinoma. Although elastic tissue staining may not visualize embedded vascular structures, a stroma rich in elastic fibers suggests the diagnosis. Immunostaining for endothelial markers may also highlight the residual vascular network.

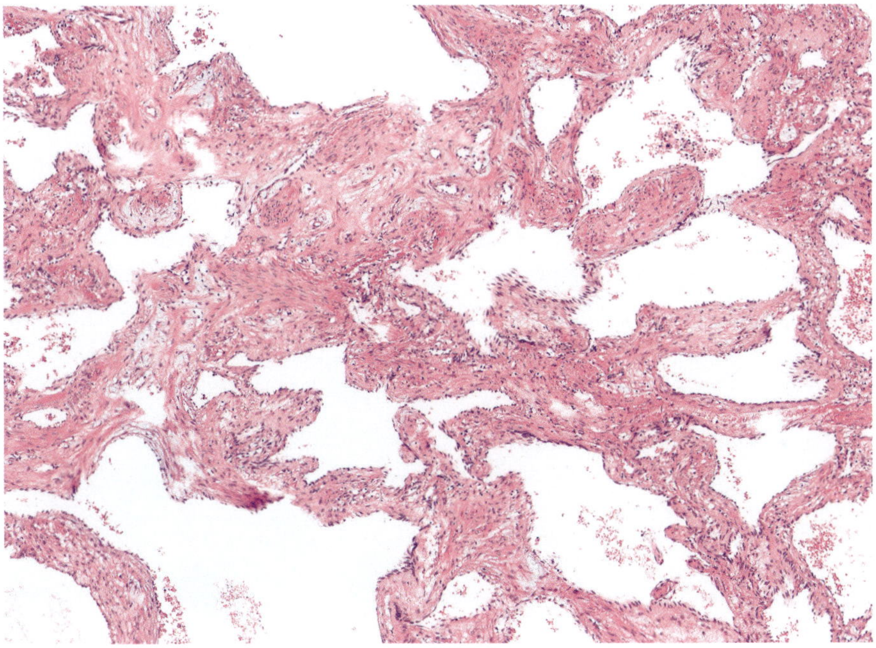

Figure 9-6

CAVERNOUS HEMANGIOMA

The fibrous septa in this case are thicker than those of classic cases.

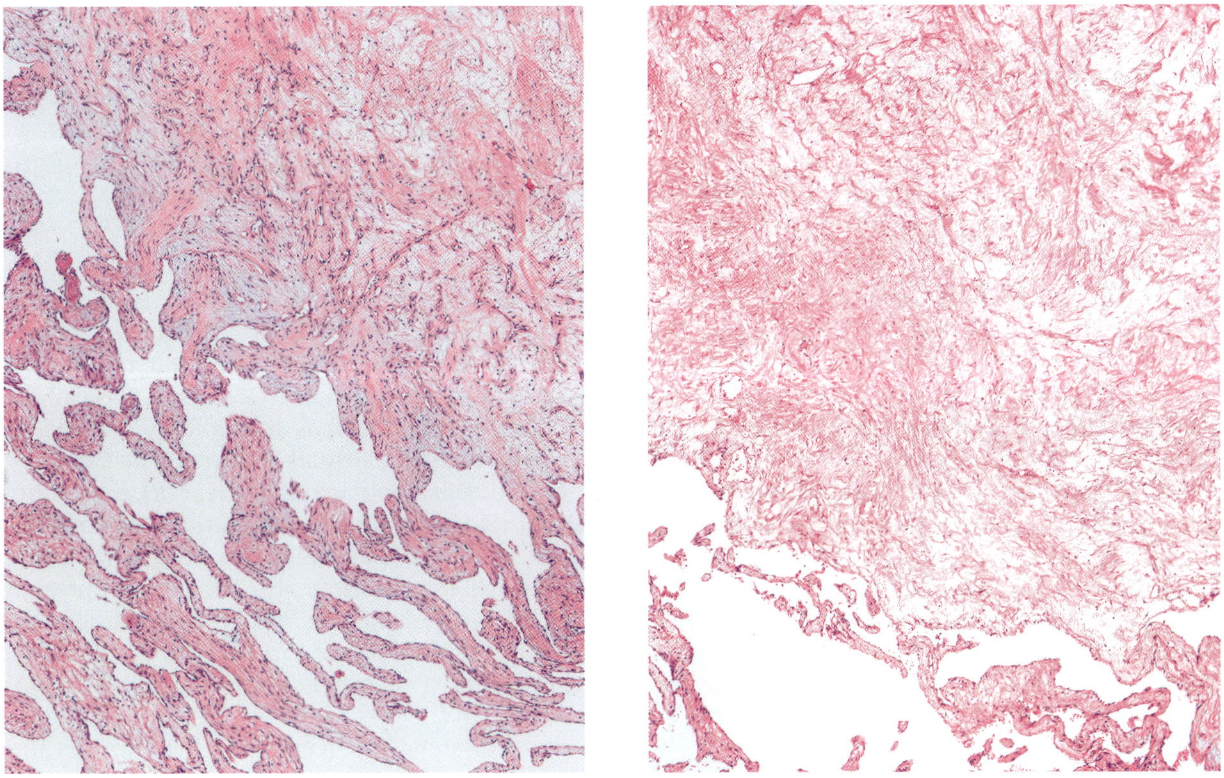

Figure 9-7

CAVERNOUS HEMANGIOMA

Left: The right upper solid area represents a central fibrous scar, in which blood vessels are narrow and angulated due to perivascular fibrosis.

Right: In an advanced central scar, vascular structures become less obvious.

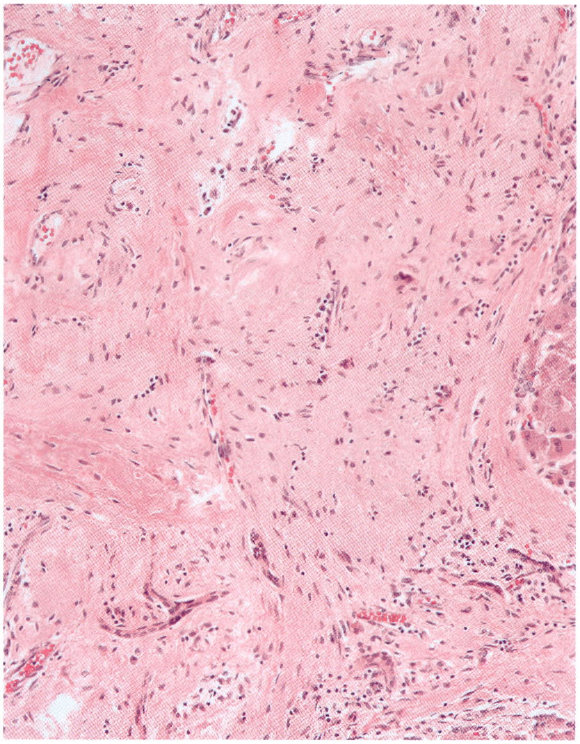

Figure 9-8

SCLEROSED HEMANGIOMA

The tumor mass consists of densely collagenized fibrous tissue and scattered small blood vessels. It is often difficult to conclude that the nodule originated from a vascular neoplasm.

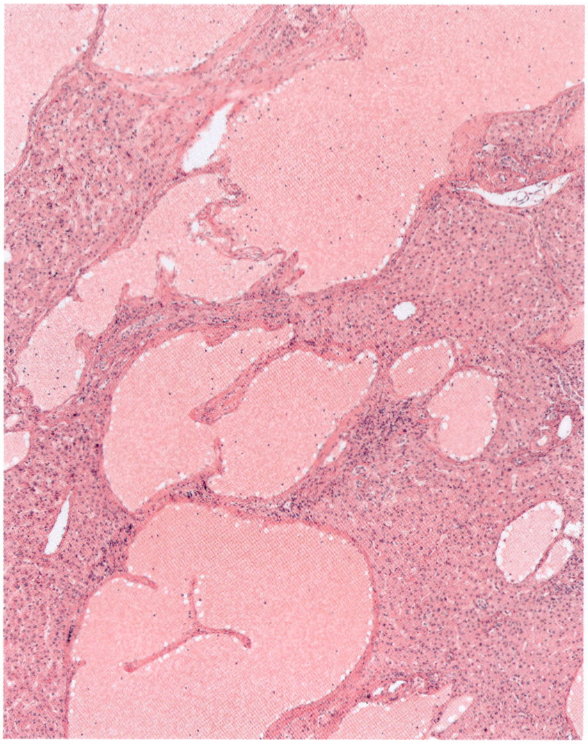

Figure 9-9

DIFFUSE HEMANGIOMATOSIS

The neoplastic process with dilated blood vessels irregularly infiltrates into the liver parenchyma.

The differential diagnosis of diffuse hemangiomatosis includes peliosis hepatis and hereditary hemorrhagic telangiectasia (Osler-Weber-Rendu disease). Unlike in hemangiomas, the spaces of peliosis hepatis lack an endothelial lining (fig. 9-10). One of the patterns observed in hereditary hemorrhagic telangiectasia mimics the extending areas of diffuse hemangiomatosis (fig. 9-11); however, the autosomal dominant genetic condition may be primarily diagnosed by clinical features and does not have accompanying cavernous hemangioma in the liver (19). Diffuse hemangiomatosis must not be misinterpreted as a malignant vascular neoplasm based solely on the infiltrating nature.

Infantile Hemangioma

Definition. *Infantile hemangioma* is a form of capillary hemangioma that is characterized by a perinatal or congenital onset and proliferation in the first year of life, followed by spontaneous regression during childhood (20). This condition was traditionally termed *infantile hemangioendothelioma* until recently (3). Similar neoplasms occurring at other anatomic sites (e.g., skin) are known as *hemangiomas of infancy*.

General and Clinical Features. The true incidence of this neoplasm is unclear because many small asymptomatic lesions supposedly regress without being diagnosed. Of those that come to clinical attention, nearly 100 percent present in the first year of life, 90 percent in the first 6 months, and 33 percent in the first month (3,4). It is the most common mesenchymal tumor of the liver in the first 2 years of life, accounting for approximately 40 percent of all liver tumors and 70 percent of benign tumors in this age group (20). Older patients have been reported, but are exceptional. Females are more commonly affected, with a male to female ratio of 1 to 2.

Hepatomegaly and abdominal masses noticed by parents or physicians are common

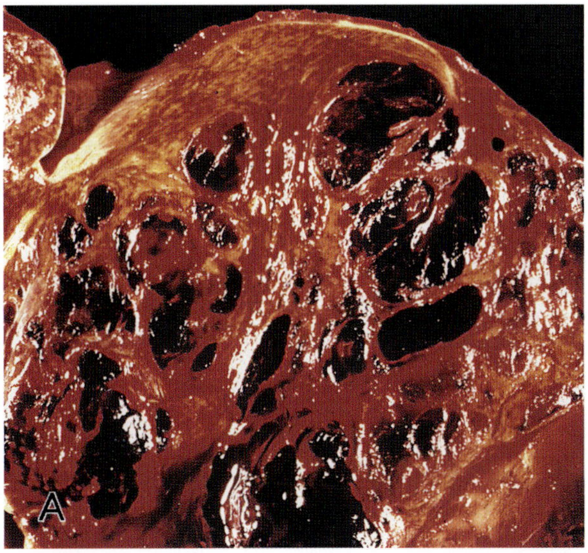

Figure 9-10

PELIOSIS HEPATIS

A: The liver section shows multiple cavities of varied size that are filled with clotted blood.

B: Three almost confluent cavities are filled with blood.

C: Higher magnification of a segment of one of the cavities shows no endothelial lining.

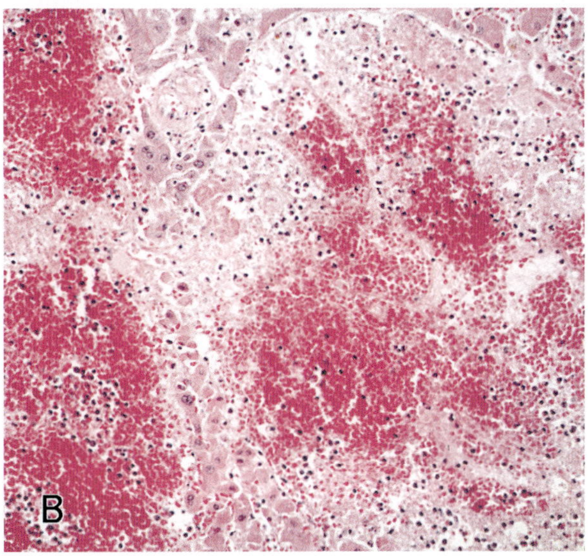

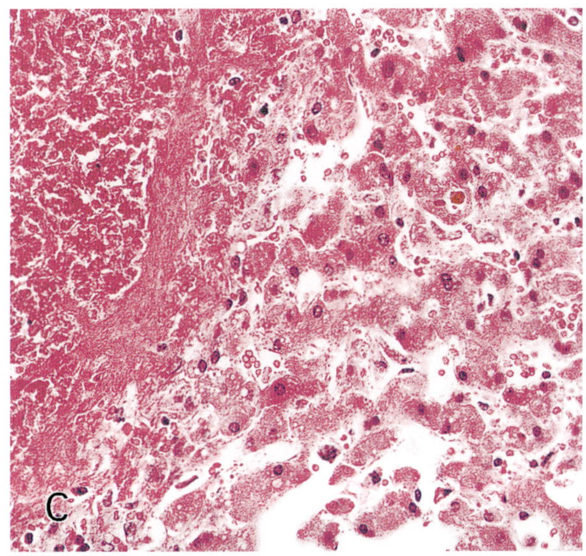

Figure 9-11

HEREDITARY HEMORRHAGIC TELANGIECTASIA (OSLER-WEBER-RENDU DISEASE)

Dilated blood vessels are present in the portal tracts and adjacent liver parenchyma.

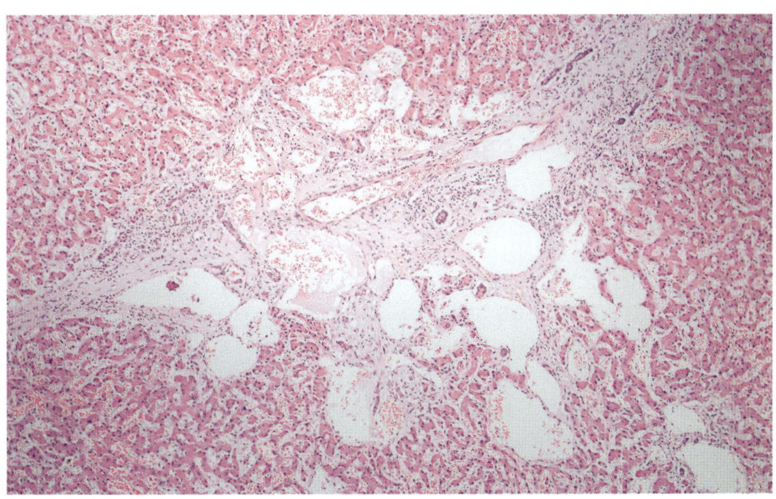

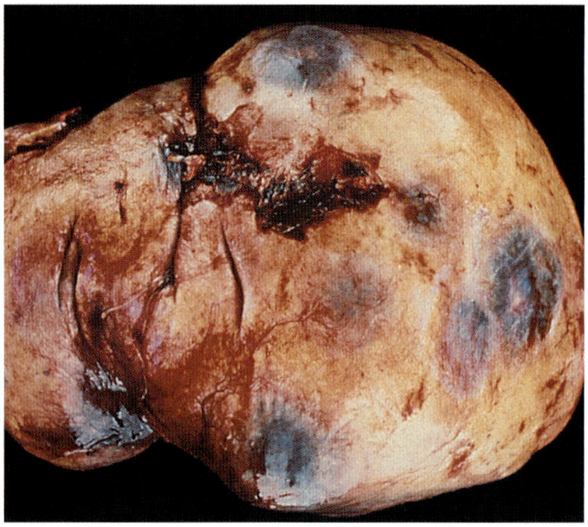

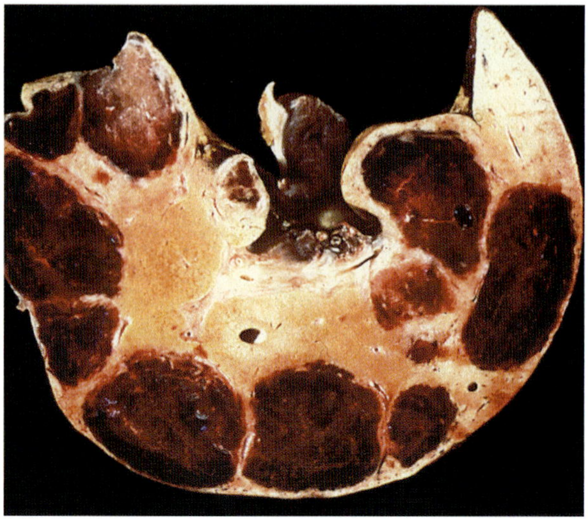

Figure 9-12

INFANTILE HEMANGIOMA

Left: Multiple, bluish subcapsular nodules.
Right: On sectioning, the nodules consist of large cavities filled with blood.

modes of presentation (4). Some patients (10 to 15 percent) have capillary hemangiomas at other anatomic sites, most commonly the skin (21). The mass effect of the tumor may lead to a symptomatic presentation such as vomiting, respiratory compromise, and jaundice. A critical complication is congestive heart failure due to arteriovenous shunting inside the tumor (22). This circulatory symptom, which is observed in up to 15 percent of patients, indicates a poor prognosis (23). Despite the benign-looking histologic appearance, up to two thirds of symptomatic patients may die due to congestive heart failure, hepatic failure, or rupture of the tumor (4).

Therapeutic approaches depend on the severity of symptoms and whether the lesion is single or multiple. Due to the potential for spontaneous regression, initial treatment needs to be conservative (using drugs such as corticosteroids, interferon, and vincristine) (24,25). Alternative therapies for nonresponders include hepatic artery ligation, embolization, and radiation (26). Surgical resection is often offered for symptomatic children with a solitary tumor. Liver transplantation may also be considered for unresectable multifocal tumors (27).

Gross Findings. Tumors are single in 55 percent and multiple in 45 percent of cases and develop anywhere in the liver (22). They form well-circumscribed nodules up to 15 cm in greatest diameter. Multiple lesions may number as many as 30 and sometimes involve both lobes (fig. 9-12). The appearance of individual lesions on cross section varies from red-brown glistening masses to whitish fibrotic nodules depending on the degree of residual vascularity and regression (fig. 9-13). Some tumors have fibrotic scarring at the center and residual red-brown vascularized areas at the periphery (fig. 9-14), suggesting that involution starts from the center. Hemorrhage and infarction may occur as a result of previous therapy.

Microscopic Findings. The "fresh" areas at the periphery consist of proliferating small vascular channels lined by plump endothelial cells (fig. 9-15) (20). Dilated cavernous vascular channels may be present in addition to capillary-type vessels (fig. 9-16). The intervening stroma is loosely fibrotic and generally scant. The stroma becomes broader and more fibrotic toward the center of the tumor (fig. 9-17) (4). Secondary changes such as hemorrhage, dystrophic calcification, and thrombosis are common (fig. 9-18). The lining endothelium is typically monolayered. A micropapillary or pseudopapillary architecture is rarely encountered, but must not be regarded as a diagnostic sign of malignancy (fig. 9-19). Neoplastic cells

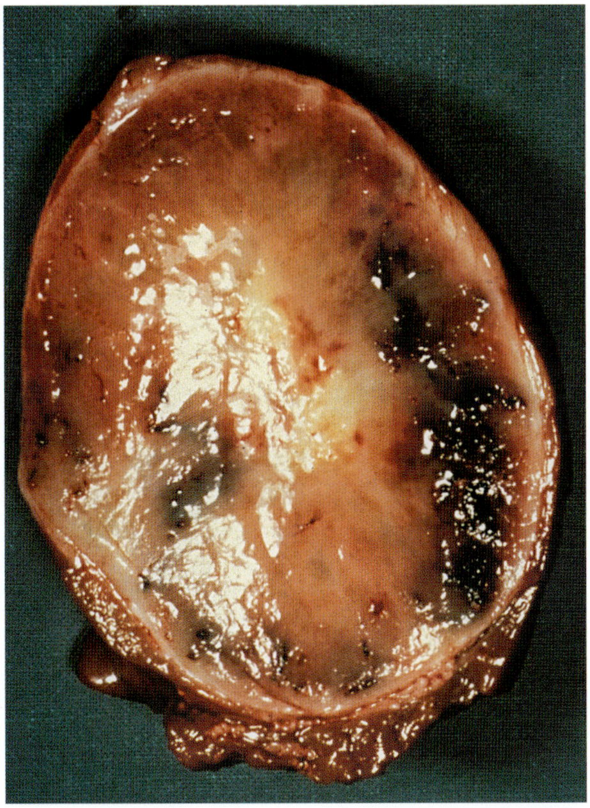

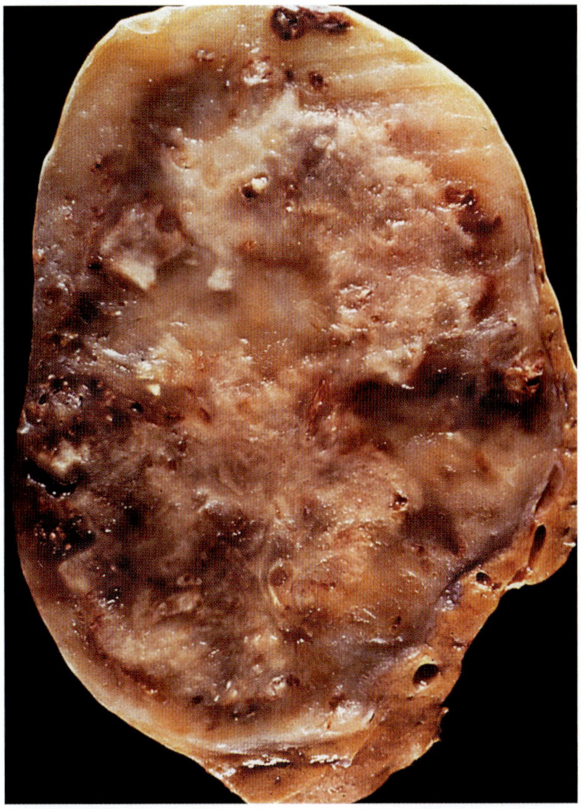

Figure 9-13

INFANTILE HEMANGIOMA

Left: This section of a single tumor shows a red to pink-brown periphery and a light tan-white center. Right: This section is mottled yellow, tan, and brown.

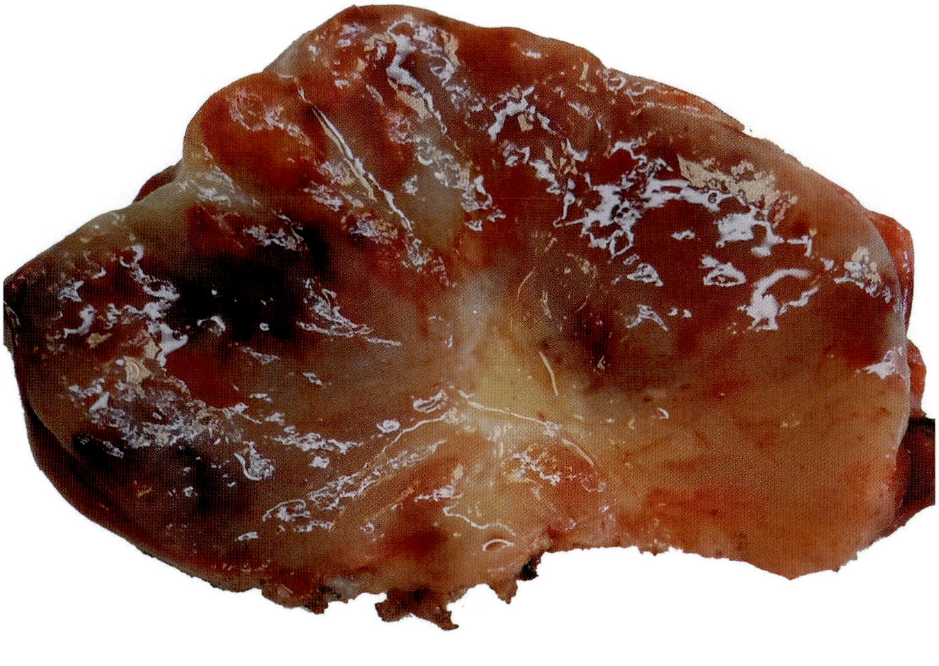

Figure 9-14

INFANTILE HEMANGIOMA

There is a red-brown glistening area at the periphery and a central fibrotic scar, the latter reflecting a regression process.

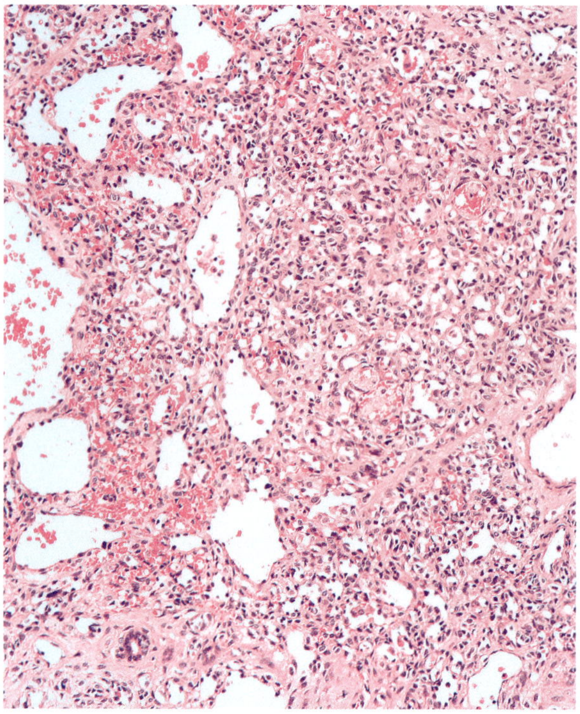

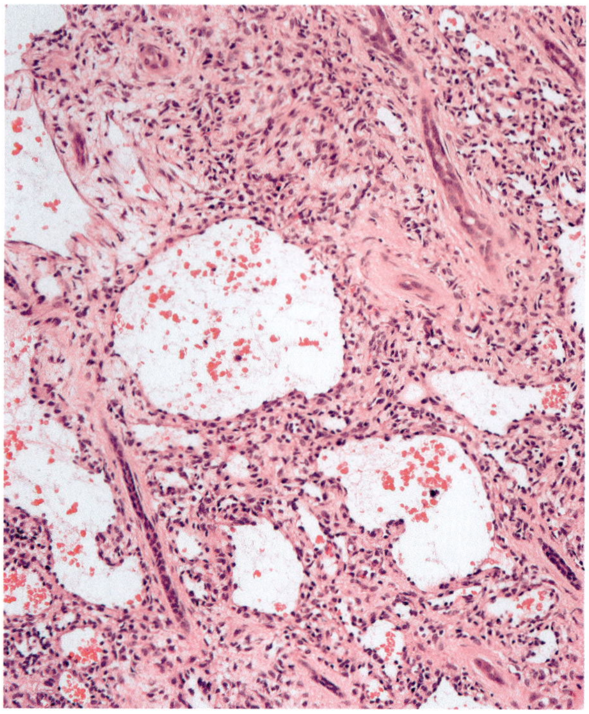

Figure 9-15

INFANTILE HEMANGIOMA

Left: The tumor consists of capillary-type small vessels, some showing slight dilatation.
Right: There are small blood vessels and narrow fibrous septa, in which entrapped bile ducts are observed.

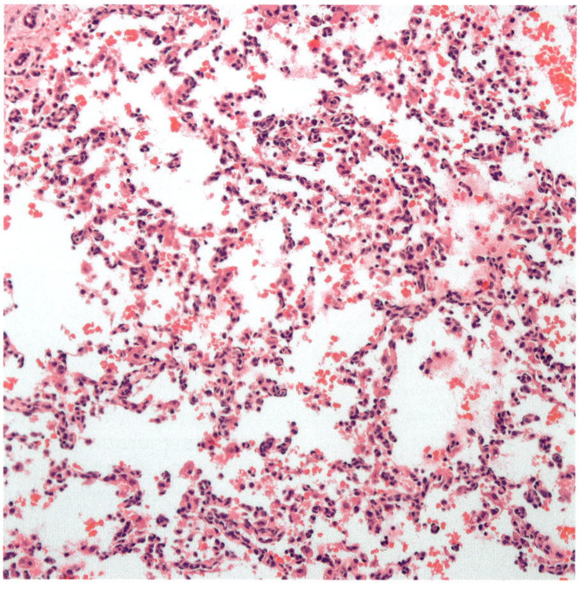

Figure 9-16

INFANTILE HEMANGIOMA

Cavernous vascular channels are seen.

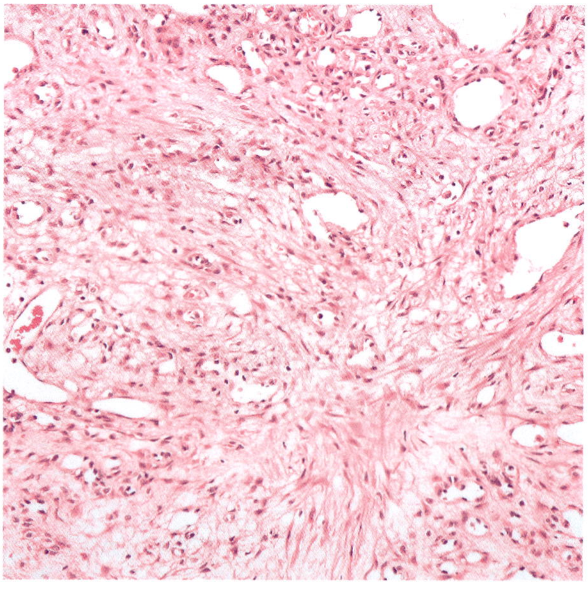

Figure 9-17

INFANTILE HEMANGIOMA

In the central part of the tumor, the stroma is fibrotic and broad, likely reflecting a regression process.

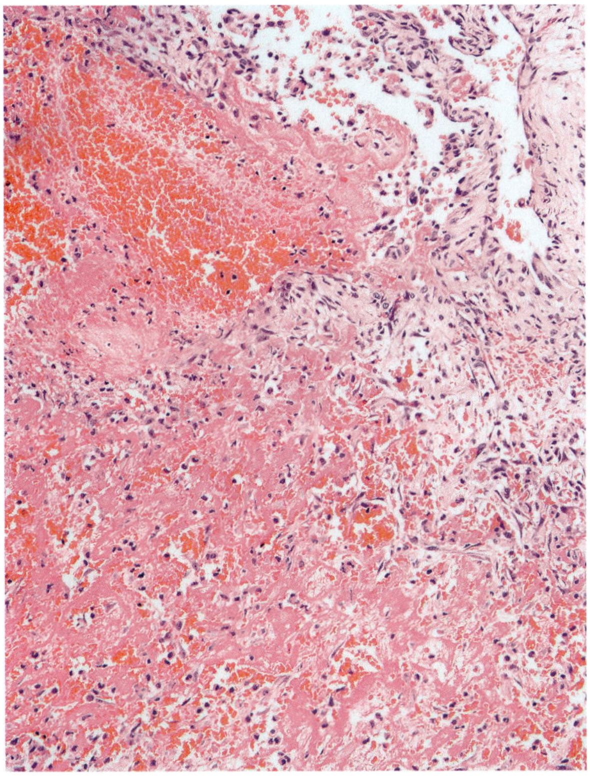

Figure 9-18

INFANTILE HEMANGIOMA

Associated hemorrhage disrupts preexisting vascular structures.

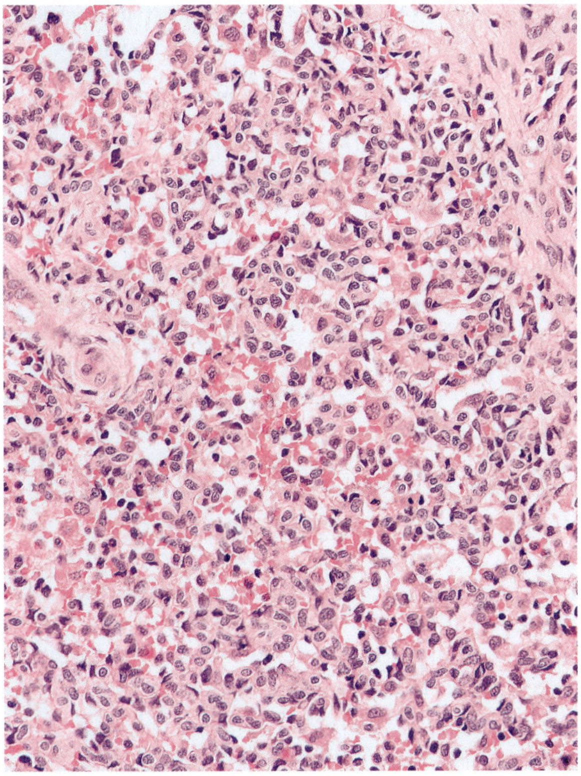

Figure 9-19

INFANTILE HEMANGIOMA

In this collapsed area, endothelial cells are arranged in a somewhat pseudopapillary architecture with high cellularity. The cells have plump nuclei but are less pleomorphic than those in angiosarcoma.

are cytologically bland with round nuclei. Mitotic figures may be present, particularly in the proliferative phase. Some cases have foci of extramedullary hematopoiesis.

Lining endothelial cells express CD31, CD34, and factor VIII. Ki-67 immunostaining is generally difficult to evaluate in this neoplasm because of the large number of other positive cells such as lymphocytes and hematopoietic cells, and the proliferation index depends on the stage of proliferation or involution. Thus, the diagnostic value of Ki-67 immunostaining in this neoplasm is low.

Histologic Types. Infantile hemangioma was previously classified into type I and type II (28). The former included the classic cases as described above, while the latter had nuclear atypia, a complex budding of the endothelial lining, and solid foci consisting of spindle cells arranged in a whorled or kaposiform architecture. Type II neoplasms are currently classified as angiosarcoma (20). Diagnostic type II changes may be focal; therefore, extensive sampling is required to exclude this possibility (21). Although some early case reports suggested that benign infantile hemangioma rarely progresses to angiosarcoma (29,30), it has not yet been established whether type II neoplasms are malignant from the beginning or transform from preexisting benign hemangioma.

Differential Diagnosis. Immunostaining for GLUT-1 is used to discriminate juvenile hemangioma from vascular malformations mimicking neoplastic lesions in extrahepatic organs (31). This approach has been tested in liver lesions in small series. An index study previously indicated that GLUT-1 was positive in infantile hemangioma, but negative in vascular malformation of the liver (32). Immunostaining for the erythrocyte-type glucose transporter may be useful for classifying congenital or infantile vascular lesions of the liver, similar to other organs.

Epithelioid Hemangioendothelioma

Definition. *Epithelioid hemangioendothelioma* is an uncommon vascular neoplasm of low-grade malignancy that is histologically characterized by the epithelioid morphology of tumor cells and abundant fibrotic stroma, which is in contrast to most of the other vascular tumors.

General Features. Similar neoplasms may develop in other organs, such as the lung and soft tissues. This uncommon neoplasm was suspected to be a carcinoma, sclerosing angiosarcoma, or even non-neoplastic fibrous lesion for decades because of its unusual histologic appearance. Ultrastructural and immunohistochemical studies eventually proved its endothelial origin, leading to the recognition of a vascular neoplasm with a clinical course between hemangioma and angiosarcoma (33,34). Since 1984, when the first series of hepatic epithelioid hemangioendotheliomas was described by Ishak et al. (35), this condition has been recognized as a distinct entity of the liver. Its annual incidence is less than 0.1 per 100,000 population (36).

Clinical Features. The mean age of patients is 42 years (range, 3 to 86 years). Although children and teenagers may be affected, patients younger than 20 years are rare (5 percent) (35). Approximately 60 percent are women. Some potential risk factors (e.g., exposure to vinyl chloride, use of contraceptive steroids, and viral hepatitis) have been suggested, but have not yet been confirmed.

Approximately 25 percent of patients are asymptomatic, while the majority of the remaining patients present with nonspecific abdominal symptoms such as right upper quadrant pain, jaundice, ascites, and hepatomegaly (37). Rarely, major vascular involvement leads to Budd-Chiari syndrome, sinusoidal obstruction syndrome/veno-occlusive disease, or portal hypertension.

Incidental liver lesions were found in about 10 percent of patients during surgery performed for other reasons; however, this presentation has become less common. Most patients have multiple liver lesions at initial presentation, and 40 percent have extrahepatic involvement (e.g., lung, lymph nodes, peritoneum, and bone) (35).

Imaging features of epithelioid hemangioendothelioma are not typical for vascular neoplasms, and often result in an incorrect diagnosis of cholangiocarcinoma or metastatic carcinoma (37). A single or few discrete nodules are observed in the early stages, and subsequently progress to bilobar multiple lesions or large confluent masses. Tumors show low density on computerized tomography (CT) scan, with heterogeneous or often ring-like enhancement (38). On magnetic resonance imaging (MRI), the central part of the tumor typically shows a low signal intensity on T1-weighted and high signal intensity on T2-weighted images (39). A multilayered targeted appearance is often observed in nonenhanced or dynamic contrast-enhanced images (40,41).

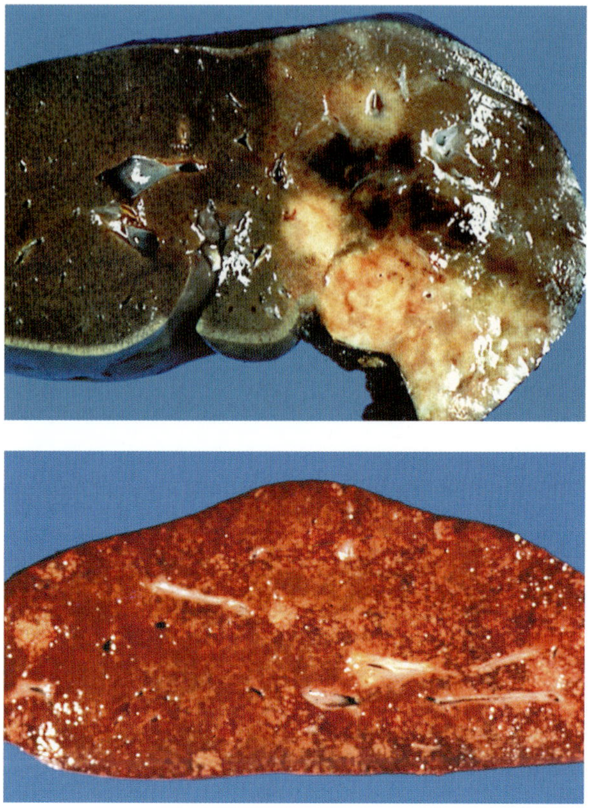

Figure 9-20

EPITHELIOID HEMANGIOENDOTHELIOMA

Top: The tumor in the right lobe is tan and gray, with a large central area of hemorrhage.

Bottom: Section of liver with tan tumor nodules of varied size scattered in both lobes.

Gross Findings. Solitary tumors (about 20 percent of cases) are less common than multiple liver nodules (over 80 percent) (fig. 9-20). Individual tumors range in size from subcentimeter

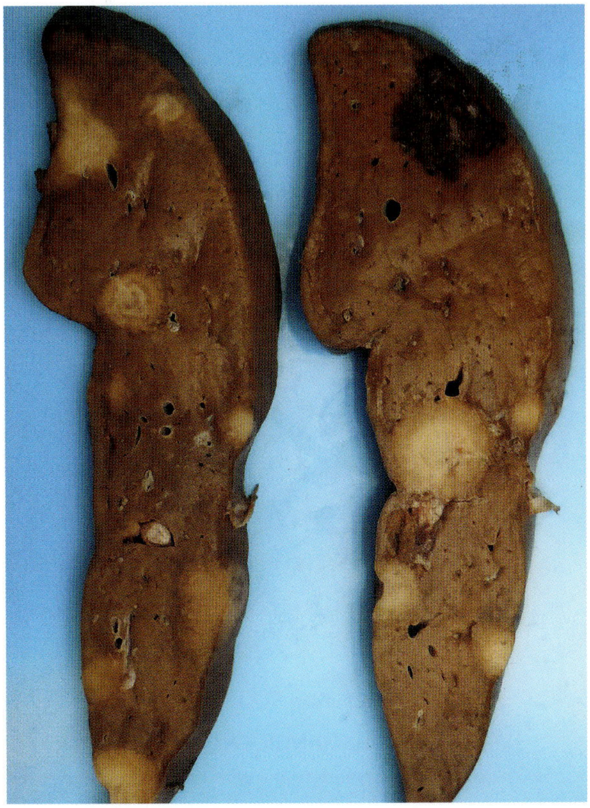

Figure 9-21

EPITHELIOID HEMANGIOENDOTHELIOMA

Cross sections of the explanted liver show multiple solid nodular lesions, some associated with the depression of the hepatic capsule. The masses are fairly uniform in size. The right upper nodule is a cavernous hemangioma.

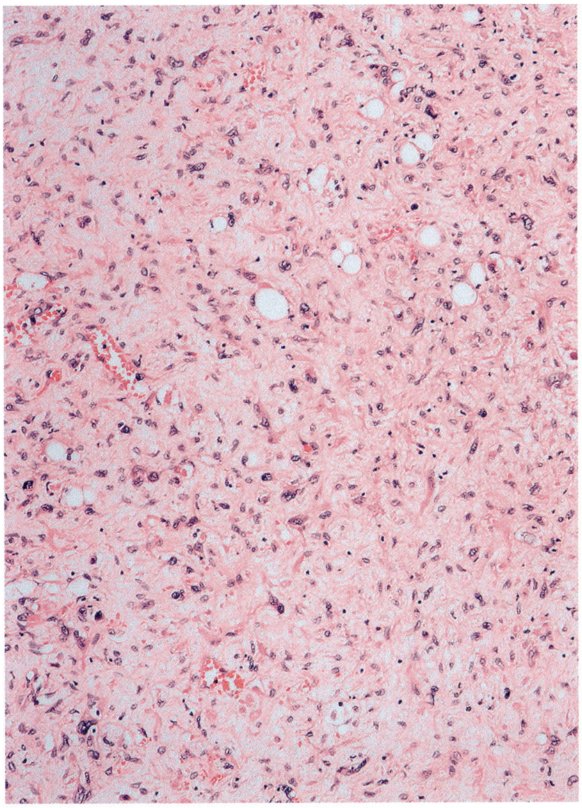

Figure 9-22

EPITHELIOID HEMANGIOENDOTHELIOMA

This low-power view shows a lightly eosinophilic appearance with scattered atypical cells, some with enlarged nuclei or vacuoles.

to 14 cm (42). Unlike other primary liver malignancies, which form a dominant mass with multiple small satellite nodules, epithelioid hemangioendothelioma sometimes consists of multiple nodules that are fairly similar in size (fig. 9-21). On cross section, the tumors are pale or whitish in color, firm or rubbery in texture, and solid in appearance with or without small calcifications. Nodules are commonly present in the peripheral parenchyma, with subcapsular lesions associated with umbilication of the hepatic capsule (42). Individual tumor masses have an infiltrative margin, but no fibrous capsule. The background liver is typically noncirrhotic.

Microscopic Findings. The tumors appear to be lightly eosinophilic at low magnification (fig. 9-22). Despite tumor extension, entrapped portal tracts and central veins are sometimes recognized inside the masses, suggesting an infiltrative nature (42). Tumor cells are arranged in single cells or small clusters against the background of a fibromyxoid stroma (fig. 9-23). The cells have a characteristic epithelioid appearance, with centrally located round nuclei and lightly eosinophilic cytoplasm. Signet ring-like cells may be present.

Two characteristic findings are intracytoplasmic lumens, with some containing erythrocytes (fig. 9-24), and papillary polypoid growth inside blood vessels or sinusoids (fig. 9-25), both of which serve as a diagnostic clue for this condition (35). Some tumor cells are less epithelioid and show spindle or stellate shapes (3).

The tumors infiltrate along sinusoidal structures, causing severe atrophy and the eventual disappearance of liver cell plates (fig. 9-26). Entrapped hepatocytes and cholangiocytes are

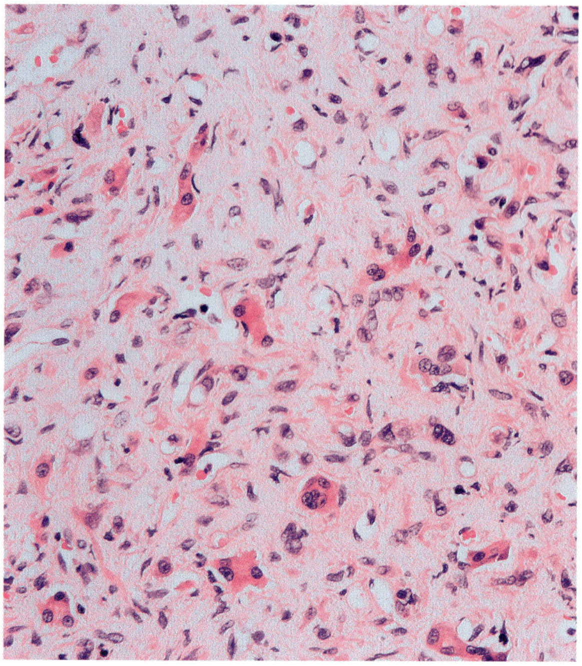

Figure 9-23

EPITHELIOID HEMANGIOENDOTHELIOMA

Spindle-shaped or epithelioid atypical cells are noted against the background of a fibromyxoid stroma. Densely eosinophilic cells are entrapped hepatocytes.

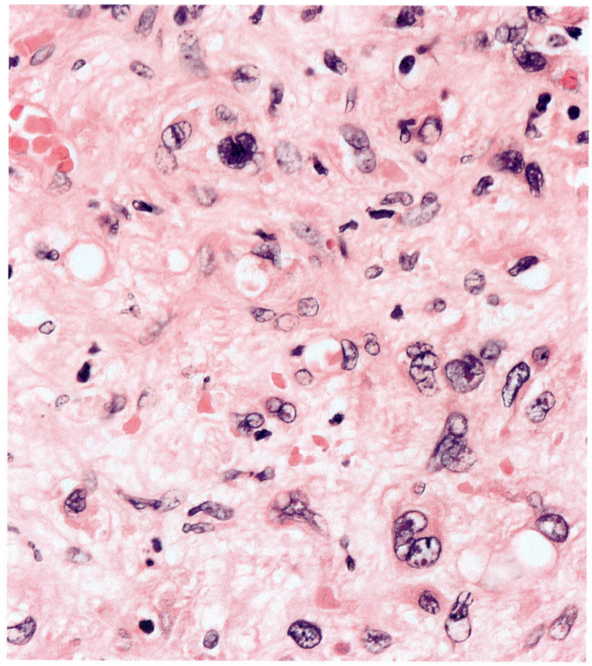

Figure 9-24

EPITHELIOID HEMANGIOENDOTHELIOMA

Neoplastic cells have vesicular nuclei and intracytoplasmic lumens.

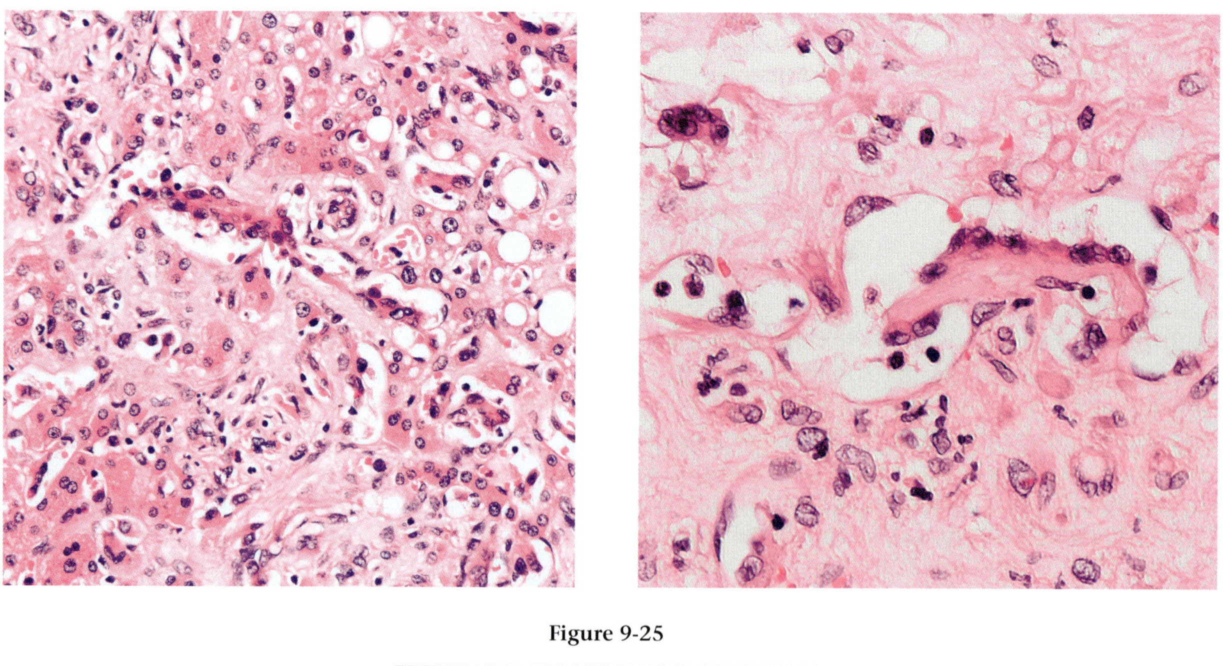

Figure 9-25

EPITHELIOID HEMANGIOENDOTHELIOMA

Left: A cell cluster infiltrating into a sinusoidal space shows a polypoid architecture.

Right: Intravascular polypoid growth is a characteristic feature of this neoplasm. This finding should not be mistaken for carcinoma.

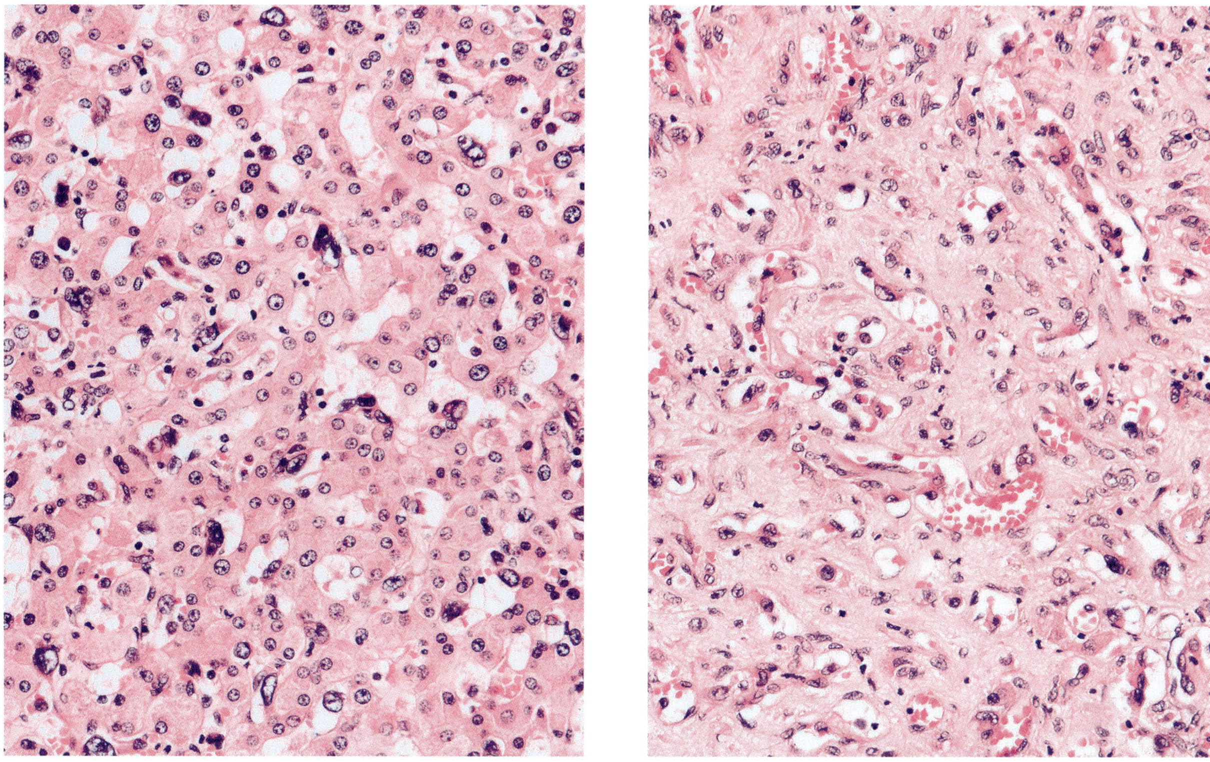

Figure 9-26

EPITHELIOID HEMANGIOENDOTHELIOMA

Left: Neoplastic cells infiltrate into sinusoidal spaces at the invasive front.

Right: Vascular structures infiltrated by tumor cells are residual sinusoidal spaces, but liver cell plates in between are extinguished.

sometimes falsely regarded as neoplastic cells (fig. 9-27), leading to the incorrect diagnosis of scirrhous hepatocellular carcinoma or cholangiocarcinoma. The cells often invade blood vessels and Glisson capsule (fig. 9-28).

The tumor produces an abundant stroma, which is initially rich in mucopolysaccharides and becomes more fibrotic with foci of hyalinization or calcification in older lesions. The fibrotic desmoplastic reaction is more pronounced at the center of the tumor. Necrotic foci may also be present (fig. 9-29). Mitotic figures are not observed in 58 percent of cases (42).

On immunolabeling, most cases express CD34, CD31, ERG, and factor VIII, at least focally (43). D2-40, a marker of the lymphatic endothelium, is also aberrantly expressed in 78 percent of cases (fig. 9-30, left) (44). Cytokeratins may be focally positive in neoplastic cells (45). Immunostaining for CK7, CK19, and HepPar1 also highlights the larger number of entrapped cholangiocytes and hepatocytes than expected on hematoxylin and eosin (H&E)-stained sections (fig. 9-30, right). These are diagnostic pitfalls because epithelioid hemangioendothelioma is sometimes mislabeled as a carcinoma based on its fibrotic morphologic appearance, epithelioid neoplastic cells, and these immunohistochemical findings. Diffuse nuclear staining of CAMTA1 (calmodulin-binding transcription activator 1) or TFE3 (transcription factor E3) indicates the presence of the *WWTR1-CAMTA1* or *YAP1-TFE3* fusion gene, respectively (see also Molecular Genetic Findings) (46,47).

Ultrastructural Findings. The cells of epithelioid hemangioendothelioma have endothelial ultrastructural features including a basal lamina, pinocytotic vesicles, and Weibel-Palade bodies (3). The amount of intracytoplasmic intermediate filament is larger than that in non-neoplastic endothelial cells, a finding that may be related to the epithelioid histologic appearance.

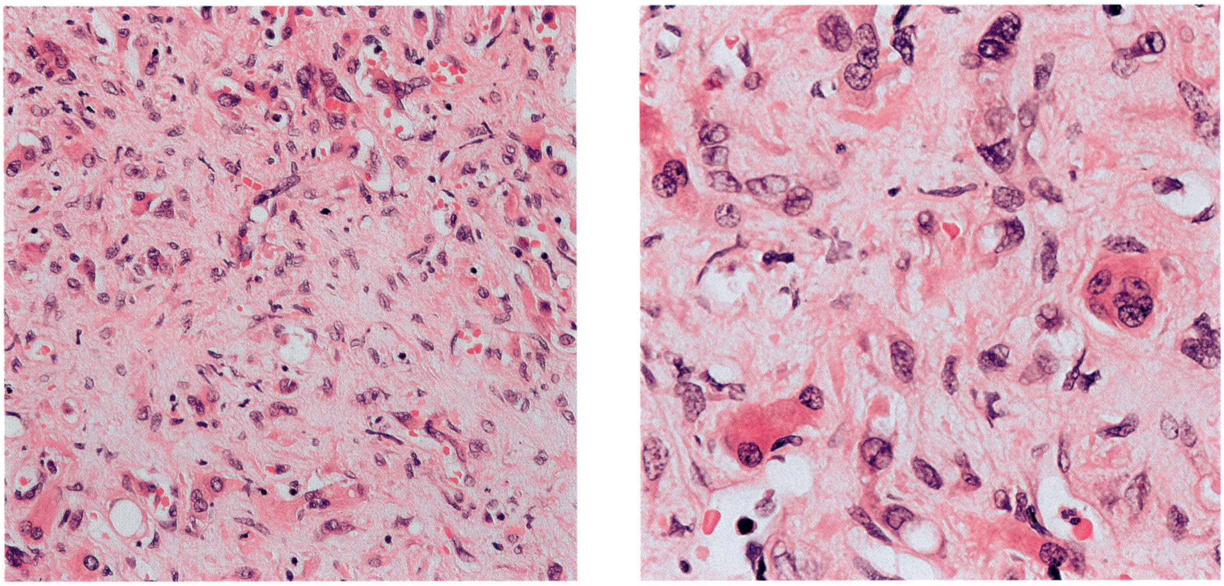

Figure 9-27

EPITHELIOID HEMANGIOENDOTHELIOMA

Left: Entrapped hepatocytes are arranged in small clusters and surrounded by a fibromyxoid stroma. This morphologic appearance is sometimes mistaken for scirrhous hepatocellular carcinoma or cholangiocarcinoma.

Right: Lightly eosinophilic cells with ill-defined border are neoplastic, while densely eosinophilic cells arranged in nests are entrapped hepatocytes. Although both have enlarged nuclei, irregularity of the nuclear membrane is more obvious in the tumor cells. The cytoplasmic appearance helps to discriminate the two types of cells.

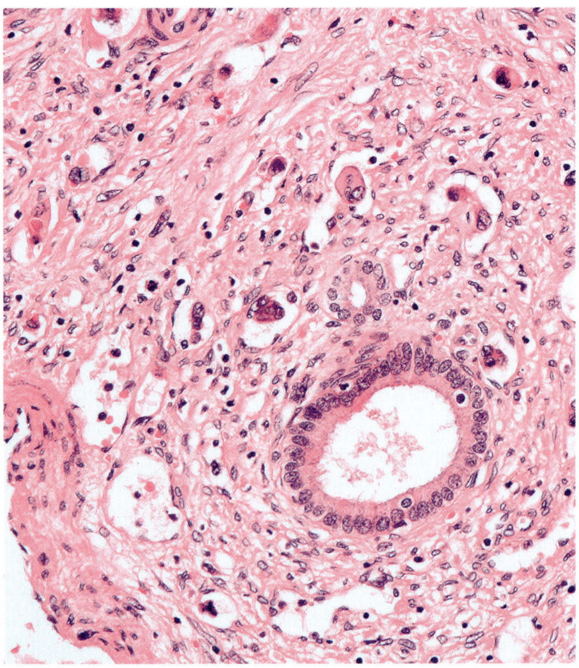

Figure 9-28

EPITHELIOID HEMANGIOENDOTHELIOMA

Tumor cells infiltrate into small vessels in a portal tract.

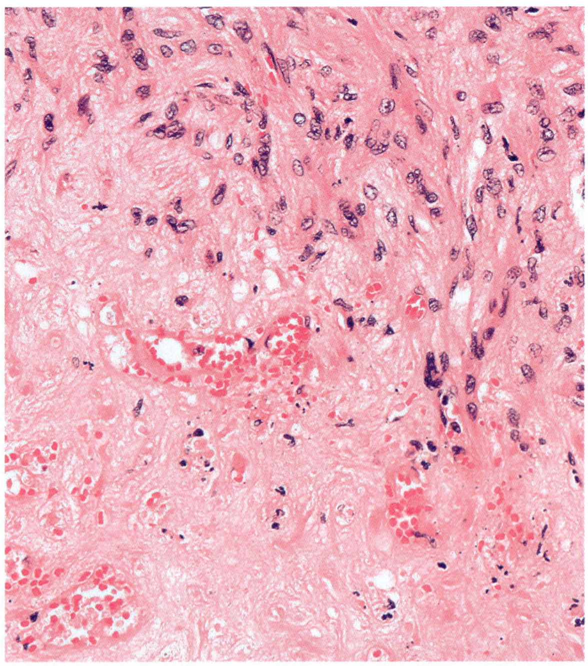

Figure 9-29

EPITHELIOID HEMANGIOENDOTHELIOMA

Necrosis is sometimes seen, particularly centrally.

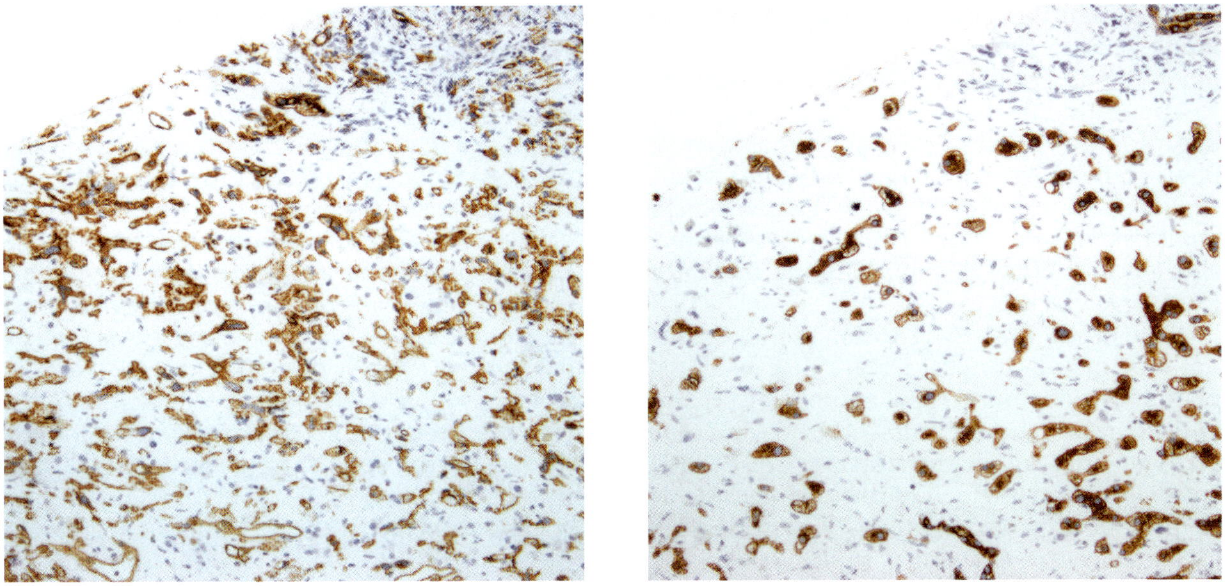

Figure 9-30

EPITHELIOID HEMANGIOENDOTHELIOMA

Left: CD34 immunostain highlights the neoplastic cells embedded in a fibrous stroma.

Right: CAM5.2 immunostain shows many entrapped hepatocytes and cholangiocytes inside a tumor mass. They should not be interpreted as neoplastic cells.

Molecular Genetic Findings. Recurrent translocations involving chromosomal regions 1p36.3 and 3q25 have been identified in epithelioid hemangioendothelioma of various organs including the liver, which eventually led to the discovery of the fusion gene *WWTR1-CAMTA1* (48,49). This gene rearrangement is found in approximately 90 percent of epithelioid hemangioendotheliomas but is exceptional in histologic mimickers (e.g., epithelioid angiosarcoma) (46,48,49). Therefore, immunostaining for CAMTA1 is not only a useful ancillary method for finding the fusion gene but is also helpful for diagnosis (46). One study (50) examined patterns of *WWTR1-CAMTA1* rearrangement in six samples from two patients with multicentric hepatic epithelioid hemangioendothelioma. An identical fusion transcript product was confirmed in different nodules in each patient, suggesting that multifocal epithelioid hemangioendothelioma is monoclonal and represents metastatic implants of the same tumor rather than a real multicentric neoplasm.

An uncommon fusion gene identified in epithelioid hemangioendothelioma is *YAP1-TFE3* (47). This genetic alteration is correlated with a distinct morphologic appearance, including the presence of focally well-formed vascular channels, solid growth pattern, voluminous eosinophilic cytoplasm, and mild to moderate nuclear atypia, all of which are atypical for conventional epithelioid hemangioendothelioma (47). Given that previous studies on *YAP1-TFE3*-rearranged epithelioid hemangioendothelioma included only a small number of hepatic neoplasms, the liver may not be the common site for this genetic variant (47,51). Although *WWTR1-CAMTA1* and *YAP1-TFE3* fusions are supposed to be mutually exclusive, a recent study has suggested that the two chromosomal rearrangements rarely coexist (51).

Differential Diagnosis. Since epithelioid hemangioendothelioma displays characteristic histologic features, awareness of its microscopic findings is critical in order to avoid a misdiagnosis. Two major entities in the differential diagnosis of epithelioid hemangioendothelioma are cholangiocarcinoma and angiosarcoma. Patients with epithelioid hemangioendothelioma are slightly younger than those with typical intrahepatic cholangiocarcinoma. The stroma in epithelioid hemangioendothelioma is more myxoid than that in cholangiocarcinoma. Immunostaining for endothelial markers is very helpful for achieving a differential diagnosis.

Angiosarcoma is a more destructive neoplasm. In this highly malignant sarcoma, neoplastic cells are less epithelioid and more spindle in shape and show considerable pleomorphism and brisk mitotic figures. Unlike angiosarcoma, epithelioid hemangioendothelioma does not form large vascular cavities.

Treatment and Prognosis. Management options include surgical resection, liver transplantation, chemotherapy, embolization, and radiotherapy. There is currently no generally accepted strategy for the treatment of hepatic epithelioid hemangioendothelioma because of its rarity, heterogeneous status, and variable clinical outcome (37). A treatment strategy is based on how extensive the liver disease and extrahepatic involvement are. Surgical resection is generally the treatment of choice for patients with monolobar disease. However, it is only possible in approximately 10 percent of cases because most patients have more advanced disease at the initial presentation (37). Liver transplantation is considered for bilobar disease with no extrahepatic involvement (52). Approximately 45 percent of patients undergo liver transplantation, with or without neoadjuvant chemotherapy. If there is extrahepatic dissemination, chemotherapy is used. Limited extrahepatic disease is not an absolute contraindication of resection or liver transplantation (52,53).

The overall 5-year survival rate is 41 to 55 percent. Liver resection and transplantation give better 5-year survival rates (75 percent and 55 percent, respectively) than chemo/radiotherapy (30 percent) and no treatment (5 percent) (37,43). Most cases of recurrence occur more than 2 years after surgery (54).

Angiosarcoma

Definition. *Angiosarcoma* is a high-grade mesenchymal malignant neoplasm showing endothelial differentiation. The tumor cells are more spindled in shape and the stroma is less fibrotic than those in epithelioid hemangioendothelioma.

General Features. Hepatic angiosarcoma is rare, but is still the most common primary sarcoma of the liver (3,4). More than 200 cases are diagnosed annually worldwide, with 10 to 20 cases in the United States and approximately 10 cases in the United Kingdom (55,56). Patients are typically adults, with the peak incidence in the sixth and seventh decades; however, rare cases occur in younger individuals, even children (4,57,58). Men are more commonly affected, with a male to female ratio of 3 to 1.

There are four known agents that increase the risk of hepatic angiosarcoma: vinyl chloride monomer, arsenic, anabolic steroids, and Thorotrast. Vinyl chloride is a gas that is used to make the plastic polyvinyl chloride (3,4). Hepatic angiosarcoma as well as hepatocellular carcinoma have been reported in workers with prolonged exposure to the vinyl chloride monomer during the manufacturing processes (3,4). Angiosarcoma was also detected in the 1950s in German vineyard workers exposed to arsenical insecticides, in those who consumed Fowler solution (potassium arsenite) medicinally for prolonged periods for asthma or psoriasis, and in a few individuals exposed to arsenic through drinking water (55,59). Thorotrast (colloidal thorium dioxide) was used as a radiographic contrast medium from the 1930s to 1950s. Once injected, nearly all the material remains permanently in the body, accumulating in the liver and to a lesser extent in the spleen, lymph nodes, and bone marrow (3,4). Twenty-five percent of patients with angiosarcoma have one of the four risk agents, while 75 percent have no apparent risk factor. The proportion of sporadic cases has increased because some of the risk agents have been less commonly used since their toxicity was widely recognized.

Clinical Features. Patients present with abdominal pain, fatigue, weight loss, anorexia, and abdominal enlargement. At the physical examination, hepatomegaly is observed in up to 70 percent of patients. Ascites and jaundice may be present. Portal hypertension with splenomegaly is a frequent finding in vinyl chloride-associated angiosarcoma. Intraabdominal hemorrhage due to tumor rupture is one cause of rapidly progressive deterioration. Although most patients have serologic liver dysfunction, no disease-specific abnormalities have been identified.

On imaging, multifocal hepatic involvement is detected in nearly all cases, with at least 10 lesions in 74 percent of cases (60). Individual nodules are typically circumscribed. Unenhanced images depict hemorrhagic areas and a markedly heterogeneous internal architecture within large tumors (61). Contrast-enhanced early phase images exhibit variable patterns, including patchy peripheral or irregular central foci of enhancement, peripheral rim enhancement, and small lesions without enhancement (62). On dynamic studies, hypervascular foci progressively expand and show blood pool (60). Although imaging features may suggest the diagnosis, tissue sampling is essential for establishing a definite diagnosis.

Gross Findings. Livers with angiosarcoma are generally enlarged and may weigh more than 3 kg. Most cases have multicentric tumors with a large number of nodules present in both lobes (fig. 9-31). A single tumor is a markedly less common presentation. The size of individual nodules ranges from subcentimeters to over 10 cm. On cross section, nodules are red or brown with hemorrhagic foci (fig. 9-32). Cystic degeneration filled with liquid blood may be observed. Thorotrast-related angiosarcoma may show variable background liver fibrosis; however, most cases of angiosarcoma develop in noncirrhotic livers (3).

Microscopic Findings. The morphologic appearance varies widely from well-formed anastomosing blood vessels to solid sheets of high-grade tumor cells without clear vascular cavity formation (fig. 9-33). Hepatic angiosarcoma, therefore, displays a solid and cystic microscopic appearance with a variable combination of the two components (fig. 9-34). The cystic area consists of largely dilated vascular cavities

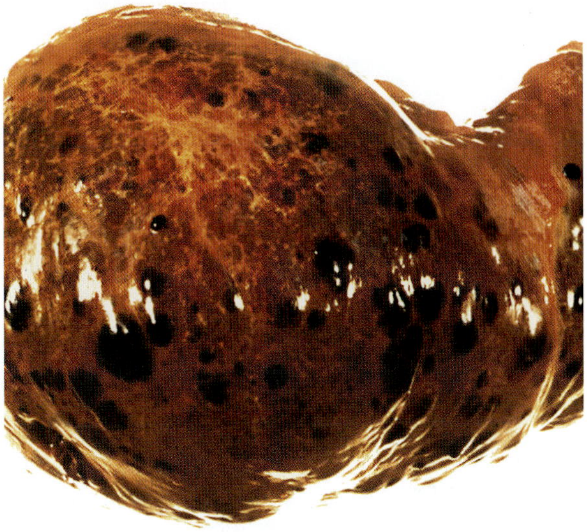

Figure 9-31

ANGIOSARCOMA

The external surface of the liver is riddled with raised, black nodules of varied size. Yellow-white reticular fibrosis is seen.

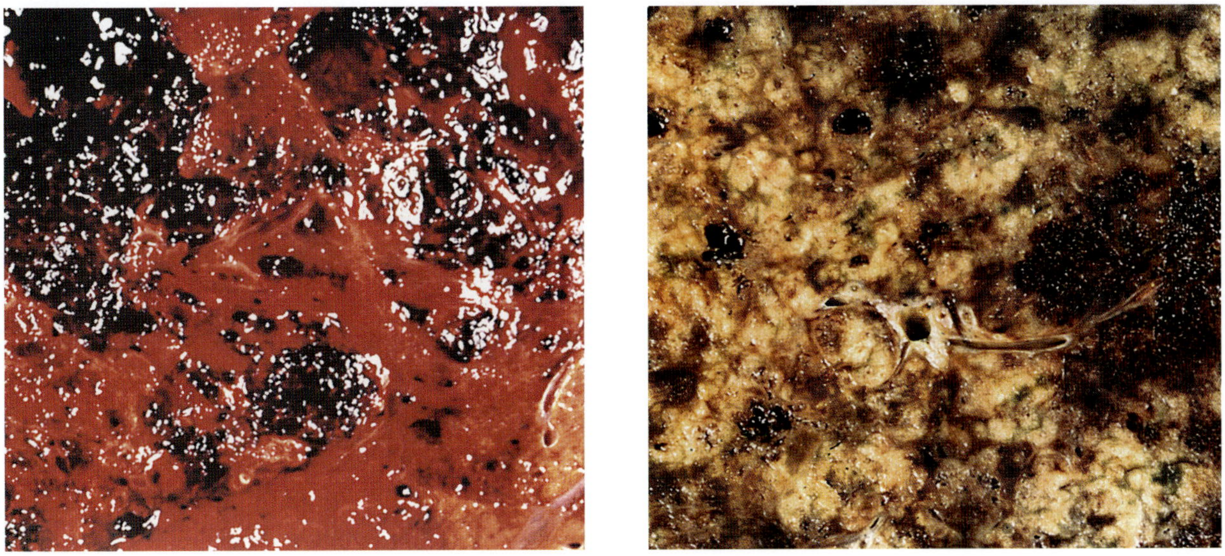

Figure 9-32

ANGIOSARCOMA

Left: Dark, red-brown cavitary lesions formed by the tumor are scattered in this close-up of a liver section. Yellowish-tan tumor foci are present.

Right: This section of the liver has a mottled tan and brown appearance.

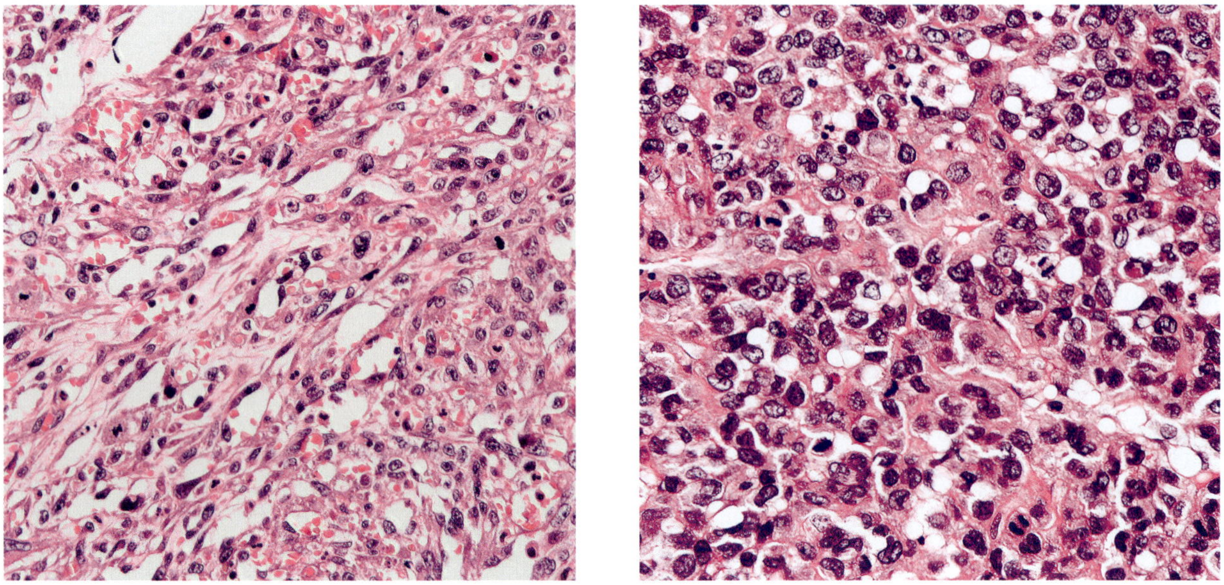

Figure 9-33

ANGIOSARCOMA

Left: Neoplastic spindle cells form small vascular structures containing red blood cells.
Right: Epithelioid atypical cells are arranged in a sheet pattern displaying high-grade nuclear atypia and brisk mitotic figures.

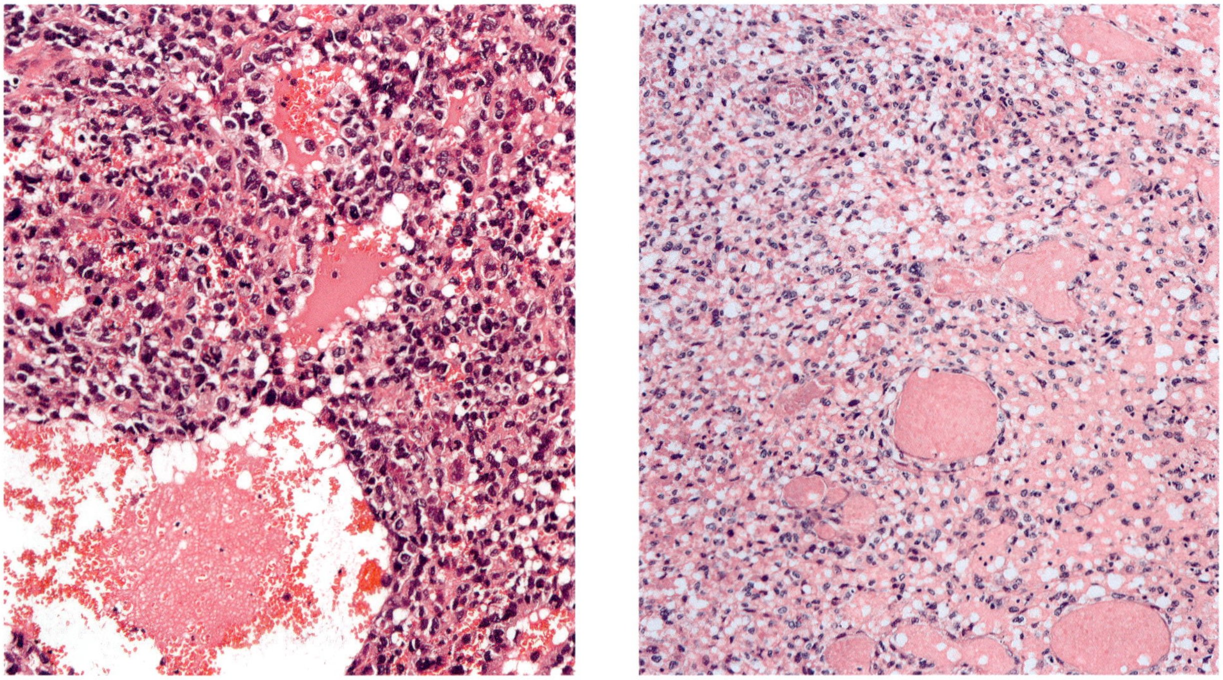

Figure 9-34

ANGIOSARCOMA

Left: This case shows a solid and cystic appearance with blood contents contained in cystic spaces.
Right: Dilated vascular spaces are formed against the background sheet of tumor cells.

filled with blood and lined by tumor cells that have enlarged and hyperchromatic nuclei; the growth pattern is often multilayered or pseudopapillary (fig. 9-35). Although the appearance may mimic cavernous hemangioma (see fig. 9-5B), cytologic atypia is more obvious than in that benign vascular neoplasm. The presence of mitotic figures also supports a diagnosis of angiosarcoma. In solid areas, epithelioid or spindle-shaped tumor cells are arranged in a sheet pattern, often associated with necrosis and hemorrhage, with the latter degeneration process sometimes leading to a reticular architecture (fig. 9-36). Cells have high-grade atypia including large vesicular nuclei with prominent nucleoli, cellular pleomorphism, and brisk mitotic figures. Tumors in which epithelioid cells predominate are often referred to as *epithelioid angiosarcoma*. They need to be carefully discriminated from carcinomas.

A characteristic feature in pediatric cases is the presence of kaposiform areas consisting of spindle cells arranged in bundles with scattered slit-like vascular spaces (fig. 9-37) (3). Kaposiform areas may also display a whorl-like arrangement of cells and numerous eosinophilic globules in the cytoplasm of the neoplastic cells (fig. 9-38) (63).

The tumor cells often spread along preexisting vascular channels and sinusoids (fig. 9-39). The nature of the endothelial origin may not be obvious on H&E-stained sections of solid areas or biopsy samples. Immunostaining assists in confirming endothelial differentiation because most cases are positive for at least one endothelial marker including CD34, CD31, and factor VIII (fig. 9-40). Cytokeratins may be positive in some cases of angiosarcoma, particularly the epithelioid variant (64). Rarely, metastatic poorly differentiated or undifferentiated carcinomas show intrasinusoidal infiltration or sinusoidal dilatation, mimicking hepatic angiosarcoma (fig. 9-41).

Molecular Genetic Findings. Two previous studies suggested that *TP53* mutation patterns are distinct between vinyl chloride-related and -nonrelated angiosarcoma. The former commonly has A to T transversion missense mutations at codons 249 and 255 (two of four cases), while only 9 percent of sporadic angiosarcomas harbor *TP53* mutations, and their mutated alleles (G to A transitions at codons at 141 and 136) differ from those observed in vinyl chloride-related angiosarcoma, suggesting that vinyl chloride-related angiosarcoma has a distinctive *TP53* mutation profile (65,66). *KRAS* is also sometimes mutated in hepatic angiosarcoma, but its frequency in vinyl chloride-related angiosarcoma (83 percent) appears to be higher than that in sporadic (26 percent) and Thorotrast-induced (40 percent) cases (67).

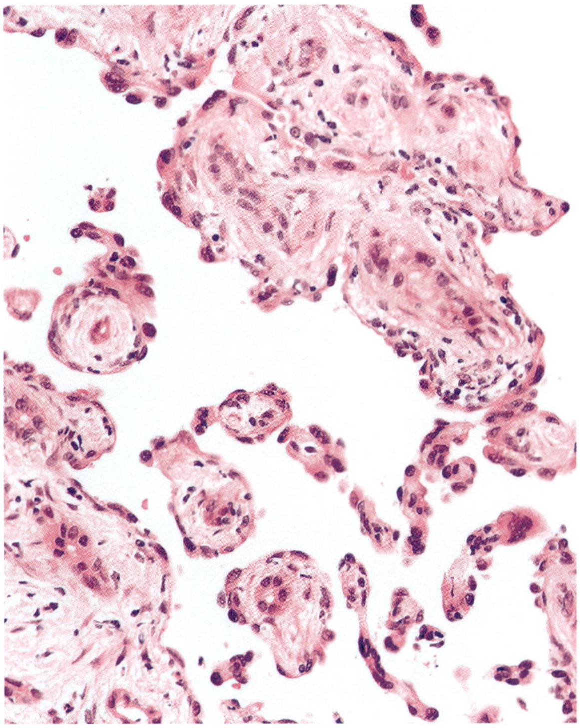

Figure 9-35

ANGIOSARCOMA

Cavernous vascular spaces have pseudopapillary projections. Lining endothelial cells are highly atypical with enlarged pleomorphic nuclei.

Treatment and Prognosis. Therapeutic approaches are limited for hepatic angiosarcoma. Although favorable responses and prolonged survival have been reported with chemotherapy, most patients die within 1 year. In autopsy series, extrahepatic metastases are commonly noted in the lungs, bone, and spleen.

Angiomyolipoma

Definition. *Angiomyolipoma* is a benign neoplasm composed of a variable admixture of adipose tissue, smooth muscle, and thick-walled

Figure 9-36

ANGIOSARCOMA

A: Spindle-shaped neoplastic cells are arranged in a reticular pattern. Note entrapped hepatocytes with bile casts.

B: At high magnification, tumor cells form slit-like spaces, probably representing early vascular formation.

C: Coagulative necrosis is often present.

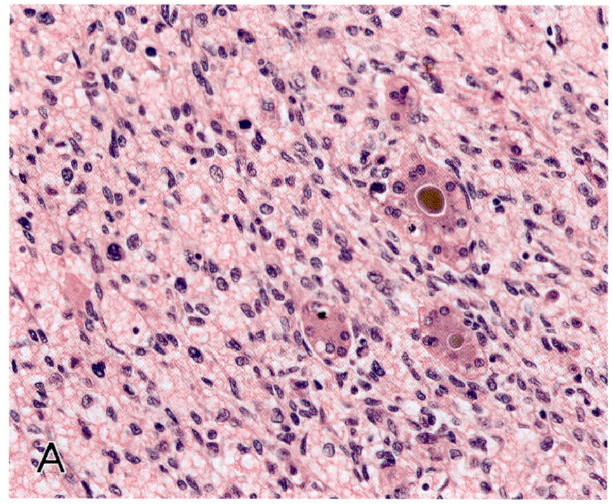

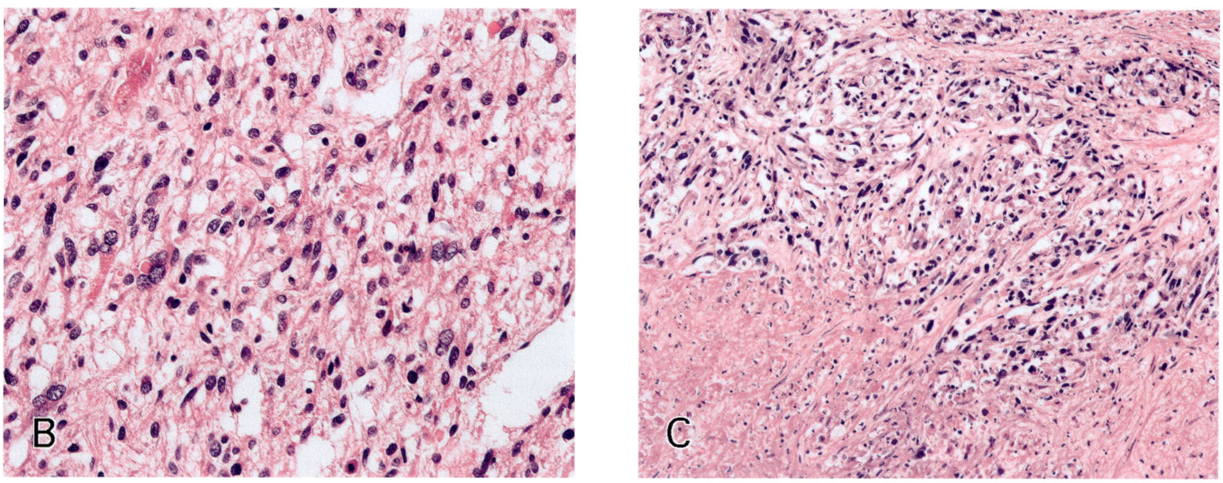

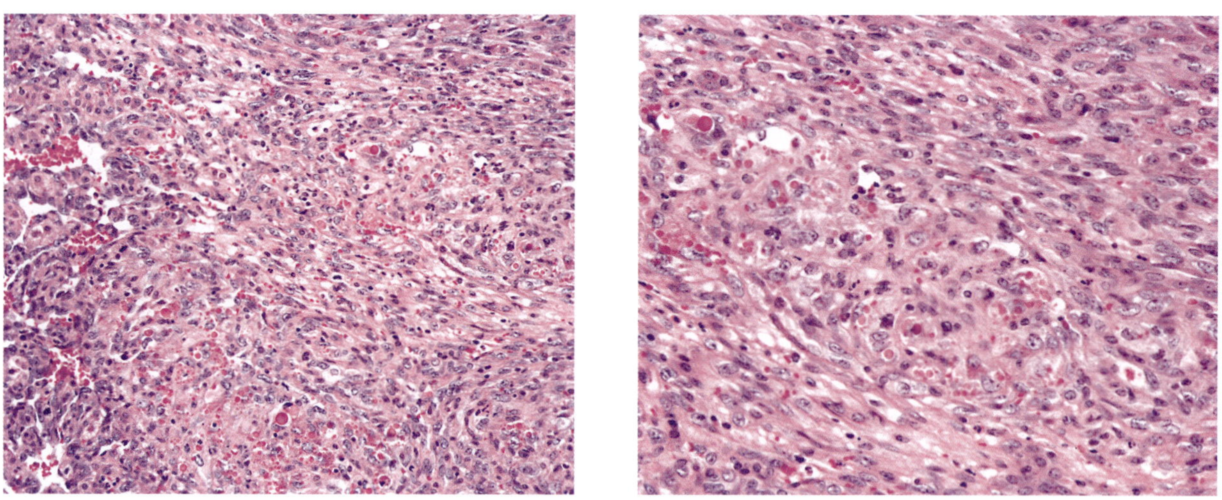

Figure 9-37

KAPOSIFORM ANGIOSARCOMA

Left: Spindle cell kaposiform area with numerous eosinophilic hyaline globules.
Right: Higher-magnification view.

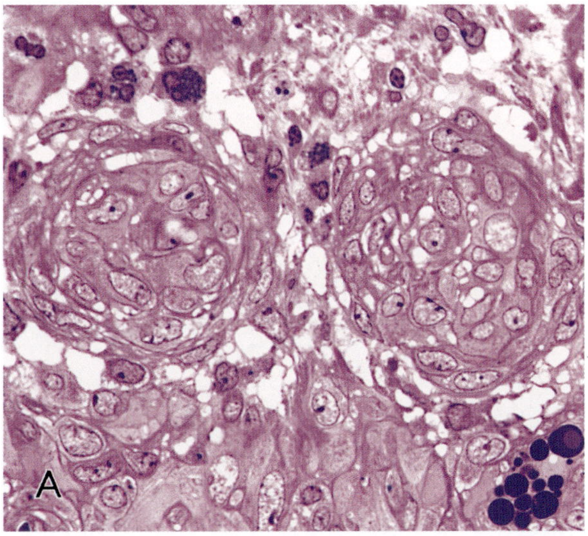

Figure 9-38

KAPOSIFORM ANGIOSARCOMA

A: Two "glomeruloid" foci have a whorled arrangement of tumor cells. Dark blue globules of varied size are seen (1 μm-thick, Epon-embedded section stained with toluidine blue).

B: Cells of a glomeruloid focus are more closely packed and have denser nuclei than the rest of the tumor.

C: Spindle cells, as well as the cells of a glomeruloid focus, strongly express CD34 (immunostain).

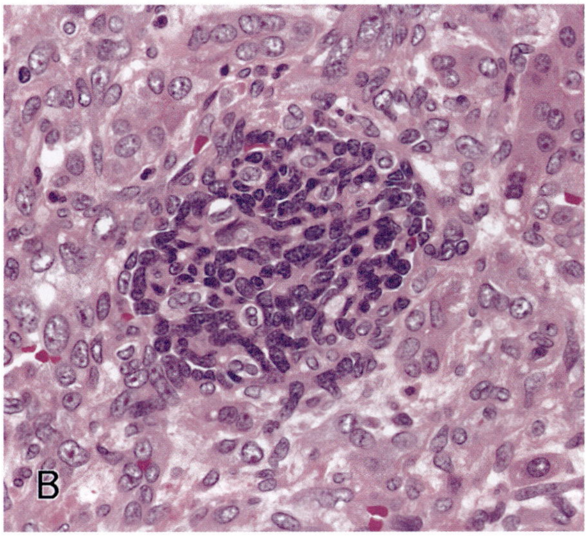

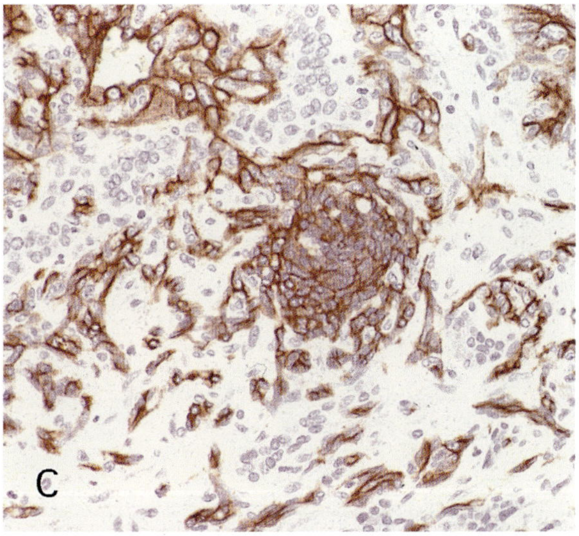

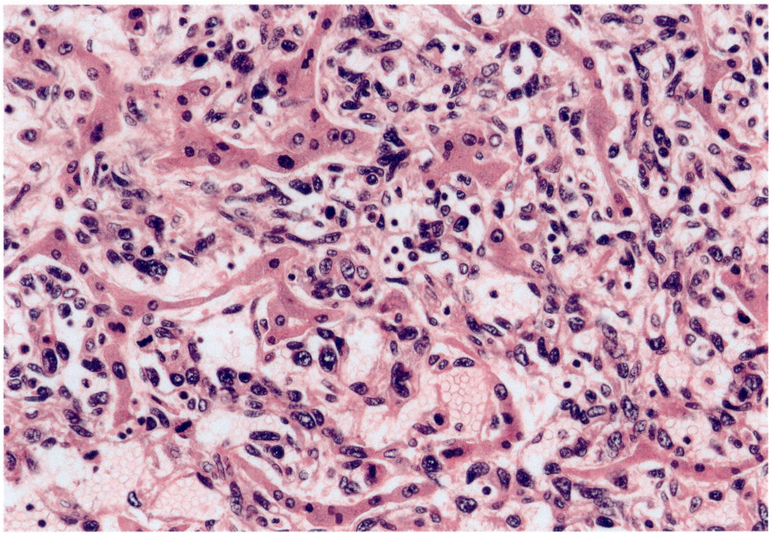

Figure 9-39

ANGIOSARCOMA

The tumor infiltrates into sinusoidal spaces and attenuates liver cell plates.

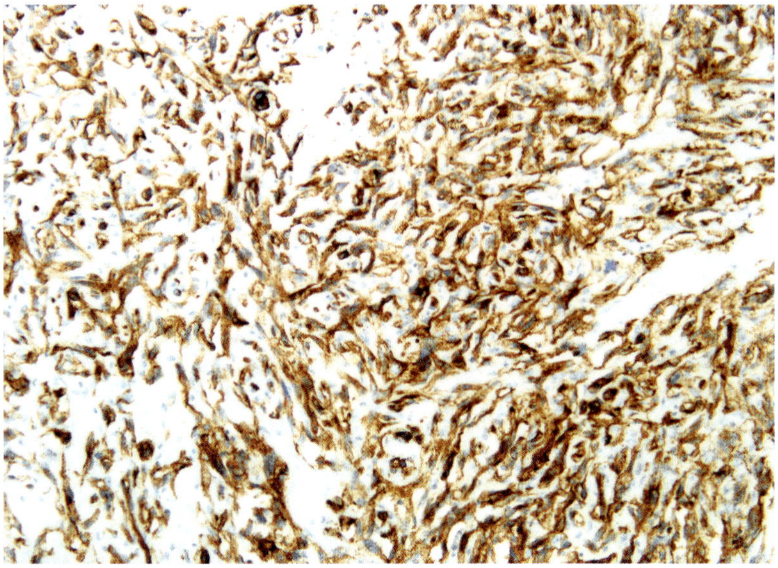

Figure 9-40

ANGIOSARCOMA

The tumor cells are diffusely positive for CD34.

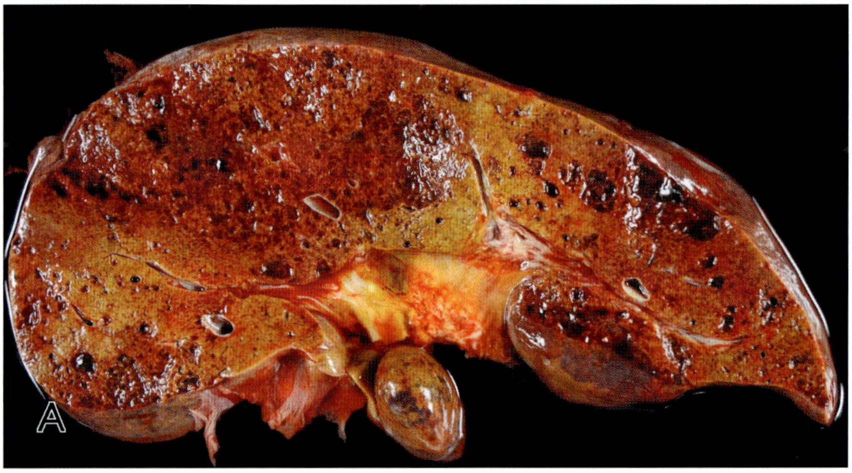

Figure 9-41

METASTATIC UNDIFFERENTIATED CARCINOMA OF PANCREATIC ORIGIN

A: The liver contains multiple blood-containing irregular nodules, a gross appearance mimicking angiosarcoma.

B: The sinusoidal spaces are dilated due to intrasinusoidal infiltration of large pleomorphic tumor cells. The growth pattern is similar to angiosarcoma.

C: The floating tumor cells in the sinusoids are strongly positive for pancytokeratin.

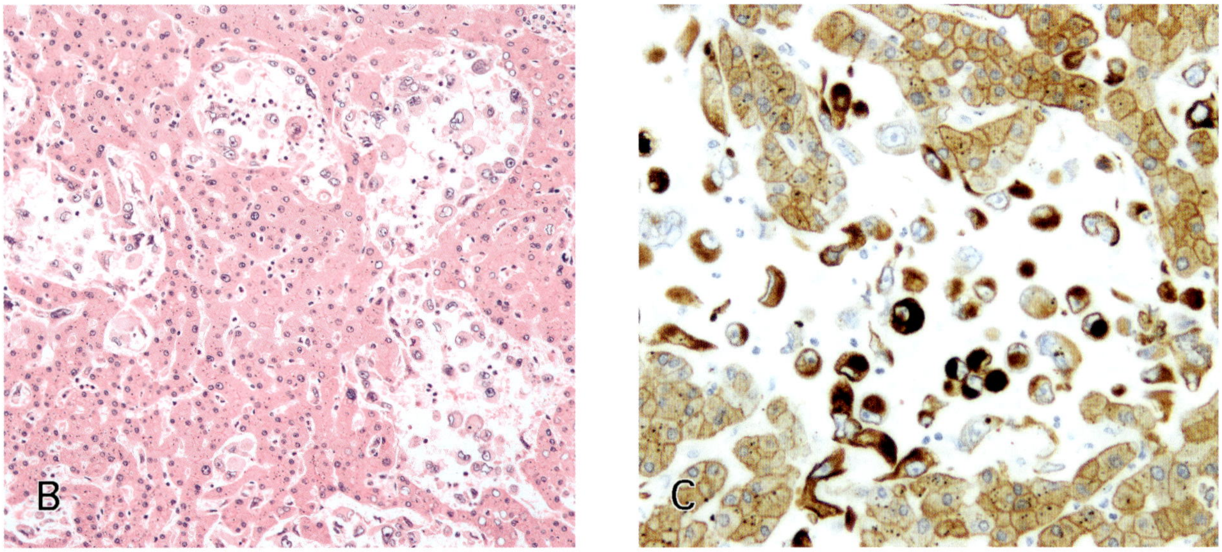

blood vessels. This entity belongs to the group of tumors derived from perivascular endothelial cells (PEComa).

General and Clinical Features. Most patients are adults with a mean age of approximately 50 years; however, rare pediatric cases have been reported (age range, 10 to 86 years). This neoplasm develops more commonly in women than men: 68 to 83 percent of patients were women in several large series (4,68,69). Approximately 5 percent of patients have a history of tuberous sclerosis complex (TSC), an autosomal dominant inherited disorder with systemic hamartomatous manifestations, but its proportion is less than that in renal angiomyolipoma (20 percent) (70).

Most patients are asymptomatic and incidentally are found to have a liver tumor. Patients with large angiomyolipomas may present with abdominal pain or rarely with hemoperitoneum due to tumor rupture. On imaging, hepatic angiomyolipoma exhibits nodular masses with variable fat content. Contrast-enhanced studies report early enhancement in more than 50 percent of cases, particularly in myomatous neoplasms (71,72). The imaging appearance of hypervascular liver tumors with fat contents is sometimes mistaken for hepatocellular carcinoma (73). Angiomyolipoma is curable with surgical resection, with small stable disease potentially not requiring treatment.

Most cases of hepatic angiomyolipoma are benign, with less than a dozen cases of "malignant" angiomyolipoma being described in the literature (74–77). Although a diagnosis of malignancy is suggested by remote metastasis, extrahepatic tumors may simply be multicentric lesions in some patients (4). Only several patients with hepatic angiomyolipoma died of tumor progression (74,75).

Gross Findings. Although hepatic angiomyolipoma is generally solitary, multiple tumors may develop, particularly in patients with TSC (fig. 9-42). Sixty-four percent of tumors occur in the right liver lobe, 30 percent in the left lobe, and 6 percent in the caudate lobe (73). Individual tumor nodules vary in size (up to 36 cm) and are typically well circumscribed, but not encapsulated. Large tumors may have foci of hemorrhage or necrosis. Color and consistency depend on the relative proportion of fat (yellow and soft) and smooth muscle (tan-white and firm), and whether there has been hemorrhaging in the tumor (fig. 9-43) (4).

Microscopic Findings. The microscopic appearance may vary from case to case and in different areas of the same tumor. Although the three histologic components of smooth muscle, adipose tissue, and blood vessels are at least focally present in most cases (fig. 9-44), the proportion of these elements varies greatly. According to the dominant component, which should account for more than 20 percent of the tumor, the most common morphologic appearance is myomatous (65 percent), followed by myoangiomatous (14 percent) and conventional triphasic (11 percent), with other combinations less common (73). Cases consisting of a predominance of one element pose a diagnostic difficulty.

Smooth muscle is the most specific diagnostic element. Four types of smooth muscle cells may be present: spindle, intermediate, epithelioid, and pleomorphic. Spindle cells show fascicular growth, resembling a true smooth muscle neoplasm (fig. 9-45). Epithelioid cells arranged in a trabecular or solid architecture have clear or eosinophilic cytoplasm (fig. 9-46) (68). Condensed cytoplasmic contents often form intracytoplasmic eosinophilic globules, which push nuclei to the periphery and are surrounded by a clear "halo," a somewhat rhabdoid change suggesting myoid differentiation (fig. 9-47). Pleomorphic cells with enlarged bizarre nuclei may mimic the high-grade neoplastic cells of sarcomas, but mitotic figures are exceptional. Abnormal blood vessels having a thick muscular or fibrotic wall are randomly distributed within these tumors (fig. 9-48). Mature adipose tissue with large lipid droplets exists to varying degrees (fig. 9-49).

Hematopoietic cells are commonly present in hepatic angiomyolipoma, and may be prominent in some cases. Some cases have a massive inflammatory infiltrate (*inflammatory angiomyolipoma*), resembling inflammatory pseudotumors (78). A complete or incomplete fibrous capsule is present in up to 10 percent of cases (73). Two thirds of cases show infiltrative growth into the adjacent liver parenchyma, into portal connective tissue, and around hepatic veins (79). These infiltrative patterns must not be considered a sign of malignancy.

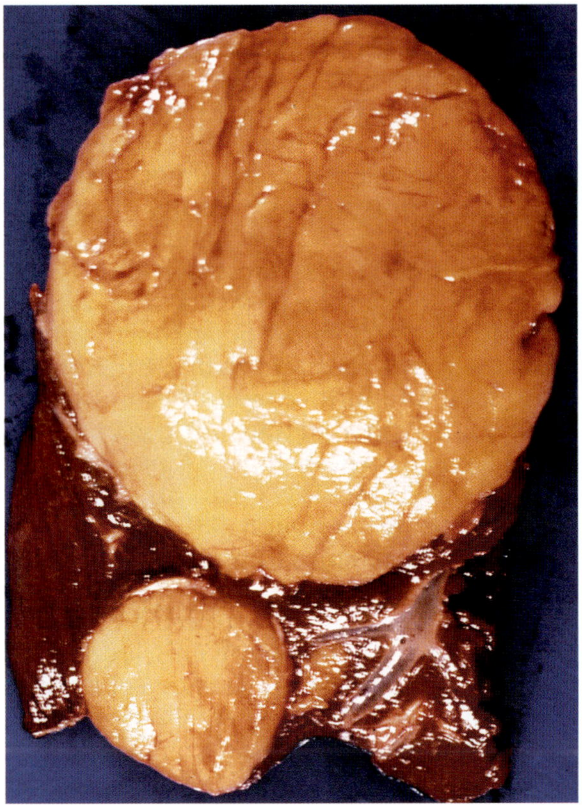

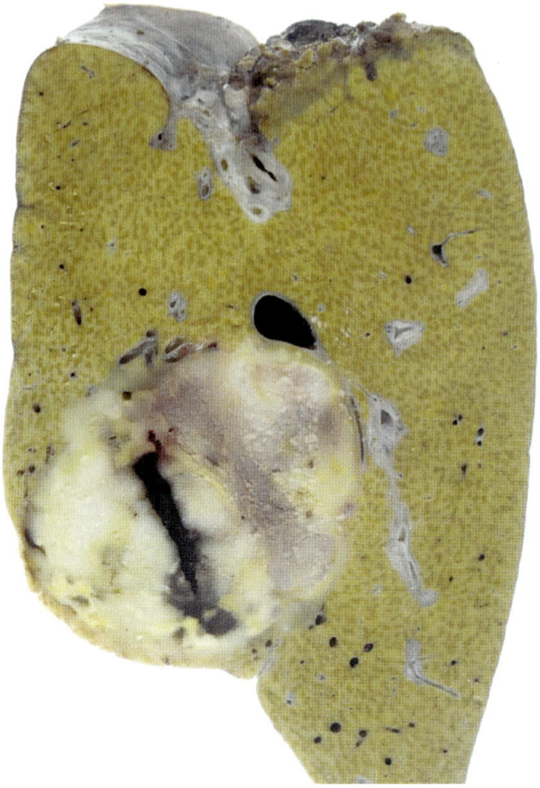

Figure 9-42

ANGIOMYOLIPOMA

Left: The section of two tumors shows them to be well circumscribed and bright yellow.
Right: This section shows a well-circumscribed mass with a partly yellowish and partly gray cut surface.

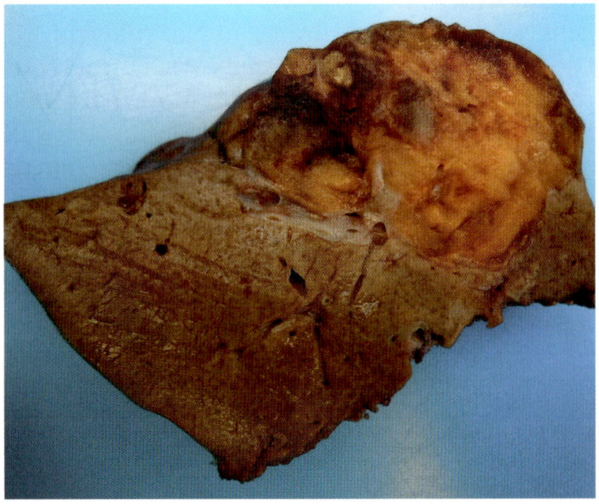

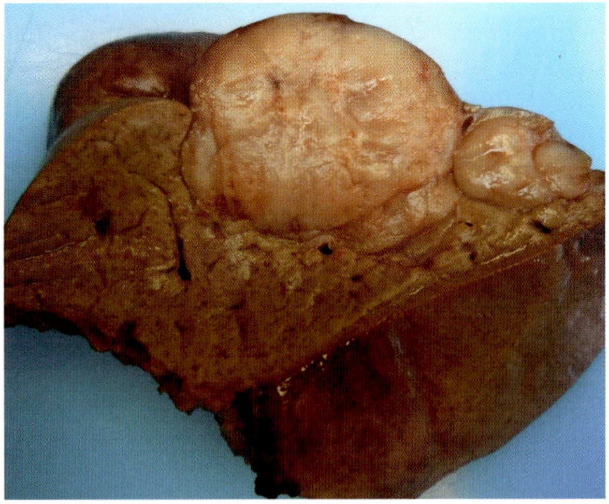

Figure 9-43

ANGIOMYOLIPOMA

Left: This tumor has a yellowish fatty gross appearance.
Right: Sectioning reveals a solid tumor with a homogeneously tan cut surface.

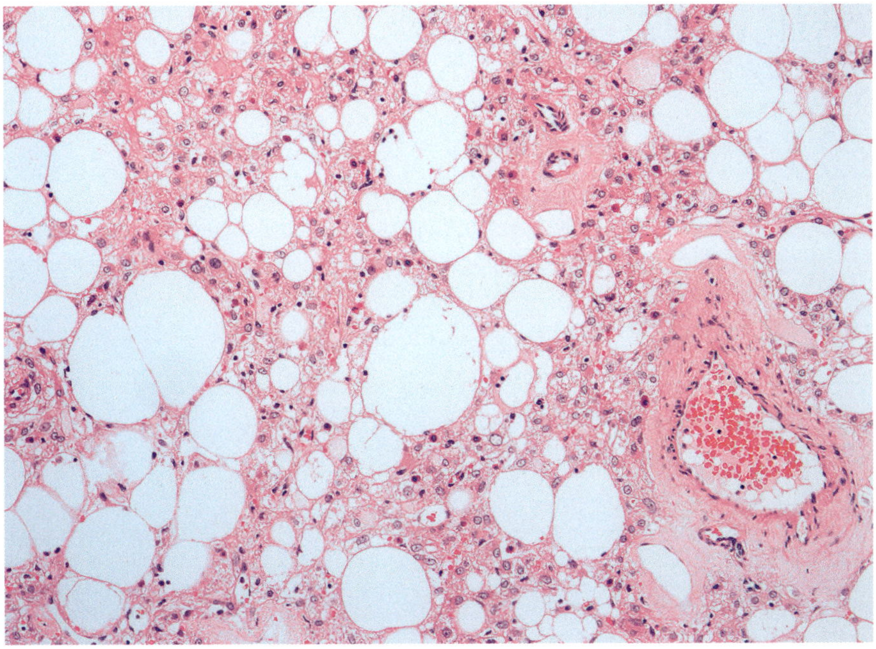

Figure 9-44

ANGIOMYOLIPOMA

The classic triphasic tumor consists of blood vessels, epithelioid smooth muscle cells, and mature fat.

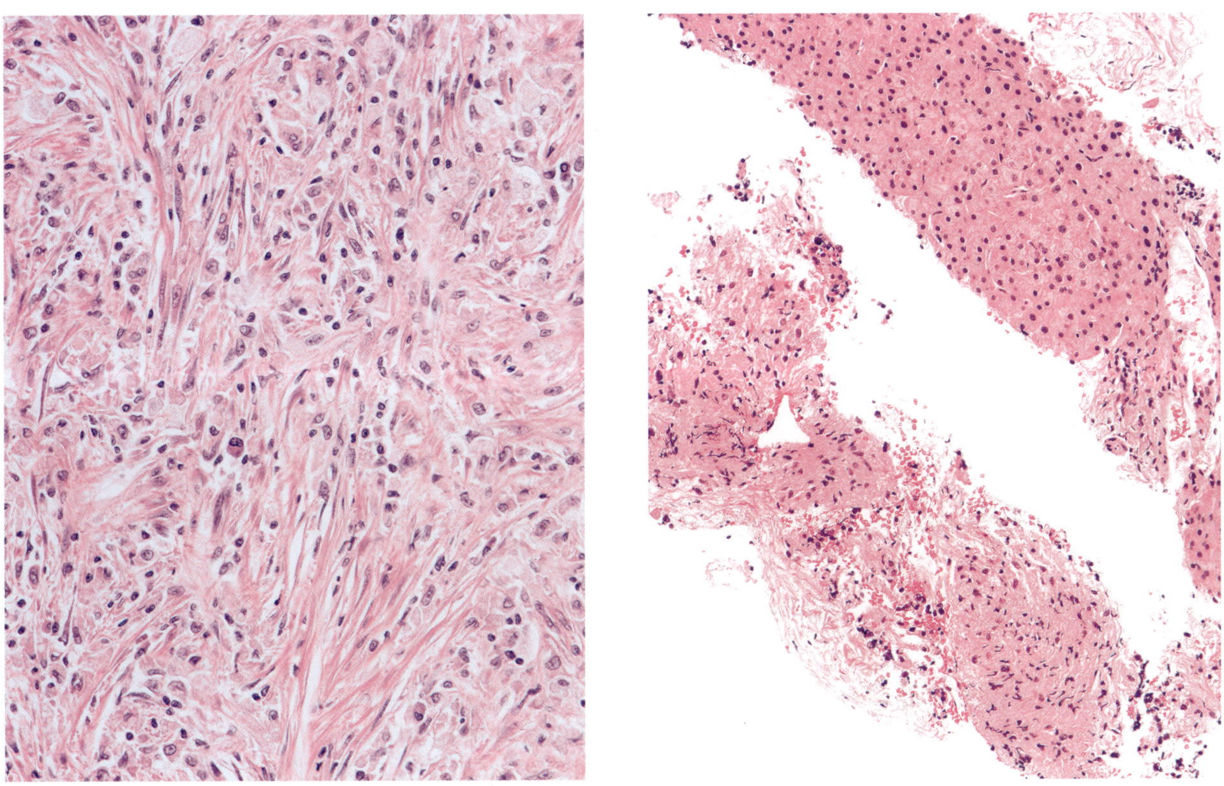

Figure 9-45

ANGIOMYOLIPOMA

Left: Spindle-shaped smooth muscle cells are arranged in a fascicular pattern.

Right: This biopsy sample contained a small piece of peculiar tissue consisting of irregularly arranged spindle cells. Angiomyolipoma needs to be considered for unusual fibrous lesions like this.

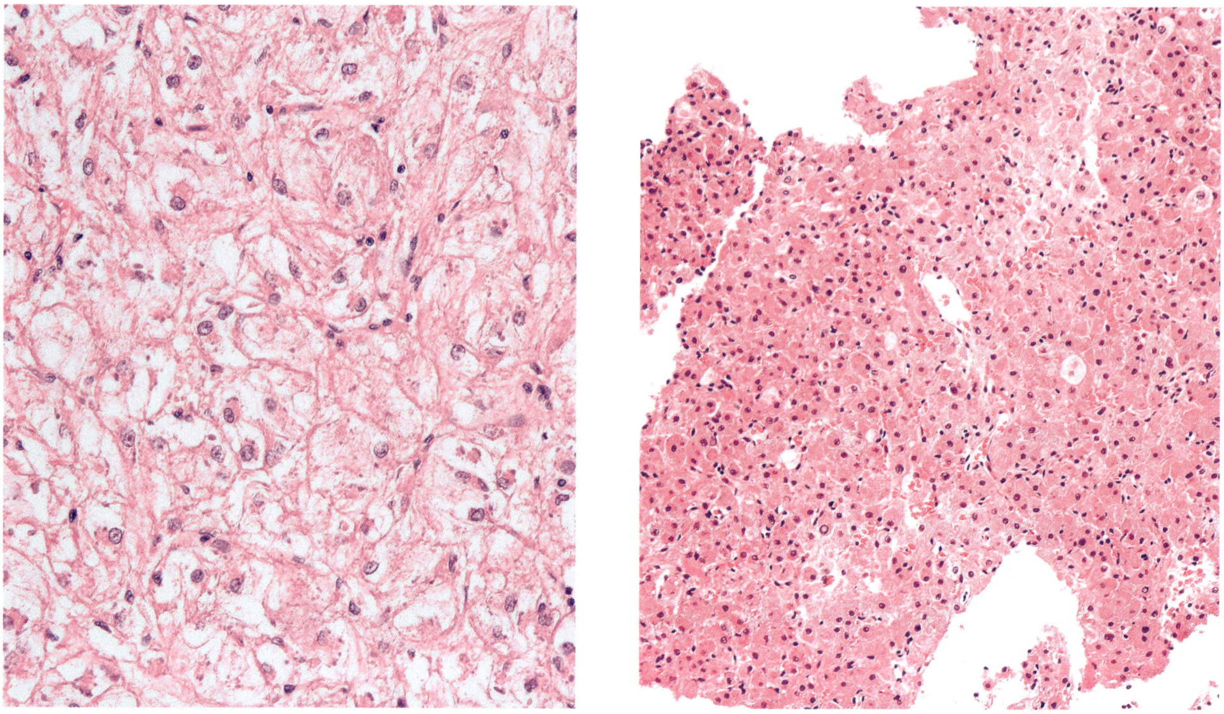

Figure 9-46

ANGIOMYOLIPOMA

Left: Epithelioid smooth muscle cells arranged in a solid pattern have clear, somewhat foamy cytoplasm.

Right: This biopsy sample shows eosinophilic polygonal cells arranged in sheets, mimicking hepatocellular carcinoma. In biopsy cases like this, the differential diagnosis between the two conditions is often challenging based on H&E-stained sections.

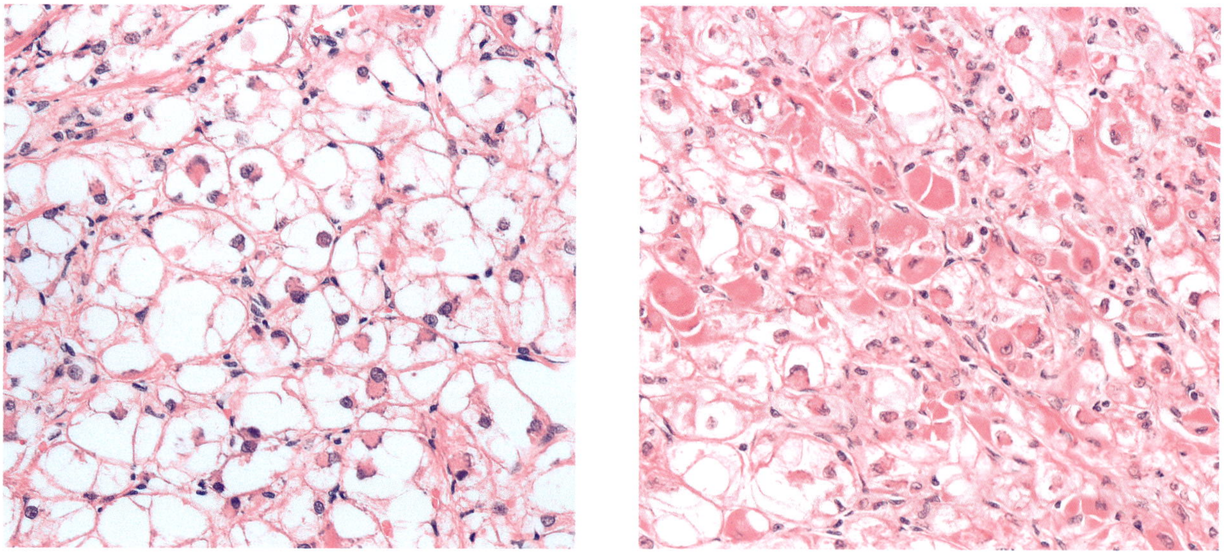

Figure 9-47

ANGIOMYOLIPOMA

Left: Condensed cytoplasmic contents next to the nuclei are characteristic for angiomyolipoma.

Right: Some cells contain intracytoplasmic eosinophilic globules surrounded by a clear "halo."

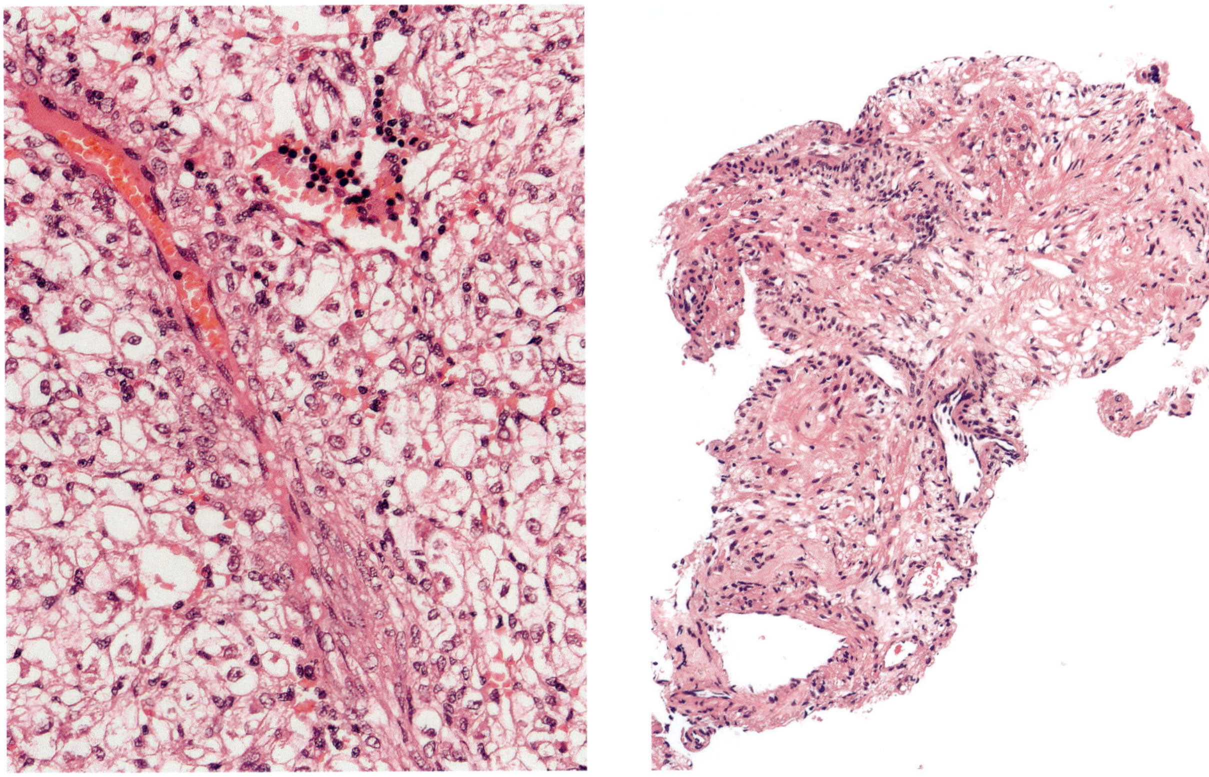

Figure 9-48

ANGIOMYOLIPOMA

Left: A blood vessel with a partly thick wall is identified. Hematopoiesis is also noted (right upper).

Right: This needle biopsy specimen contains abnormal blood vessels surrounded by smooth muscle cells that are irregular in shape and arrangement, an appearance suggesting angiomyolipoma.

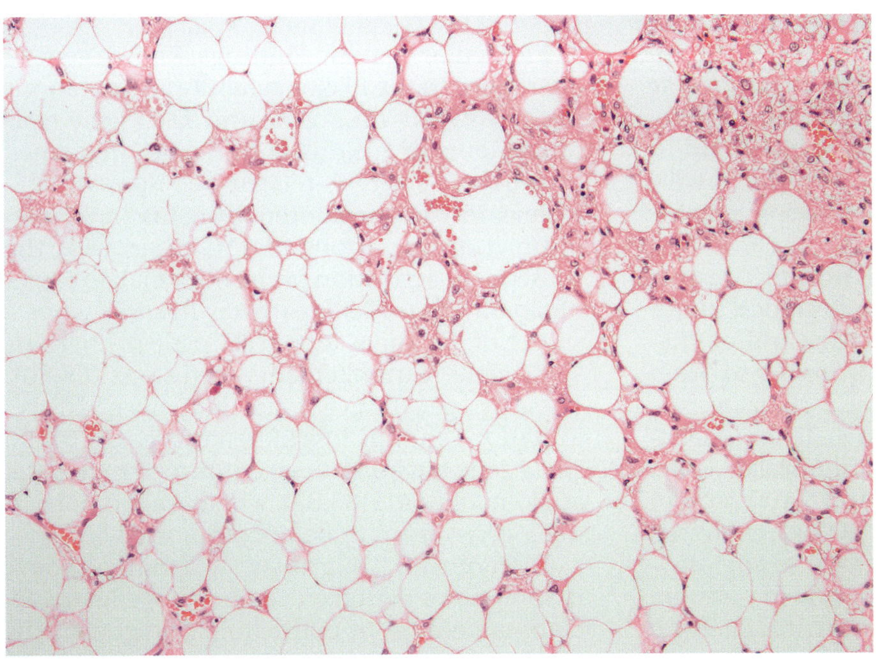

Figure 9-49

ANGIOMYOLIPOMA

There is a component of well-differentiated adipose tissue. Epithelioid smooth muscle cells are also present (right upper).

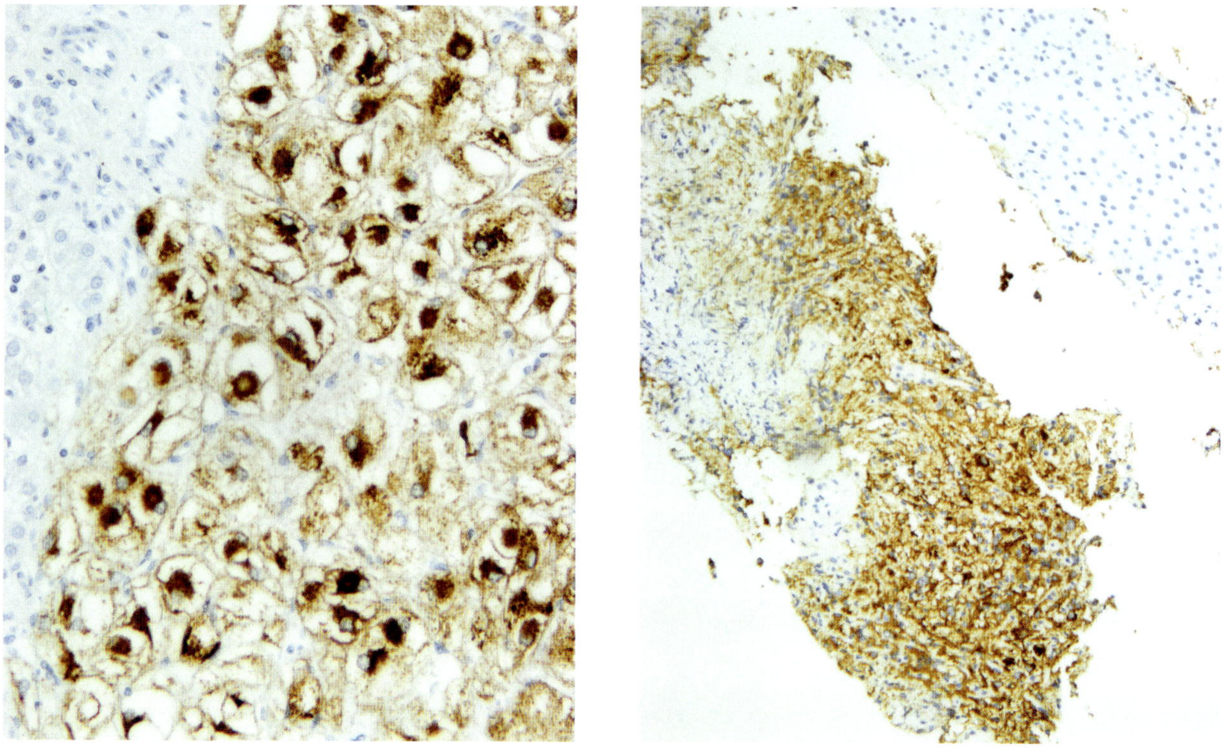

Figure 9-50

ANGIOMYOLIPOMA

Left: Epithelioid smooth muscle cells are positive for HMB-45. The signal is particularly strong in condensed cytoplasmic contents.

Right: Melan-A is expressed in the spindle-shaped smooth muscle components. (Same case as fig. 9-45, right.)

The presence of coagulative necrosis and the lack of CD117 expression were previously reported in four cases of malignant hepatic angiomyolipoma (74). However, it is impossible to establish a diagnosis of malignant angiomyolipoma purely on morphologic grounds. An aggressive clinical course with progressive extrahepatic dissemination is the sole reliable indicator of malignancy.

Immunohistochemical Findings. Despite the epithelioid morphologic appearance, tumor cells are negative for cytokeratins and epithelial membrane antigen (EMA). Similar to other tumors of the PEComa family, a characteristic feature is immunoreactivity to melanoma-related antigens including HMB-45 and Melan-A (fig. 9-50) (68,80). CD117 (c-kit) and S-100 protein are also commonly expressed. SOX10, expressed in melanocyte lineages, is negative in angiomyolipoma (81). Spindle-shaped myoid cells are more commonly positive for vimentin, desmin, and smooth muscle actin than epithelioid cells (fig. 9-51) (82).

Molecular Genetic Findings. Known genetic alterations in the PEComa family are mutations in the *TSC1* or *TSC2* gene and *TFE3* gene rearrangements or fusions (83). A high frequency of tuberous sclerosis-related and sporadic PEComas in extrahepatorenal organs have loss-of-function mutations in *TSC* genes with the subsequent activation of the mammalian target of rapamycin (mTOR) pathway (84, 85), while a subset of PEComas (about 23 percent) harbors *TFE3* gene rearrangements or fusions (83,86). These two genetic events are mutually exclusive. Mutations and the loss of heterozygosity in the *TSC2* gene have also been confirmed in hepatic angiomyolipoma (83,87), whereas alterations in *TFE3* genes seem to be uncommon (87a).

Differential Diagnosis. Angiomyolipoma is sometimes mistaken for hepatocellular carcinoma because of epithelioid polygonal cells

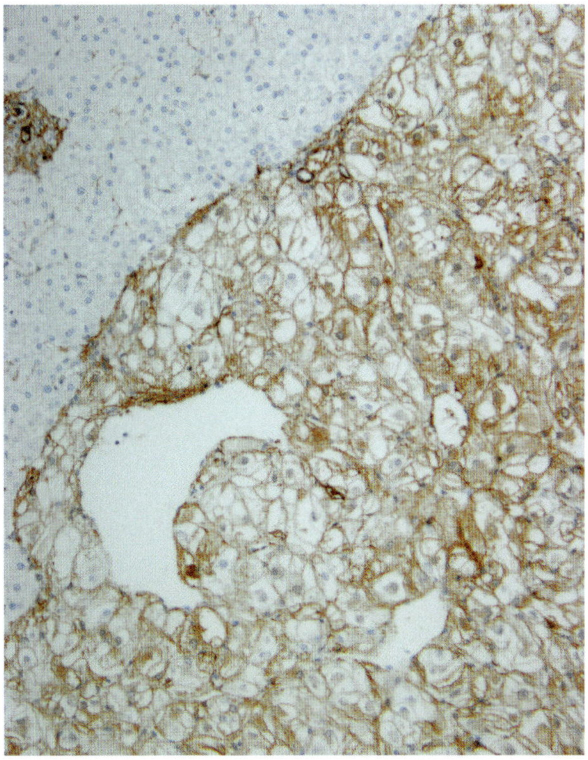

Figure 9-51

ANGIOMYOLIPOMA

Smooth muscle actin is positive in epithelioid neoplastic cells, but is negative in adjacent liver parenchyma (left upper).

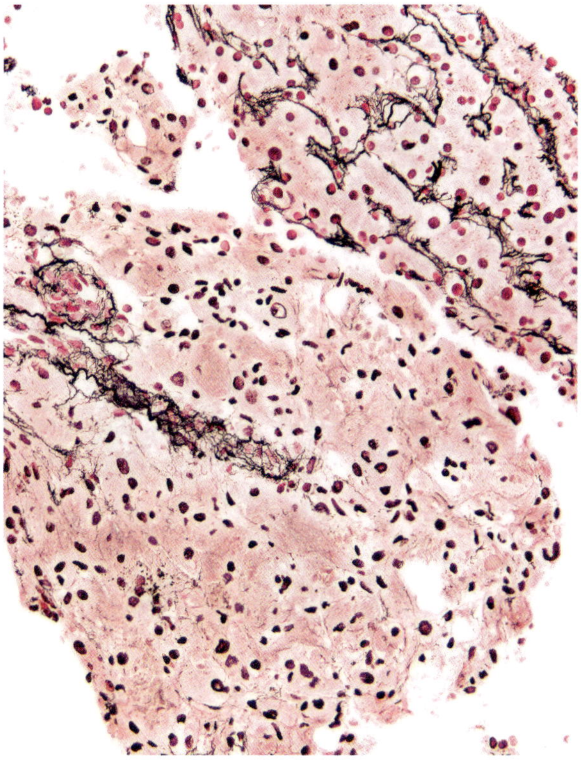

Figure 9-52

ANGIOMYOLIPOMA

This biopsy sample consists of pieces of background liver (top) and tumor tissue (bottom). Angiomyolipoma is epithelioid in appearance but has little intercellular reticulin (reticulin stain).

arranged in a trabecular pattern. In addition to immunohistochemistry, reticulin staining may assist in this differential diagnosis. Epithelioid angiomyolipoma completely lacks intercellular reticulin fibers (fig. 9-52). In contrast, although hepatocellular carcinoma is known to have reticulin loss, residual fibers are at least focally present.

Angiomyolipoma composed predominantly of spindle cells may mimic leiomyosarcoma in morphology and immunohistochemistry. Lipomatous angiomyolipoma may also be mistaken for lipoma. Since true hepatic lipoma is extremely uncommon, the possibility of angiomyolipoma needs to be considered for lipomatous lesions in the liver.

A rare morphologic variant of angiomatous angiomyolipoma may have abnormal large vessels resembling vascular malformation. Fat-containing solitary fibrous tumor may also mimic angiomyolipoma (see below). Immunostaining for HMB-45 and Melan-A is always useful for those differential diagnoses. Both of these markers need to be stained in biopsy samples because their focal expression may cause a false-negative result.

Kaposi Sarcoma

Kaposi sarcoma is a malignant vascular neoplasm that is characterized by spindle cells arranged in a mesh pattern, with occasional slit-like vascular spaces. The most common initial presentation is a skin lesion, and other organs including the liver are subsequently affected as a part of visceral or systemic dissemination. Hepatic involvement is incidentally found in approximately 20 percent of cases at autopsy (88). Although it is strongly associated with acquired immunodeficiency syndrome (AIDS), and hepatic involvement most commonly occurs in AIDS patients, Kaposi sarcoma unrelated

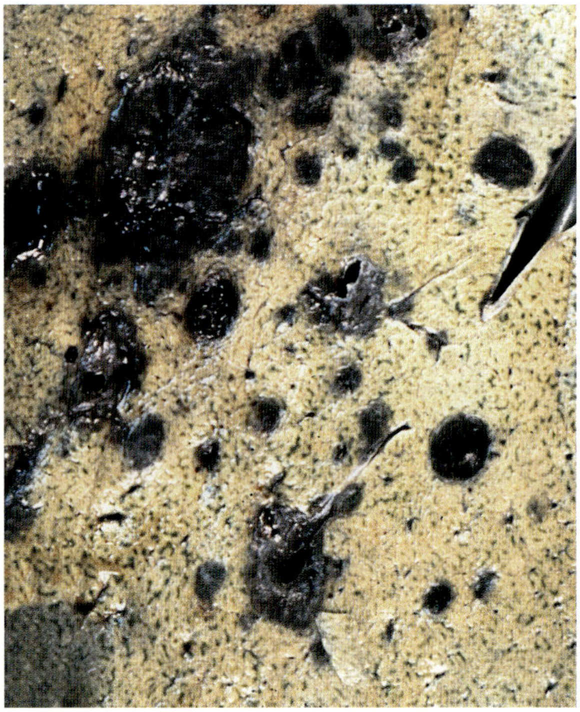
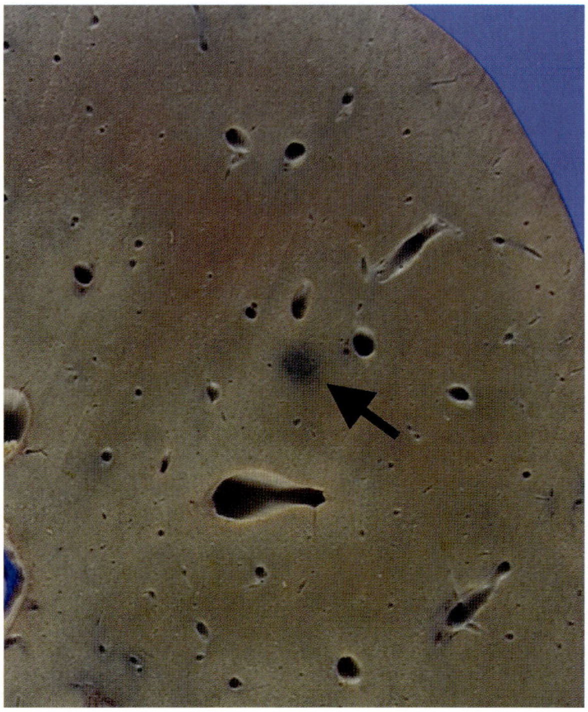

Figure 9-53

KAPOSI SARCOMA

Left: Blue-black tumor foci are present in large portal areas, with confluence of some of the larger foci.

Right: The autopsied liver contains a dark brown spot (arrow), representing a metastatic Kaposi sarcoma from the stomach. (Courtesy of Dr. Y. Kodama, Kyoto, Japan.)

to AIDS may develop in those of Mediterranean/East European descent and middle-aged men or children in equatorial Africa (89–91). Some cases may be associated with iatrogenic immunosuppression (e.g., post-transplantation) (92,93). Human herpesvirus 8 (HHV8) is detectable in all clinical forms of Kaposi sarcoma (94-96). Liver lesions themselves do not directly contribute to morbidity and mortality (97).

Grossly, hepatic Kaposi sarcoma typically involves portal and periportal areas, which are grossly identified as dark red spots (fig. 9-53). There may also be capsular deposits of the tumor, measuring 5 to 10 mm in diameter, appearing as dark red blebs (98).

Microscopically, the lesions consist of spindle cells with plump nuclei proliferating in portal connective tissue (fig. 9-54). These cells form slit-like spaces containing red blood cells (fig. 9-55), similar to Kaposi sarcoma in other organs. Intracytoplasmic hyaline globules and hemosiderin deposition are commonly observed.

On immunostaining, cells are positive for CD34, CD31, D2-40, and FLI1 (a transcription factor involved in endothelial differentiation) (fig. 9-56, left) (99–101). The immunohistochemical detection of HHV8 in the nuclei of tumor cells is useful for reaching a diagnosis (fig. 9-56, right) (102,103).

Lymphangioma

Lymphangioma is a benign neoplastic condition of lymphatic endothelial origin displaying hemangioma-like fluid-containing lesions. Hepatic lymphangioma rarely occurs in isolation and more commonly develops in association with similar lesions in other organs such as the spleen and skeleton (*lymphangiomatosis*).

The extent of liver involvement varies. Hepatic lesions are solitary at one end of the spectrum of manifestations, while the affected liver may be markedly enlarged with multiple lesions at the opposite end. Lesions are cystic on sections and contain clear or chylous milky fluid.

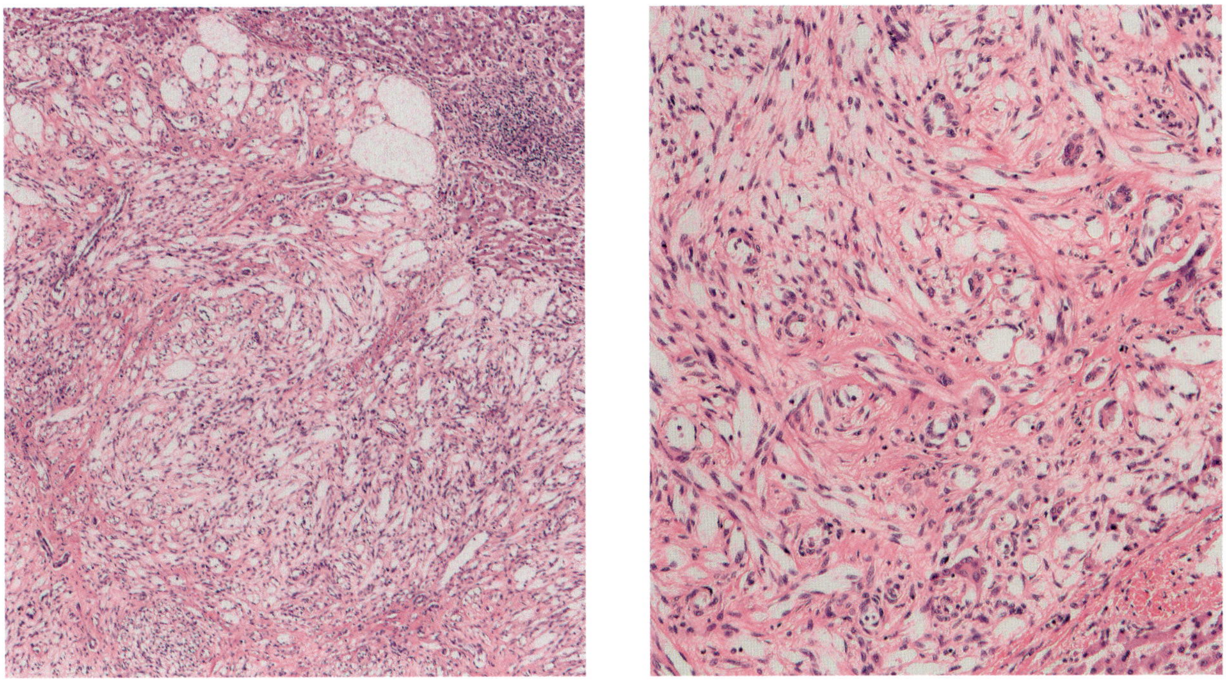

Figure 9-54

KAPOSI SARCOMA

Left: The tumor forms a lobulated mass involving the portal tracts. Slit-like spaces are present throughout the tumor. Right: Atypical spindle cells form slender vascular spaces. Entrapped bile ducts are also noted. (Left, right: courtesy of Dr. Y. Kodama, Kyoto, Japan.)

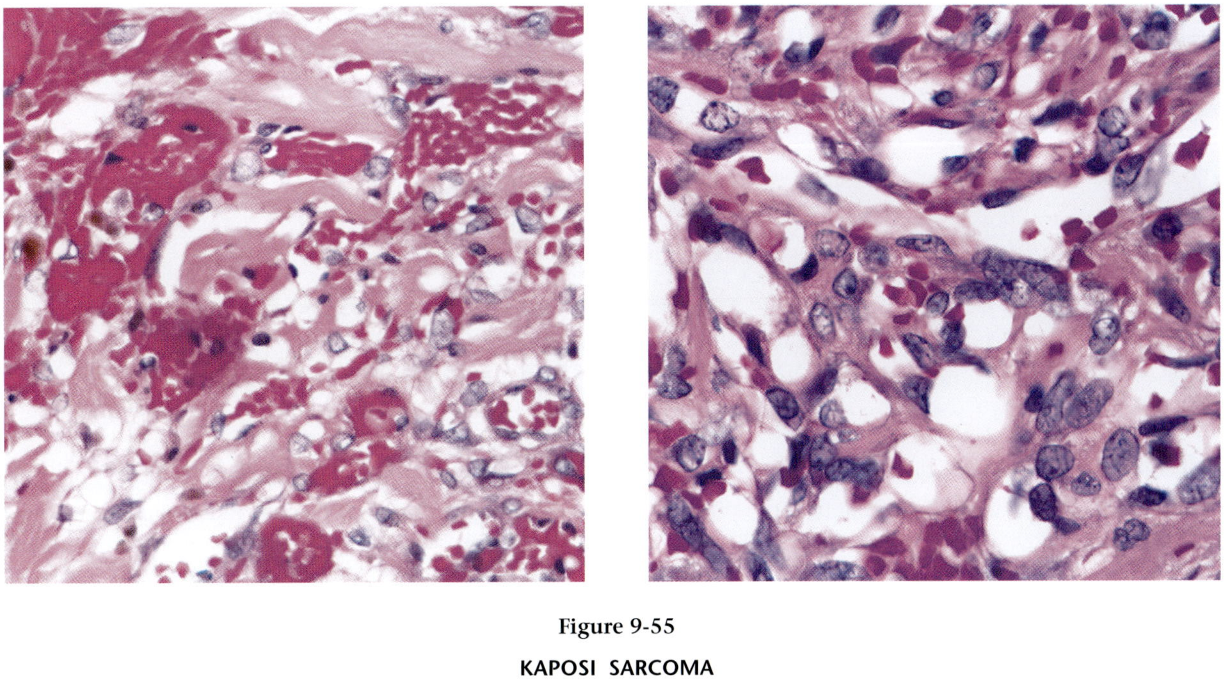

Figure 9-55

KAPOSI SARCOMA

Left: High magnification of the spindle cells, some collagen fibers, and red blood cells in slit-like spaces. Right: The spindle cells have ill-defined outlines and vesicular, round or ovoid nuclei.

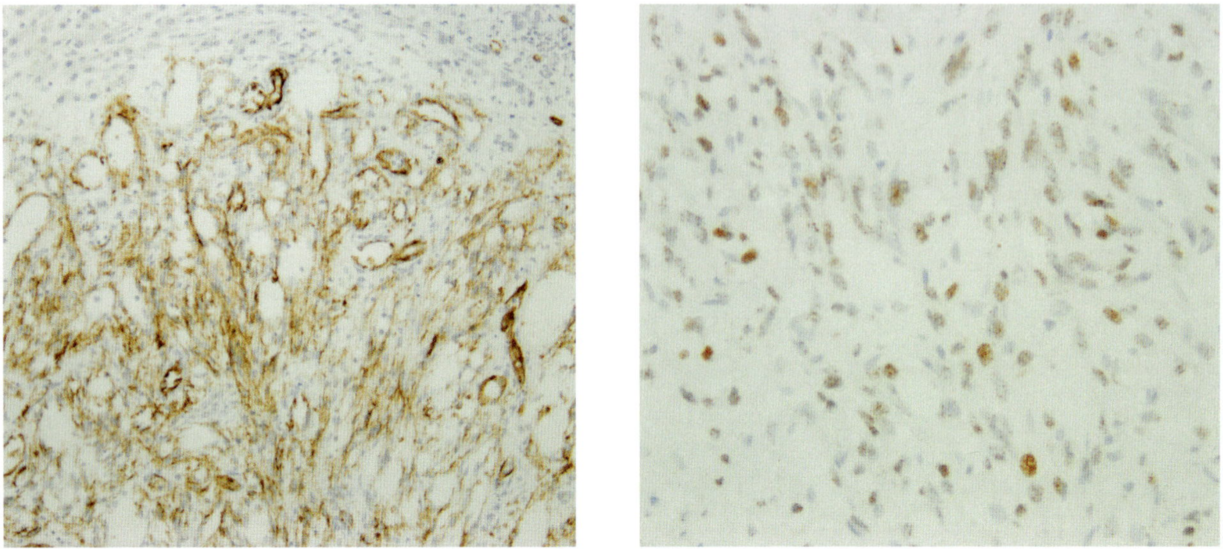

Figure 9-56

KAPOSI SARCOMA

Left: Tumor cells are positive for CD34.

Right: Immunostaining for HHV8 shows positive signals in the nuclei of tumor cells. (Left, right: courtesy of Dr. Y. Kodama, Kyoto, Japan.)

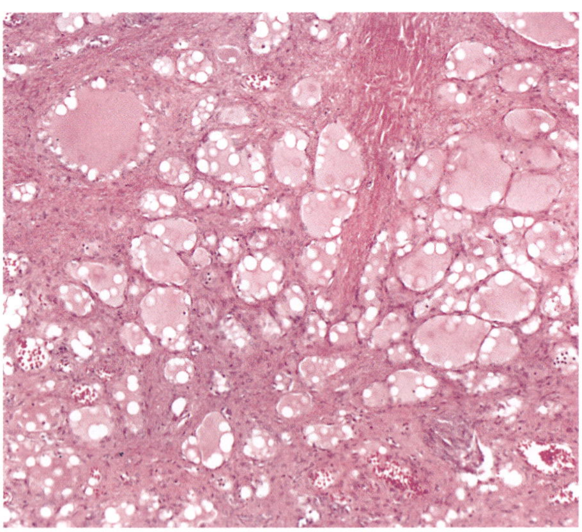

Figure 9-57

LYMPHANGIOMA

The vascular spaces contain lymph.

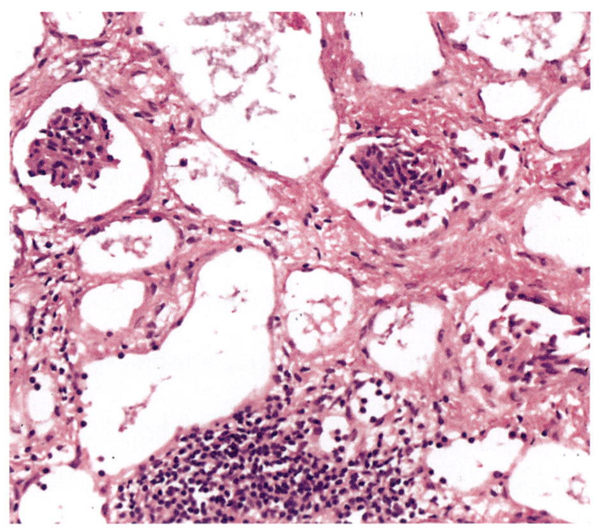

Figure 9-58

LYMPHANGIOMA

The vascular spaces are empty and are lined by a single layer of flat endothelial cells. Three of the spaces show papillary proliferation of the endothelial lining.

Lymphangioma microscopically consists of multiple endothelial-lined spaces that vary in size from small channels to large cystic spaces containing clear pink-staining lymph (fig. 9-57). The surrounding stroma may contain lymphoid tissue (fig. 9-58). The lymphatic endothelial origin is confirmed by immunoreactivity to CD34, CD31, and D2-40.

Prognosis depends on how extensively the liver and other organs are involved. Localized lesions are generally curable with liver resection.

PEDIATRIC MESENCHYMAL TUMORS

Mesenchymal Hamartoma

Definition. *Mesenchymal hamartoma* is a benign lesion that presumably develops before birth, and is characterized by a multicystic and loosely fibrotic mass. Despite its name, its exact pathogenesis is unknown, with proposed theories on its etiology including an unusual form of ductal plate malformation, an ischemic source, an imprinting defect due to chromosomal abnormalities, and a genuine neoplastic lesion (4).

General and Clinical Features. Mesenchymal hamartoma accounts for 8 percent of all liver tumors and 18 percent of benign tumors in patients from birth to 21 years of age. During the first 2 years of life, these proportions slightly increase to 12 percent of liver tumors and 22 percent of benign tumors (3,104). Nearly 80 percent of cases are diagnosed in the first 2 years of life, and another 17 percent in the next 3 years. Although rare, adult cases have also been reported (105–107). Males are slightly more commonly affected than females with a male to female ratio of 3 to 2.

Children with mesenchymal hamartoma typically present with abdominal distention and an upper abdominal nontender mass, which may increase in size rapidly over a period of only a few days to weeks due to cystic degeneration and fluid accumulation inside the mass. Large lesions may cause respiratory distress. Congestive heart failure, described in infants with highly vascular lesions, may be due to arteriovenous shunts, although this presentation is more often associated with infantile hemangioendothelioma (108). A rare presentation is ascites caused by tumor rupture. Some cases are associated with extrahepatic congenital anomalies including diaphragmatic hernia, placental mesenchymal dysplasia, and Beckwith-Wiedemann syndrome (109–113). Mesenchymal hamartoma may also develop in an intrathoracic ectopic liver in patients with diaphragmatic hernia (114,115).

The findings of liver tests are generally unremarkable; however, serum levels of alpha-fetoprotein (AFP) may be slightly elevated owing to AFP production by regenerating hepatocytes located around the tumor mass (116–118). Infantile liver masses with AFP elevations are sometimes mistaken for hepatoblastoma, particularly in patients with risk factors for malignant neoplasms (e.g., Beckwith-Wiedemann syndrome) (109,110).

Some cases of mesenchymal hamartoma are detected prenatally by fetal ultrasonography or CT in the last trimester of pregnancy (119,120). The imaging appearance of the mass after birth depends on the proportion of stromal (mesenchymal) to cystic components (121). On unenhanced CT, mesenchymal hamartoma typically shows as a complex solid and cystic mass, in which stromal elements appear hypoattenuating, whereas the cystic component has water attenuation (121–123). After the intravenous administration of contrast material, the septa and stromal components are enhanced (121). The MRI appearance varies depending on the presence of stromal elements and the protein content of the fluid (122,124).

Gross Findings. Mesenchymal hamartoma forms a solitary circumscribed mass. It involves the right lobe in 75 percent of cases, the left lobe in 22 percent, and both lobes in 3 percent (3). About 20 percent of patients present with a pedunculated mass at the inferior surface of the liver (3). Lesions vary in size from a few centimeters to more than 30 cm in diameter, and they typically contain multiple cysts of variable sizes (fig. 9-59). The cysts are slightly larger in older patients, while young infants may have solid lesions without grossly visible cysts, suggesting that the cysts develop in parallel with progressive tumor growth. Cysts are filled with a watery fluid or gelatinous material, and do not communicate with the bile duct. The septa and solid components are whitish to tan in color and glistening (fig. 9-60). Hemorrhage and necrosis are rare.

Microscopic Findings. Mesenchymal hamartoma consists of a mixture of loose mesenchyme, bile ducts, hepatocyte nests, and clusters of vessels in variable proportions (fig. 9-61) (104). The mesenchyme consists of spindle- or stellate-shaped cells, loosely arranged collagen fibers, and a myxoid stroma (figs. 9-62). Extramedullary hematopoiesis and scarce inflammatory infiltrates may also be present.

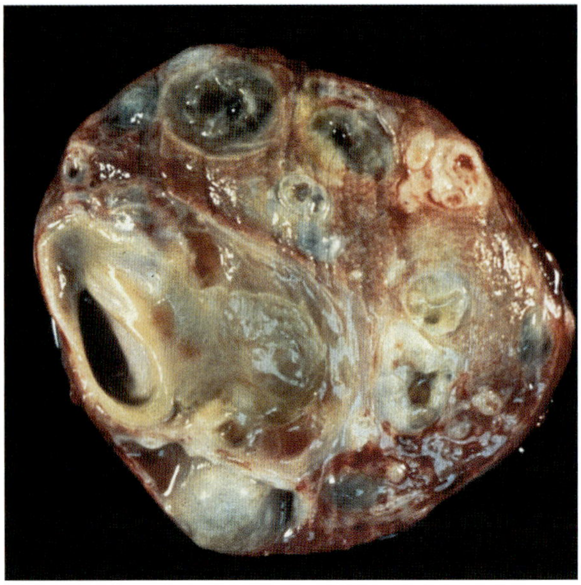

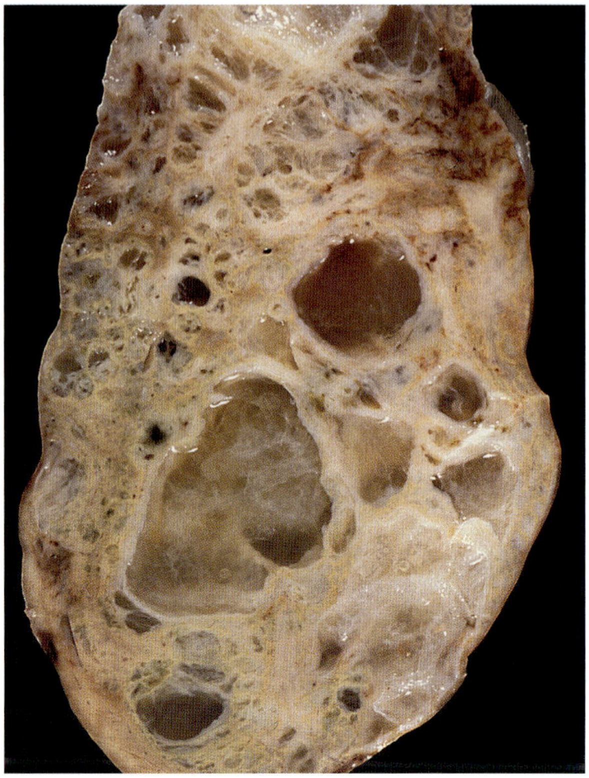

Figure 9-59

MESENCHYMAL HAMARTOMA

Left: There are cysts of varied size with a smooth lining, as well as solid tan-brown tissue.

Right: The tumor is composed largely of cysts.

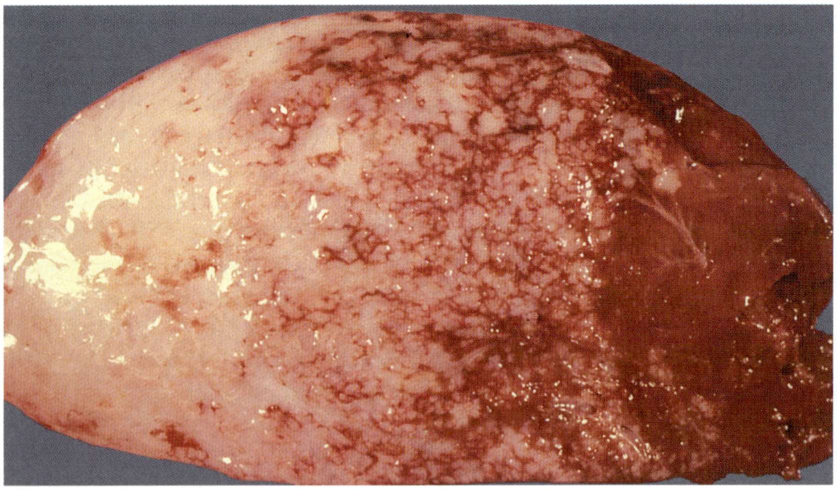

Figure 9-60

MESENCHYMAL HAMARTOMA

Cut section shows solid, glistening, pink tissue in one area, and mottled pink and red-brown tissue in another. Small separate ("satellite") nodules at the junction with the nontumor parenchyma.

Fluid accumulation in the fibromyxoid stroma undergoes cystic degeneration, a characteristic finding of mesenchymal hamartoma (fig. 9-63). The cyst walls only contain mesenchymal tissue with no apparent epithelial lining, while cystic dilatation of the bile duct element is rarely encountered, particularly in older patients (3).

The bile ducts in mesenchymal hamartoma are irregular in shape and sometimes arranged in a ductal-plate malformation pattern (fig. 9-64). The lining epithelium is often attenuated by periductal loose or fibrotic fibrosis. Small nests of hepatocytes are also scattered within the lesion. The cells are mature in appearance, but the lobular architecture is unclear. Vascular components may be conspicuous in places, and variably thick vessels are surrounded by fibrous stroma.

Molecular Genetic Findings. Chromosomal aberrations in mesenchymal hamartoma have been confirmed in multiple studies, with most

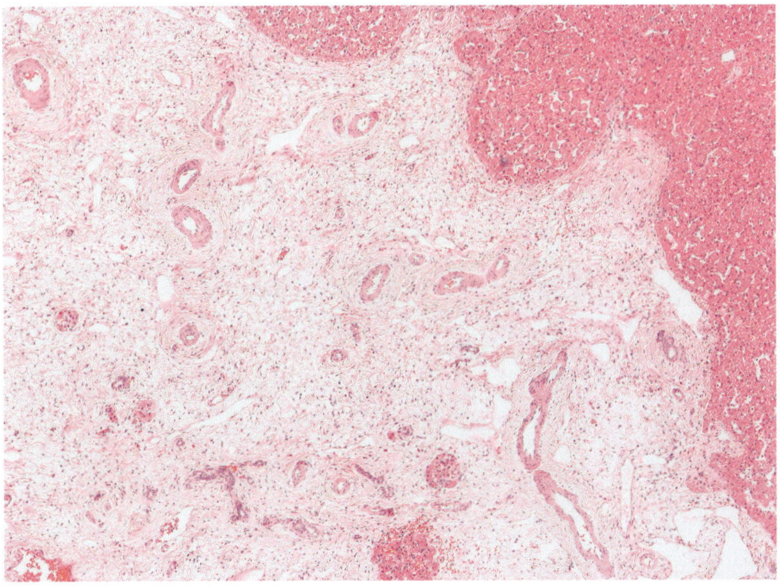

Figure 9-61

MESENCHYMAL HAMARTOMA

The tumor consists mainly of loose fibrous mesenchyme and occasional blood vessels.

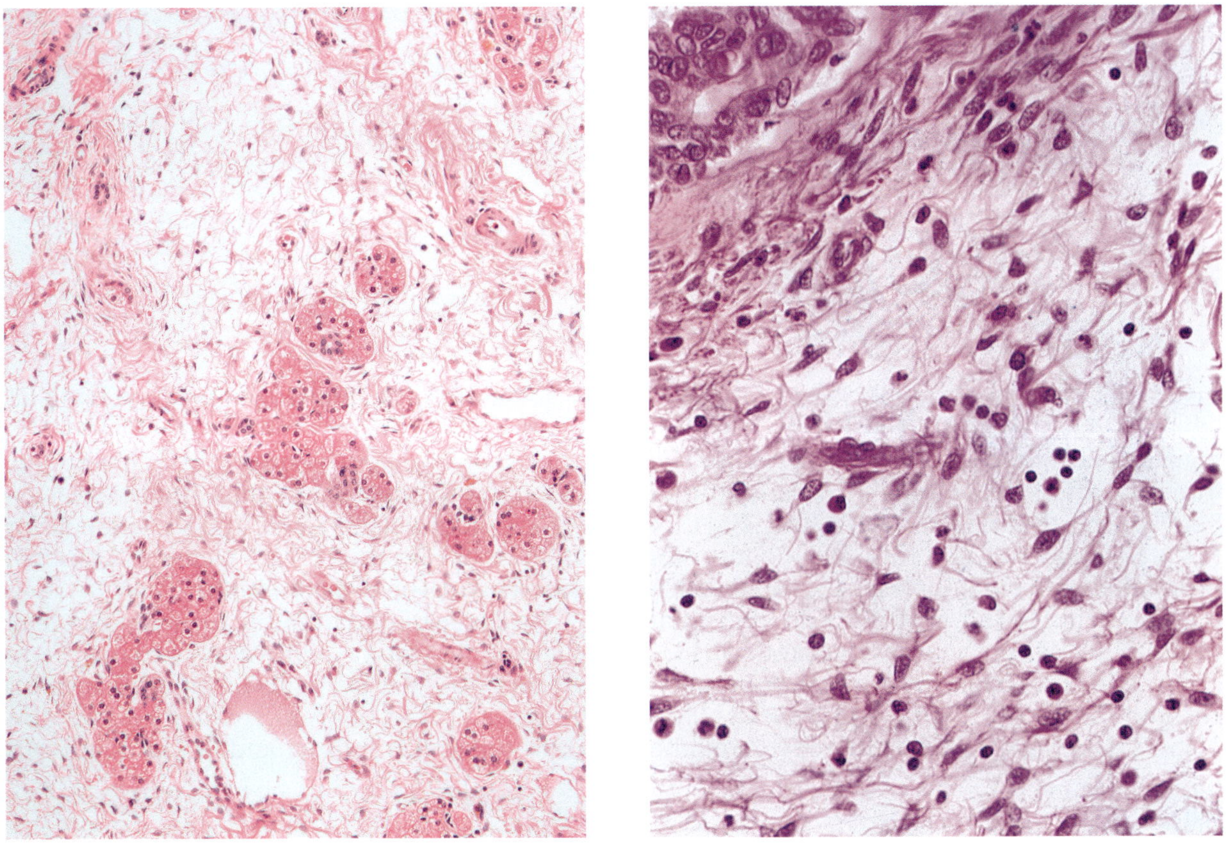

Figure 9-62

MESENCHYMAL HAMARTOMA

Left: Small nests of hepatocytes are present inside the tumor. The background stroma is hypocellular with several plumped spindle cells.

Right: At higher magnification, the mesenchyme consists of stellate-shaped cells in a loose matrix.

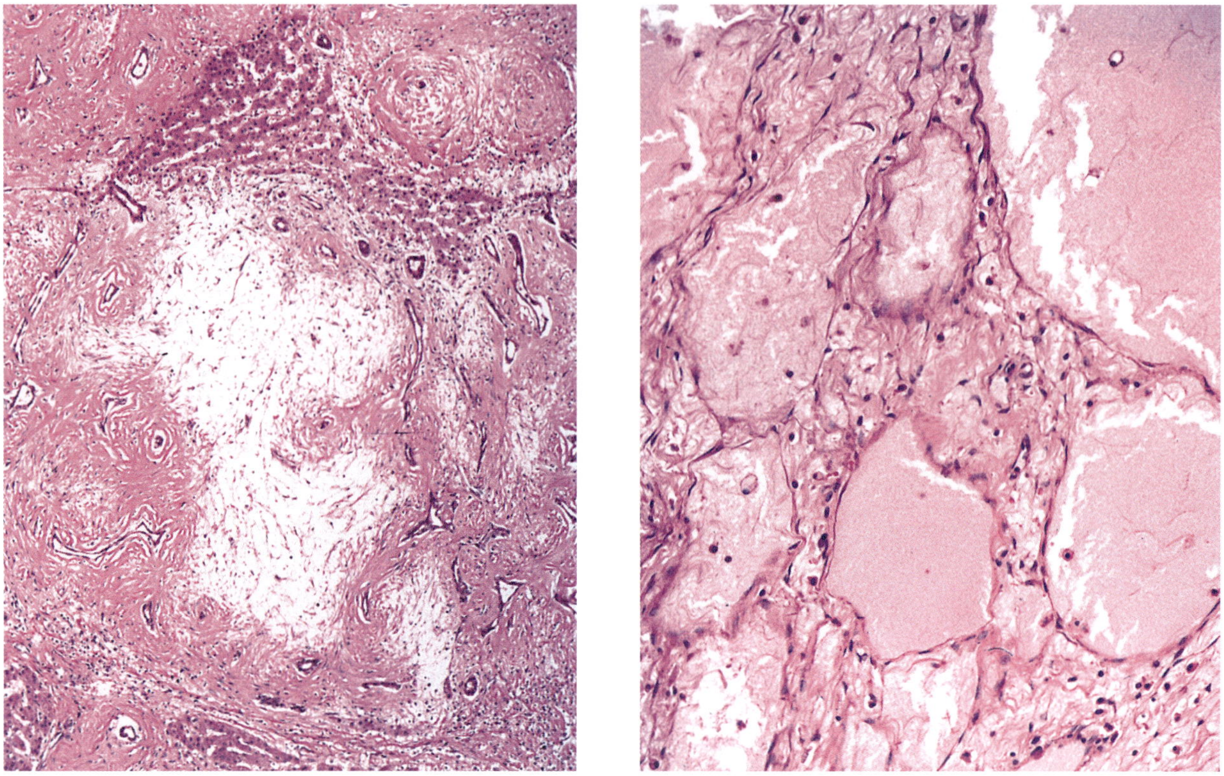

Figure 9-63

MESENCHYMAL HAMARTOMA

Left: Early cyst formation.
Right: Higher magnification of fully developed cysts. An endothelial lining is absent.

involving the chromosome band 19q13.4, which is often termed MHLB1 (mesenchymal hamartoma of the liver breakpoint 1) (128). The initially confirmed abnormality is translocation between chromosomes 15q15 and 19q13.4 (129). Subsequent studies also identify translocations between chromosomes 11 and 19 with a breakpoint at 19q13.4 (130–132), an interstitial deletion involving chromosome band 19q13.4 (133), and a complex translocation between chromosomes 11q2, 17p11, and 19q13.3 (134). Therefore, genetic abnormalities involving the long arm of chromosome 19 appear to be important in the development of mesenchymal hamartoma; however, whether these abnormalities are sufficient to confirm its neoplastic nature continues to be debated. Some cases of embryonal sarcoma arising in mesenchymal hamartoma have rearrangements involving chromosome 19q13.4 (126–128).

Differential Diagnosis. Multiple cysts with no epithelial lining may be mistaken for lymphangioma. Lymphangioma, however, is far less fibrotic than mesenchymal hamartoma. Immunoreactivity for endothelial markers and the presence or absence of torturous biliary elements also help differentiate the two conditions.

Focally regressed infantile hemangioma may share some features with mesenchymal hamartoma. Vascular elements in infantile hemangioma are derived from smaller vessels, and thus, the wall is thinner and less muscular. An anastomosing capillary network may vaguely remain in regressed hemangioma.

Treatment and Prognosis. Surgical resection is the treatment of choice for mesenchymal hamartoma. It does not recur after resection. In some patients, complete resection cannot be achieved because of the large size of the lesion and the involvement of vital structures such as

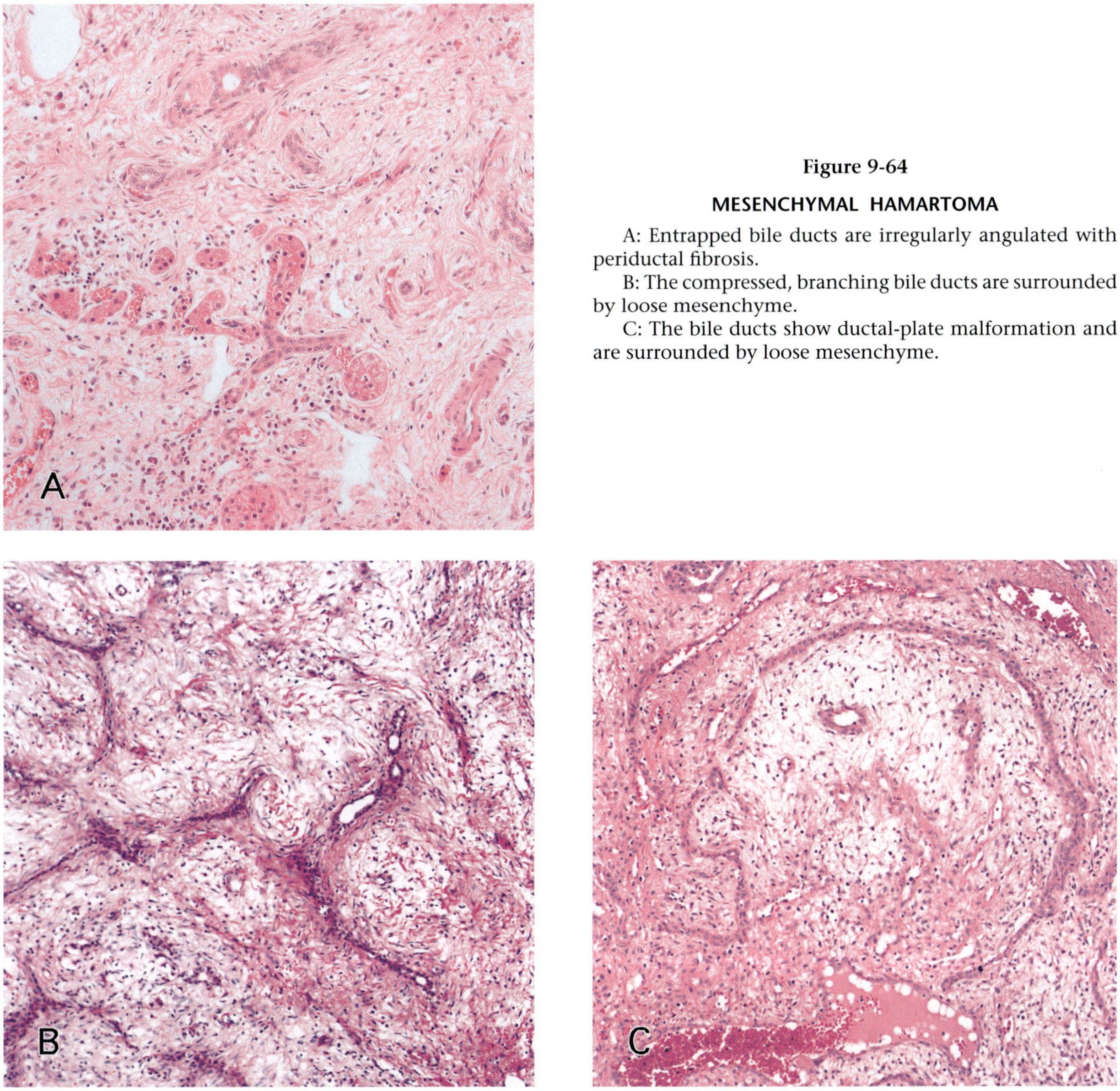

Figure 9-64

MESENCHYMAL HAMARTOMA

A: Entrapped bile ducts are irregularly angulated with periductal fibrosis.

B: The compressed, branching bile ducts are surrounded by loose mesenchyme.

C: The bile ducts show ductal-plate malformation and are surrounded by loose mesenchyme.

the inferior vena cava and porta hepatis. Even if there are residual tumors, the prognosis is good. Rare cases evolve into embryonal sarcoma (125–127).

Embryonal Sarcoma

Definition. *Embryonal sarcoma* is a primitive neoplasm unique to the liver, with characteristic clinical and histologic features (3). It is composed of undifferentiated mesenchymal cells, with no consistent differentiation into particular cellular lineages. Other terms that have been used for this tumor include *undifferentiated sarcoma, mesenchymal sarcoma,* and *malignant mesenchymoma.*

General and Clinical Features. This neoplasm chiefly occurs in children and teenagers: 16 percent of cases are diagnosed at 0 to 5 years of age, 52 percent at 6 to 10 years, and 20 percent at 11 to 15 years (135). Only 7 percent of patients are older than 20 years, with a limited number of middle-aged or older patients reported (136–138). Embryonal sarcoma ranks as the third most common primary malignant pediatric liver tumor after hepatoblastoma and hepatocellular carcinoma (135). Patients generally

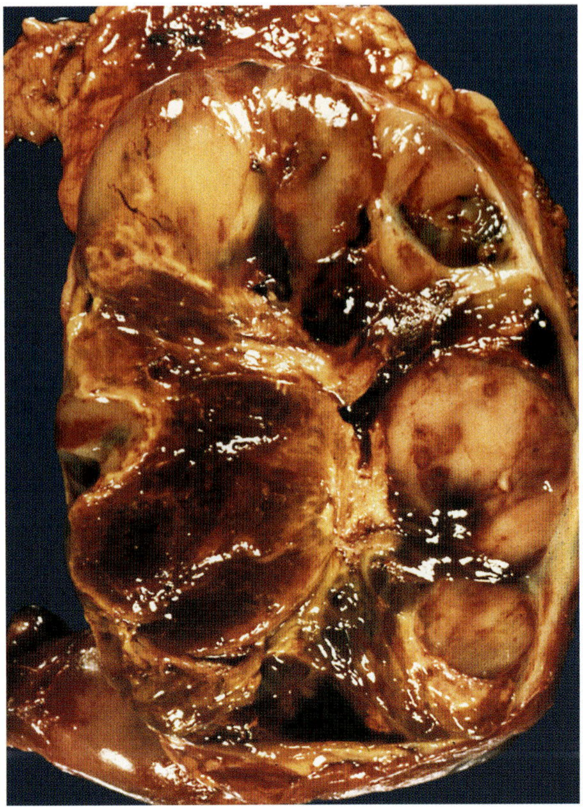

Figure 9-65

EMBRYONAL SARCOMA

This tumor is lobulated and shows solid, yellow-tan areas as well as necrotic and hemorrhagic foci.

lack preexisting liver diseases or extrahepatic associated lesions, except for rare cases of embryonal sarcoma developing in mesenchymal hamartoma (125–127).

Tumors grow rapidly and become large, with areas of cystic degeneration and necrosis, and abdominal enlargement and pain, with or without a palpable mass, are the usual presenting findings. Other less specific symptoms are fever and weight loss. Some patients may be severely ill at presentation with systemic signs of malignancy (20). Rarely, tumors invade the inferior vena cava and grow into the right atrium, presenting clinically as a primary intracardiac tumor (139). Liver tests are abnormal in up to 50 percent of patients; however, the findings are nonspecific. Serum concentrations of AFP are within the normal range or slightly increased due to the regeneration of non-neoplastic hepatocytes.

Imaging studies reveal a spectrum of solid and cystic findings with the characteristic feature being a predominantly solid appearance at ultrasonography yet cystic at CT and MRI due to the high water content of the prominent myxoid stroma (140,141). CT predominantly reveals water attenuation representing the myxoid stroma with occasional solid foci generally at the periphery or forming septa of variable thickness (140–143). On MRI, embryonal sarcoma is predominantly of the cerebrospinal fluid signal intensity on T1- and T2-weighted images. The heterogeneous enhancement of the peripheral and solid portions of the mass is observed after the intravenous administration of contrast material (140,141,144). At ultrasonography, the tumor typically appears solid and isoechoic to hyperechoic relative to a normal liver, with small anechoic spaces correlating with foci of necrosis, old hemorrhage, and cystic degeneration (140–142). Although differentiation from mesenchymal hamartoma may be difficult based purely on imaging findings, a diagnosis of embryonal sarcoma is strongly suspected in the clinical setting of a child with a large, rapidly growing cystic liver mass (4).

Gross Findings. Seventy-four percent of tumors are located in the right lobe, 10 percent in the left, and 16 percent in both (135). Tumor masses are generally 10 to 20 cm at their greatest diameter, globular in shape, and well-demarcated from the background liver, but are nonencapsulated. The cut surface is variegated gelatinous or glistening, ranging in color from yellowish gray to tan (fig. 9-65). Multiple cystic spaces containing necrotic debris and clotted blood are observed in more than 50 percent of cases; these degenerative changes may become more extensive after neoadjuvant chemotherapy (fig. 9-66).

Microscopic Findings. Embryonal sarcoma consists of stellate, spindle, pleomorphic, and giant cells that grow against the background of fibromyxoid stroma (fig. 9-67) (135). The cells are compactly or loosely arranged with variable cellularity; however, highly cellular areas are at least focally present in most cases. Tumor cells often display prominent anisonucleosis with hyperchromasia. Giant cells with bizarre nuclei are scattered or aggregated in places (fig. 9-68), and may show emperipolesis.

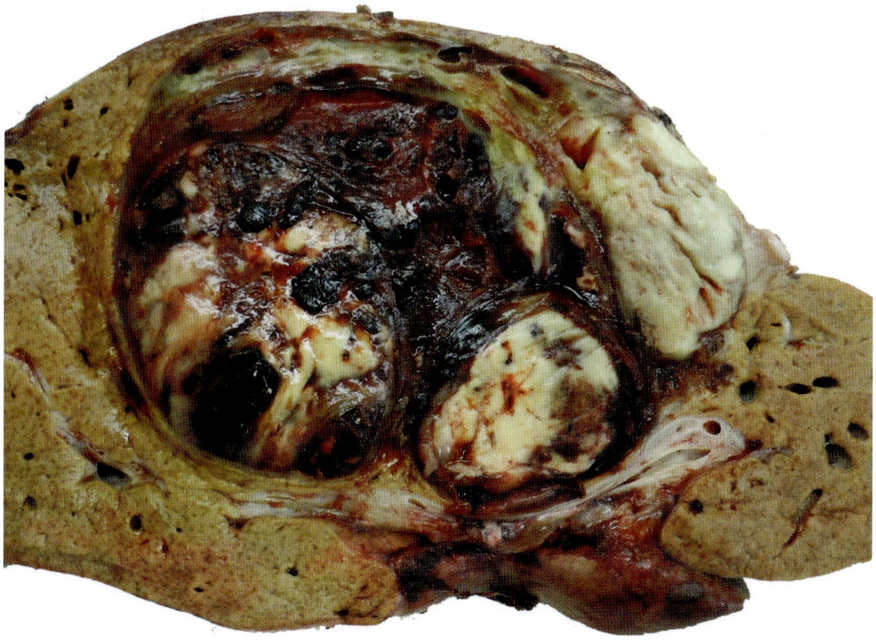

Figure 9-66

EMBRYONAL SARCOMA

The bulky mass has a heterogeneous cut surface with hemorrhagic foci. This tumor was resected after chemotherapy.

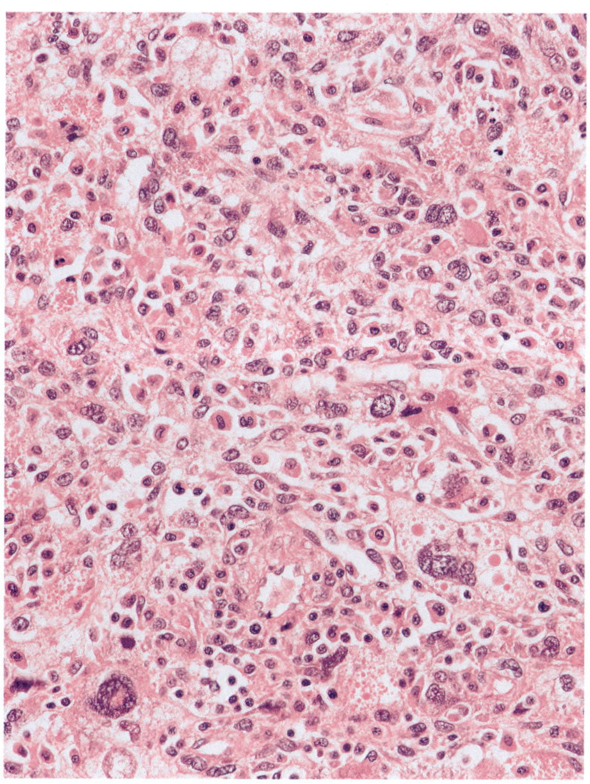

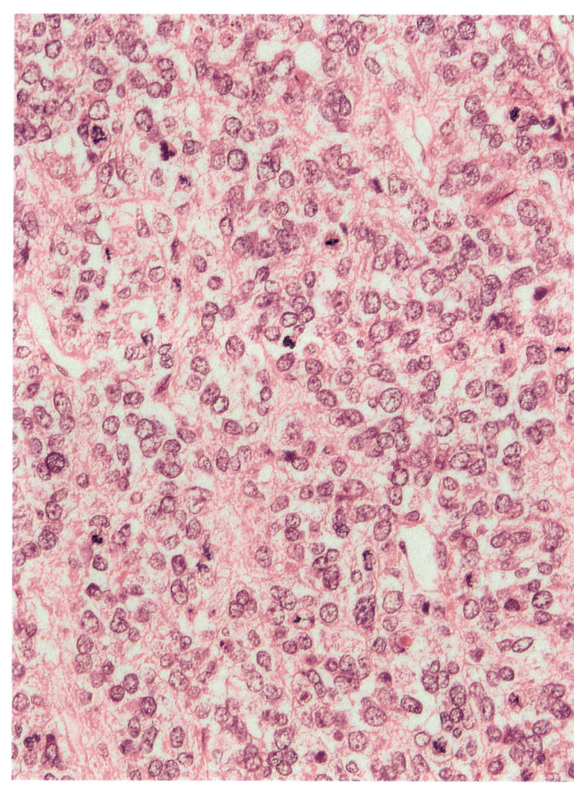

Figure 9-67

EMBRYONAL SARCOMA

Left: Pleomorphic tumor cells are diffusely arranged with occasional bizarre cells.
Right: Some parts show less pleomorphic features with fairly uniform small round cells.

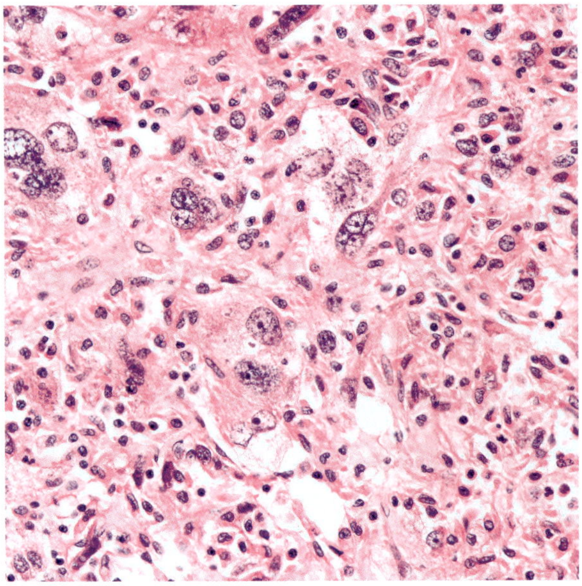

Figure 9-68

EMBRYONAL SARCOMA

Giant cells with one or multiple bizarre nuclei are noted.

A characteristic feature is the presence of eosinophilic intracytoplasmic globules of variable sizes that are periodic acid-Schiff (PAS) positive and diastase resistant (fig. 9-69). These globules are immunoreactive to alpha-1-antitrypsin, alpha-1-antichymotripsin, vimentin, immunoglobulins, and albumin, and likely represent electron dense lysosomes with dense precipitates (145,146). Mitotic figures are easily found throughout the tumor. Foci of hemorrhage, necrosis, and cystic degeneration are commonly observed (fig. 9-70). Peripheral parts of the tumor may entrap hepatocytes and bile ducts (146,147).

Uncommon histologic findings that may be encountered in embryonal sarcoma include a storiform pattern, trabecular architecture (fig. 9-71), hemangiopericytoma-like areas, and osteoid formation (145,148). Spindle cells with the features of myoid differentiation or small cells resembling hepatoblastoma or rhabdoid tumor may also be present (149). In cases of embryonal

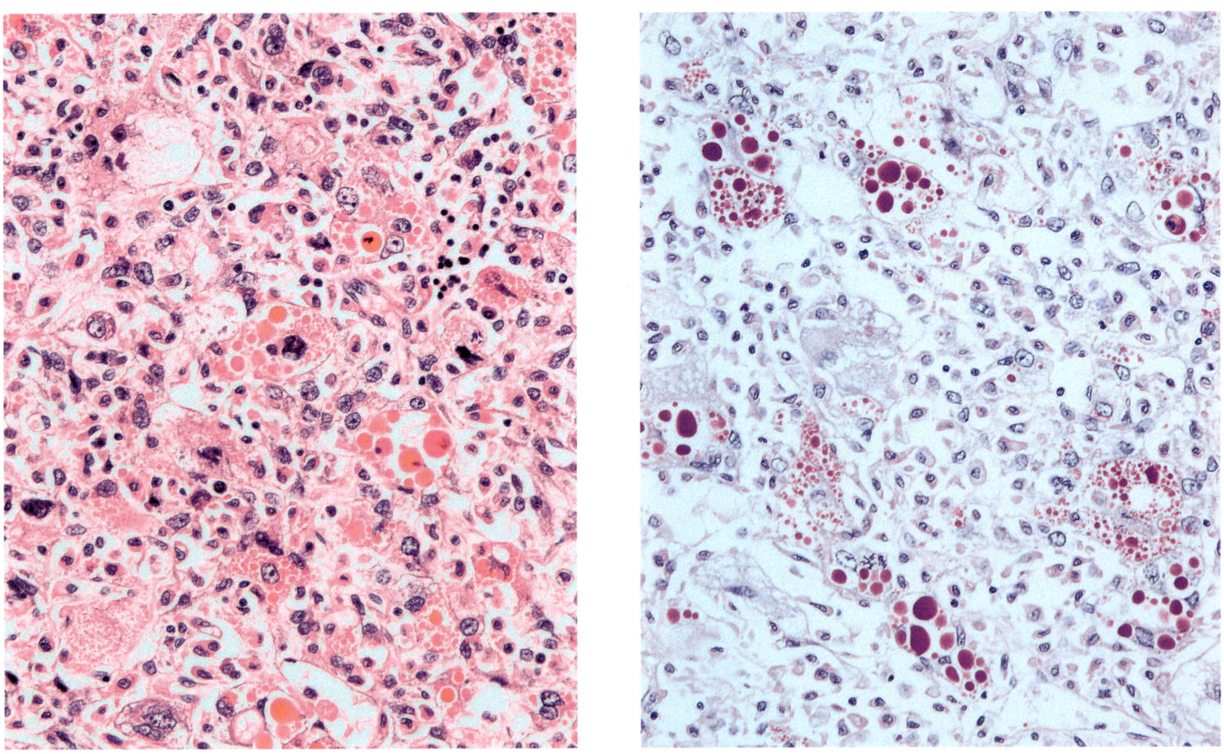

Figure 9-69

EMBRYONAL SARCOMA

Left: Some tumor cells contain eosinophilic intracytoplasmic globules.
Right: The intracytoplasmic globules are positive for the periodic acid–Schiff (PAS) diastase-resistant stain.

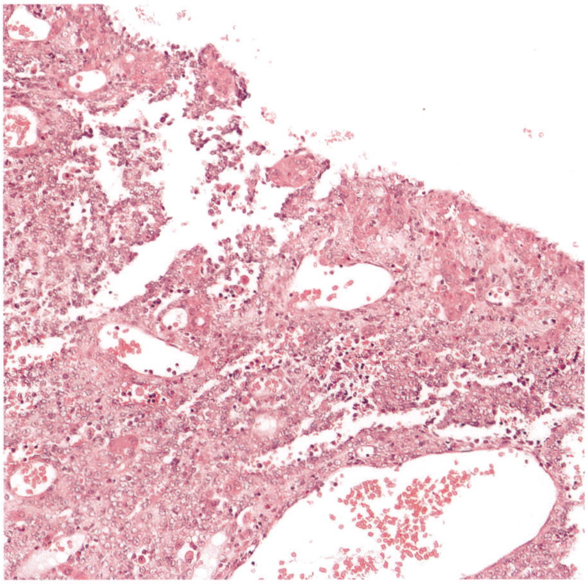

Figure 9-70

EMBRYONAL SARCOMA

There is cystic degeneration with no epithelial or endothelial lining.

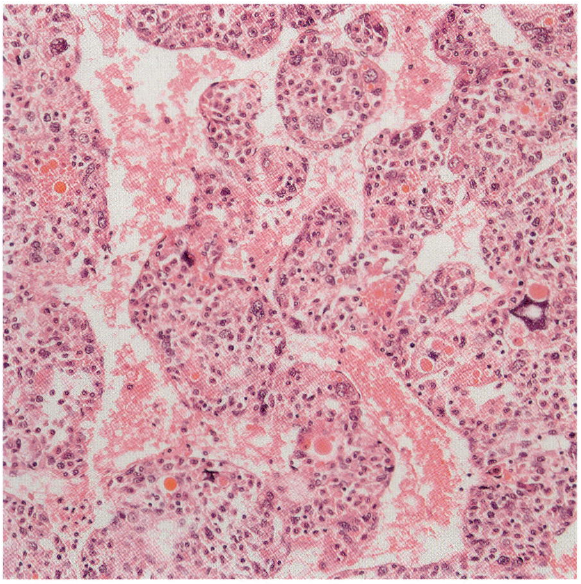

Figure 9-71

EMBRYONAL SARCOMA

The tumor cells are arranged in a thick trabecular pattern with sinusoidal spaces.

sarcoma arising from mesenchymal hamartoma, benign hamartomatous changes are confirmed in the periphery.

Immunohistochemical Findings. Embryonal sarcoma does not have a specific immunophenotype. Tumors variably express mesenchymal, epithelial, and histiocytic markers including vimentin, desmin, smooth muscle actin, calponin, cytokeratins, CD10, CD68, BCL-2, and alpha-1-antitrypsin (148,150–153). Glypican-3 is positive in a subset (58 percent) of cases (154) and is not a reliable marker for differentiating embryonal sarcoma from hepatoblastoma and hepatocellular carcinoma. Since HepPar1, myogenin, myogenic regulatory protein D1 (MyoD1), CD34, CD117 (c-kit), anaplastic lymphoma kinase 1 (ALK-1), and S-100 protein are negative in most cases, these markers are useful for excluding hepatoblastoma, hepatocellular carcinoma, rhabdomyosarcoma, gastrointestinal stromal tumor, inflammatory myofibroblastic tumors, and neuronal neoplasms (152,155,156). In contrast to hepatoblastoma, embryonal sarcoma does not show the nuclear expression of β-catenin.

Molecular Genetic Findings. Cytogenetically, embryonal sarcoma is diploid or aneuploid with extensive chromosomal rearrangements (157,158). Comparative genomic hybridization has revealed several chromosomal gains and deletions, suggesting underlying progressive genomic instability (159,160). Nevertheless, there is no known particular genetic alteration specific for this neoplasm. Similar to pure mesenchymal hamartoma, embryonal sarcoma arising from mesenchymal hamartoma has a chromosomal translocation at 19q13.4 (126–128); this genetic event, however, has not been confirmed in de novo embryonal sarcoma (160,161). These findings suggest that secondary embryonal sarcoma has distinct molecular features, and additional genetic alterations besides the translocation at 19q13.4 may lead to malignant transformation in mesenchymal hamartoma. *TP53* is often mutated in embryonal sarcoma (159,161,162).

Treatment and Prognosis. The prognosis for patients with embryonal sarcoma was previously very poor, with a median survival time of less than 1 year after diagnosis. However, modern multimodal treatments and supportive therapies have improved survival (163). Treatment regimens combining surgical resection and postoperative adjuvant chemotherapy yield long-term, disease-free survival (164).

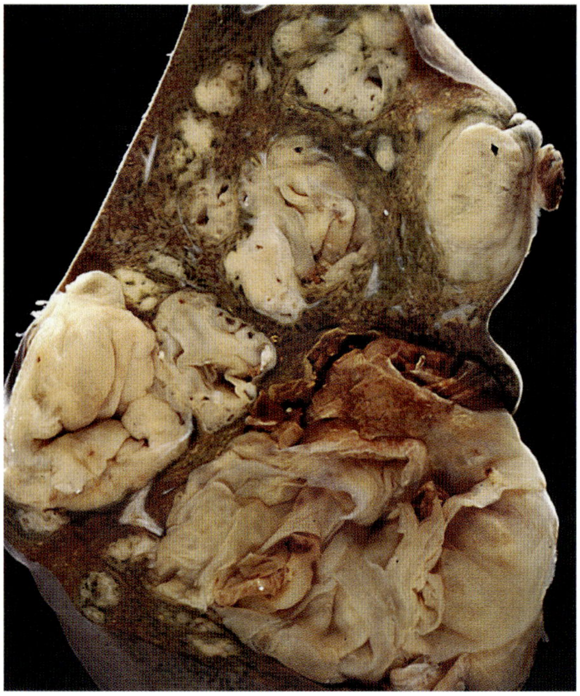

Figure 9-72

EMBRYONAL RHABDOMYOSARCOMA

Cross section of liver shows multiple foci of a light tan tumor. The billowy appearance is due to luminal projections and folds of the affected bile ducts. The green discoloration of the liver between the tumor masses is due to cholestasis.

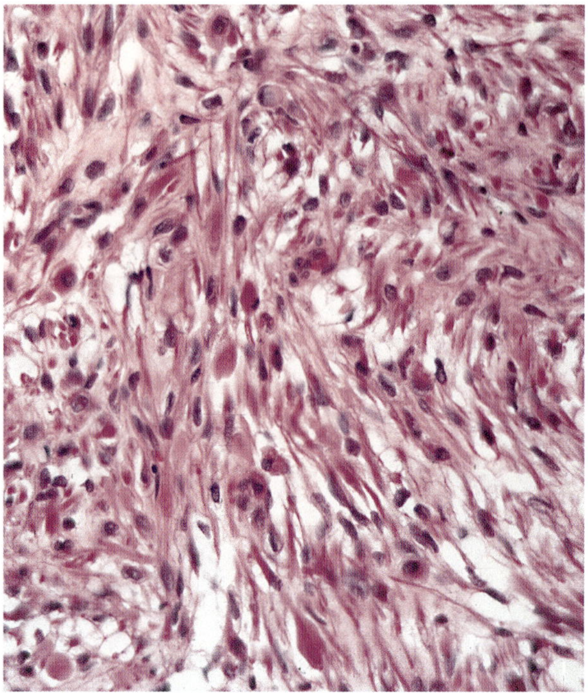

Figure 9-73

EMBRYONAL RHABDOMYOSARCOMA

The tumor cells are spindle or elongated and have eosinophilic cytoplasm.

Preoperative neoadjuvant chemotherapy may also be considered, and sometimes allows for the complete resection of tumors that were initially considered to be unresectable (165). This multidisciplinary approach often leads to complete remission for years (166).

Rhabdomyosarcoma

Definition. *Rhabdomyosarcoma* of the hepatobiliary system is basically similar to that of other sites (20,167). It shows an embryonal histology and grows along the biliary tract.

General and Clinical Features. Although most patients are less than 5 years of age (median, 3 years) (167,168), tumors have sometimes been diagnosed in older children and adults (169–171). Lesions are rarely present at birth. Males are more commonly affected, with a male to female ratio of approximately 2 to 1 (168). Rhabdomyosarcoma in liver is rare, but it is the most common biliary tumor in children, accounting for 1 percent of all pediatric cases of rhabdomyosarcoma (172). Intermittent obstructive jaundice, with or without abdominal distention, fever, and loss of appetite, is the typical presentation (172).

Gross Findings. Rhabdomyosarcoma forms soft tan masses that extend along the biliary tree (fig. 9-72) and sometimes protrude into the lumen (botryoid growth) (173). The affected ducts have thick walls.

Microscopic Findings. Hepatobiliary rhabdomyosarcoma is histologically of the embryonal type and is characterized by tumor cells arranged against a background of loose fibromyxoid stroma (fig. 9-73). The cells are round, stellate, or spindle in shape, and have hyperchromatic nuclei and occasional mitotic figures (fig. 9-74). Cross-striation may be observed (fig. 9-75). Botryoid masses are lined by an unremarkable biliary epithelium with occasional foci of erosion (fig. 9-76). A characteristic finding is that the cellularity of tumor cells is particularly high beneath the lining epithelium (cambium layer), while it decreases in the deep stroma.

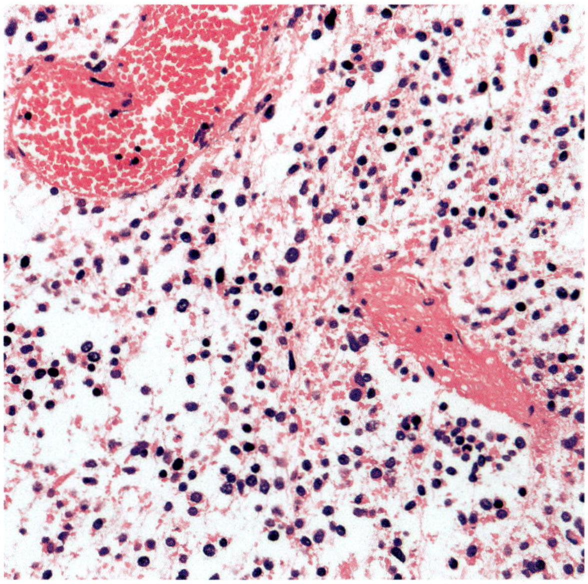

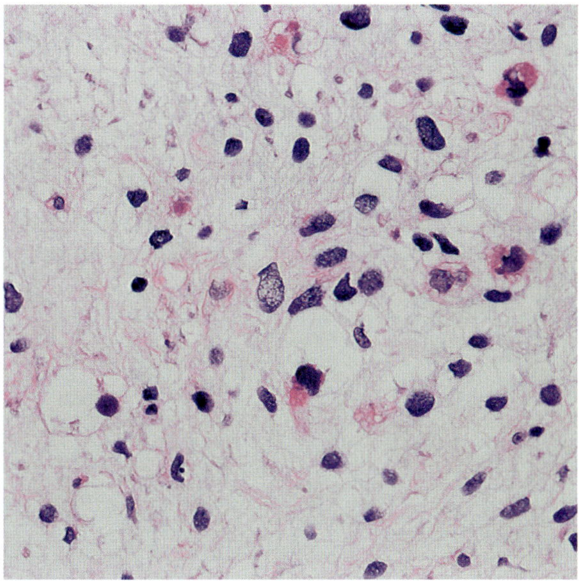

Figure 9-74

EMBRYONAL RHABDOMYOSARCOMA

Left: This biopsy sample consists of small atypical cells arranged against a background of loose connective tissue.
Right: At high magnification, the tumor cells show a high nuclear to cytoplasmic ratio and dark nuclei. Some cells also have eosinophilic cytoplasm.

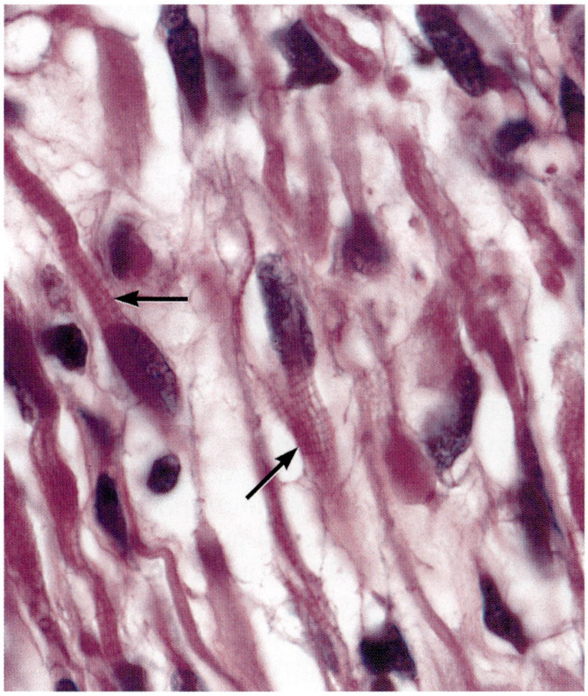

Figure 9-75

EMBRYONAL RHABDOMYOSARCOMA

Cross striations are clearly visible in the cytoplasm of some cells (arrows).

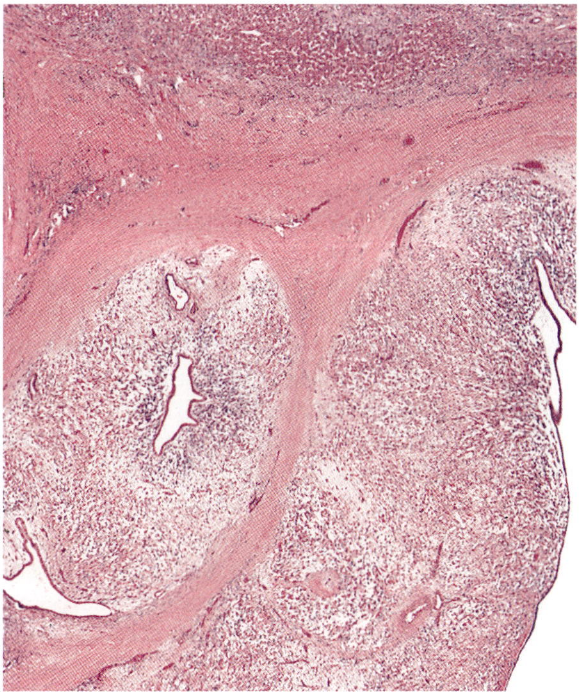

Figure 9-76

EMBRYONAL RHABDOMYOSARCOMA

The wall of the bile duct is extensively infiltrated by tumor, with marked narrowing of the lumen.

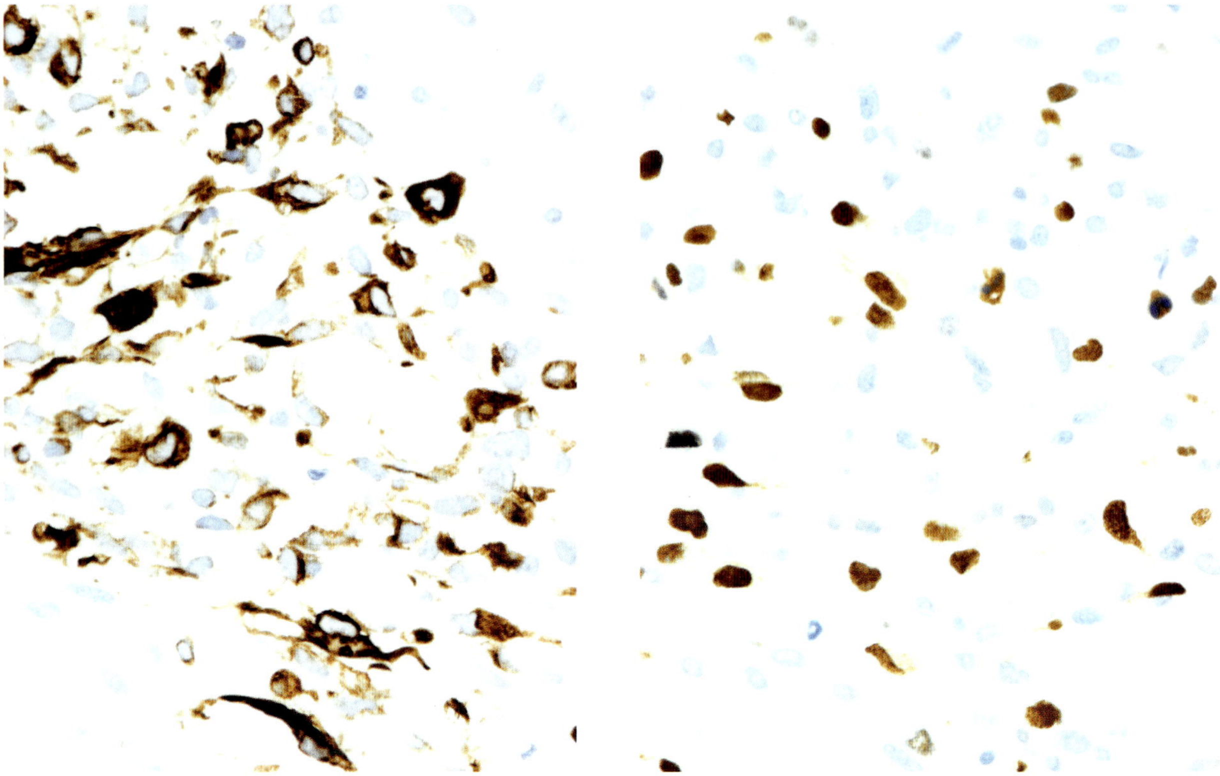

Figure 9-77

EMBRYONAL RHABDOMYOSARCOMA

Left: Desmin is positive in the cytoplasm of the tumor cells.
Right: Nuclear expression of myogenin is highly specific for this neoplasm.

On immunostaining, the tumor cells are positive for desmin (fig. 9-77, left), muscle-specific actin, myogenin (fig. 9-77, right), and MyoD1. Myogenin and MyoD1 are particularly useful for differentiating rhabdomyosarcoma from embryonal sarcoma because the latter may be positive for desmin and actin, but does not express myogenin or MyoD1 (160,168).

Treatment and Prognosis. Similar to those with rhabdomyosarcoma of other organs, patients are treated using a multidisciplinary approach, including multidrug chemotherapy, surgery, and radiotherapy. The 5-year survival rate of patients with biliary rhabdomyosarcoma has been improved to 66 percent (168).

Malignant Rhabdoid Tumor

Definition. *Malignant rhabdoid tumor* of the liver is a rare and highly aggressive tumor consisting of undifferentiated tumor cells with a rhabdoid cytomorphologic appearance. Identical tumors were initially identified in the kidney and subsequently found in other organs including the brain, soft tissue, and liver. A characteristic molecular feature is inactivation of the *SMARCB1/INI1* gene at 22q11.2. Synonyms include *rhabdoid tumor* and *extrarenal rhabdoid tumor.*

General and Clinical Features. The loss of SMARCB1/INI1 expression is currently nearly essential for the diagnosis of malignant rhabdoid tumor. Since the SMARCB1/INI1 status was not confirmed in earlier reported cases of hepatic rhabdoid tumor, some may not be true malignant rhabdoid tumors (174). According to a recent review of 53 cases of hepatic rhabdoid tumor previously reported in the literature (SMARCB1/INI1 negativity confirmed in 20 cases) (175), most patients presented in the first 3 years of life, with 66 percent diagnosed in the first year and an additional 23 percent in the next 2 years (median age at diagnosis, 8 months). Both males and females are affected almost equally.

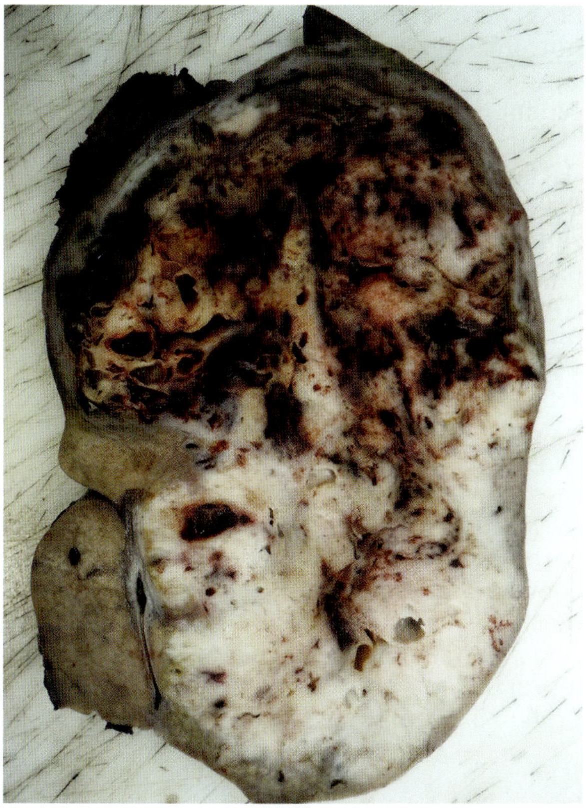

Figure 9-78

MALIGNANT RHABDOID TUMOR

A bulky mass with a whitish cut surface, hemorrhagic foci, and small cystic degeneration are seen.

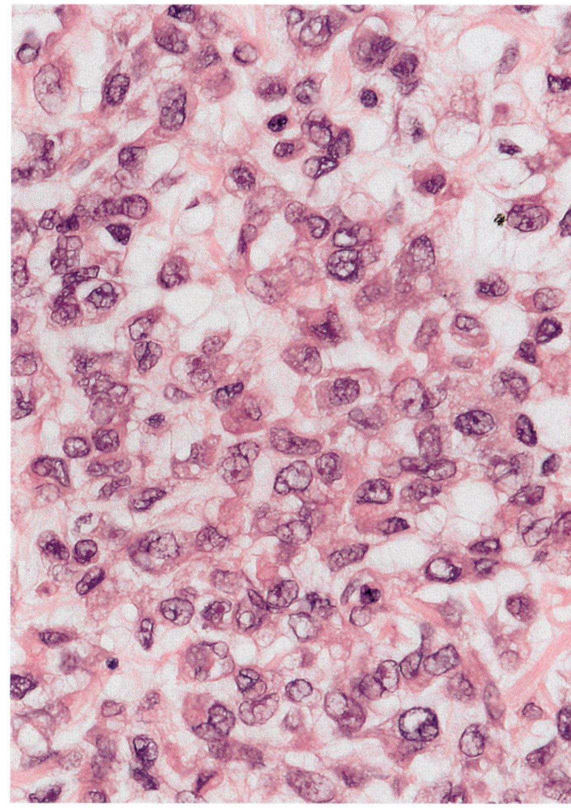

Figure 9-79

MALIGNANT RHABDOID TUMOR

The tumor consists of small round cells with clear to eosinophilic cytoplasm. Nuclei are irregular in shape and contain distinct nucleoli.

Similar to other pediatric liver tumors, common presenting symptoms are an abdominal mass or distention, fever, vomiting, and pain. Up to 17 percent of patients also present with tumor rupture (174). Laboratory tests show normal or slightly increased serum AFP levels (174).

Metastatic disease is identified in 76 percent of patients at initial presentation, with common sites of metastasis including the lungs, lymph nodes, central nervous system, skin, and bone; only 5 out of 53 patients were alive at the time of reporting (175). Deaths occur early, with nearly 50 percent of patients dying within 1 month and most prior to 1 year after diagnosis (174). Although the number of survivors is limited, clinical factors supposedly related to a better prognosis are age over 1 year, female gender, no metastasis at presentation, and the achievement of complete resection (175).

Gross Findings. Most tumors are larger than 5 cm at the greatest diameter, and are solid. The cut surface is gray to tan and commonly associated with necrosis and hemorrhage (fig. 9-78). Multiple nodules, often involving both liver lobes, may be present.

Microscopic Findings. Malignant rhabdoid tumor consists of small to medium-sized round cells with vesicular nuclei and distinct nucleoli (fig. 9-79). The cells are arranged in a solid sheet pattern (fig. 9-80) and show infiltrative growth with no obvious fibrous capsule (fig. 9-81). Cystic degeneration or a somewhat trabecular architecture may be encountered (fig. 9-82). Some tumor cells have distinct paranuclear spherical inclusions composed of intracellular filamentous aggregates, leading to a rhabdoid cytomorphologic appearance (fig. 9-83) (20). Cytoplasmic eosinophilic inclusions are PAS

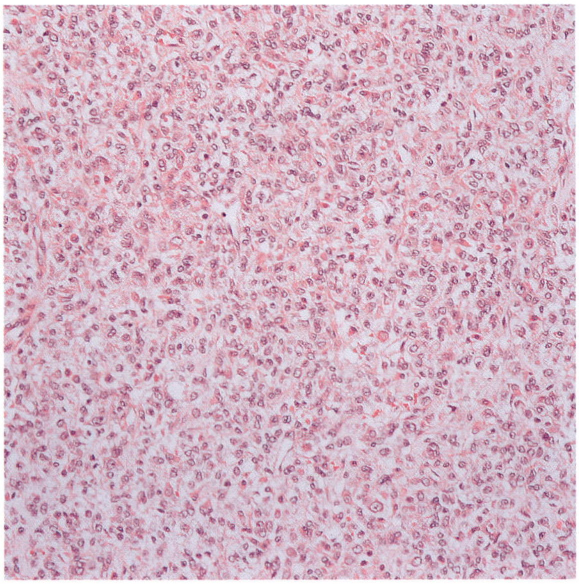

Figure 9-80

MALIGNANT RHABDOID TUMOR

Diffusely arranged tumor cells give a fairly homogeneous appearance.

positive. Rhabdoid cells are characteristic, but not entirely specific for this neoplasm, with similar cells present in other sarcomas and carcinomas.

A molecular or immunohistochemical analysis of SMARCB1/INI1 is essential for an accurate diagnosis. The loss of SMARCB1/INI1 expression is confirmed by immunohistochemistry using the BAF47 antibody (fig. 9-84). Immunoreactivity to other antibodies is variable, with most tumors coexpressing mesenchymal (e.g., vimentin) and epithelial (e.g., cytokeratins and EMA) markers. AFP is negative.

Molecular Genetic Findings. A characteristic genetic feature of malignant rhabdoid tumor is the homozygous inactivation of the *SMARCB1/INI1* gene in chromosome band 22q11.2. This pathognomonic genomic event occurs in both copies of the gene as a consequence of various mechanisms, including coding-sequence mutations, partial or whole gene deletions, and the loss of heterozygosity (176). The SMARCB1/INI1 protein is a component of the mammalian SWI/

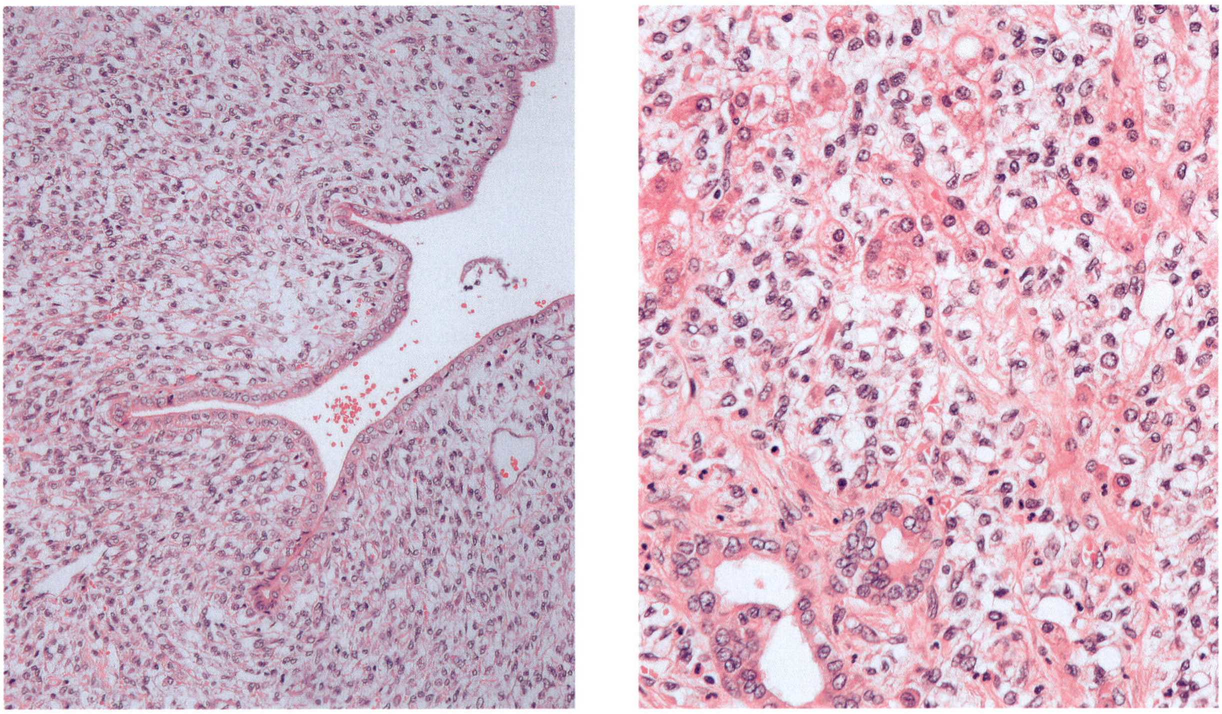

Figure 9-81

MALIGNANT RHABDOID TUMOR

Left: An entrapped bile duct is slightly dilated. Despite diffuse tumor infiltration, the lining epithelium is intact. Right: Because of an infiltrative growth, bile ducts and liver cells are observed inside the tumor mass.

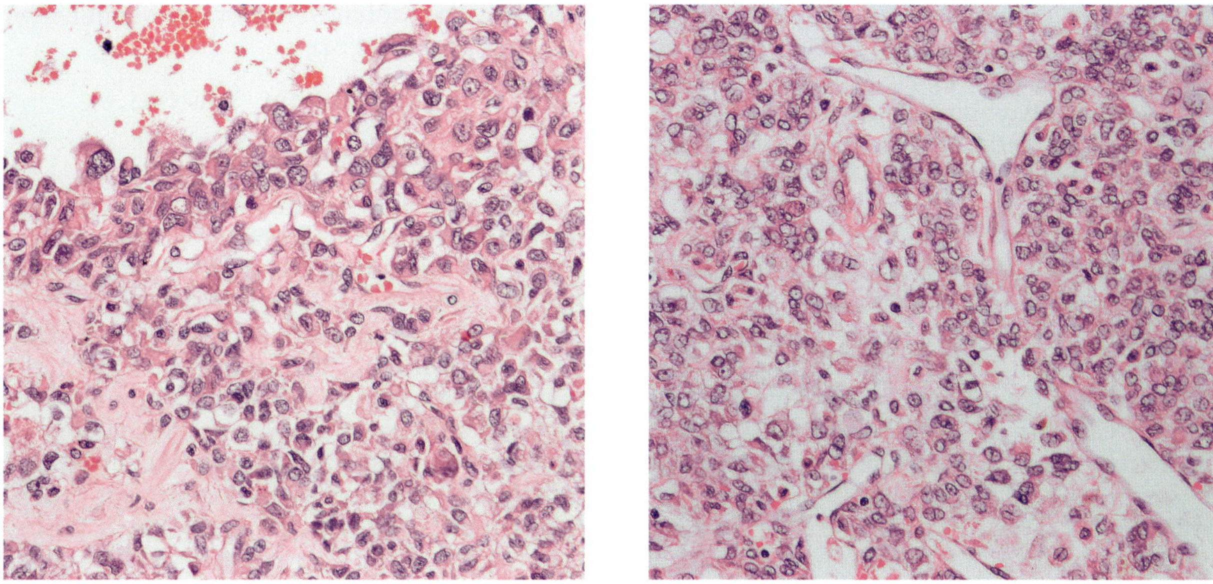

Figure 9-82

MALIGNANT RHABDOID TUMOR

Left: This area is associated with cystic degeneration.
Right: The combination of sheet-pattern growth and intervening thin vessels results in a trabecular architecture.

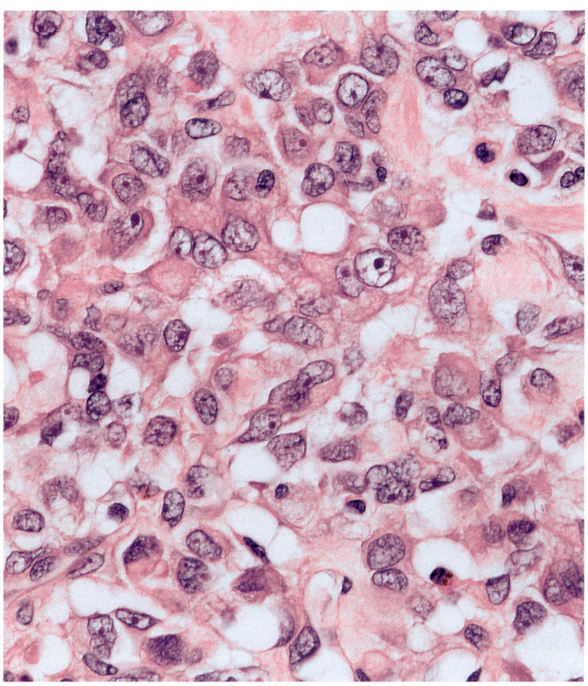

Figure 9-83

MALIGNANT RHABDOID TUMOR

Tumor cells have distinct paranuclear spherical inclusions with a rhabdoid cytomorphologic appearance.

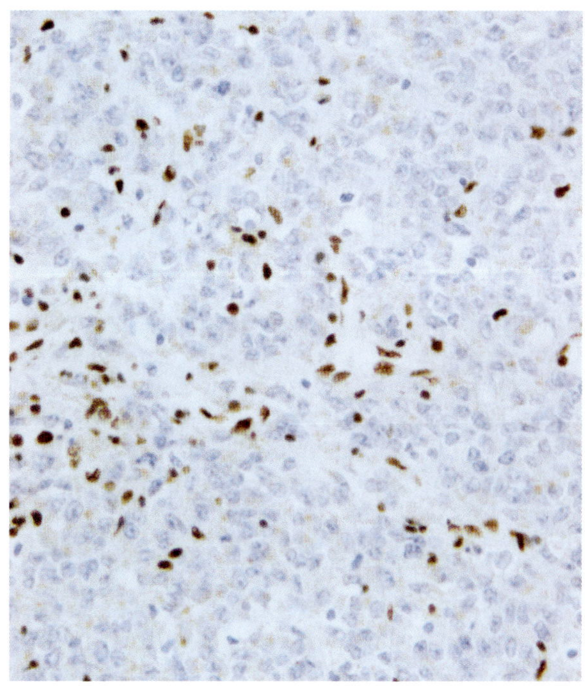

Figure 9-84

MALIGNANT RHABDOID TUMOR

On immunohistochemistry using the BAF47 antibody, SMARCB1/INI1 is positive in background non-neoplastic cells, but negative in malignant rhabdoid tumor cells.

SNF complex, which functions in an ATP-dependent manner to alter the chromatin structure. Familial cases, described as *rhabdoid tumor predisposition syndrome*, have been linked to heterozygous *SMARCB1/INI1* germline mutations. Mutations in and/or the loss of the *SMARCA4/BRG1* gene in 19p13.2 has been reported in rare cases of rhabdoid tumor, with retained SMARCB1/INI1 expression that developed in extrahepatic organs (177,178); these genetic alterations, however, have not been confirmed in liver neoplasms

Mutations in the *KRT8* gene coding for CK8 have also been identified in malignant rhabdoid tumors. Conformational changes in CK8 filaments caused by these genetic events may lead to the formation of intracytoplasmic inclusion bodies (179).

Differential Diagnosis. The overlap of clinicopathologic features between malignant rhabdoid tumor and small cell undifferentiated hepatoblastoma poses diagnostic difficulty (180). When small cell undifferentiated elements constitute a small proportion of an otherwise typical hepatoblastoma, they are generally positive for SMARCB1/INI1 immunostaining, supporting the diagnosis of hepatoblastoma. This discrimination becomes more challenging for neoplasms entirely or predominantly showing a small cell undifferentiated histology.

Trobaugh-Lotrario et al. (181) reviewed 11 cases of unresectable small cell undifferentiated hepatoblastoma from this aspect. The patients examined were younger than those with typical hepatoblastoma, and AFP levels were normal or only slightly elevated. All 6 patients who were tested for SMARCB1/INI1 status were negative for INI1 immunostaining. In addition, none of the patients survived: 10 died of disease progression, and 1 died from treatment complications. Another study also suggested that the prognosis of patients with INI1-negative small cell undifferentiated "hepatoblastoma" was worse than that of INI1-retained cases (182).

Although similarities and differences in the two conditions have not yet been clarified in detail, some of the cases classified as small cell undifferentiated hepatoblastoma behaved as malignant rhabdoid tumor. Therefore, immunohistochemical and molecular analyses for SMARCB1/INI need to be conducted for undifferentiated infantile liver neoplasms that lack the classic fetal/embryonal elements of hepatoblastoma (174).

MESENCHYMAL TUMORS

Leiomyosarcoma

Primary hepatic *leiomyosarcoma* is extremely uncommon. Leiomyosarcoma of the inferior vena cava presenting as a dominant liver mass may be mistaken for a primary liver tumor. Although smooth muscle neoplasms observed in the liver frequently turn out to be metastatic, one exception is the Epstein-Barr virus (EBV)-associated smooth muscle tumor occurring in immunocompromised patients. Acquired and iatrogenic immunosuppression and congenital immunodeficiency are potential predisposing conditions of EBV-driven leiomyosarcoma (183). In addition to the liver, various organs including the central nervous system, skin, gastrointestinal tract, pharynx, larynx, and lung are potentially involved. About 60 percent of patients may have multiorgan involvement but it does not necessarily indicate metastasis. In patients with transplantations (e.g., kidney, liver, heart, and lung transplantation), the liver or liver allograft is the main site of tumor occurrence (56 percent). Tumors occur late after transplantation, with a median interval of 4 years (range, 0.5 to 30 years) and develop earlier in children than in adults (184).

Microscopically, EBV-driven smooth muscle tumors typically display a well-differentiated histology, with mild cellular atypia and low mitotic activity. Unlike classic leiomyosarcomas, they lack significant pleomorphism, but frequently have foci of primitive round cells and the prominent intratumoral infiltration of T lymphocytes (185). EBV-encoded RNA (EBER) in situ hybridization is useful for reaching an accurate diagnosis (186). There is no consistent relationship between the histologic features and clinical outcome. On immunohistochemistry, all cases express smooth muscle actin, and in about 50 percent of cases, desmin (185).

Patients are treated by surgical resection, reduced immunosuppression, and/or chemotherapy. Multiorgan involvement, particularly with intracranial disease, is a poor prognostic factor; the clinical course, however, is generally difficult to predict (183,184).

Solitary Fibrous Tumor

Solitary fibrous tumor is characterized by its histology, which consists of spindle cells, intervening collagen bundles, and a hemangiopericytoma-like branching vascular network. Patients are generally adults and, more commonly, women, with a male to female ratio of 3 to 7 (187). Symptoms are typically due to the compression of nearby structures. Some patients (about 8 percent) present with hypoglycemia, which is presumably due to the paraneoplastic production of insulin-like growth factor (187).

Similar to its pleural counterpart, hepatic solitary fibrous tumor may form intraparenchymal or exophytic pedunculated masses, ranging from 2 to 20 cm in diameter (188). Sections reveal a lightly tan to gray-white cut surface with a whorled texture (fig. 9-85). Although solid tumors are common, small foci of cystic degeneration may be observed.

Microscopically, typical cases consist of a combination of hypocellular and hypercellular areas with a "patternless" architecture. Branching, occasionally dilated blood vessels also display a hemangiopericytoma-like pattern (fig. 9-86) (188). The tumor cells are spindle or oval in shape, with mildly atypical vesicular nuclei, and are surrounded by delicate collagen fibers or thin-walled blood vessels (fig. 9-87). Myxoid changes may be encountered.

Although it is generally difficult to predict the behavior of solitary fibrous tumors, the diagnosis of malignancy is considered for cases showing increased mitoses (over 4 mitotic figures per 10 high-power fields), variable cytologic atypia, tumor necrosis, and infiltrative growth, among which mitoses appear to be the most prognostic (189). In a literature review, 6 out of 61 reported cases (10 percent) of hepatic solitary fibrous tumor were diagnosed as malignant, with 4 having extrahepatic metastases either at initial presentation or during follow-up (187).

CD34, BCL-2, and CD99 have traditionally been used to diagnose this neoplasm (fig. 9-88). More recently, STAT6 has been identified as a highly specific diagnostic marker because recurrent somatic fusions of the two genes, *NAB2* and *STAT6*, located at the chromosomal region 12q13, have been proposed as the presumable tumor-initiating events of this neoplasm (fig. 9-89) (190,191).The differential diagnosis is wide, comprising reactive conditions (e.g., inflammatory pseudotumor) to benign or malignant mesenchymal tumors (e.g., sclerosed hemangioma, sarcomatoid carcinoma, leiomyosarcoma, and mesothelioma). Some cases of solitary fibrous tumor, particularly those developing in the retroperitoneum or soft tissues, contain mature adipocytes (fat-forming solitary fibrous tumors) (fig. 9-90) (189). If that variant form occurs in the liver, its appearance may mimic angiomyolipoma.

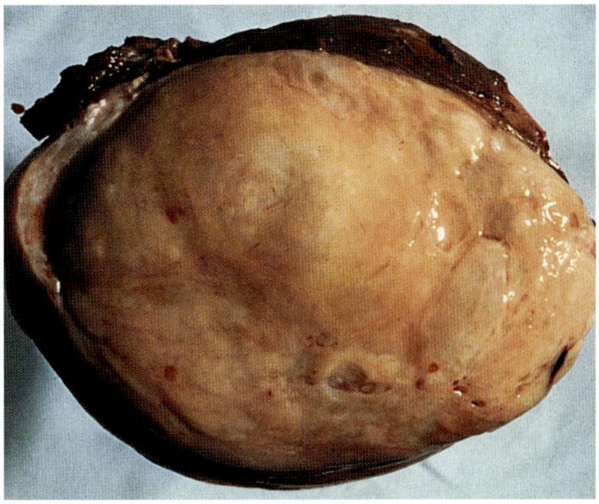

Figure 9-85

SOLITARY FIBROUS TUMOR

A bulging well-circumscribed tumor with a vaguely nodular tan surface is seen.

Mesothelioma

Hepatic mesothelioma is generally a secondary involvement of diffuse peritoneal mesothelioma. In rare cases, primary hepatic mesothelioma forms a localized intrahepatic mass with no apparent diffuse peritoneal involvement and thus mimics primary liver cancers. Although less than a dozen cases have been reported in the literature (192–199), this rare manifestation of a mesothelial neoplasm may be under-recognized.

Patients are adults, with a male to female ratio of approximately 2 to 1. The association with asbestos exposure is markedly weaker than that in classic mesothelioma, with only one patient proven to have such an occupational history (192). Tumors are generally solitary, 3 to 16 cm in size, and most commonly form a

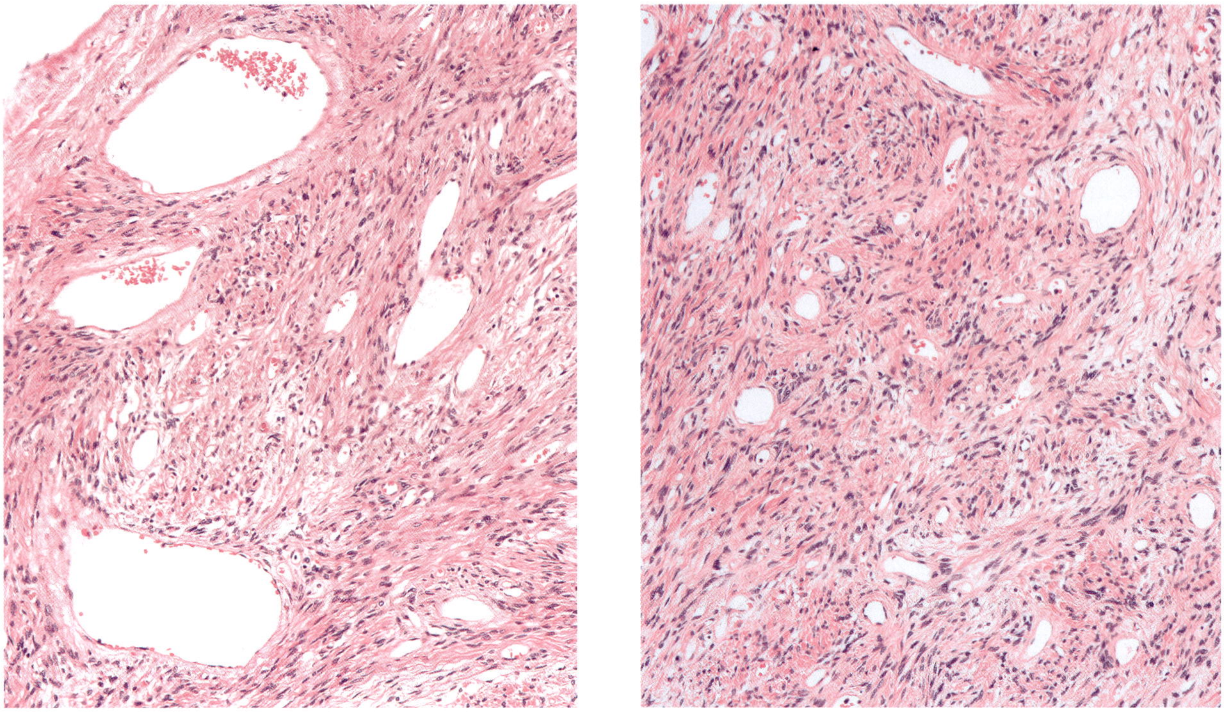

Figure 9-86

SOLITARY FIBROUS TUMOR

Left: The spindle cells are arranged in a "patternless" pattern, with occasional dilated blood vessels.
Right: A hemangiopericytomatous pattern is observed.

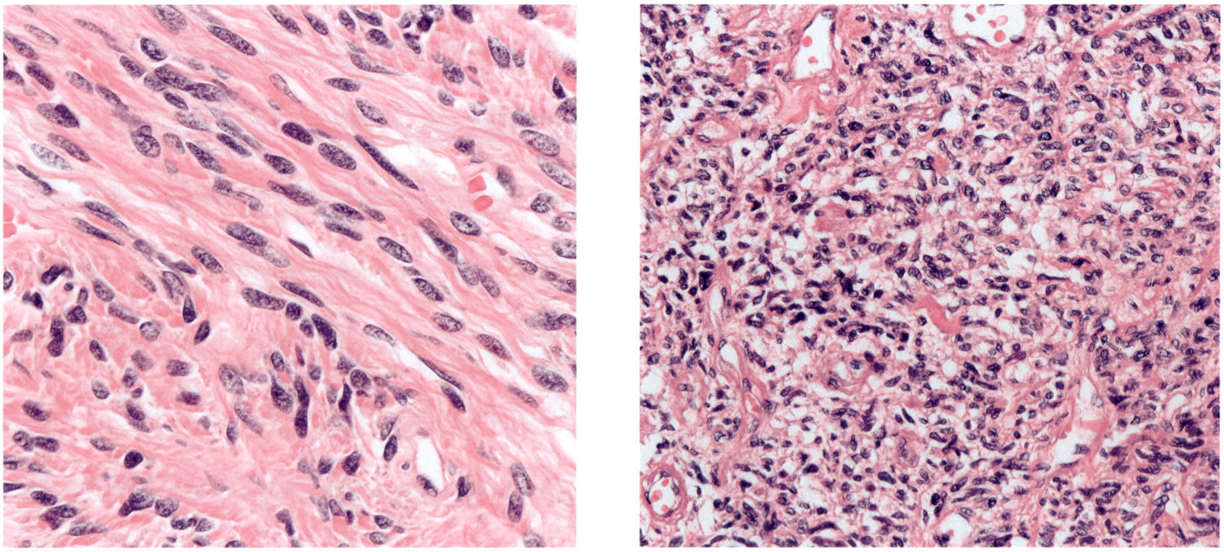

Figure 9-87

SOLITARY FIBROUS TUMOR

Left: Wavy collagen fibers are present between tumor cells.
Right: In this area, tumor cells are less spindle in shape, but irregularly arranged blood vessels with perivascular fibrosis gives a hemangiopericytomatous pattern.

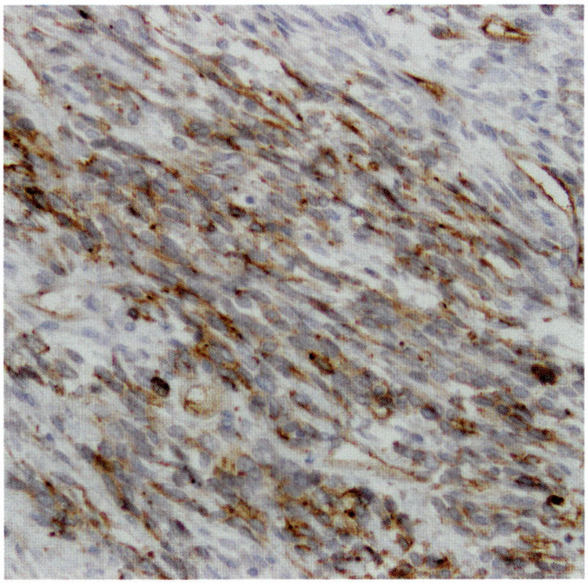

Figure 9-88

SOLITARY FIBROUS TUMOR

Tumor cells are positive for CD34.

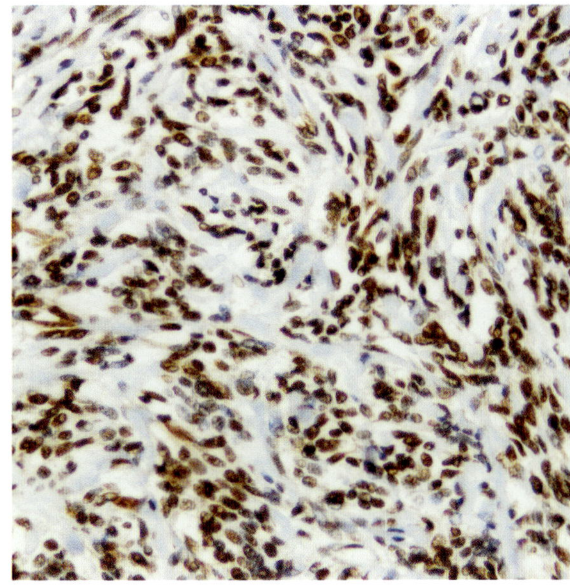

Figure 9-89

SOLITARY FIBROUS TUMOR

Nuclear expression of STAT6 is characteristic for this neoplasm.

subcapsular mass (fig. 9-91). Malignant ascites is an uncommon presentation.

Microscopically, the tumors are epithelioid (70 percent) or biphasic (30 percent), with no cases of pure sarcomatoid mesothelioma reported (fig. 9-92) (195). Epithelioid tumor cells are arranged in a tubulopapillary, gland-like, or sheet pattern in various proportions. The cells have clear or eosinophilic cytoplasm and round nuclei (fig. 9-93). A characteristic finding is a gland-like architecture with flat cells, sometimes associated with periglandular fibrosis, which is reminiscent of adenomatoid tumors (fig. 9-94). Spindle cells predominate in sarcomatoid areas, but the cells verge on an epithelioid configuration in places.

Sarcomatoid mesothelioma is cytologically blander than sarcomatoid cholangiocarcinoma or hepatocellular carcinoma. An important entity in the differential diagnosis is small duct intrahepatic cholangiocarcinoma. Mesothelioma is less desmoplastic and tumor cells are more cuboidal or flatter in appearance, with less pleomorphic nuclei, than cholangiocarcinoma.

The immunophenotype of primary hepatic mesothelioma is similar to that of classic diffuse mesothelioma. Calretinin, thrombomodulin, WT1, cytokeratin 5/6, D2-40, and mesothelin are positive (fig. 9-95), while CEA, BerEP4,

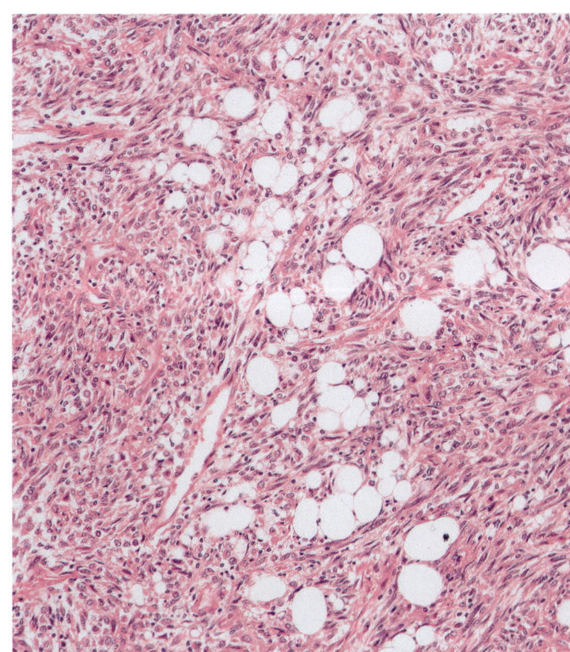

Figure 9-90

FAT-FORMING SOLITARY FIBROUS TUMOR IN THE RETROPERITONEUM

Mature adipose tissue is incorporated in the tumor. If similar tumors develop in the liver, the appearance may mimic angiomyolipoma.

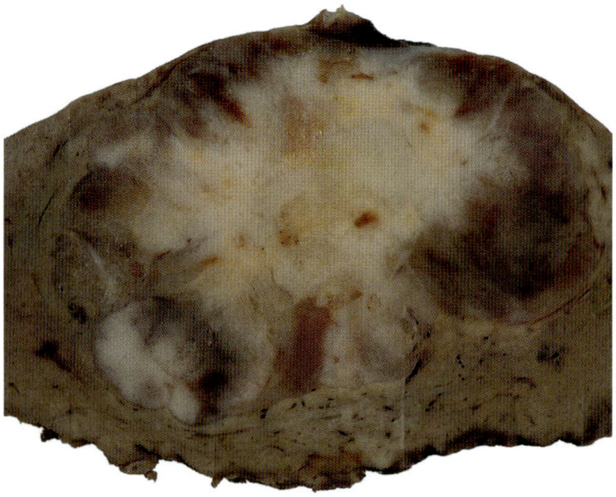

Figure 9-91

MESOTHELIOMA

A lobular liver mass has a white to slightly brown cut surface. The tumor is located just beneath the hepatic capsule and is well circumscribed with a pushing border.

CD15, and MOC31 are typically negative; if positive, adenocarcinoma is suggested.

Inflammatory Myofibroblastic Tumor

Inflammatory pseudotumor was originally considered to be a heterogeneous condition that included neoplastic and reactive processes. *Inflammatory myofibroblastic tumor* was isolated from this group since the neoplastic nature of proliferating myofibroblasts was suggested. Inflammatory myofibroblastic tumor most frequently occurs in the soft tissues of the mesentery, omentum, retroperitoneum, pelvis, and abdomen. It may also develop in parenchymal organs including the lung and liver (200,201). Although aged adults may be affected, patients are more commonly children and young adults, with occasional infantile cases. After surgical resection, local recurrence may occur, but the risk of remote metastasis is low (about 5 percent).

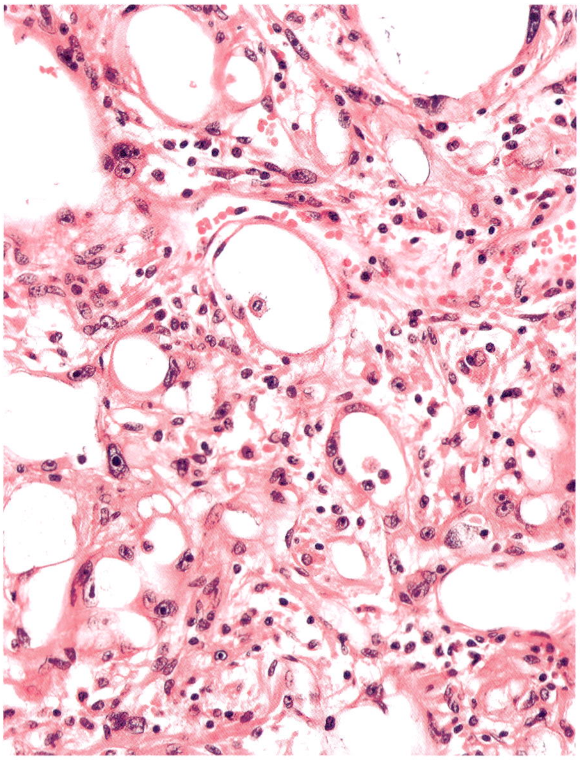

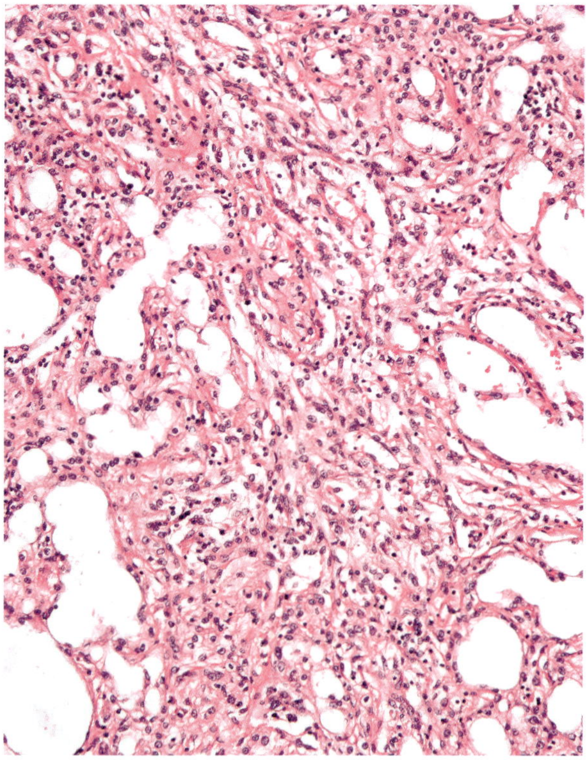

Figure 9-92

MESOTHELIOMA

Left: The tumor consists of cuboidal cells forming glandular structures and spindle-shaped cells.
Right: A biphasic growth pattern is noted.

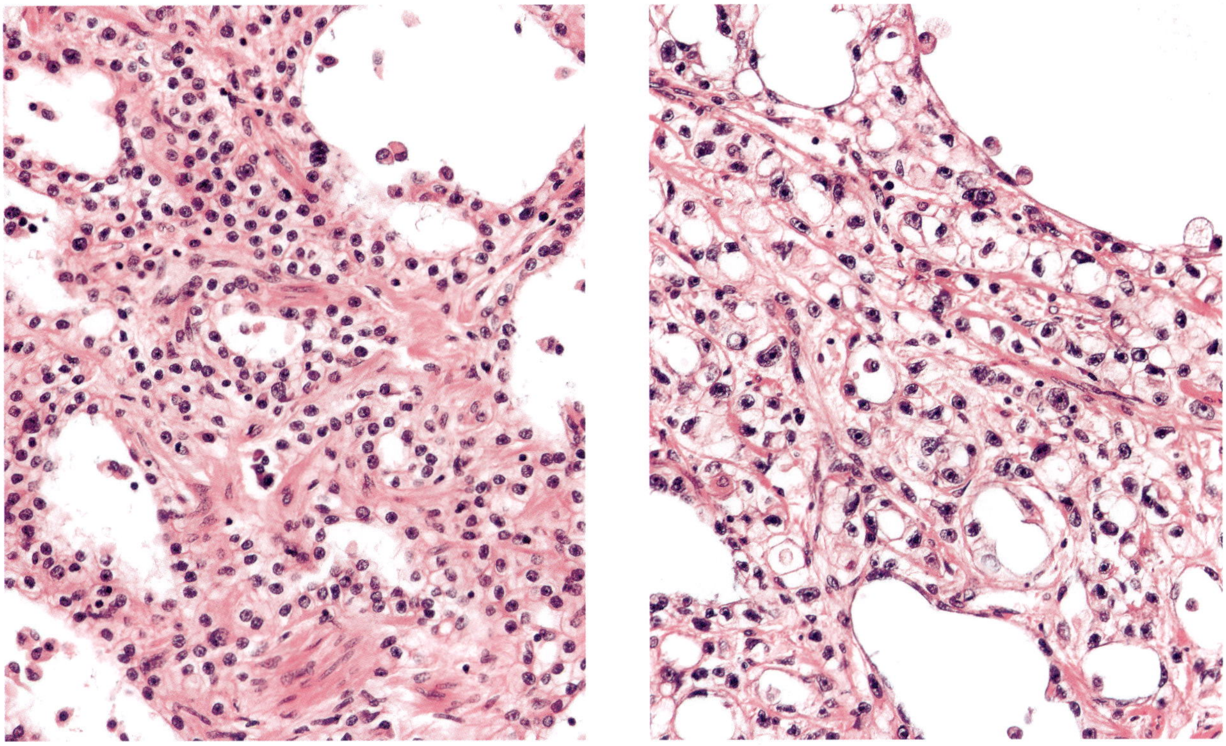

Figure 9-93

MESOTHELIOMA

Left: Cuboidal epithelioid cells have clear cytoplasm.
Right: This area shows high-grade dysplastic changes. The cells are cuboidal to polygonal.

This uncommon neoplasm forms solitary, or rarely, multiple solid tumors of up to 10 cm. Microscopically, the tumor consists of fibroblastic or myofibroblastic spindle cells proliferating in an inflammatory infiltrate that includes lymphocytes, plasma cells, and eosinophils. The neoplastic cells have plump or vesicular nuclei and distinct nucleoli, and are arranged in a fascicular or dispersed pattern in a variably fibromyxoid stroma (fig. 9-96) (202). Ganglion-like large cells may also be present. Mitotic activity varies, but is generally low. Necrosis is uncommon.

The tumor cells show immunohistochemical myofibroblastic differentiation, such as the expression of smooth muscle actin and, less commonly, desmin. *ALK* fusions are identified in about 60 percent of cases, particularly in patients younger than 40 years. Another 10 percent of cases have *ROS1* rearrangements (203–205). Immunohistochemistry for ALK and ROS1 is useful for predicting genetic alterations (203–206).

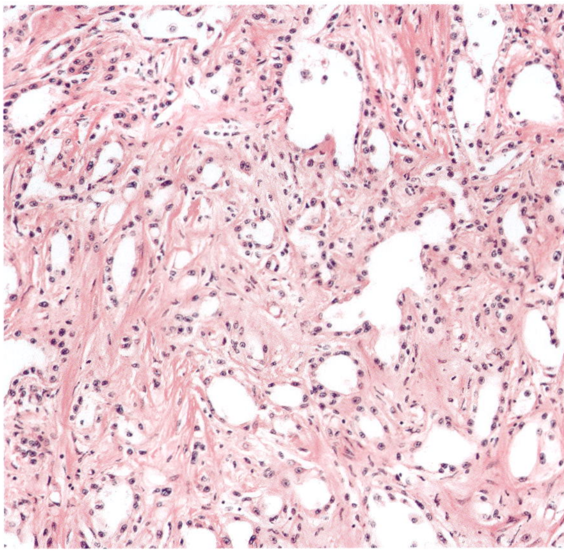

Figure 9-94

MESOTHELIOMA

Gland-like structures embedded in a fibrotic stroma mimic adenomatoid tumor.

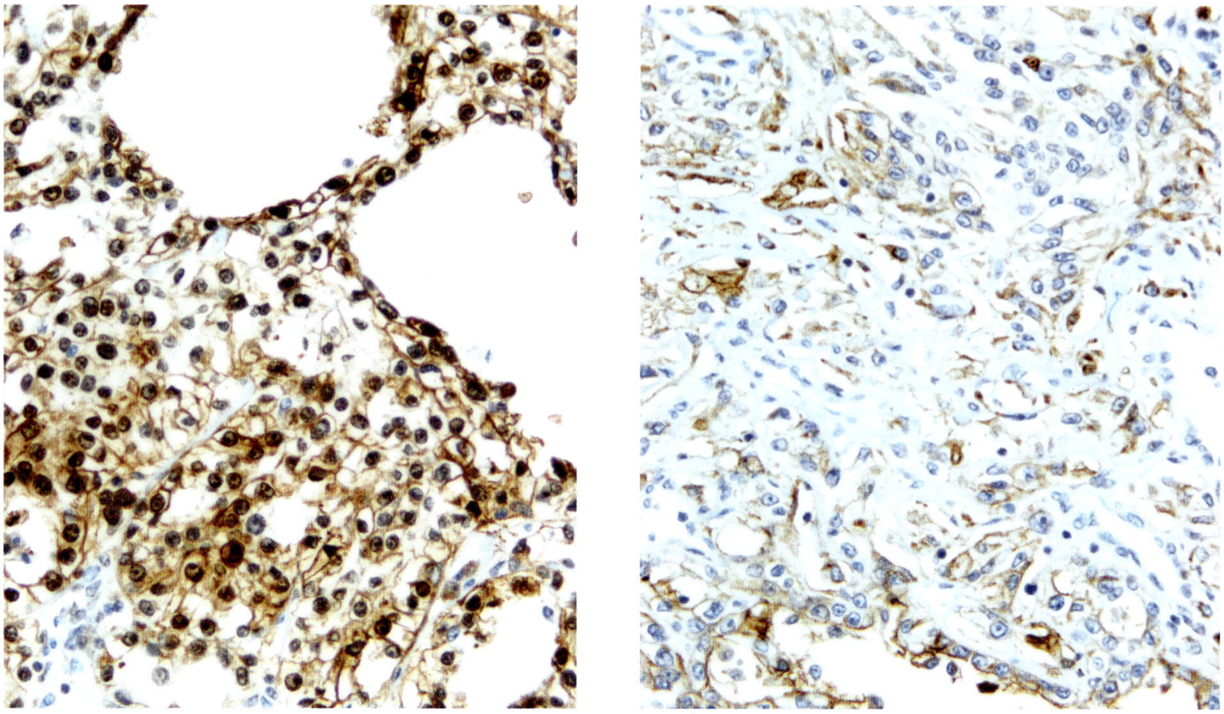

Figure 9-95

MESOTHELIOMA

Left: Calretinin is strongly expressed.
Right: D2-40 is expressed in both epithelioid and sarcomatoid cells.

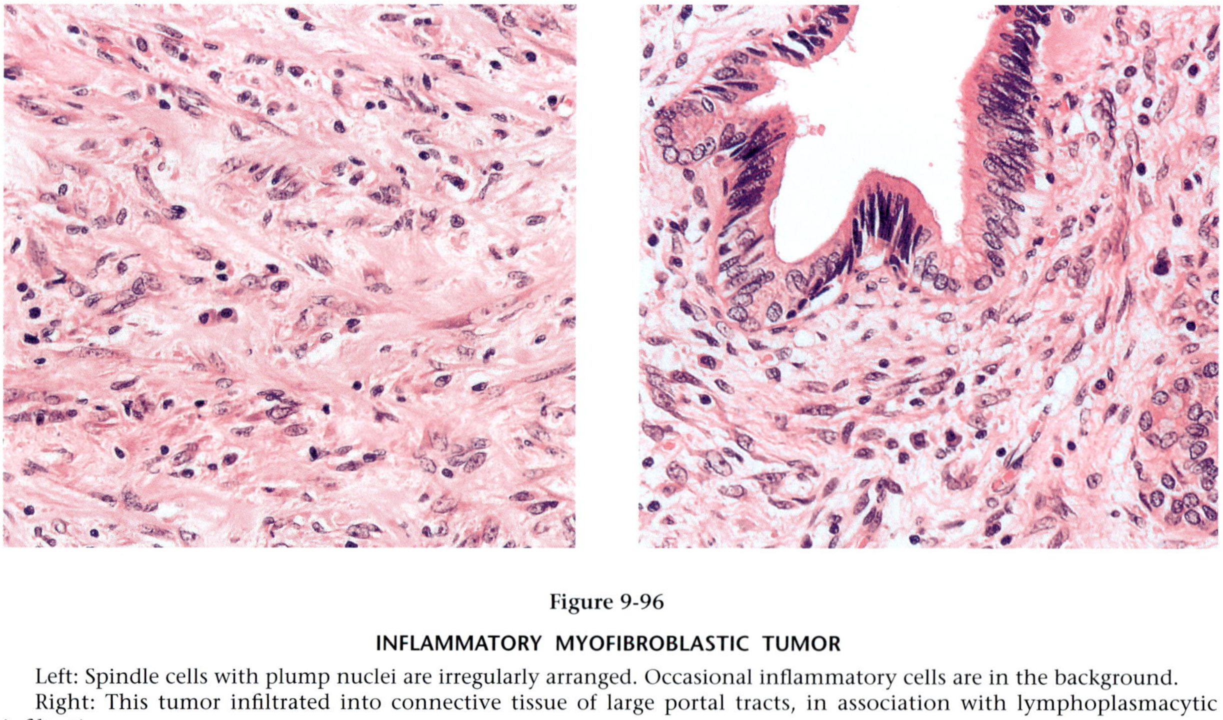

Figure 9-96

INFLAMMATORY MYOFIBROBLASTIC TUMOR

Left: Spindle cells with plump nuclei are irregularly arranged. Occasional inflammatory cells are in the background.
Right: This tumor infiltrated into connective tissue of large portal tracts, in association with lymphoplasmacytic infiltration.

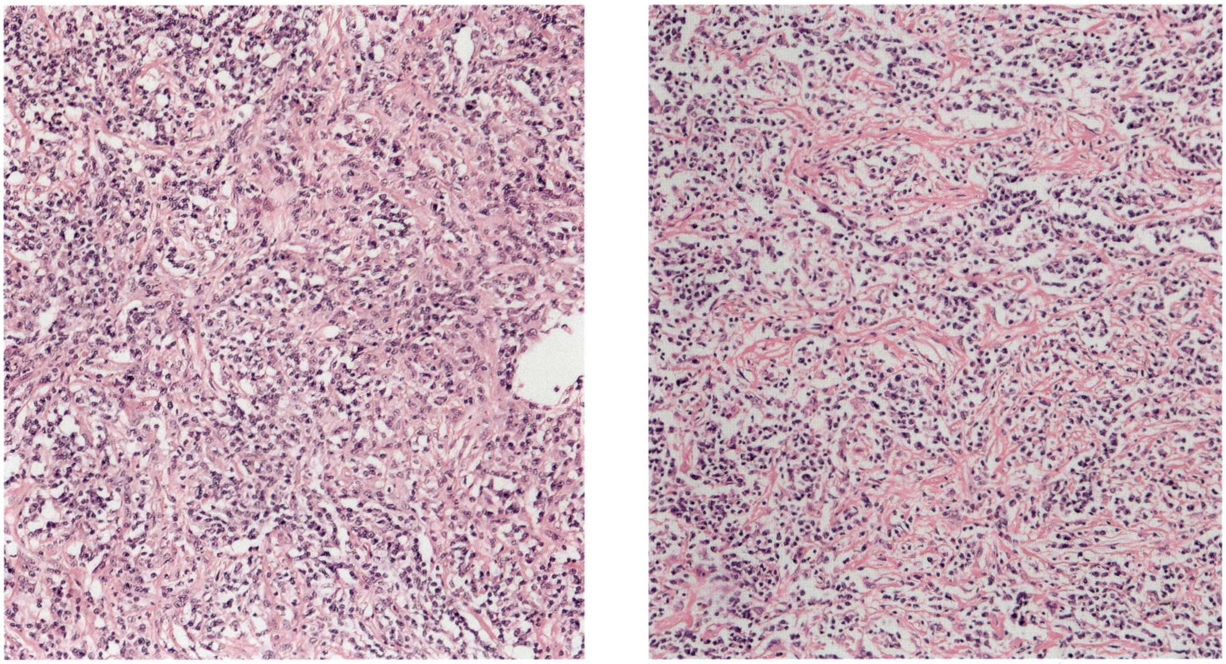

Figure 9-97

INFLAMMATORY PSEUDOTUMOR-LIKE FOLLICULAR DENDRITIC CELL TUMOR

Left: This tumor mass consists mainly of fibrous stroma and dense inflammatory infiltrates. At this magnification, neoplastic cells are difficult to identify.

Right: This area is more fibrotic than on the left.

Inflammatory Pseudotumor-Like Follicular Dendritic Cell Tumor

Inflammatory pseudotumor-like follicular dendritic cell tumor is another condition that was originally included in the group of inflammatory pseudotumors, but was subsequently proven to be a distinct entity. This rare entity is an EBV-driven neoplastic proliferation of follicular dendritic cells that occurs exclusively in the liver and spleen. The presence of EBV in a subset of "inflammatory pseudotumors" was confirmed in 1995 (207). In the following year, the expression of a follicular dendritic cell marker in EBV-positive hepatic "inflammatory pseudotumor" was almost simultaneously described in two studies (208,209).

The clinicopathologic features of this rare entity were characterized in a series of six cases reported in 2001 (210). Most cases occur in women aged between 30 and 60 years. Patients may present with weight loss, fever, or malaise.

The liver tumors are solitary and range between 4 and 20 cm in diameter. The tumor may recur or even metastasize after surgical resection; however, its biologic behavior and risk factors for recurrence have not yet been characterized.

Microscopically, these tumors consist of variably fibrotic stroma and a dense inflammatory infiltrate that includes lymphocytes and plasma cells (fig. 9-97). Because of the massive inflammatory infiltrate, the neoplastic cells may be difficult to identify at low magnification. Higher magnification reveals oval or spindle cells with vesicular nuclei and distinct nucleoli (fig. 9-98). The overall appearance may suggest malignant lymphoma, particularly Hodgkin lymphoma, rather than a mesenchymal neoplasm (210).

The cells express follicular dendritic cell markers such as CD21 and CD35, while CD23 is weakly positive. EBER in situ hybridization shows strong nuclear labeling in the tumor cells (fig. 9-99), which may occur in combination with the focal expression of EBV-LMP1 in some cases. ALK1 is negative.

Compared to classic follicular dendritic cell tumors in the lymph node, the inflammatory pseudotumor-like variant is unique in its hepatosplenic anatomic location, dispersed distribution

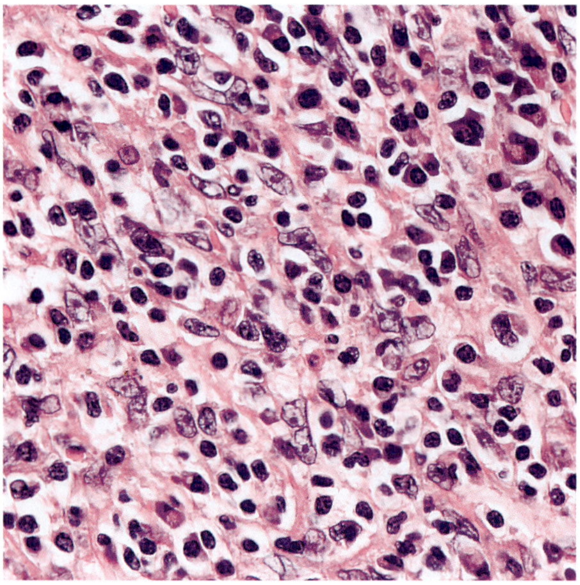

Figure 9-98

INFLAMMATORY PSEUDOTUMOR-LIKE FOLLICULAR DENDRITIC CELL TUMOR

A high-magnification view reveals spindle-shaped tumor cells that have enlarged nuclei and distinct nucleoli.

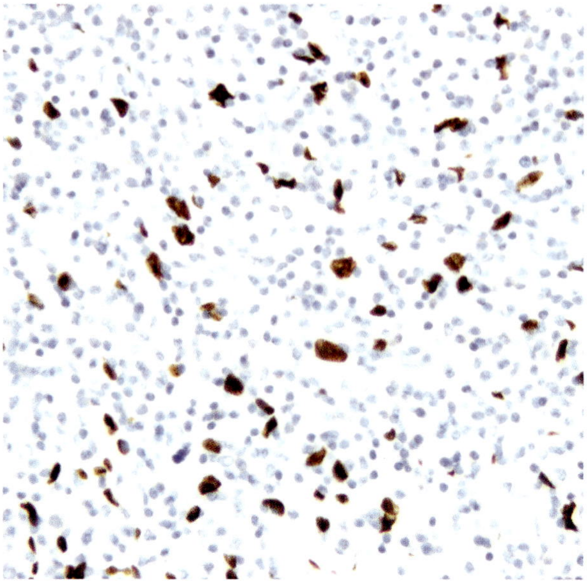

Figure 9-99

INFLAMMATORY PSEUDOTUMOR-LIKE FOLLICULAR DENDRITIC CELL TUMOR

The neoplastic cells are strongly positive for Epstein-Barr virus (EBV) encoded RNA (EBER).

of neoplastic cells, prominent lymphoplasmacytic infiltration, and consistent association with EBV (210). Areas of conventional follicular dendritic cell tumors may focally coexist.

Inflammatory Pseudotumor

Since the exclusion of inflammatory myofibroblastic and follicular dendritic cell tumors, *inflammatory pseudotumors* have become a less heterogeneous group than before. This group consists of two conditions with distinct clinicopathologic features (Table 9-1) (211).

Lymphoplasmacytic-type inflammatory pseudotumor is a hepatobiliary manifestation of IgG4-related disease and generally develops in patients over 50 years of age, with a male predominance (212,213). It is located inside the periportal connective tissue of hilar or intrahepatic large bile ducts, with little involvement of the liver parenchyma. More than 80 percent of patients have IgG4-related disease in other organs including autoimmune pancreatitis, sclerosing sialodacryoadenitis, retroperitoneal fibrosis, and tubulointerstitial nephritis (214). Similar inflammatory pseudotumors may also be present in the lungs. Serum IgG4 elevations (greater than 135 mg/dL) have been observed in approximately 70 percent of patients (214). Steroid therapy is very useful, and unnecessary surgeries are sometimes performed because of imaging features reminiscent of perihilar cholangiocarcinoma, particularly in patients with isolated liver disease.

Grossly, there is a well-circumscribed mass found along the biliary tree with a homogeneously white or tan cut surface (fig. 9-100). Microscopically, mass-forming lesions located inside periportal connective tissue consist of a massive lymphoplasmacytic infiltration and occasional eosinophils but no neutrophils (fig. 9-101). Intervening fibroblasts and myofibroblasts are sparse and not dysplastic. Although the bile duct and peribiliary glands are deeply involved in the fibroinflammatory process, the lining epithelium is typically intact (fig. 9-102). Characteristic histologic features are obliterative phlebitis and storiform fibrosis (fig. 9-103) (211,215).

Immunostaining shows a massive infiltration of IgG4-positive plasma cells with over 50 positive cells per high-power field and a greater than 40 percent IgG4/IgG-positive plasma cell ratio (fig. 9-104) (216). CD68-positive macrophages are few in number, while CD168 immunostaining

Table 9-1

CLASSIFICATION AND CLINICOPATHOLOGIC FEATURES OF HEPATIC INFLAMMATORY PSEUDOTUMOR

	Lymphoplasmacytic Type	Fibrohistiocytic Type
Age	>50 years	>30 years
Gender	Male >80%	Male 60%
Serology	IgG4 elevation (~80%)	None
Location	Periductal masses in perihilar or intrahepatic large portal tracts	Intraparenchymal nodular lesions (80%) or perihilar nodules (20%)
Histology	Plasma cell-rich inflammation Storiform fibrosis Obliterative phlebitis	Xanthogranulomatous change Suppurative inflammation Microabscess
IgG4+ plasma cells	Diffusely present Many (>50 cells/high-power field)	Patchy Few to occasionally present
IgG4+/IgG+ cell ratio	>40%	<40%
Extrahepatic lesions	Autoimmune pancreatitis Retroperitoneal fibrosis Sclerosing sialodacryoadenitis Other IgG4-related diseases	None

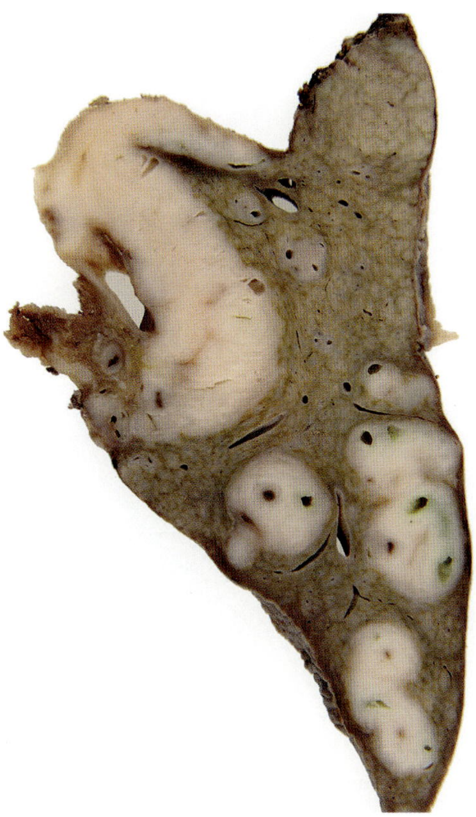

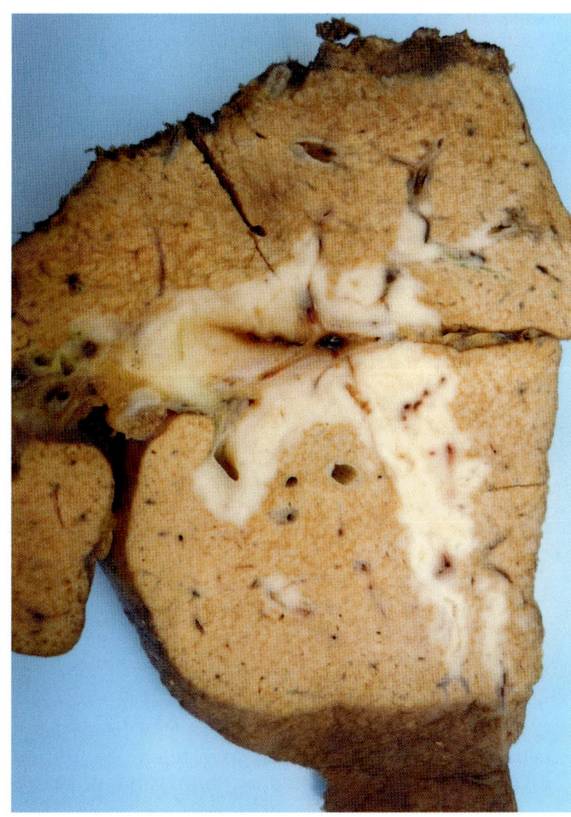

Figure 9-100

LYMPHOPLASMACYTIC-TYPE INFLAMMATORY PSEUDOTUMOR

Left: An irregularly shaped mass with a homogeneously white cut surface extends along the portal tract. Right: This lesion is extensively distributed from perihilar connective tissue to peripheral small portal tracts.

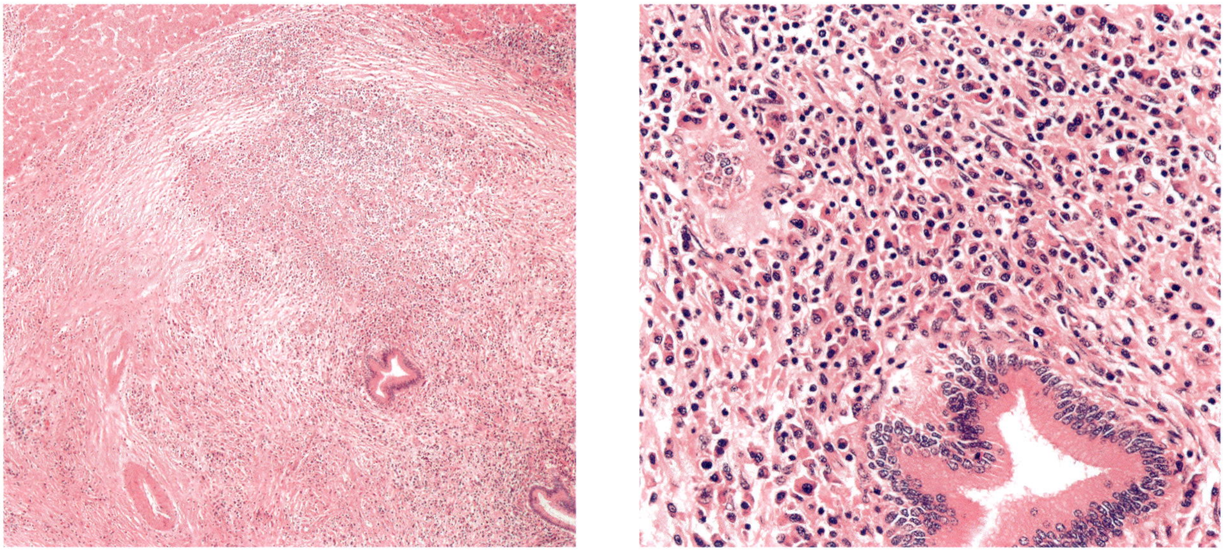

Figure 9-101

LYMPHOPLASMACYTIC-TYPE INFLAMMATORY PSEUDOTUMOR

Left: The portal tract is expanded by a massive inflammatory infiltrate and fibrosis. The adjacent liver parenchyma is less affected.

Right: The infiltrating inflammatory cells are mainly lymphocytes and plasma cells.

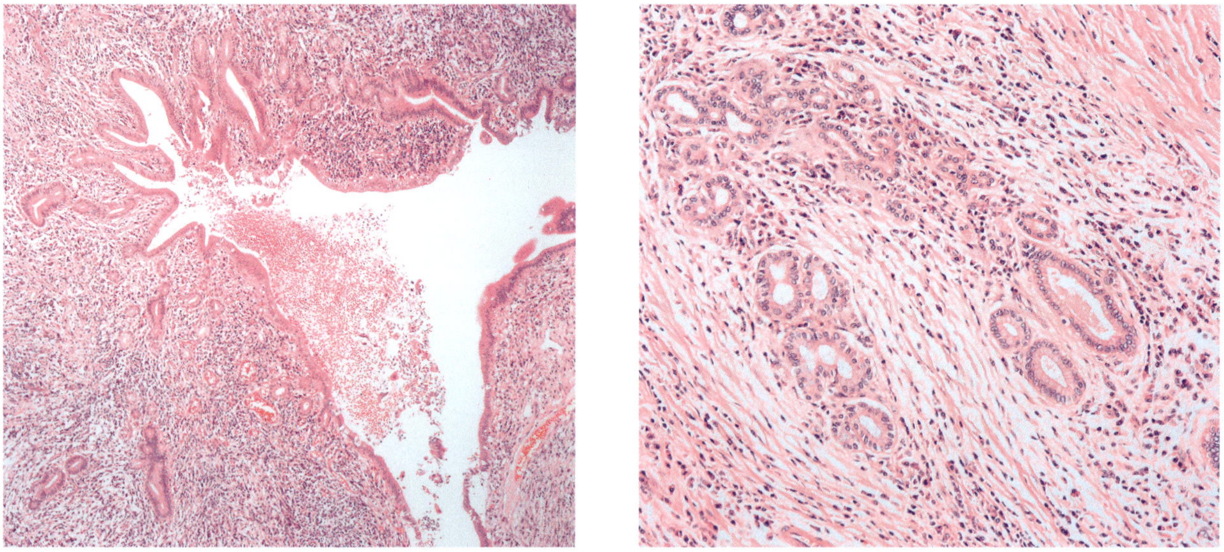

Figure 9-102

LYMPHOPLASMACYTIC-TYPE INFLAMMATORY PSEUDOTUMOR

Left: A large bile duct is deeply involved in the fibroinflammatory process, but the lining epithelium is well preserved.

Right: Despite the periglandular fibrosis and inflammation, the epithelium of the peribiliary glands is intact.

highlights the presence of a large number of M2-type macrophages in the mass (217).

Fibrohistiocytic-type inflammatory pseudotumor of the liver is a mass-forming lesion that is histologically characterized by the presence of suppurative or xanthogranulomatous inflammation in addition to lymphoplasmacytic infiltration (fig. 9-105) (211). Unlike the lymphoplasmacytic type,

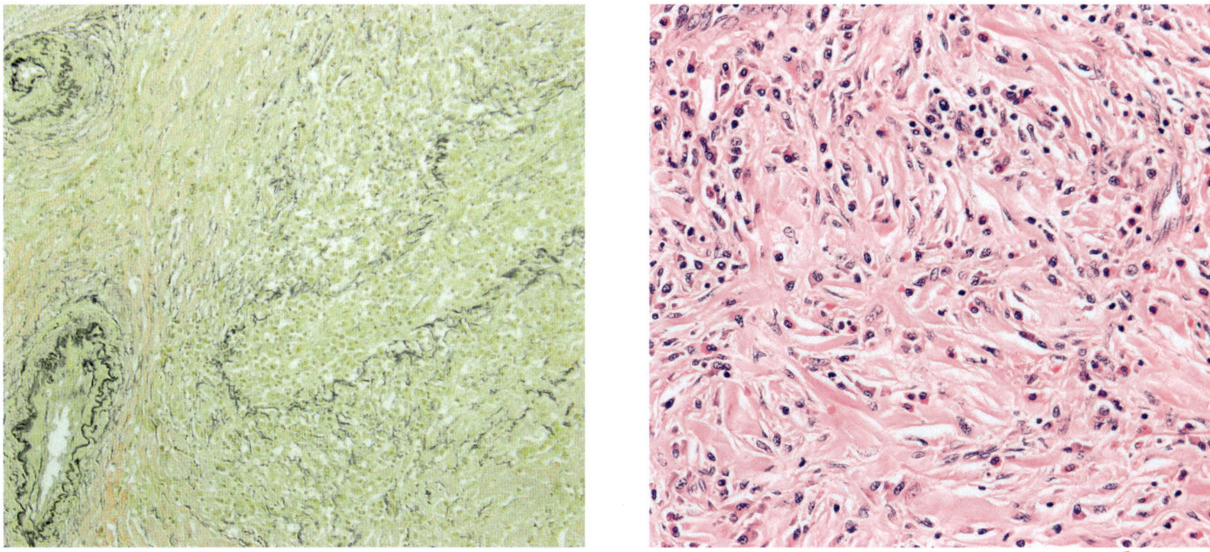

Figure 9-103

LYMPHOPLASMACYTIC-TYPE INFLAMMATORY PSEUDOTUMOR

Left: Elastica staining shows a small vein completely obliterated by the fibroinflammatory process (obliterative phlebitis). Right: Collagen fibers are arranged in a storiform pattern. Many eosinophils are in the background.

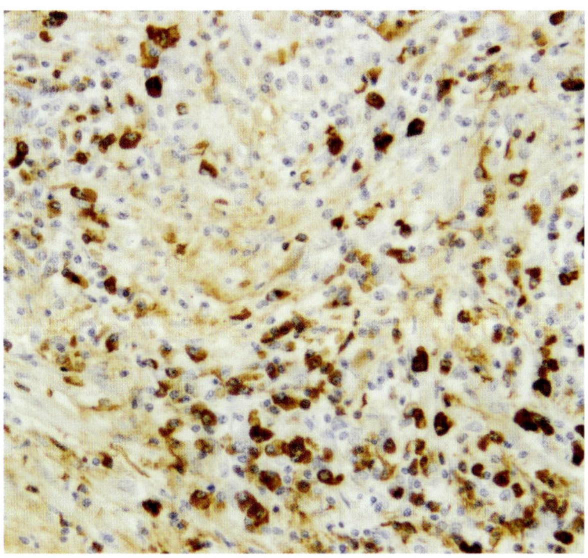

Figure 9-104

LYMPHOPLASMACYTIC-TYPE INFLAMMATORY PSEUDOTUMOR

Many plasma cells are IgG4 positive.

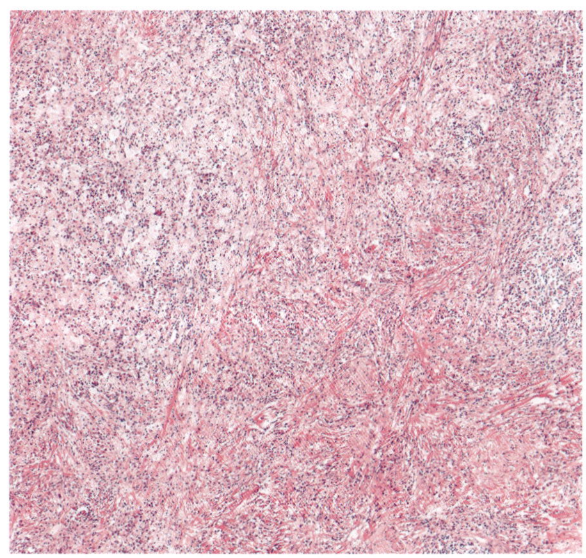

Figure 9-105

FIBROHISTIOCYTIC-TYPE INFLAMMATORY PSEUDOTUMOR

In addition to irregular fibrosis, there are foci of xanthogranulomatous inflammation.

this subtype occurs equally in both genders and more commonly exhibits nodular masses in the peripheral liver parenchyma (211). Although there is no known associated extrahepatic condition, some patients may have obstructive cholangiopathy due to cholangiocarcinoma or an ampullary neoplasm.

Grossly, the lesions are irregular in shape and may have necrotic foci or multiple liver nodules.

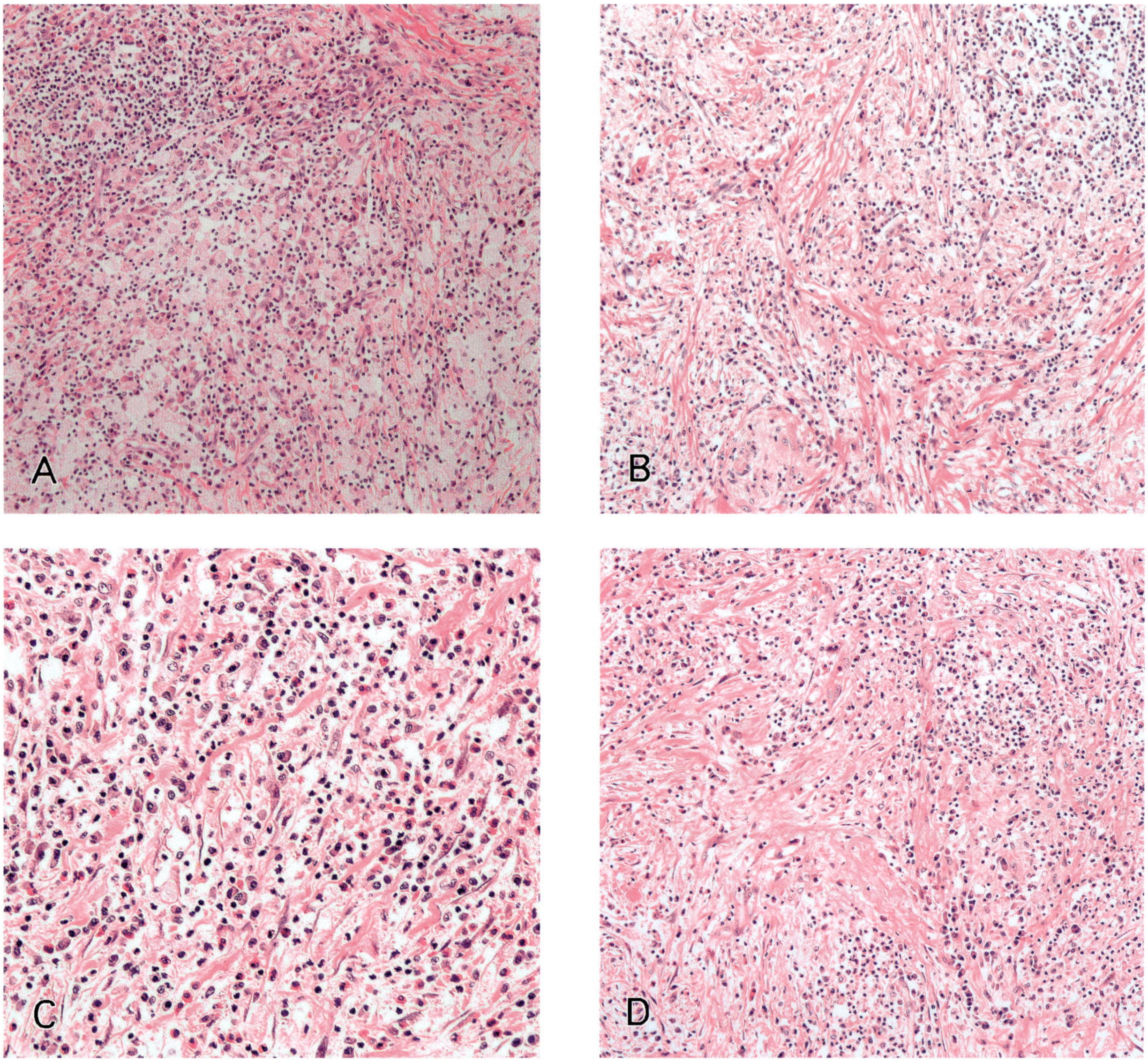

Figure 9-106

FIBROHISTIOCYTIC-TYPE INFLAMMATORY PSEUDOTUMOR

A: Many foamy macrophages are aggregated in this area.
B: Xanthogranulomatous inflammation is associated with irregular fibrosis.
C: In addition to lymphocytes, plasma cells, and eosinophils, there are many neutrophils.
D: Small clusters of neutrophils (microabscess) are noted.

Microscopically, the nodules consist of a mixed inflammatory infiltrate with aggregated foamy macrophages and neutrophils against the background of variable fibrosis (fig. 9-106). Multinucleated giant cells may also be present.

CD68 highlights the infiltration of macrophages (211). IgG4-positive plasma cells may be observed, but are fewer in number and their distribution is less diffuse than those in the lymphoplasmacytic type (213). The IgG4/IgG-positive plasma cell ratio is generally less than 40 percent. Some cases are caused by infection and culture studies may assist in the identification of causative agents such as *Escherichia coli*, *Actinomyces*, and *Klebsiella pneumoniae*.

REFERENCES

1. Miettinen M, Fetsch JF, Antonescu CR, Folpe AL, Wakely PE, Jr. Tumors of the soft tissues. AFIP Atlas of Tumor Pathology, 4th Series, Fascicle 20. Washington, DC: American Registry of Pathology; 2014.
2 Fletcher CD, Bridge JA, Hogendoorn PC, Mertens F. World Health Organization classification of tumours of soft tissue and bone, 4th ed. Lyon: IARC Press; 2013.
3. Ishak KG, Goodman ZD, Stocker JT. Tumors of the liver and intrahepatic bile ducts. AFIP Atlas of Tumor Pathology, 3rd Series, Fascicle 31. Washington, DC: American Registry of Pathology; 1999.
4. Goodman ZD, Luigi MT, Wee A. Tumours and tumour-like lesios of the liver. In: Burt A, Portmann B, Ferrell L, eds. MacSween's pathology of the liver, 6th ed. Edinburgh: Elsevier; 2012:761-851.
5. Bioulac-Sage P, Laumonier H, Laurent C, Blanc JF, Balabaud C. Benign and malignant vascular tumors of the liver in adults. Semin Liver Dis 2008;28:302-314.
6. Karhunen PJ. Benign hepatic tumours and tumour like conditions in men. J Clin Pathol 1986;39:183-188.
7. Iwatsuki S, Todo S, Starzl TE. Excisional therapy for benign hepatic lesions. Surg Gynecol Obstet 1990;171:240-246.
8. Yamamoto T, Kawarada Y, Yano T, Noguchi T, Mizumoto R. Spontaneous rupture of hemangioma of the liver: treatment with transcatheter hepatic arterial embolization. Am J Gastroenterol 1991;86:1645-1649.
9. Hotokezaka M, Kojima M, Nakamura K, et al. Traumatic rupture of hepatic hemangioma. J Clin Gastroenterol 1996;23:69-71.
10. Shimizu M, Miura J, Itoh H, Saitoh Y. Hepatic giant cavernous hemangioma with microangiopathic hemolytic anemia and consumption coagulopathy. Am J Gastroenterol 1990;85:1411-1413.
11. Makhlouf HR, Ishak KG. Sclerosed hemangioma and sclerosing cavernous hemangioma of the liver: a comparative clinicopathologic and immunohistochemical study with emphasis on the role of mast cells in their histogenesis. Liver 2002;22:70-78.
12. Doyle DJ, Khalili K, Guindi M, Atri M. Imaging features of sclerosed hemangioma. AJR Am J Roentgenol 2007;189:67-72.
13. Mathieu D, Rahmouni A, Vasile N, et al. Sclerosed liver hemangioma mimicking malignant tumor at MR imaging: pathologic correlation. J Magn Reson Imaging 1994;4:506-508.
14. Aibe H, Hondo H, Kuroiwa T, et al. Sclerosed hemangioma of the liver. Abdom Imaging 2001; 26:496-499.
15. Lehmann FS, Beglinger C, Schnabel K, Terracciano L. Progressive development of diffuse liver hemangiomatosis. J Hepatol 1999;30:951-954.
16. Feurle GE. Arteriovenous shunting and cholestasis in hepatic hemangiomatosis associated with metoclopramide. Gastroenterology 1990;99:258-262.
17. Frangides C, Kounis NG, Papadaki PJ, Goudevenos J, Zavras GM. Diffuse hepatic haemangiomatosis in the elderly. Br J Clin Pract 1995;49:215-216.
18. Kim GE, Thung SN, Tsui WM, Ferrell LD. Hepatic cavernous hemangioma: underrecognized associated histologic features. Liver Int 2006;26:334-338.
19. Garcia-Tsao G, Korzenik JR, Young L, et al. Liver disease in patients with hereditary hemorrhagic telangiectasia. N Engl J Med 2000;343:931-936.
20. Miettinen M, Fletcher CD, Kindblom LG, Zimmermann A, Tsui WM. Mesenchymal tumours of the liver. In: Bosman FT, Carneiro F, Hruban RH, Theise ND, eds. World Health Organization classification of tumours of the digestive system. Lyon: IARC; 2010:241-250.
21. Linda F, Kakar S. Tumors of the liver, gallbladder, and biliary tree. In: Fletcher CD, ed. Diagnostic histopathology of tumors, 3rd ed. Edinburg: Elsevier; 2007:417-461.
22. Selby DM, Stocker JT, Waclawiw MA, Hitchcock CL, Ishak KG. Infantile hemangioendothelioma of the liver. Hepatology 1994;20:39-45.
23. Shah KD, Beck AR, Jhaveri MK, Keohane M, Weinberg B, Gerber MA. Infantile hemangioendothelioma of heterotopic intrathoracic liver associated with diaphragmatic hernia. Hum Pathol 1987;18:754-756.
24. Sciveres M, Marrone G, Pipitone S, et al. Successful first-line treatment with propranolol of multifocal infantile hepatic hemangioma with high-flow cardiac overload. J Pediatr Gastroenterol Nutr 2011;53:693-695.
25. Perez Payarols J, Pardo Masferrer J, Gomez Bellvert C. Treatment of life-threatening infantile hemangiomas with vincristine. N Engl J Med 1995;333:369.
26. Kuroda T, Kumagai M, Nosaka S, et al. Critical infantile hepatic hemangioma: results of a nationwide survey by the Japanese Infantile Hepatic Hemangioma Study Group. J Pediatr Surg 2011;46:2239-2243.
27. Kasahara M, Kiuchi T, Haga H, et al. Monosegmental living-donor liver transplantation for infantile hepatic hemangioendothelioma. J Pediatr Surg 2003;38:1108-1111.
28. Dehner LP, Ishak KG. Vascular tumors of the liver in infants and children. A study of 30 cases and review of the literature. Arch Pathol 1971;92:101-111.

29. Kirchner SG, Heller RM, Kasselberg AG, Greene HL. Infantile hepatic hemangioendothelioma with subsequent malignant degeneration. Pediatr Radiol 1981;11:42-45.
30. Awan S, Davenport M, Portmann B, Howard ER. Angiosarcoma of the liver in children. J Pediatr Surg 1996;31:1729-1732.
31. North PE, Waner M, Mizeracki A, Mihm MC Jr. GLUT1: a newly discovered immunohistochemical marker for juvenile hemangiomas. Hum Pathol 2000;31:11-22.
32. Mo JQ, Dimashkieh HH, Bove KE. GLUT1 endothelial reactivity distinguishes hepatic infantile hemangioma from congenital hepatic vascular malformation with associated capillary proliferation. Hum Pathol 2004;35:200-209.
33. Weiss SW, Enzinger FM. Epithelioid hemangioendothelioma: a vascular tumor often mistaken for a carcinoma. Cancer 1982;50:970-981.
34. Weiss SW, Ishak KG, Dail DH, Sweet DE, Enzinger FM. Epithelioid hemangioendothelioma and related lesions. Semin Diagn Pathol 1986;3:259-287.
35. Ishak KG, Sesterhenn IA, Goodman ZD, Rabin L, Stromeyer FW. Epithelioid hemangioendothelioma of the liver: a clinicopathologic and follow-up study of 32 cases. Hum Pathol 1984;15:839-852.
36. Hertl M, Cosimi AB. Liver transplantation for malignancy. Oncologist 2005;10:269-281.
37. Mehrabi A, Kashfi A, Fonouni H, et al. Primary malignant hepatic epithelioid hemangioendothelioma: a comprehensive review of the literature with emphasis on the surgical therapy. Cancer 2006;107:2108-2121.
38. Zhou L, Cui MY, Xiong J, et al. Spectrum of appearances on CT and MRI of hepatic epithelioid hemangioendothelioma. BMC Gastroenterol 2015;15:69.
39. Paolantonio P, Laghi A, Vanzulli A, et al. MRI of hepatic epithelioid hemangioendothelioma (HEH). J Magn Reson Imaging 2014;40:552-558.
40. Economopoulos N, Kelekis NL, Argentos S, et al. Bright-dark ring sign in MR imaging of hepatic epithelioid hemangioendothelioma. J Magn Reson Imaging 2008;27:908-912.
41. Paolantonio P, Rengo M, Ferrari R, Vecchietti F, Vasselli F, Laghi A. Hepatic epithelioid hemangioendothelioma (HEH) at MRI using reticuloendothelial system (RES)-specific contrast agent: the "bright-bright sign" rather than the "bright-dark sign." J Magn Reson Imaging 2009;29:994-995; author reply 5.
42. Makhlouf HR, Ishak KG, Goodman ZD. Epithelioid hemangioendothelioma of the liver: a clinicopathologic study of 137 cases. Cancer 1999;85:562-582.
43. Lauffer JM, Zimmermann A, Krahenbuhl L, Triller J, Baer HU. Epithelioid hemangioendothelioma of the liver. A rare hepatic tumor. Cancer 1996;78:2318-2327.
44. Fujii T, Zen Y, Sato Y, et al. Podoplanin is a useful diagnostic marker for epithelioid hemangioendothelioma of the liver. Mod Pathol 2008;21:125-130.
45. Miettinen M, Fetsch JF. Distribution of keratins in normal endothelial cells and a spectrum of vascular tumors: implications in tumor diagnosis. Hum Pathol 2000;31:1062-1067.
46. Doyle LA, Fletcher CD, Hornick JL. Nuclear Expression of CAMTA1 distinguishes epithelioid hemangioendothelioma from histologic mimics. Am J Surg Pathol 2016;40:94-102.
47. Antonescu CR, Le Loarer F, Mosquera JM, et al. Novel YAP1-TFE3 fusion defines a distinct subset of epithelioid hemangioendothelioma. Genes Chromosomes Cancer 2013;52:775-784.
48. Tanas MR, Sboner A, Oliveira AM, et al. Identification of a disease-defining gene fusion in epithelioid hemangioendothelioma. Sci Transl Med 2011;3:98ra82.
49. Errani C, Zhang L, Sung YS, et al. A novel WWTR1-CAMTA1 gene fusion is a consistent abnormality in epithelioid hemangioendothelioma of different anatomic sites. Genes Chromosomes Cancer 2011;50:644-653.
50. Errani C, Sung YS, Zhang L, Healey JH, Antonescu CR. Monoclonality of multifocal epithelioid hemangioendothelioma of the liver by analysis of WWTR1-CAMTA1 breakpoints. Cancer Genet 2012;205:12-17.
51. Lee SJ, Yang WI, Chung WS, Kim SK. Epithelioid hemangioendotheliomas with TFE3 gene translocations are compossible with CAMTA1 gene rearrangements. Oncotarget 2016;7:7480-488.
52. Lerut JP, Orlando G, Sempoux C, et al. Hepatic haemangioendothelioma in adults: excellent outcome following liver transplantation. Transpl Int 2004;17:202-207.
53. Ben-Haim M, Roayaie S, Ye MQ, et al. Hepatic epithelioid hemangioendothelioma: resection or transplantation, which and when? Liver Transpl Surg 1999;5:526-531.
54. Penn I. Hepatic transplantation for primary and metastatic cancers of the liver. Surgery 1991;110:726-34; discussion 734-735.
55. Falk H, Herbert J, Crowley S, et al. Epidemiology of hepatic angiosarcoma in the United States: 1964-1974. Environ Health Perspect 1981;41: 107-113.
56. Baxter PJ, Anthony PP, Macsween RN, Scheuer PJ. Angiosarcoma of the liver: annual occurrence and aetiology in Great Britain. Br J Ind Med 1980;37:213-221.
57. Dannaher CL, Tamburro CH, Yam LT. Occupational carcinogenesis: the Louisville experience with vinyl chloride-associated hepatic angiosarcoma. Am J Med 1981;70:279-287.

58. Locker GY, Doroshow JH, Zwelling LA, Chabner BA. The clinical features of hepatic angiosarcoma: a report of four cases and a review of the English literature. Medicine (Baltimore) 1979;58:48-64.
59. Falk H, Caldwell GG, Ishak KG, Thomas LB, Popper H. Arsenic-related hepatic angiosarcoma. Am J Ind Med 1981;2:43-50.
60. Pickhardt PJ, Kitchin D, Lubner MG, Ganeshan DM, Bhalla S, Covey AM. Primary hepatic angiosarcoma: multi-institutional comprehensive cancer centre review of multiphasic CT and MR imaging in 35 patients. Eur Radiol 2015;25:315-322.
61. Koyama T, Fletcher JG, Johnson CD, Kuo MS, Notohara K, Burgart LJ. Primary hepatic angiosarcoma: findings at CT and MR imaging. Radiology 2002;222:667-673.
62. Bruegel M, Muenzel D, Waldt S, Specht K, Rummeny EJ. Hepatic angiosarcoma: cross-sectional imaging findings in seven patients with emphasis on dynamic contrast-enhanced and diffusion-weighted MRI. Abdom Imaging 2013;38:745-754.
63. Zukerberg LR, Nickoloff BJ, Weiss SW. Kaposiform hemangioendothelioma of infancy and childhood. An aggressive neoplasm associated with Kasabach-Merritt syndrome and lymphangiomatosis. Am J Surg Pathol 1993;17:321-328.
64. Meis-Kindblom JM, Kindblom LG. Angiosarcoma of soft tissue: a study of 80 cases. Am J Surg Pathol 1998;22:683-697.
65. Hollstein M, Marion MJ, Lehman T, et al. p53 mutations at A:T base pairs in angiosarcomas of vinyl chloride-exposed factory workers. Carcinogenesis 1994;15:1-3.
66. Soini Y, Welsh JA, Ishak KG, Bennett WP. p53 mutations in primary hepatic angiosarcomas not associated with vinyl chloride exposure. Carcinogenesis 1995;16:2879-2881.
67. Przygodzki RM, Finkelstein SD, Keohavong P, et al. Sporadic and Thorotrast-induced angiosarcomas of the liver manifest frequent and multiple point mutations in K-ras-2. Lab Invest 1997;76:153-159.
68. Tsui WM, Colombari R, Portmann BC, et al. Hepatic angiomyolipoma: a clinicopathologic study of 30 cases and delineation of unusual morphologic variants. Am J Surg Pathol 1999;23:34-48.
69. Nonomura A, Mizukami Y, Kadoya M. Angiomyolipoma of the liver: a collective review. J Gastroenterol 1994;29:95-105.
70. Nelson CP, Sanda MG. Contemporary diagnosis and management of renal angiomyolipoma. J Urol 2002;168:1315-1325.
71. Zhu Z, Yang L, Zhao XM, Luo DQ, Zhang HT, Zhou CW. Myomatous hepatic angiomyolipoma: imaging findings in 14 cases with radiological-pathological correlation and review of the literature. Br J Radiol 2014;87:20130712.
72. Hogemann D, Flemming P, Kreipe H, Galanski M. Correlation of MRI and CT findings with histopathology in hepatic angiomyolipoma. Eur Radiol 2001;11:1389-1395.
73. Nonomura A, Enomoto Y, Takeda M, Takano M, Morita K, Kasai T. Angiomyolipoma of the liver: a reappraisal of morphological features and delineation of new characteristic histological features from the clinicopathological findings of 55 tumours in 47 patients. Histopathology 2012;61:863-880.
74. Nguyen TT, Gorman B, Shields D, Goodman Z. Malignant hepatic angiomyolipoma: report of a case and review of literature. Am J Surg Pathol 2008;32:793-798.
75. Dalle I, Sciot R, de Vos R, et al. Malignant angiomyolipoma of the liver: a hitherto unreported variant. Histopathology 2000;36:443-450.
76. Deng YF, Lin Q, Zhang SH, Ling YM, He JK, Chen XF. Malignant angiomyolipoma in the liver: a case report with pathological and molecular analysis. Pathol Res Pract 2008;204:911-918.
77. Parfitt JR, Bella AJ, Izawa JI, Wehrli BM. Malignant neoplasm of perivascular epithelioid cells of the liver. Arch Pathol Lab Med 2006;130:1219-1222.
78. Shi H, Cao D, Wei L, Sun L, Guo A. Inflammatory angiomyolipomas of the liver: a clinicopathologic and immunohistochemical analysis of 5 cases. Ann Diagn Pathol 2010;14:240-246.
79. Nonomura A, Enomoto Y, Takeda M, et al. Invasive growth of hepatic angiomyolipoma; a hitherto unreported ominous histological feature. Histopathology 2006;48:831-835.
80. Tsui WM, Yuen AK, Ma KF, Tse CC. Hepatic angiomyolipomas with a deceptive trabecular pattern and HMB-45 reactivity. Histopathology 1992;21:569-573.
81. Miettinen M, McCue PA, Sarlomo-Rikala M, et al. Sox10—a marker for not only schwannian and melanocytic neoplasms but also myoepithelial cell tumors of soft tissue: a systematic analysis of 5134 tumors. Am J Surg Pathol 2015;39:826-835.
82. Nonomura A, Mizukami Y, Takayanagi N, et al. Immunohistochemical study of hepatic angiomyolipoma. Pathol Int 1996;46:24-32.
83. Agaram NP, Sung YS, Zhang L, et al. Dichotomy of genetic abnormalities in PEComas with therapeutic implications. Am J Surg Pathol 2015;39:813-825.
84. Pan CC, Chung MY, Ng KF, et al. Constant allelic alteration on chromosome 16p (TSC2 gene) in perivascular epithelioid cell tumour (PEComa): genetic evidence for the relationship of PEComa with angiomyolipoma. J Pathol 2008;214:387-393.
85. Qin W, Bajaj V, Malinowska I, et al. Angiomyolipoma have common mutations in TSC2 but no other common genetic events. PLoS One 2011;6:e24919.

86. Argani P, Aulmann S, Illei PB, et al. A distinctive subset of PEComas harbors TFE3 gene fusions. Am J Surg Pathol 2010;34:1395-1406.
87. Huang SC, Chuang HC, Chen TD, et al. Alterations of the mTOR pathway in hepatic angiomyolipoma with emphasis on the epithelioid variant and loss of heterogeneity of TSC1/TSC2. Histopathology 2015;66:695-705.
87a. Jimbo N, Nishigami T, Noguchi M, et al. Hepatic angiomyolipomas may overexpress TFE3, but have no relevant genetic alterations. Hum Pathol 2017;61:41-48.
88. Guarda LA, Luna MA, Smith JL, Jr., Mansell PW, Gyorkey F, Roca AN. Acquired immune deficiency syndrome: postmortem findings. Am J Clin Pathol 1984;81:549-557.
89. Kaldor JM, Coates M, Vettom L, Taylor R. Epidemiological characteristics of Kaposi's sarcoma prior to the AIDS epidemic. Br J Cancer 1994;70: 674-676.
90. Franceschi S, Geddes M. Epidemiology of classic Kaposi's sarcoma, with special reference to mediterranean population. Tumori 1995;81:308-14.
91. Cottoni F, De Marco R, Montesu MA. Classical Kaposi's sarcoma in north-east Sardinia: an overview from 1977 to 1991. Br J Cancer 1996;73: 1132-1133.
92. Vijgen S, Wyss C, Meylan P, et al. Fatal outcome of multiple clinical presentations of human herpesvirus 8-related disease after solid organ transplantation. Transplantation 2016;100:134-140.
93. Marcelin AG, Roque-Afonso AM, Hurtova M, et al. Fatal disseminated Kaposi's sarcoma following human herpesvirus 8 primary infections in liver-transplant recipients. Liver Transpl 2004;10: 295-300.
94. Chang Y, Cesarman E, Pessin MS, et al. Identification of herpesvirus-like DNA sequences in AIDS-associated Kaposi's sarcoma. Science 1994;266:1865-1869.
95. Chang Y, Moore PS. Kaposi's Sarcoma (KS)-associated herpesvirus and its role in KS. Infect Agents Dis 1996;5:215-222.
96. Noel JC, Hermans P, Andre J, et al. Herpesvirus-like DNA sequences and Kaposi's sarcoma: relationship with epidemiology, clinical spectrum, and histologic features. Cancer 1996;77:2132-2136.
97. Antinori S, Ridolfo AL, Esposito R, Vago L, Moroni M. Liver involvement in AIDS-associated malignancies. J Hepatol. 1994;21:1145-1146.
98. Lucas SB, Zaki SR, Portmann B. Other viral and infectious diseases and HIV-related liver disease. In: Burt A, Portmann B, Ferrell L, eds. MacSween's pathology of the liver, 6th ed. Edinburgh: Elsevier; 2012:403-466.
99. Rossi S, Orvieto E, Furlanetto A, Laurino L, Ninfo V, Dei Tos AP. Utility of the immunohistochemical detection of FLI-1 expression in round cell and vascular neoplasm using a monoclonal antibody. Mod Pathol 2004;17:547-552.
100. Folpe AL, Chand EM, Goldblum JR, Weiss SW. Expression of Fli-1, a nuclear transcription factor, distinguishes vascular neoplasms from potential mimics. Am J Surg Pathol 2001;25:1061-1066.
101. Russell Jones R, Orchard G, Zelger B, Wilson Jones E. Immunostaining for CD31 and CD34 in Kaposi sarcoma. J Clin Pathol 1995;48:1011-1016.
102 Schwartz EJ, Dorfman RF, Kohler S. Human herpesvirus-8 latent nuclear antigen-1 expression in endemic Kaposi sarcoma: an immunohistochemical study of 16 cases. Am J Surg Pathol 2003;27:1546-1550.
103. Robin YM, Guillou L, Michels JJ, Coindre JM. Human herpesvirus 8 immunostaining: a sensitive and specific method for diagnosing Kaposi sarcoma in paraffin-embedded sections. Am J Clin Pathol 2004;121:330-334.
104. Stocker JT, Ishak KG. Mesenchymal hamartoma of the liver: report of 30 cases and review of the literature. Pediatr Pathol 1983;1:245-267.
105. Drachenberg CB, Papadimitriou JC, Rivero MA, Wood C. Distinctive case. Adult mesenchymal hamartoma of the liver: report of a case with light microscopic, FNA cytology, immunohistochemistry, and ultrastructural studies and review of the literature. Mod Pathol 1991;4:392-395.
106. Gramlich TL, Killough BW, Garvin AJ. Mesenchymal hamartoma of the liver: report of a case in a 28-year-old. Hum Pathol 1988;19:991-992.
107. Chau KY, Ho JW, Wu PC, Yuen WK. Mesenchymal hamartoma of liver in a man: comparison with cases in infants. J Clin Pathol 1994;47:864-866.
108. Alkalay AL, Puri AR, Pomerance JJ, et al. Mesenchymal hamartoma of the liver responsive to cyclophosphamide therapy: therapeutic approach. J Pediatr Surg 1985;20:125-128.
109. Cajaiba MM, Sarita-Reyes C, Zambrano E, Reyes-Mugica M. Mesenchymal hamartoma of the liver associated with features of Beckwith-Wiedemann syndrome and high serum alpha-fetoprotein levels. Pediatr Dev Pathol 2007;10:233-238.
110. Abrahao-Machado LF, de Macedo FC, Dalence C, et al. Mesenchymal hamartoma of the liver in an infant with Beckwith-Wiedemann syndrome: a rare condition mimicking hepatoblastoma. ACG Case Rep J 2015;2:258-260.
111. Carta M, Maresi E, Giuffre M, et al. Congenital hepatic mesenchymal hamartoma associated with mesenchymal stem villous hyperplasia of the placenta: case report. J Pediatr Surg 2005;40: e37-39.

112. Kitano Y, Ruchelli E, Weiner S, Adzick NS. Hepatic mesenchymal hamartoma associated with mesenchymal stem villous hyperplasia of the placenta. Fetal Diagn Ther 2000;15:134-138.
113. Mack-Detlefsen B, Boemers TM, Groneck P, Bald R. Multiple hepatic mesenchymal hamartomas in a premature associated with placental mesenchymal dysplasia. J Pediatr Surg 2011;46:e23-25.
114. Ortiz Otero A, de Prada Vicente I, Gutierrez Herrera J, Azorin Cuadrilleros D. Hepatic mesenchymal hamartoma in a neonate with a Bochdalek diaphragmatic hernia: a case report. J Pediatr Surg 2012;47:e45-48.
115. Antoniou D, Soutis M, Karentzou O. Cystic mesenchymal hamartoma arising in intrathoracic heterotopic liver: a case report. J Pediatr Surg 2012;47:e49-51.
116. Boman F, Bossard C, Fabre M, Diab N, Bonnevalle M, Boccon-Gibod L. Mesenchymal hamartomas of the liver may be associated with increased serum alpha foetoprotein concentrations and mimic hepatoblastomas. Eur J Pediatr Surg 2004;14:63-66.
117. Fretzayas A, Moustaki M, Kitsiou S, Nychtari G, Alexopoulou E. Long-term follow-up of a multifocal hepatic mesenchymal hamartoma producing a-fetoprotein. Pediatr Surg Int 2009;25:381-384.
118. Gunes D, Uysal KM, Cecen E, et al. Stromal-predominant mesenchymal hamartoma of the liver with elevated serum alpha-fetoprotein level. Pediatr Hematol Oncol 2008;25:685-692.
119. Hirata GI, Matsunaga ML, Medearis AL, Dixon P, Platt LD. Ultrasonographic diagnosis of a fetal abdominal mass: a case of a mesenchymal liver hamartoma and a review of the literature. Prenat Diagn 1990;10:507-512.
120. Tovbin J, Segal M, Tavori I, Lotan G, Maymon R. Hepatic mesenchymal hamartoma: a pediatric tumor that may be diagnosed prenatally. Ultrasound Obstet Gynecol 1997;10:63-65.
121. Chung EM, Cube R, Lewis RB, Conran RM. From the archives of the AFIP: pediatric liver masses: radiologic-pathologic correlation part 1. Benign tumors. Radiographics 2010;30:801-826.
122. Horton KM, Bluemke DA, Hruban RH, Soyer P, Fishman EK. CT and MR imaging of benign hepatic and biliary tumors. Radiographics 1999; 19:431-451.
123. Ros PR, Goodman ZD, Ishak KG, et al. Mesenchymal hamartoma of the liver: radiologic-pathologic correlation. Radiology 1986;158: 619-624.
124. Helmberger TK, Ros PR, Mergo PJ, Tomczak R, Reiser MF. Pediatric liver neoplasms: a radiologic-pathologic correlation. Eur Radiol 1999;9: 1339-1347.
125. de Chadarevian JP, Pawel BR, Faerber EN, Weintraub WH. Undifferentiated (embryonal) sarcoma arising in conjunction with mesenchymal hamartoma of the liver. Mod Pathol 1994;7:490-493.
126. Lauwers GY, Grant LD, Donnelly WH, et al. Hepatic undifferentiated (embryonal) sarcoma arising in a mesenchymal hamartoma. Am J Surg Pathol 1997;21:1248-1254.
127. O'Sullivan MJ, Swanson PE, Knoll J, Taboada EM, Dehner LP. Undifferentiated embryonal sarcoma with unusual features arising within mesenchymal hamartoma of the liver: report of a case and review of the literature. Pediatr Dev Pathol 2001;4:482-489.
128. Rajaram V, Knezevich S, Bove KE, Perry A, Pfeifer JD. DNA sequence of the translocation breakpoints in undifferentiated embryonal sarcoma arising in mesenchymal hamartoma of the liver harboring the t(11;19)(q11;q13.4) translocation. Genes Chromosomes Cancer 2007;46:508-513.
129. Speleman F, De Telder V, De Potter KR, et al. Cytogenetic analysis of a mesenchymal hamartoma of the liver. Cancer Genet Cytogenet 1989;40:29-32.
130. Rakheja D, Margraf LR, Tomlinson GE, Schneider NR. Hepatic mesenchymal hamartoma with translocation involving chromosome band 19q13.4: a recurrent abnormality. Cancer Genet Cytogenet 2004;153:60-63.
131. Mascarello JT, Krous HF. Second report of a translocation involving 19q13.4 in a mesenchymal hamartoma of the liver. Cancer Genet Cytogenet 1992;58:141-142.
132. Bove KE, Blough RI, Soukup S. Third report of t(19q)(13.4) in mesenchymal hamartoma of liver with comments on link to embryonal sarcoma. Pediatr Dev Pathol 1998;1:438-442.
133. Talmon GA, Cohen SM. Mesenchymal hamartoma of the liver with an interstitial deletion involving chromosome band 19q13.4: a theory as to pathogenesis? Arch Pathol Lab Med 2006;130:1216-1218.
134. Murthi GV, Paterson L, Azmy A. Chromosomal translocation in mesenchymal hamartoma of liver: what is its significance? J Pediatr Surg 2003;38:1543-1545.
135. Stocker JT, Ishak KG. Undifferentiated (embryonal) sarcoma of the liver: report of 31 cases. Cancer 1978;42:336-348.
136. Tokunaga Y, Ryo J, Hoppou T, et al. Hepatic undifferentiated (embryonal) sarcoma in an adult: a case report and review of the literature. Eur J Gastroenterol Hepatol 2000;12:1247-1251.
137. McFadden DW, Kelley DJ, Sigmund DA, Barrett WL, Dickson B, Aron BS. Embryonal sarcoma of the liver in an adult treated with preoperative chemotherapy, radiation therapy, and hepatic lobectomy. Cancer 1992;69:39-44.

138. Johnson JA 3rd, White JG, Thompson AR. Undifferentiated (embryonal) sarcoma of the liver in adults. Am Surg 1995;61:285-287.
139. Gallivan MV, Lack EE, Chun B, Ishak KG. Undifferentiated ("embryonal") sarcoma of the liver: ultrastructure of a case presenting as a primary intracardiac tumor. Pediatr Pathol 1983;1:291-300.
140. Buetow PC, Buck JL, Pantongrag-Brown L, et al. Undifferentiated (embryonal) sarcoma of the liver: pathologic basis of imaging findings in 28 cases. Radiology 1997;203:779-783.
141. Chung EM, Lattin GE Jr, Cube R, et al. From the archives of the AFIP: Pediatric liver masses: radiologic-pathologic correlation. Part 2. Malignant tumors. Radiographics 2011;31:483-507.
142. Ros PR, Olmsted WW, Dachman AH, Goodman ZD, Ishak KG, Hartman DS. Undifferentiated (embryonal) sarcoma of the liver: radiologic-pathologic correlation. Radiology 1986;161:141-145.
143. Joshi SW, Merchant NH, Jambhekar NA. Primary multilocular cystic undifferentiated (embryonal) sarcoma of the liver in childhood resembling hydatid cyst of the liver. Br J Radiol 1997;70:314-316.
144. Yoon W, Kim JK, Kang HK. Hepatic undifferentiated embryonal sarcoma: MR findings. J Comput Assist Tomogr 1997;21:100-102.
145. Keating S, Taylor GP. Undifferentiated (embryonal) sarcoma of the liver: ultrastructural and immunohistochemical similarities with malignant fibrous histiocytoma. Hum Pathol 1985;16:693-699.
156. Agaram NP, Baren A, Antonescu CR. Pediatric and adult hepatic embryonal sarcoma: a comparative ultrastructural study with morphologic correlations. Ultrastruct Pathol 2006;30:403-408.
157. Walker NI, Horn MJ, Strong RW, et al. Undifferentiated (embryonal) sarcoma of the liver. Pathologic findings and long-term survival after complete surgical resection. Cancer 1992;69:52-59.
158. Lack EE, Schloo BL, Azumi N, Travis WD, Grier HE, Kozakewich HP. Undifferentiated (embryonal) sarcoma of the liver. Clinical and pathologic study of 16 cases with emphasis on immunohistochemical features. Am J Surg Pathol 1991;15:1-16.
159. Nishio J, Iwasaki H, Sakashita N, et al. Undifferentiated (embryonal) sarcoma of the liver in middle-aged adults: smooth muscle differentiation determined by immunohistochemistry and electron microscopy. Hum Pathol 2003;34:246-252.
150. Putra J, Ornvold K. Undifferentiated embryonal sarcoma of the liver: a concise review. Arch Pathol Lab Med. 2015;139:269-273.
151. Aoyama C, Hachitanda Y, Sato JK, Said JW, Shimada H. Undifferentiated (embryonal) sarcoma of the liver. A tumor of uncertain histogenesis showing divergent differentiation. Am J Surg Pathol 1991;15:615-624.
152. Kiani B, Ferrell LD, Qualman S, Frankel WL. Immunohistochemical analysis of embryonal sarcoma of the liver. Appl Immunohistochem Mol Morphol 2006;14:193-197.
153. Parham DM, Kelly DR, Donnelly WH, Douglass EC. Immunohistochemical and ultrastructural spectrum of hepatic sarcomas of childhood: evidence for a common histogenesis. Mod Pathol 1991;4:648-653.
154. Levy M, Trivedi A, Zhang J, et al. Expression of glypican-3 in undifferentiated embryonal sarcoma and mesenchymal hamartoma of the liver. Hum Pathol 2012;43:695-701.
155. Wei ZG, Tang LF, Chen ZM, Tang HF, Li MJ. Childhood undifferentiated embryonal liver sarcoma: clinical features and immunohistochemistry analysis. J Pediatr Surg 2008;43:1912-1919.
156. Dias P, Parham DM, Shapiro DN, Webber BL, Houghton PJ. Myogenic regulatory protein (MyoD1) expression in childhood solid tumors: diagnostic utility in rhabdomyosarcoma. Am J Pathol 1990;137:1283-1291.
157. Chou P, Mangkornkanok M, Gonzalez-Crussi F. Undifferentiated (embryonal) sarcoma of the liver: ultrastructure, immunohistochemistry, and DNA ploidy analysis of two cases. Pediatr Pathol 1990;10:549-562.
158. Leuschner I, Schmidt D, Harms D. Undifferentiated sarcoma of the liver in childhood: morphology, flow cytometry, and literature review. Hum Pathol 1990;21:68-76.
159. Hu X, Chen H, Jin M, et al. Molecular cytogenetic characterization of undifferentiated embryonal sarcoma of the liver: a case report and literature review. Mol Cytogenet 2012;5:26.
160. Sowery RD, Jensen C, Morrison KB, Horsman DE, Sorensen PH, Webber EM. Comparative genomic hybridization detects multiple chromosomal amplifications and deletions in undifferentiated embryonal sarcoma of the liver. Cancer Genet Cytogenet 2001;126:128-133.
161. Lepreux S, Rebouissou S, Le Bail B, et al. Mutation of TP53 gene is involved in carcinogenesis of hepatic undifferentiated (embryonal) sarcoma of the adult, in contrast with Wnt or telomerase pathways: an immunohistochemical study of three cases with genomic relation in two cases. J Hepatol 2005;42:424-429.
162. Sangkhathat S, Kusafuka T, Nara K, Yoneda A, Fukuzawa M. Non-random p53 mutations in pediatric undifferentiated (embryonal) sarcoma of the liver. Hepatol Res 2006;35:229-234.

163. Bisogno G, Pilz T, Perilongo G, et al. Undifferentiated sarcoma of the liver in childhood: a curable disease. Cancer 2002;94:252-257.
164. May LT, Wang M, Albano E, Garrington T, Dishop M, Macy ME. Undifferentiated sarcoma of the liver: a single institution experience using a uniform treatment approach. J Pediatr Hematol Oncol 2012;34:e114-116.
165. Kim DY, Kim KH, Jung SE, Lee SC, Park KW, Kim WK. Undifferentiated (embryonal) sarcoma of the liver: combination treatment by surgery and chemotherapy. J Pediatr Surg 2002;37:1419-1423.
166. Ismail H, Dembowska-Baginska B, Broniszczak D, et al. Treatment of undifferentiated embryonal sarcoma of the liver in children—single center experience. J Pediatr Surg 2013;48:2202-2206.
167. Davis GL, Kissane JM, Ishak KG. Embryonal rhabdomyosarcoma (sarcoma botryoides) of the biliary tree. Report of five cases and a review of the literature. Cancer 1969;24:333-342.
168. Nicol K, Savell V, Moore J, et al. Distinguishing undifferentiated embryonal sarcoma of the liver from biliary tract rhabdomyosarcoma: a Children's Oncology Group study. Pediatr Dev Pathol 2007;10:89-97.
169. McArdle JP, Hawley I, Shevland J, Brain T. Primary rhabdomyosarcoma of the adult liver. Am J Surg Pathol 1989;13:961-965.
170. Aldabagh SM, Shibata CS, Taxy JB. Rhabdomyosarcoma of the common bile duct in an adult. Arch Pathol Lab Med 1986;110:547-550.
171. Schoofs G, Braeye L, Vanheste R, Verswijvel G, Debiec-Rychter M, Sciot R. Hepatic rhabdomyosarcoma in an adult: a rare primary malignant liver tumor. Case report and literature review. Acta Gastroenterol Belg 2011;74:576-581.
172. Ruymann FB, Raney RB Jr, Crist WM, Lawrence W Jr, Lindberg RD, Soule EH. Rhabdomyosarcoma of the biliary tree in childhood. A report from the Intergroup Rhabdomyosarcoma Study. Cancer 1985;56:575-581.
173. Lack EE, Perez-Atayde AR, Schuster SR. Botryoid rhabdomyosarcoma of the biliary tract. Am J Surg Pathol 1981;5:643-652.
174. Trobaugh-Lotrario AD, Finegold MJ, Feusner JH. Rhabdoid tumors of the liver: rare, aggressive, and poorly responsive to standard cytotoxic chemotherapy. Pediatr Blood Cancer 2011;57:423-428.
175. Oita S, Terui K, Komatsu S, et al. Malignant rhabdoid tumor of the liver: a case report and literature review. Pediatr Rep 2015;7:5578.
176. Jackson EM, Sievert AJ, Gai X, et al. Genomic analysis using high-density single nucleotide polymorphism-based oligonucleotide arrays and multiplex ligation-dependent probe amplification provides a comprehensive analysis of INI1/SMARCB1 in malignant rhabdoid tumors. Clin Cancer Res 2009;15:1923-1930.
177. Schneppenheim R, Fruhwald MC, Gesk S, et al. Germline nonsense mutation and somatic inactivation of SMARCA4/BRG1 in a family with rhabdoid tumor predisposition syndrome. Am J Hum Genet 2010;86:279-284.
178. Hasselblatt M, Gesk S, Oyen F, et al. Nonsense mutation and inactivation of SMARCA4 (BRG1) in an atypical teratoid/rhabdoid tumor showing retained SMARCB1 (INI1) expression. Am J Surg Pathol 2011;35:933-935.
179. Shiratsuchi H, Saito T, Sakamoto A, et al. Mutation analysis of human cytokeratin 8 gene in malignant rhabdoid tumor: a possible association with intracytoplasmic inclusion body formation. Mod Pathol 2002;15:146-153.
180. Wagner LM, Garrett JK, Ballard ET, et al. Malignant rhabdoid tumor mimicking hepatoblastoma: a case report and literature review. Pediatr Dev Pathol 2007;10:409-415.
181. Trobaugh-Lotrario AD, Tomlinson GE, Finegold MJ, Gore L, Feusner JH. Small cell undifferentiated variant of hepatoblastoma: adverse clinical and molecular features similar to rhabdoid tumors. Pediatr Blood Cancer 2009;52:328-334.
182. Zhou S, Gomulia E, Mascarenhas L, Wang L. Is INI1-retained small cell undifferentiated histology in hepatoblastoma unfavorable? Hum Pathol 2015;46:620-624.
183. Hussein K, Rath B, Ludewig B, Kreipe H, Jonigk D. Clinico-pathological characteristics of different types of immunodeficiency-associated smooth muscle tumours. Eur J Cancer 2014;50:2417-2424.
184. Jonigk D, Laenger F, Maegel L, et al. Molecular and clinicopathological analysis of Epstein-Barr virus-associated posttransplant smooth muscle tumors. Am J Transplant 2012;12:1908-1917.
185. Deyrup AT, Lee VK, Hill CE, et al. Epstein-Barr virus-associated smooth muscle tumors are distinctive mesenchymal tumors reflecting multiple infection events: a clinicopathologic and molecular analysis of 29 tumors from 19 patients. Am J Surg Pathol 2006;30:75-82.
186. Rogatsch H, Bonatti H, Menet A, Larcher C, Feichtinger H, Dirnhofer S. Epstein-Barr virus-associated multicentric leiomyosarcoma in an adult patient after heart transplantation: case report and review of the literature. Am J Surg Pathol 2000;24:614-621.
187. Debs T, Kassir R, Amor IB, Martini F, Iannelli A, Gugenheim J. Solitary fibrous tumor of the liver: report of two cases and review of the literature. Int J Surg 2014;12:1291-1294.

188. Moran CA, Ishak KG, Goodman ZD. Solitary fibrous tumor of the liver: a clinicopathologic and immunohistochemical study of nine cases. Ann Diagn Pathol 1998;2:19-24.
189. Fletcher CD, Bridge JA, Lee JC. Extrapleural solitary fibrous tumour. In: Fletcher CD, Bridge JA, Hogendoorn PC, Mertens F, eds. World Health Organization classification of tumours of soft tissue and bone, 4th ed. Lyon: IARC; 2013:86-90.
190. Robinson DR, Wu YM, Kalyana-Sundaram S, et al. Identification of recurrent NAB2-STAT6 gene fusions in solitary fibrous tumor by integrative sequencing. Nat Genet 2013;45:180-185.
191. Chmielecki J, Crago AM, Rosenberg M, et al. Whole-exome sequencing identifies a recurrent NAB2-STAT6 fusion in solitary fibrous tumors. Nat Genet 2013;45:131-132.
192. Sasaki M, Araki I, Yasui T, et al. Primary localized malignant biphasic mesothelioma of the liver in a patient with asbestosis. World J Gastroenterol 2009;15:615-621.
193. Perysinakis I, Nixon AM, Spyridakis I, Kakiopoulos G, Zorzos C, Margaris I. Primary intrahepatic malignant epithelioid mesothelioma. Int J Surg Case Rep 2014;5:1098-1101.
194. Kim DS, Lee SG, Jun SY, Kim KW, Ha TY, Kim KK. Primary malignant mesothelioma developed in liver. Hepatogastroenterology 2008;55:1081-1084.
195. Inagaki N, Kibata K, Tamaki T, Shimizu T, Nomura S. Primary intrahepatic malignant mesothelioma with multiple lymphadenopathies due to non-tuberculous mycobacteria: A case report and review of the literature. Oncol Lett 2013;6:676-680.
196. Imura J, Ichikawa K, Takeda J, et al. Localized malignant mesothelioma of the epithelial type occurring as a primary hepatic neoplasm: a case report with review of the literature. APMIS 2002;110:789-794.
197. Dong A, Dong H, Zuo C. Multiple primary hepatic malignant mesotheliomas mimicking cystadenocarcinomas on enhanced CT and FDG PET/CT. Clin Nucl Med 2014;39:619-622.
198. Leonardou P, Semelka RC, Kanematsu M, Braga L, Woosley JT. Primary malignant mesothelioma of the liver: MR imaging findings. Magn Reson Imaging 2003;21:1091-1093.
199. Gutgemann I, Standop J, Fischer HP. Primary intrahepatic malignant mesothelioma of epithelioid type. Virchows Arch 2006;448:655-658.
200. Chen ST, Lee JC. An inflammatory myofibroblastic tumor in liver with ALK and RANBP2 gene rearrangement: combination of distinct morphologic, immunohistochemical, and genetic features. Hum Pathol 2008;39:1854-1858.
201. Al-Hussaini H, Azouz H, Abu-Zaid A. Hepatic inflammatory pseudotumor presenting in an 8-year-old boy: A case report and review of literature. World J Gastroenterol 2015;21:8730-8738.
202. Coffin CM, Fletcher JA. Inflammatory myofibroblastic tumour. In: Fletcher CD, Bridge JA, Hogendoorn PC, Mertens F, eds. World Health Organization classification of tumours of soft tissue and bone. Lyon: IARC; 2013.
203. Yamamoto H, Yoshida A, Taguchi K, et al. ALK, ROS1 and NTRK3 gene rearrangements in inflammatory myofibroblastic tumors. Histopathology 2015;69:72-83.
204. Hornick JL, Sholl LM, Dal Cin P, Childress MA, Lovly CM. Expression of ROS1 predicts ROS1 gene rearrangement in inflammatory myofibroblastic tumors. Mod Pathol 2015;28:732-739.
205. Antonescu CR, Suurmeijer AJ, Zhang L, et al. Molecular characterization of inflammatory myofibroblastic tumors with frequent ALK and ROS1 gene fusions and rare novel RET rearrangement. Am J Surg Pathol 2015;39:957-967.
206. Chan JK, Cheuk W, Shimizu M. Anaplastic lymphoma kinase expression in inflammatory pseudotumors. Am J Surg Pathol 2001;25:761-768.
207. Arber DA, Kamel OW, van de Rijn M, et al. Frequent presence of the Epstein-Barr virus in inflammatory pseudotumor. Hum Pathol 1995;26:1093-1098.
208. Selves J, Meggetto F, Brousset P, et al. Inflammatory pseudotumor of the liver. Evidence for follicular dendritic reticulum cell proliferation associated with clonal Epstein-Barr virus. Am J Surg Pathol 1996;20:747-753.
209. Shek TW, Ho FC, Ng IO, Chan AC, Ma L, Srivastava G. Follicular dendritic cell tumor of the liver. Evidence for an Epstein-Barr virus-related clonal proliferation of follicular dendritic cells. Am J Surg Pathol 1996;20:313-324.
210. Cheuk W, Chan JK, Shek TW, et al. Inflammatory pseudotumor-like follicular dendritic cell tumor: a distinctive low-grade malignant intra-abdominal neoplasm with consistent Epstein-Barr virus association. Am J Surg Pathol 2001;25:721-731.
211. Zen Y, Fujii T, Sato Y, Masuda S, Nakanuma Y. Pathological classification of hepatic inflammatory pseudotumor with respect to IgG4-related disease. Mod Pathol 2007;20:884-894.
212. Stone JH, Zen Y, Deshpande V. IgG4-related disease. N Engl J Med 2012;366:539-551.
213. Zen Y, Nakanuma Y, Portmann B. Immunoglobulin G4-related sclerosing cholangitis: pathologic features and histologic mimics. Semin Diagn Pathol 2012;29:205-211.

214. Zen Y, Kawakami H, Kim JH. IgG4-related sclerosing cholangitis: all we need to know. J Gastroenterol 2016;51:295-312.
215. Zen Y, Harada K, Sasaki M, et al. IgG4-related sclerosing cholangitis with and without hepatic inflammatory pseudotumor, and sclerosing pancreatitis-associated sclerosing cholangitis: do they belong to a spectrum of sclerosing pancreatitis? Am J Surg Pathol 2004;28:1193-203.
216. Deshpande V, Zen Y, Chan JK, et al. Consensus statement on the pathology of IgG4-related disease. Mod Pathol 2012;25:1181-1192.
217. Zen Y, Britton D, Mitra V, Pike I, Heaton N, Quaglia A. A global proteomic study identifies distinct pathological features of IgG4-related and primary sclerosing cholangitis. Histopathology 2016;68:796-809.

10 METASTATIC DISEASE

The word metastasis is derived from the Greek word for displacement. Metastatic liver disease is defined as a malignant neoplasm originating from an extrahepatic organ that has spread to the liver via angiolymphatic routes or by direct extension.

DEMOGRAPHICS

Carcinomas and melanomas are more likely than sarcomas to metastasize to the liver. For adults, autopsy studies show the most frequent carcinomas to metastasize to the liver are from the colon, breast, lung, pancreas adenocarcinoma, stomach, neuroendocrine tumors, and cervix (1). In children, metastases are most likely to be from neuroblastomas, Wilms tumors, or sarcomas (2).

Most individuals with metastatic liver disease present with nonspecific findings such as abdominal pain and weight loss. Some individuals have jaundice and most have nonspecific elevations in transaminases and alkaline phosphatase levels. The primary signs and symptoms are related more often to the primary cancer than to the liver metastases. For example, colorectal cancer with widespread liver metastases often presents with symptoms of colonic obstruction or of rectal bleeding and not liver disease. On the other hand, individuals with functioning neuroendocrine tumors typically do not develop the carcinoid syndrome until there are liver metastases. Finally, some individuals are completely asymptomatic and metastatic cancer is an unexpected finding during evaluation for other disease symptoms.

Types of Neoplasms that Metastasize to the Liver

Overall, 60 percent of all metastatic tumors eventually involve the liver (3). These are the most common carcinomas metastatic to the liver from autopsy studies: colorectal, breast, lung, pancreas, and neuroendocrine (1,3). In part, this is a reflection of their frequency. However, when these tumors do metastasize, the liver is at increased risk for involvement compared to other organs (3). By way of contrast, when kidney cancers metastasize, the liver has a lower risk of metastatic deposits than do other organs (3). Of note, the patterns seen in autopsy studies are different from those seen in surgical pathology biopsy specimens, as surgical pathology specimens are enriched for cases for which the primary tumor is uncertain based on imaging studies.

Metastases to Cirrhotic Livers

Cirrhotic livers are at a much lower risk than non-cirrhotic livers for metastatic disease. However, there is a common misconception that cirrhotic livers do not harbor metastatic disease; this is not true. For example, one study examined nonliver carcinomas in the distribution of the portal vein and found that 48 percent of noncirrhotic livers developed metastatic disease versus 30 percent of cirrhotic livers (4). Sometimes there is a related misconception that hepatocellular carcinomas arise almost exclusively in cirrhotic livers, yet about 20 percent of hepatocellular carcinomas occur in noncirrhotic livers.

Cancer of Unknown Primary

A primary site is not identified in approximately 2 percent of metastatic carcinomas, despite full clinical, serologic, imaging, and histologic evaluations (fig. 10-1). This group of tumors is often referred to as CUP (cancer of unknown primary). In about 40 percent of CUP cases, the liver is the only metastatic site (5). Most CUPs are adenocarcinomas (45 percent), undifferentiated carcinomas (35 percent), or squamous cell carcinomas (10 percent) (5,6). Neuroendocrine neoplasms and sarcomas make up most of the remainder. Even at autopsy, in only about one third of patients is the primary site identified (6). When identified, the most common primary sites are the lung, pancreas, and gastrointestinal tract (5).

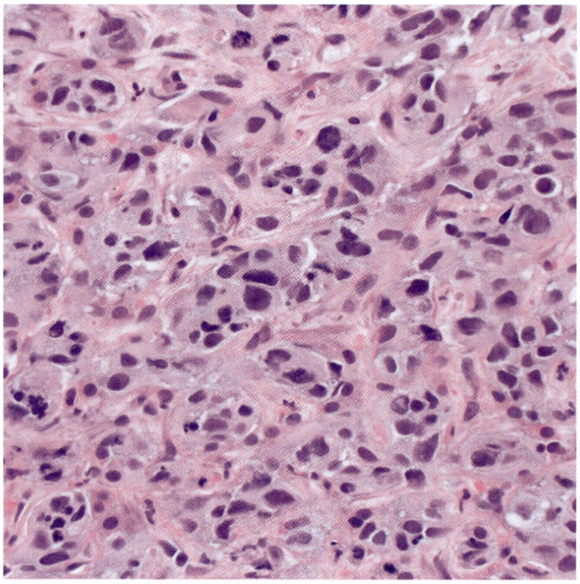

Figure 10-1

CANCER OF UNKNOWN PRIMARY

Imaging studies were negative for a primary, but there were numerous metastatic deposits in the liver, lung, and bone. The tumor was CK7 positive, CK20 negative, and negative for all other markers of differentiation.

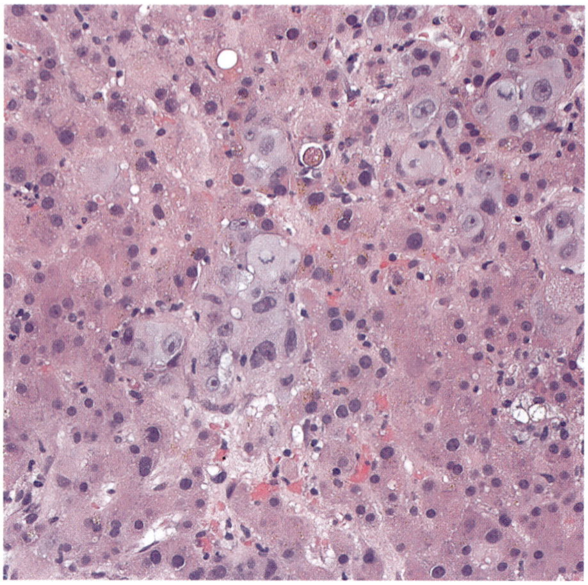

Figure 10-2

PANCREAS CARCINOMA: METASTATIC TO LIVER

This poorly differentiated carcinoma infiltrates the liver sinusoids without forming a discrete mass.

SERUM FINDINGS

Serum markers for various malignancies have been avidly sought for decades. These efforts have met with much success, and numerous serum tumor markers are used clinically. Table 10-1 focuses on the markers most commonly encountered in clinical practice, although many more have been reported. While these markers have been advocated as tools for screening, diagnosis, and prognosis, none have sufficient sensitivity or specificity to replace imaging studies and biopsies. In specific settings, however, they are a very useful part of patient management, most commonly when following a patient with known cancer for recurrent disease.

GROSS FINDINGS

The gross findings in metastatic tumors vary considerably. The classic setting is numerous tumors involving both lobes of a noncirrhotic liver. In many cases, however, metastatic deposits are single or few in number.

In most cases, metastatic deposits are not resected and the pathology evaluation is from biopsy material. Nevertheless, resection of isolated or small numbers of metastatic tumors (sometimes referred to as "metastasectomy") is becoming more common, in particular for metastatic colon carcinomas, but also occasionally for lung, stomach, and other metastatic tumors. In these surgical cases, the primary diagnosis is commonly known before surgery, so gross examination focuses on size, margin status, percent necrosis, and macroscopic vascular involvement.

Gross examination can reflect the tumor's histology. For example, mucinous adenocarcinomas can show a gelatinous, glistening cut surface; melanomas can be brown; and squamous cell carcinomas can be firm, white, and granular. In rare cases, metastatic tumors show diffuse sinusoidal infiltration of the liver, with imaging studies showing either no mass lesion or ill-defined lesions. This pattern is also commonly associated with elevated liver enzymes, and the biopsy may have been performed to evaluate for causes of acute hepatitis (fig. 10-2). The most common malignancies with this rare presentation are lymphomas and leukemias (7,8). For solid tumors, the most common tumor type with this presentation is breast carcinoma, but this pattern can also be seen with melanoma (9,10), small cell (11–13) and non-small cell

Table 10-1

SERUM TUMOR MARKERS IN ADULTS

Serum Tumor Markers	Associated Tumors
Alpha-fetoprotein (AFP)	Hepatocellular carcinoma, germ cell tumors. Rarely: cholangiocarcinoma, acinar cell carcinomas, neuroendocrine tumors
Alpha-fetoprotein L3 (AFP-L3)	Hepatocellular carcinoma, germ cell tumors, acinar cell carcinomas (rare)
Beta unit of human chorionic gonadotropin (beta-HCG)	Germ cell tumors
Calcitonin	Medullary thyroid carcinoma; also can be elevated in lung and neuroendocrine tumors
CA15-3	Breast carcinoma
CA19-9	Pancreatic adenocarcinoma, cholangiocarcinoma, colon adenocarcinoma, gastric adenocarcinoma
CA 27-29	Breast carcinoma
CA125	Ovarian and other carcinomas
Carcinoembryonic antigen (CEA)	Colorectal carcinoma and other carcinomas
Chromogranin A (CgA)	Neuroblastoma, neuroendocrine tumors
Des-gamma-carboxyprothrombin (DCP)	Hepatocellular carcinoma
Inhibin A and B	Granulosa cell tumor
Neuron-specific enolase (NSE)	Neuroblastoma, neuroendocrine tumors
Gastrin	Neuroendocrine tumor, most arising in the duodenum or pancreas
Glucagon	Glucagon-producing neuroendocrine tumors
Human epididymis protein 4	Most serous and endometrioid ovarian carcinomas; about 50% of clear cell ovarian carcinomas
Metanephrines	Catecholamine-secreting pheochromocytomas or paragangliomas
Pancreatic polypeptide	Pancreatic polypeptide-producing neuroendocrine tumor, most arising in the pancreas
Prostate-specific antigen (PSA)	Prostate carcinoma
Serotonin	Neuroendocrine tumors, particularly rectum
Squamous cell carcinoma antigen (SCC)	Squamous cell carcinoma
Thyroglobulin	Follicular thyroid carcinoma
Vasoactive intestinal polypeptide (VIP)	VIP-producing neuroendocrine tumor, most arising in the pancreas

lung carcinoma (14), stomach carcinoma (11), pancreas adenocarcinoma (11), colon adenocarcinoma (7,11), and urothelial carcinoma.

MICROSCOPIC FINDINGS INCLUDING IMMUNOHISTOCHEMISTRY

The hematoxylin and eosin (H&E) findings can strongly suggest the tumor's origin, but in most cases immunostains are needed to accurately classify the tumor.

Morphologic Clues

Although not specific, the H&E morphologic findings can suggest a differential (Table 10-2). Gland formation (fig. 10-3) suggests an adenocarcinoma, but true glands must be separated from pseudoglands, which are commonly present in hepatocellular carcinomas (fig. 10-4) and neuroendocrine tumors, and from the acinar structures seen in acinar cell carcinomas. Glassy, eosinophilic cytoplasm with distinct cell membranes can indicate squamous differentiation and suggest a primary squamous or urothelial carcinoma (fig. 10-5). Squamous differentiation can also be a component of adenosquamous carcinomas of the lung and biliary tree, and of pancreatoblastomas.

Nuclear changes that suggest a possible primary include nuclear grooves and prominent

Table 10-2

POTENTIAL MORPHOLOGIC CLUES TO DIAGNOSIS

Histologic Finding	Possible Tumors
Nuclear Changes	
Prominent nuclear grooves	Carcinoma: some solid pseudopapillary tumors of pancreas, papillary thyroid carcinoma, granulosa cell tumor
Prominent nucleoli	Fibrolamellar carcinoma, melanoma, prostate carcinoma, acinar cell carcinoma, yolk sac tumor
Cytoplasmic Changes	
Rhabdoid morphology	Rhabdoid tumors of various sites (INI-1 or BRG1 loss in tumor), large cell carcinoma of the lung, neuroendocrine carcinoma, mesothelioma, urothelial carcinoma, renal carcinoma, melanoma, gastrointestinal stromal tumor, desmoplastic small round cell tumor, Ewing sarcoma
Hyaline globules	Carcinoma: hepatocellular carcinoma (up to 50%), clear cell carcinoma of ovary, renal carcinoma (clear cell and chromophobe), adrenal cortical carcinoma, neuroendocrine tumors (about 5%), pheochromocytoma, yolk sac tumor Sarcoma: embryonal sarcoma, angiosarcoma, Kaposi sarcoma Neural: secretory meningioma
Clear cytoplasm	Hepatocellular carcinoma, clear cell variant; renal clear cell carcinoma; clear cell carcinoma of ovary; clear cell neuroendocrine tumor; adrenal carcinoma
Squamous differentiation	Squamous carcinoma, adenosquamous carcinoma, pancreatoblastoma
Fatty change	Benign: focal nodular hyperplasia, hepatocellular adenoma, angiomyolipoma, adrenal rest tumors, pseudolipoma, Malignant: hepatocellular carcinoma, adrenal cortical carcinoma, lipid-rich variant of breast carcinoma, lipid-rich variant of neuroendocrine tumor, lipid-rich follicular carcinoma, lipid-rich mammary analogue secretory carcinoma of parotid gland Liposarcoma
Other Findings	
Bile production	Hepatocellular carcinoma, hepatoid carcinoma
Mucinous carcinoma	Most are colon, but other possible sites include stomach, pancreas, appendix, ampulla of Vater, lung, breast, bladder, ovary, endometrium, cervix
Schiller–Duval body	Yolk sac tumor

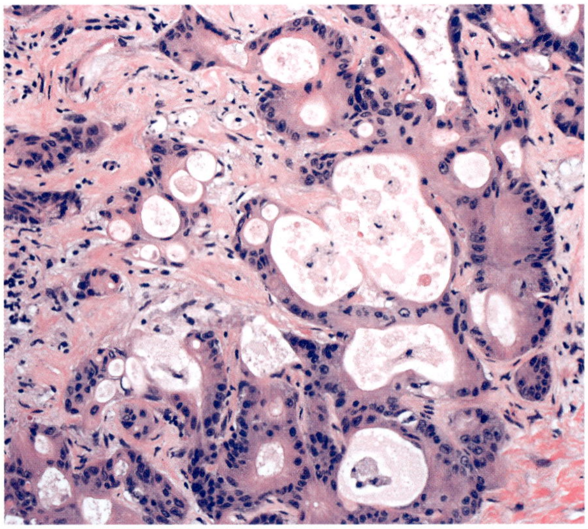

Figure 10-3

ADENOCARCINOMA: METASTATIC TO LIVER

This metastatic colon carcinoma shows definite gland formation.

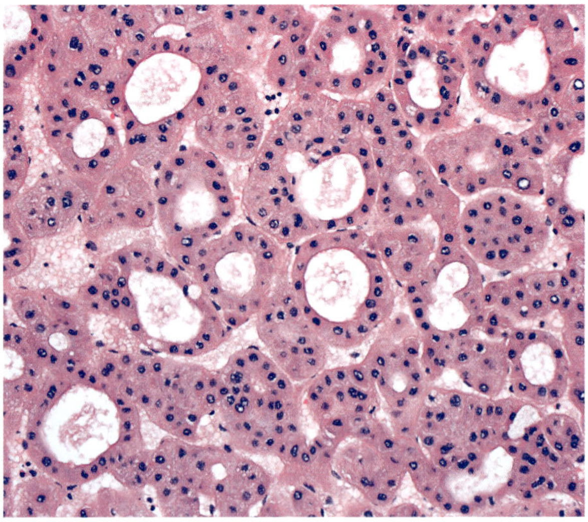

Figure 10-4

HEPATOCELLULAR CARCINOMA: PSEUDOGLANDS

This pattern of growth can sometimes mimic adenocarcinoma.

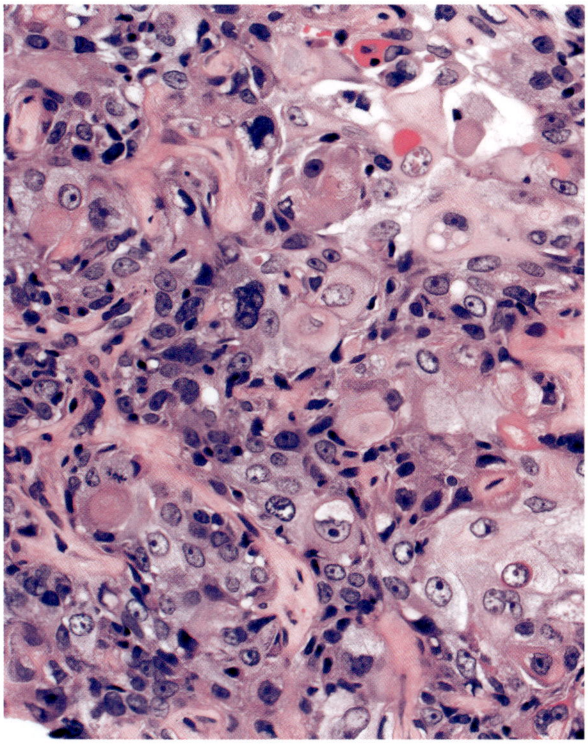

Figure 10-5

SQUAMOUS CARCINOMA: METASTATIC TO LIVER

A squamous carcinoma metastatic to the liver shows abundant eosinophilic cytoplasm with distinct cell borders.

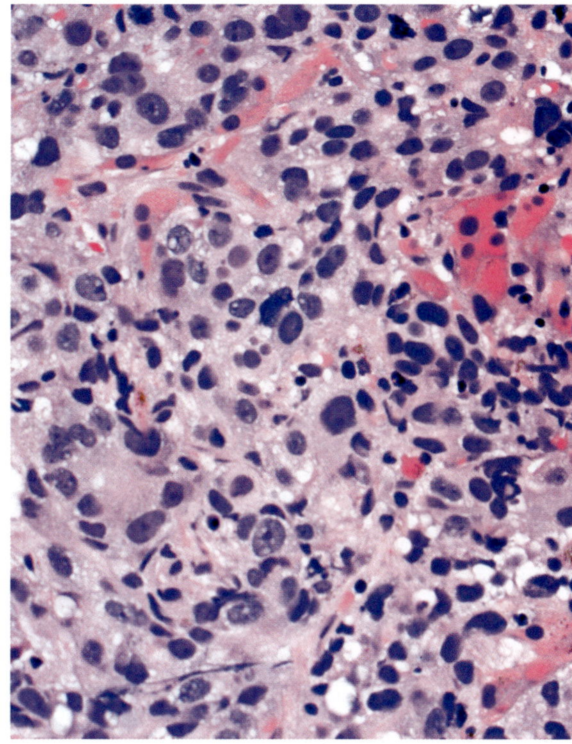

Figure 10-6

PROMINENT NUCLEOLI

This metastatic prostate carcinoma shows prominent nucleoli.

nucleoli (fig. 10-6). Nuclear grooves, although sometimes best seen in books and not active cases, can be prominent in solid pseudopapillary tumors, papillary thyroid carcinoma, and granulosa cell tumors. Unusually large eosinophilic nucleoli are often found in fibrolamellar carcinoma, conventional hepatocellular carcinoma, melanoma, and prostate carcinoma. Finely stippled chromatin suggests a neuroendocrine tumor, especially when the nuclei are uniform and regularly spaced. Small cell carcinomas have nuclear molding, smudgy chromatin, and inconspicuous nucleoli.

Eosinophilic hyaline inclusions can be a prominent component, at least focally, of a number of both carcinomas and sarcomas. The globules can represent a number of different proteins and many globules are positive for alpha-1-antitrypsin, fibrinogen, p62, and/or ubiquitin. The most common carcinoma with hyaline bodies is hepatocellular carcinoma (fig. 10-7), but they are also found in hepatoid carcinomas from other organs, solid pseudopapillary tumors, and cholangiocarcinomas, among others. The most common sarcoma with hyaline bodies is embryonal sarcoma, but rarely angiosarcomas can show similar inclusions (fig. 10-8).

Steatosis within the tumor cytoplasm is most often seen in hepatocellular carcinomas (fig. 10-9), where the changes can be sufficiently striking to suggest the diagnosis of steatohepatitis. Lesser degrees of steatosis can be seen in adrenal cortical carcinomas and solid pseudopapillary tumors of the pancreas (fig. 10-10). Other organs also have lipid-rich variants of carcinoma (Table 10-2). In most lipid-rich carcinomas, the cytoplasm has a predominately microvesicular pattern of steatosis (fig. 10-11), but macrovesicular steatosis can also be seen, and rarely, can be prominent.

A rhabdoid morphology (fig. 10-12) can be seen in carcinomas, melanoma, and anaplastic large cell lymphoma (Table 10-2). Immunostains are typically required to arrive at the diagnosis. As part of this workup, INI-1 and

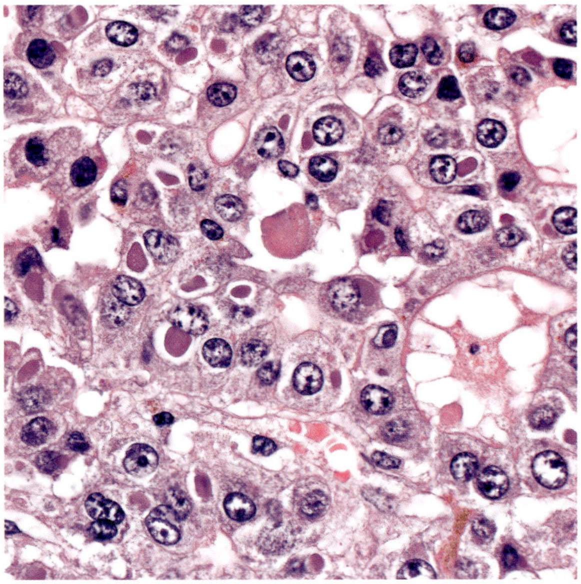

Figure 10-7

HYALINE BODIES

Big, pink globules are seen in the cytoplasm of a hepatocellular carcinoma

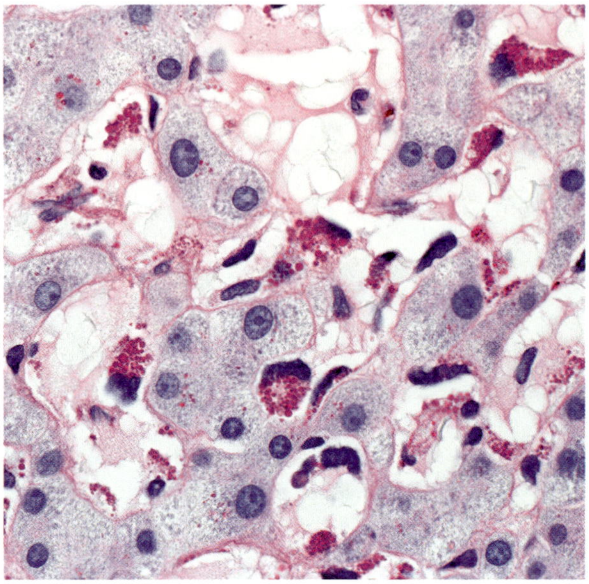

Figure 10-8

HYALINE BODIES

This angiosarcoma metastatic to the liver (growing in the sinusoids) has small, round, eosinophilic and periodic acid–Schiff, diastase positive (PASD) hyaline bodies.

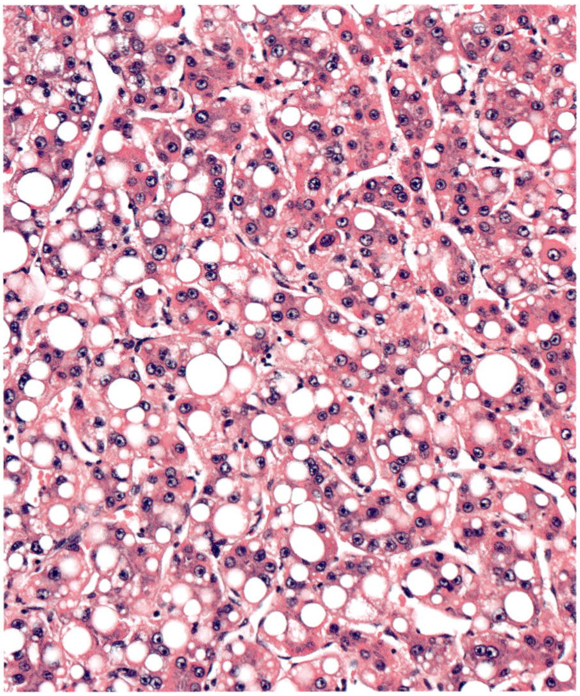

Figure 10-9

HEPATOCELLULAR CARCINOMA: STEATOSIS

This hepatocellular carcinoma shows macrovesicular steatosis.

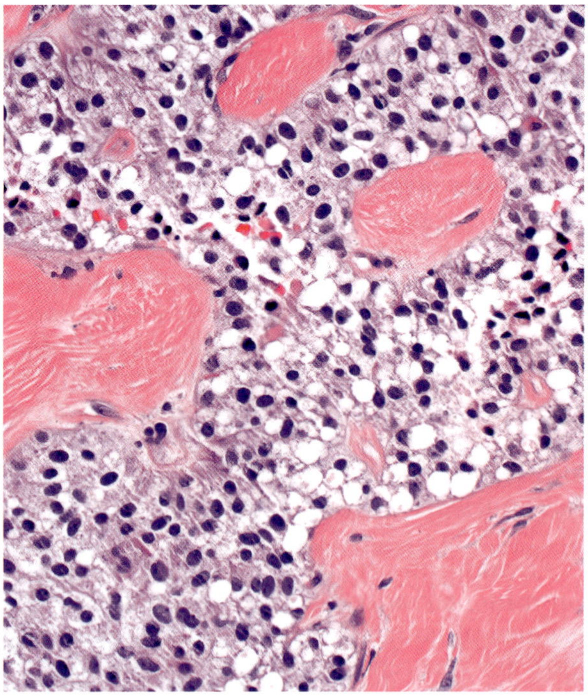

Figure 10-10

SOLID PSEUDOPAPILLARY TUMOR OF PANCREAS: STEATOSIS

Patchy fatty change is seen.

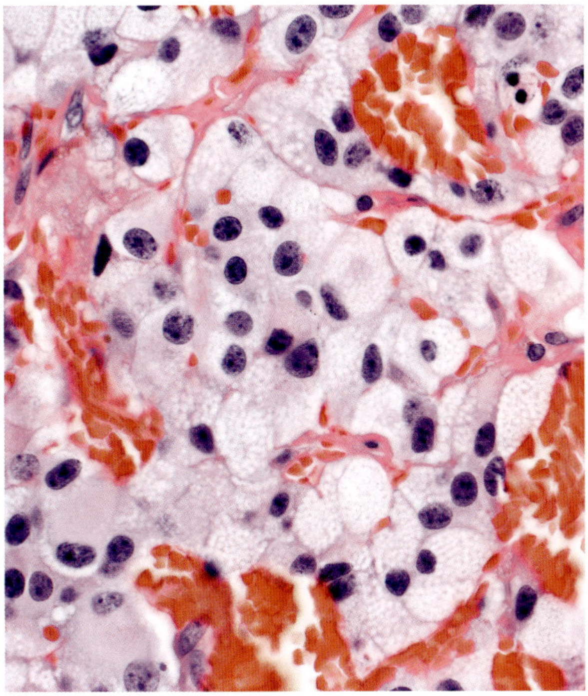

Figure 10-11

LIPID-RICH CARCINOMA

This lipid-rich neuroendocrine tumor shows microvesicular steatosis.

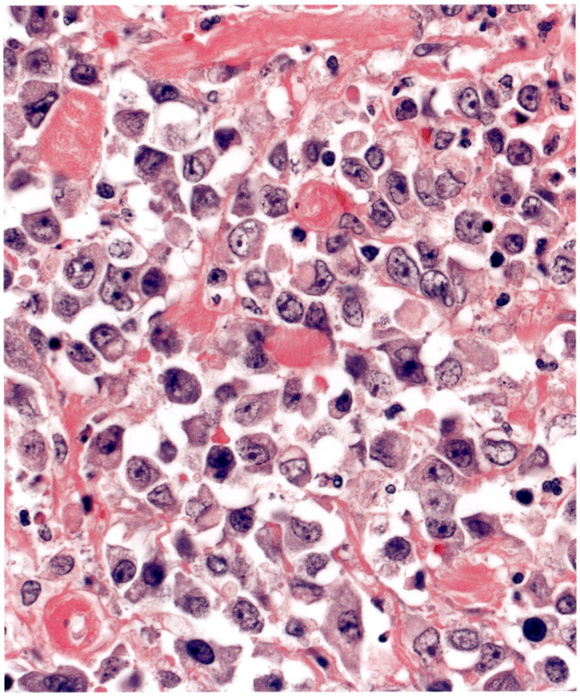

Figure 10-12

RHABDOID MORPHOLOGY

The carcinoma is growing as discohesive cells with eccentric, densely eosinophilic cytoplasm and prominent nucleoli. Occasional eosinophilic inclusions are seen in the cytoplasm.

BRG-1 immunostains are helpful to rule out rhabdoid tumors, which can be primary to the liver or metastatic.

Bile production indicates hepatocytic differentiation and in most cases is essentially diagnostic of hepatocellular carcinoma. However, hepatoid carcinomas from other organs also produce bile (15). When bile is abundant on the slide, it is confidently recognized (fig. 10-13). However, other nonhepatoid carcinomas can produce material that focally suggests bile, but is not true bile (fig. 10-14). For this reason, additional immunostains are often warranted to confirm hepatocytic differentiation. Histochemical stains for bile, such as the Hall bile stain, are often challenging to interpret and generally not as helpful as immunostains confirming hepatocytic differentiation, such as HepPar1, arginase, and glypican 3.

Mucinous carcinomas can arise from many organs (Table 10-2; fig. 10-15). In these cases, extracellular mucin is a dominant feature of the histology (a commonly used definition is greater than 50 percent). Overall, metastases

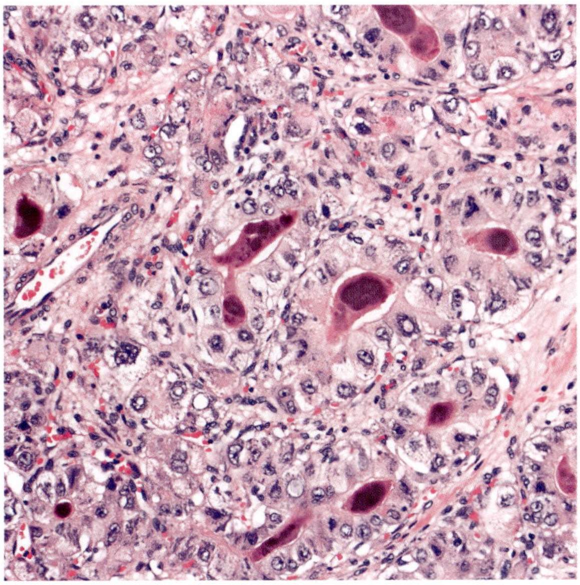

Figure 10-13

HEPATOCELLULAR CARCINOMA: BILE

There is abundant bile production.

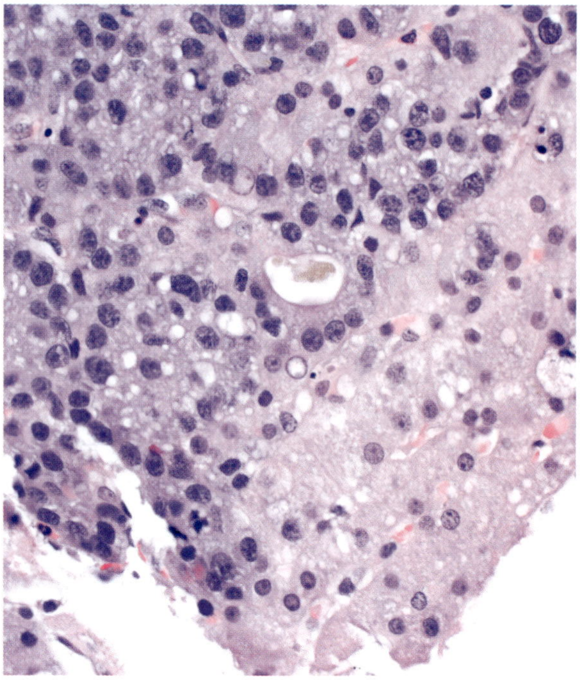

Figure 10-14

HEPATOCELLULAR CARCINOMA: BILE MIMIC

The material in this metastatic prostate carcinoma resembles bile.

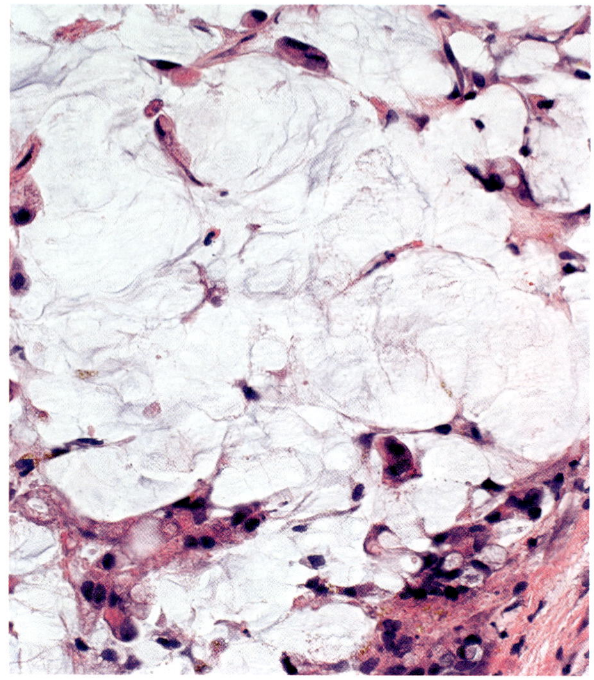

Figure 10-15

MUCINOUS CARCINOMA

This mucinous carcinoma is metastatic from the pancreas.

from gastrointestinal primaries are the most commonly encountered in surgical pathology. An immunostain panel of CK7, CK20, CDX2, estrogen receptor (ER), and PAX8 will allow classification of most cases.

General Approach

There are several general approaches for the workup of a liver tumor of unknown origin. A number of instructive immunostain algorithms have been published, in which the results of an initial stain or panel of stains leads to certain possibilities, which can be further explored with additional stains. In clinical practice, most pathologists use a more comprehensive approach, incorporating clinical findings, H&E morphology, and a stepwise approach to immunostain selection.

A useful comprehensive approach relies on following the 10 steps. This approach has the advantage of being practical and, when followed, can arrive at a diagnosis in most cases. This approach also has the advantage of widespread application in clinical care, being used by numerous pathologists over a long period of time in many different situations, all of which has made this approach extremely robust. Many times, pathologists struggle unnecessarily with a case because they forgot to perform one or more of these simple steps.

1. History. Is there relevant clinical history, such as a prior surgical resection of a tumor? If so, the specimen slides should be reviewed, if possible, especially if the surgery was within the prior 5 years.

2. Imaging. Have there been imaging studies (e.g., magnetic resonance imaging [MRI], computerized tomography [CT], etc.) and, if so, were any mass lesions noted? The clinical information provided with the pathology specimen is often not very forthcoming about imaging findings, and sometimes some phone work before ordering stains can pay off.

3. Liver disease. Is there a history of chronic liver disease and/or advanced fibrosis? If so, this would favor hepatocellular carcinoma or cholangiocarcinoma.

4. Serum markers. Serum markers typically have modest sensitivity and specificity, but can be useful starting points (Table 10-1).

Table 10-3

CK7 AND CK20 GENERAL STAINING PATTERNS IN VARIOUS NEOPLASMS[a]

Cytokeratin Stains	CK20 positive	CK20 variable	CK20 negative
CK7 positive	Ovarian, mucinous	Cholangiocarcinoma, intrahepatic Cholangiocarcinoma, extrahepatic Endocervical adenocarcinoma Esophageal adenocarcinoma Pancreas carcinoma Small bowel adenocarcinoma Transitional cell urothelial carcinoma	Breast, ductal Breast, lobular Cervical, squamous cell Endometrial Lung adenocarcinoma Ovarian, clear cell Ovarian, serous Ovarian, endometrioid Salivary gland Thyroid, follicular Thyroid, papillary
CK7 variable	Appendix, adenocarcinoma Rectum	Colon, MSI[b] high Gastric carcinoma Prostate	Hepatocellular carcinoma Mesothelioma Renal clear cell carcinoma Renal chromophobe carcinoma Squamous cell, head and neck Squamous cell, lung Squamous cell, esophagus
CK7 negative	Appendix, goblet cell Colon Merkel cell		Adrenal Germ cell tumors Neuroendocrine tumor Pancreas, solid pseudopapillary Pancreas, acinar Small cell carcinoma

[a]Many exceptions exist.
[b]MSI = microsatellite instability.

5. Establish the main tumor lineage. On light microscopy, establish the broad lineage of the tumor, either by morphology (Table 10-2) or by immunostains: carcinoma versus sarcoma versus lymphoma versus melanoma.

6. If carcinoma, rule out hepatocellular carcinoma. For nongland-forming carcinomas, follow-up with a battery of stains to rule out hepatocellular carcinoma. A panel of HepPar1, arginase, and glypican 3 works well.

7. Organ suggestive markers. Once hepatocellular carcinoma has been excluded, carcinomas can be further evaluated with a panel of immunostains that suggest site of origin (Tables 10-3, 10-4).

8. Lymphoma. Lymphomas can be worked up based on morphology. The most common primary lymphoma of the liver is diffuse large B-cell lymphoma.

9. Sarcomas. The most common metastatic sarcomas seen in biopsy material are leiomyosarcomas from the uterus, gastrointestinal stromal tumors, and angiosarcomas. Essentially all other sarcomas can also metastasize to the liver, but typically there is a known history of sarcoma and biopsies of metastatic deposits in the liver are not performed.

10. Morphology and immunostains: use together. Both the morphology and the immunohistochemical findings should support the diagnosis. If one disagrees with the other, this conflict should be resolved with additional sampling (in resection specimens) and/or additional immunohistochemical or molecular studies. Repeating the discrepant stain can also be helpful to ensure the staining is not a false positive/false negative.

Broad Lineage Markers

In some cases, the morphology is sufficient to determine lineage and immunostains are not needed for that purpose. As one example, a mucinous adenocarcinoma does not benefit from broad-spectrum keratin markers to prove it is a carcinoma. In contrast, less well

Table 10-4

IMMUNOHISTOCHEMICAL STAINING PATTERNS FOR COMMON PRIMARY AND METASTATIC CARCINOMAS OF THE LIVER[a]

Tumor	CK7/20 Profile and Typically Positive Stains	Notes
Adrenal cortical	CK7 negative CK20 negative Inhibin MelA Calretinin	
Cholangio-carcinoma	CK7 positive CK20 variable CK19 MOC31 CDX2 (30%), often focal	CK20 and CDX2 positivity is more common in hilar and extrahepatic tumors
Breast	CK7 positive CK20 negative GATA3 (up to 90%) Mammaglobin (up to 75%) GCDFP (up to 75%) ER	ER can be helpful, but other tumors can also be positive, such as gynecologic tumors, salivary gland tumors, and thyroid tumors. Most carcinomas of the stomach, small intestine, colon, and appendix are ER negative. S-100 protein can be positive, an important diagnostic pitfall. GATA3 is sensitive but not specific
Colorectal	CK7 negative CK20 positive CDX2	MSI-H[b] carcinomas can show reduced staining for CK20 and CK7 positivity. Rectal carcinomas are CK7 variable
Endometrial carcinoma	CK7 positive CK20 negative Pax8 Vimentin ER PR	Breast carcinomas are PAX8 negative
Germ cell tumor, seminoma/ dysgerminoma	CK7 negative CK20 negative SALL4 OCT4 D2-40 C-KIT PLAP	Negative for CD30, AFP, glypican 3, GATA3, and HCG Keratins are negative or may have focal staining including dot-like staining
Germ cell tumor, embryonal	CK7 negative CK20 negative SALL4 OCT4 CD30 SOX2 PLAP Keratins, low molecular weight	Negative for C-KIT, AFP, D2-40 (or weak, apical staining), glypican 3 (or weak staining), and HCG.
Germ cell tumor, choriocarcinoma	CK7 negative CK20 negative SALL4 (variable, about 70%) GATA3 HCG Glypican 3, variable Keratins, low molecular weight CD10 PLAP (variable, about 50%)	Negative: OCT4, D2-40, CD30, C-KIT, SOX2

Table 10-4, continued

Tumor	CK7/20 Profile and Typically Positive Stains	Notes
Germ cell tumor, yolk sac tumor (endodermal sinus tumor)	CK7 negative CK20 negative SALL4 Glypican 3 Alpha-fetoprotein (but staining often focal) C-KIT Keratins, low molecular weight PLAP (variable, about 50%)	Negative: OCT4, D2-40, SOX2, CD30
Hepatocellular carcinoma	CK7 variable CK20 negative HepPar1 Arginase Glypican 3 (only 50% in well differentiated HCC) ALB-ISH CD10 or pCEA (canalicular pattern)	MOC31 is positive in 35% CDX2 can be positive in 5%, typically focal CK7 positive in 30%, mostly focal, can be diffuse CK20 positive in10% CK19 positive in 15%
Lung adeno-carcinoma	CK7 positive CK20 negative Napsin TTF1	Napsin is also positive in about 3/4 of papillary renal cell carcinomas and about 1/3 of clear cell renal carcinomas. Most (95%) of thyroid tumors are napsin negative.
Mesothelioma	CK7 variable CK20 negative CK5/6 WT1 Calretinin D2-40	GATA3 is positive in about 50% Negative for MOC 31, CEA, BerEP4
NUT midline carcinoma	CK7 positive CK20 negative NUT1 CD34 (about 50% of cases)	
Neuroendocrine tumor/carcinoma	CK7 negative CK20 negative Synaptophysin Chromogranin CD56	Synaptophysin can be positive in many other tumors.
Ovarian, endo-metrioid	CK7 positive CK20 negative CEA PAX8	
Ovarian, clear cell	CK7 positive CK20 negative PAX8 HNF-1 beta Napsin A VHL	Negative for WT1, ER, PR
Ovarian, mucinous	CK7 positive CK20 positive CK7 CK20 CEA	PAX8 usually negative CK20 staining is typically not diffuse
Ovarian, serous	CK7 positive CK20 negative PAX8 P53 WT1 CA125	Mesothelioma is PAX8 negative

Table 10-4, continued

Tumor	CK7/20 Profile and Typically Positive Stains	Notes
Pancreas, acinar	CK7 negative CK20 negative CK8, 18 (CAM5.2) Trypsin Chymotrypsin Synaptophysin, variable Chromogranin, variable Alpha-1-antitrypsin Alpha-1-antichymotrypsin	If >25% of cells show positive staining for synaptophysin or chromogranin, classify as mixed acinar-endocrine carcinoma. 60% of tumors are glypican 3 positive.
Pancreas, ductal	CK7 positive CK20 variable CK19 MOC31 CDX2, variable Loss of DPC4 (50%)	DPC4 loss is also seen in 50% of cholangiocarcinomas and 30% of carcinomas of the ampulla of Vater
Pancreas, solid pseudopapillary	CK7 negative CK20 negative Beta-catenin, nuclear CD10 Progesterone receptor Vimentin Alpha-1-antitrypsin CD56 Neuron-specific enolase	
Prostate	CK7 variable CK20 variable PSA PSAP ERG (positive in 50%)	PSA can also stain some salivary gland tumors PSAP can stain many rectal NET[b]
Renal, chromophobe	CK7 positive CK20 negative PAX8 CKIT E-cadherin	50% of chromophobe carcinomas are GATA3 positive vimentin negative or weak RCC negative CD10 negative
Renal, clear cell	CK7 positive CK20 negative PAX8 PAX2 RCC CD10 Vimentin	PAX8 overall performs best. E-cadherin negative
Renal, papillary	CK7 positive CK20 negative PAX8 PAX2 RCC Vimentin	E-cadherin negative
Small bowel	CK7 (often focal) CK20 (positive in jejunum and ileum) CDX2	CK20 is negative in duodenum HepPar 1 is positive in 2/3 of nonampullary adenocarcinomas and 2/3 of ampullary carcinomas with an intestinal phenotype. Arginase is positive in about 5% of cases.
Stomach	CK7 variable CK20 variable CDX2 variable	CDX2 staining frequency varies by morphology: about 80% of intestinal type and 50% of diffuse; CK7 is positive in about 80% of cases; CK20 in about 50%. ER staining is negative.

Table 10-4, continued

Tumor	CK7/20 Profile and Typically Positive Stains	Notes
Squamous cell carcinoma	CK7 variable CK20 negative CK5/6 P40 P63	20% are glypican 3 positive (106) HPV[b] positivity suggests cervical or oropharynx primary GATA3 is positive in 80% of skin squamous cell carcinomas, 30% of cervical, and 20% of lung/larynx
Thyroid carcinoma	CK7 positive CK20 negative TTF1 Thyroglobulin PAX8 Calcitonin (medullary)	TTF1 is routinely positive in small cell carcinomas and also can be positive in biliary carcinomas and some endometrial carcinomas
Transitional cell	CK7 positive CK20 variable CK5/6 P40 P63 GATA3 Uroplakin	GATA3 is sensitive for urothelial differentiation, but lacks specificity. Uroplakin is insensitive, but has good specificity for bladder
Leiomyosarcoma	Smooth muscle actin Desmin Caldesmon	
Rhabdomyosarcoma	Desmin Myogenin MyoD1	
Solitary fibrous tumor	CD34 CD99 BCL2 Factor 8a	
Gastrointestinal stromal tumor	CKIT DOG1 CD34 SMA SDHB	CKIT is also positive in melanoma and some carcinomas DOG1 has best sensitivity in spindle cell tumors CD34 is positive in about 2/3 of cases SMA is positive in about 1/3 of cases SDHB loss is seen in a small subset of pediatric GIST
Angiosarcoma	ERG FLI1 CD31 Factor 8 CD34	About 50% of prostate carcinomas are ERG positive.
Melanoma	S-100 protein HMB45 MelA MITF	Breast carcinoma can be S-100 protein positive.
Synovial Sarcoma	CD99 BCL2 CEA	Molecular testing for *SYT-SSX1* or *SYT-SSX2*

[a]Exceptions to these patterns exist.
[b]MSI-H = microsatellite instability-high; NET = neuroendocrine tumor; HPV = human papillomavirus.

differentiated malignancies often require lineage markers as the foundation for subsequent evaluation. Even in these cases, the morphology can suggest a line of differentiation and guide stain selection. If the morphology suggests a lymphoma, then lymphoid markers are the best place to start and carcinoma and melanoma markers may be needed only if the stains for lymphoid differentiation are negative.

Carcinoma

Overall, the most commonly used markers of epithelial differentiation are cytokeratin stains and epithelial membrane antigen (EMA). There are a number of pankeratin stains available, which have excellent performance characteristics in well- and moderately differentiated carcinomas. However, in poorly differentiated carcinomas, single pankeratin stains can be negative and a panel of cytokeratins is useful. One potential panel is cytokeratin AE1/AE3 (broad spectrum), CAM5.2 (low molecular weight), and CK903 or CK5/6 (both high molecular weight). An important point to consider when evaluating the keratin stains is the strength of the immunopositivity. Keratin staining in carcinomas should be strong and bright, even if it is focal. Also of note, focal staining has to be interpreted cautiously, as focal staining is seen occasionally in mesotheliomas, sarcomas such as angiosarcomas (16) and epithelioid hemangioendotheliomas (17), and anaplastic large cell lymphomas (18). In addition, correlation with the H&E morphology is important to ensure positive staining, even when strong, does not represent entrapped hepatocytes or bile ducts.

Some carcinomas have a distinctive dot-like staining pattern with cytokeratin stains, especially with low molecular weight cytokeratins. This pattern is found most commonly in neuroendocrine tumors, ranging from small cell carcinomas to well-differentiated neuroendocrine tumors. Not all neuroendocrine tumors have a dot-like keratin staining pattern, but overall this pattern is most common in small cell carcinoma. Merkel cell carcinomas also show this pattern with keratin stains, although usually with somewhat larger dots and a distinctive perinuclear staining pattern. Merkel cell carcinomas are also CK20 positive, a very useful clue, as most other neuroendocrine carcinomas are CK20 negative. Other tumors with occasional dot-like keratin staining include renal oncocytomas, seminomas, and granulosa cell tumors (19,20). Rarely, sarcomas show dot-like keratin staining, including gastrointestinal stromal tumors, leiomyosarcomas, synovial sarcomas, and desmoplastic small round cell tumors (21,22).

Metastatic melanomas can be challenging tumors to recognize, both because they can closely mimic carcinomas and because a history of a melanotic skin lesion is often not known or not available at the time of sign out. A single negative marker is not enough to rule out melanoma. One useful panel includes multiple stains from this list: S-100 protein, melan-A, HMB-45, SOX10, and microphthalmia transcription factor 1 (MITF1).

For sarcomas, a useful starting panel includes C-KIT, DOG1, S-100 protein, desmin, and ERG or other vascular markers. Using isolated stains can lead to diagnostic missteps. For example, C-KIT is less useful as an isolated stain because it is positive in a number of different carcinomas as well as melanomas.

DISTINGUISHING PRIMARY LIVER CARCINOMA FROM METASTATIC CARCINOMA

Hepatocellular Carcinoma versus Metastatic Disease

For poorly differentiated carcinomas, the H&E differential diagnosis commonly includes both hepatocellular carcinoma and metastatic disease, and immunostains should be used to exclude hepatocellular carcinoma. An excellent panel for this purpose is composed of HepPar1, arginase, and glypican 3. Albumin in situ hybridization is less commonly available, but is also helpful. If all of these stains are negative, then the tumor is unlikely to have hepatocytic differentiation. A single negative stain is insufficient to exclude hepatocellular carcinoma when the malignancy is poorly differentiated. Likewise, no immunostain for hepatocytic differentiation is perfectly specific, and this is unlikely to change within the span of our careers. Thus, a single positive stain is best interpreted in the context of the morphology and clinical findings. Of these three key stains for hepatocytic differentiation, glypican 3 is the least specific.

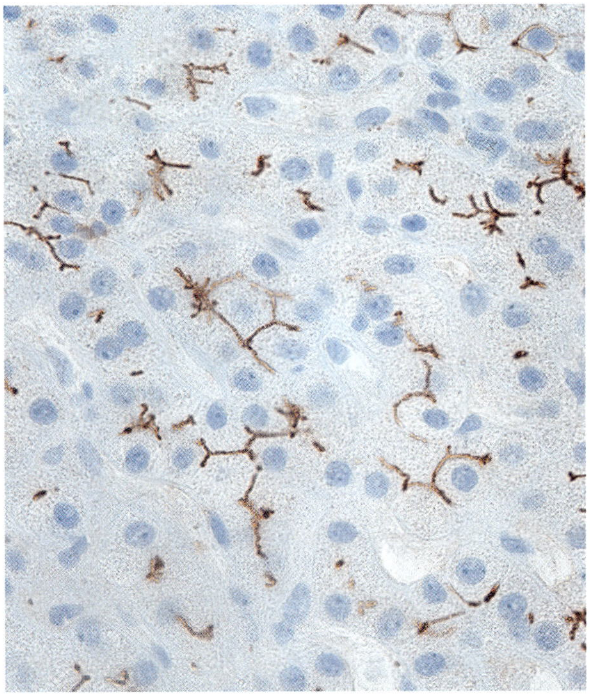

Figure 10-16

HEPATOCELLULAR CARCINOMA: CD10 CANALICULAR STAINING

This pattern is very specific for hepatocellular carcinoma, but is almost never present in poorly differentiated hepatocellular carcinomas.

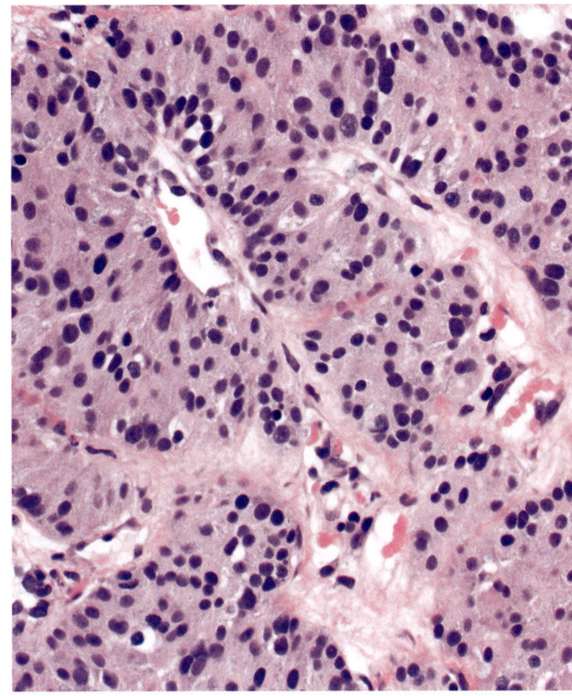

Figure 10-17

METASTATIC NEUROENDOCRINE TUMOR

The neuroendocrine tumor is growing in trabeculae. The cytology is bland, but the Ki-67 index was higher, making it a World Health Organization (WHO) grade 3 tumor.

CD10 and pCEA stains are essentially never helpful as markers of hepatocytic differentiation in poorly differentiated carcinomas: poorly differentiated hepatocellular carcinomas almost never have the canalicular structures needed to give the distinctive "canalicular" staining that is typical of well and moderately differentiated hepatocellular carcinomas (fig. 10-16). Interpretation is further compounded by the challenge of deciding if little bits of linear staining that might be seen here and there in a poorly differentiated carcinoma are sufficient for a "canalicular" staining pattern.

Positive staining for either CK19 or MOC31 does not exclude hepatocellular carcinoma, as both are positive in 15 or 35 percent of hepatocellular carcinomas, respectively (see chapter 3). The positivity in hepatocellular carcinomas tends to be less strong and less diffuse than in adenocarcinomas, a distinction that is best appreciated on full sections of tumor and can be less evident on biopsy specimens.

Well-differentiated hepatocellular carcinomas can also pose diagnostic challenges. At times they can be even trickier to diagnose than poorly differentiated hepatocellular carcinomas because the cytology of a well-differentiated carcinoma can lull the pathologist into a false sense of a straightforward diagnosis. In fact, a number of well-differentiated metastatic tumors have a trabecular growth pattern, closely mimicking the cytology and architectural growth of hepatocellular carcinoma. The most common culprits are neuroendocrine tumors (fig. 10-17), renal carcinoma (fig. 10-18), and adrenal cortical carcinoma. This potential diagnostic pitfall becomes even more prominent when relying on single markers of hepatocytic differentiation, in particular, arginase or glypican 3, as both can be negative in a subset of well-differentiated hepatocellular carcinomas (figs. 10-19, 10-20), whereas HepPar1 and pCEA tend to be more reliable in this setting.

The final diagnosis needs to be firmly anchored to the morphologic findings. None of

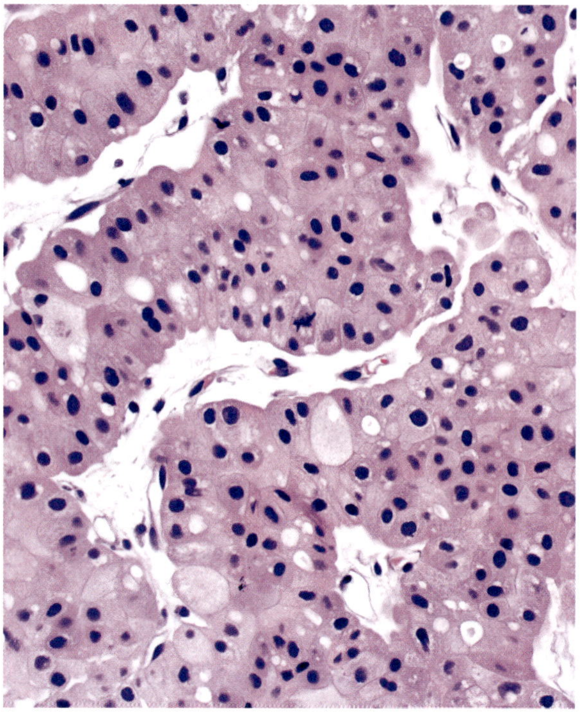

Figure 10-18

METASTATIC CHROMOPHOBE CARCINOMA

This metastatic renal chromophobe carcinoma closely mimics the cytology and architecture of well-differentiated hepatocellular carcinoma.

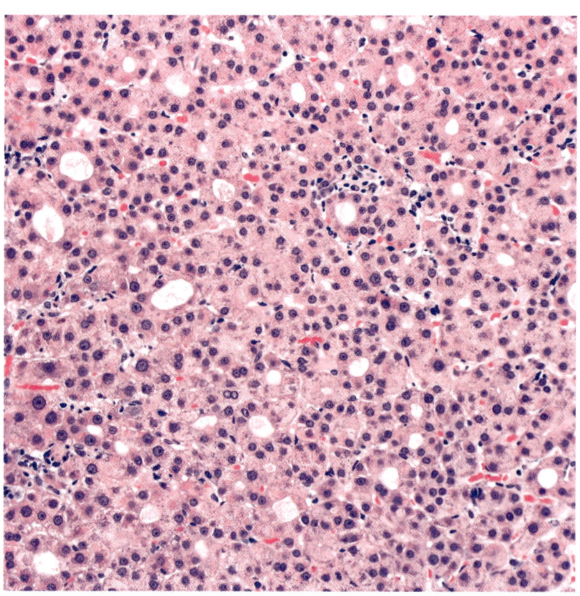

Figure 10-19

HEPATOCELLULAR CARCINOMA

The hepatocellular carcinoma is well differentiated.

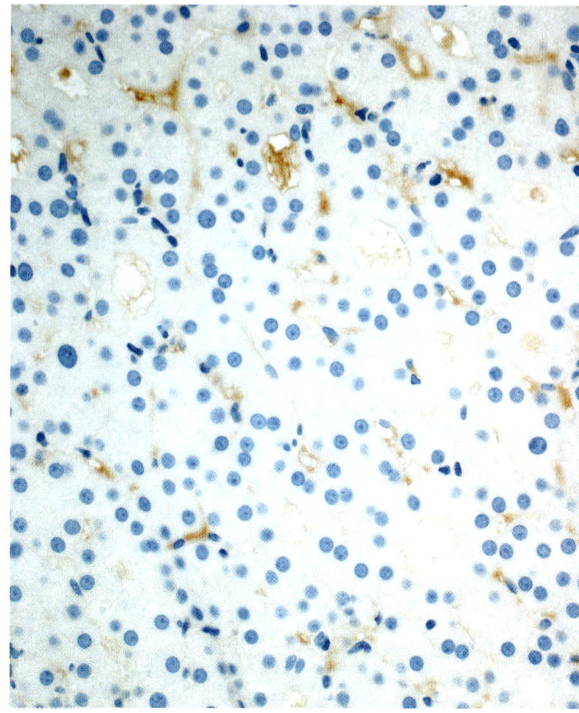

Figure 10-20

HEPATOCELLULAR CARCINOMA: ARGINASE STAIN

An immunostain for arginase is negative (same case as shown in fig. 10-19).

the immunohistochemical stains now, and perhaps ever, will be perfectly sensitive or specific. For this reason, interpreting immunostains in isolation from the morphology is strongly discouraged. As one example, small intestinal adenocarcinomas are frequently positive for HepPar1 (about two thirds) and can be positive for arginase (about 5 percent) (23). However, the distinction from hepatocellular carcinoma is readily made in almost all cases by incorporating the morphologic findings.

Cholangiocarcinoma versus Metastatic Disease

Classically, cholangiocarcinomas show a pattern of moderately differentiated adenocarcinoma with an abundant and diffuse desmoplastic response. However, cholangiocarcinomas have a much wider spectrum of growth patterns, ranging from solid to trabecular to glandular, and can have varying degrees of intratumoral fibrosis, ranging from little fibrosis to the more classic pattern of abundant and diffuse fibrosis. Rare cases of intrahepatic cholangiocarcinoma have a growth pattern that closely resembles thyroid carcinoma (24,25). For these reasons, the H&E findings in cholangiocarcinomas are not diagnostic and should be followed by immunostains. These immunostains can exclude other potential primary sites and confirm a typical immunostaining pattern within the tumor. The diagnosis of cholangiocarcinoma at this time is fundamentally one of exclusion, where a diagnosis is secured by compatible histology (H&E findings and immunohistochemical findings) plus imagining studies that show no other potential primary site.

While precursor lesions are not identified in most cases, when present they can indicate the proper diagnosis of cholangiocarcinoma. For example, mucinous cystic neoplasms and intraductal papillary neoplasms of the bile duct can have foci of invasive carcinoma. Another clue is nearby bile ducts with high-grade biliary intraepithelial neoplasia (BilIN-3). In these cases immunostains are still important as some metastatic adenocarcinomas grow along the bile ducts, a pattern called "cancerization of the bile ducts." When growing in this manner, these metastatic carcinomas can closely mimic BilIN-3. Colorectal adenocarcinomas are the most likely to have this rare growth pattern (seen in up to 4 percent of cases) but other carcinomas that colonize the bile ducts include stomach, pancreas, and breast cancers (26). Either the small ducts or the large ducts can be colonized and there may be significant secondary changes to the background liver, changes that can mimic primary sclerosing cholangitis. Radiologic findings in this setting can also suggest a cholangiocarcinoma (27). However, in most cases, the surgical specimen shows more typical areas of tumor morphology and growth, which, along with immunostains, will lead to the correct diagnosis.

Cholangiocarcinomas are positive for CK7 (85 to 95 percent) and CK19 (90 percent) but negative for strong diffuse CK20 (28–30). CDX2 is positive in 30 to 50 percent of cases, especially in hilar tumors (31,32). However, this staining pattern is not very sensitive or specific for cholangiocarcinoma, as not all cholangiocarcinomas show this pattern of staining and metastatic disease from other organs can have this pattern. Unfortunately, there currently are no validated immunohistochemical stains available in routine practice that accurately distinguish intrahepatic cholangiocarcinoma from metastatic adenocarcinoma. In fact, the lack of positive, affirmative immunostains or molecular assays that indicate biliary differentiation is a major weakness in our diagnostic armamentarium, one that is a research interest of many groups and will hopefully be rectified in the future. Some possible markers or techniques that have been published but await larger, independent studies, include albumin in situ hybridization, ANXA1, ANXA10, S-100 protein, and pVHL (33–35), with albumin in situ hybridization appearing the most promising.

At this point, available immunostains can support a diagnosis of cholangiocarcinoma by fairly effectively ruling out many other carcinomas, including lung, breast, hepatocellular, neuroendocrine, renal, adrenal, mullerian, squamous, and prostate. There are some important and common diagnostic pitfalls, however: 1) thyroid transcription factor (TTF1) nuclear staining in an adenocarcinoma should not be used in isolation to diagnose metastatic lung carcinoma, as TTF1 can be positive in 50 percent of extrahepatic cholangiocarcinomas (36); 2) glypican 3 is positive in about 5 percent of cholangiocarcinomas (37); 3) HepPar1 is positive in 10 percent of cholangiocarcinomas (38,39); and 4) CK20 staining is seen in 10 to 40 percent of cholangiocarcinomas (30,32), in particular, hilar tumors (29), although it tends to be more patchy than in colon carcinoma. Also of note, right-sided colon carcinomas can be CK20 negative (40–42).

Adenocarcinomas arising from the upper gastrointestinal tract, pancreas, and extrahepatic biliary tree can have similar morphologic findings and a similar basic immunohistochemical profile to intrahepatic cholangiocarcinoma (CK7 positive, CK20 negative to focally positive, CDX2 either positive or negative). In fact, the histologic findings do not adequately separate these types of tumors. For this reason, a typical approach for biopsy specimens is to indicate the diagnosis of adenocarcinoma or carcinoma in the diagnostic line of the surgical pathology report, and then to include a prioritized differential in the surgical pathology comment, one that includes intrahepatic cholangiocarcinoma, carcinoma of the extrahepatic biliary tree, pancreas ductal adenocarcinoma, and adenocarcinoma of the upper gastrointestinal tract. In some cases, imaging studies

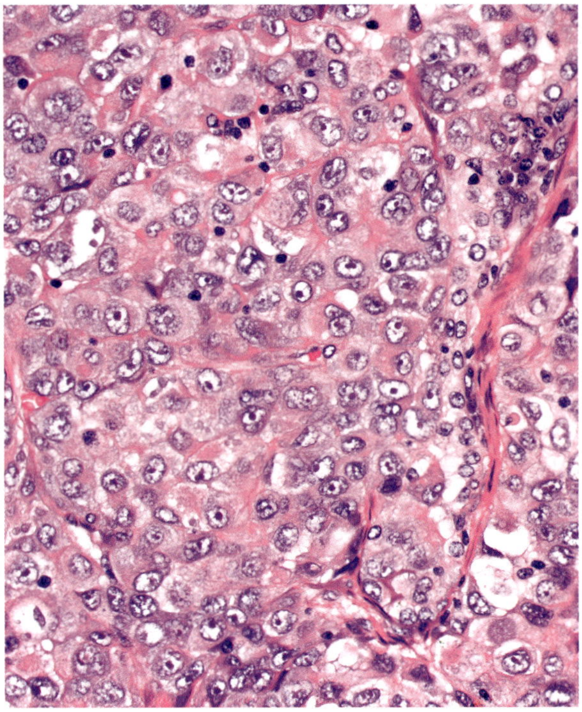

Figure 10-21

HEPATOID CARCINOMA

This hepatoid carcinoma originated in the lung.

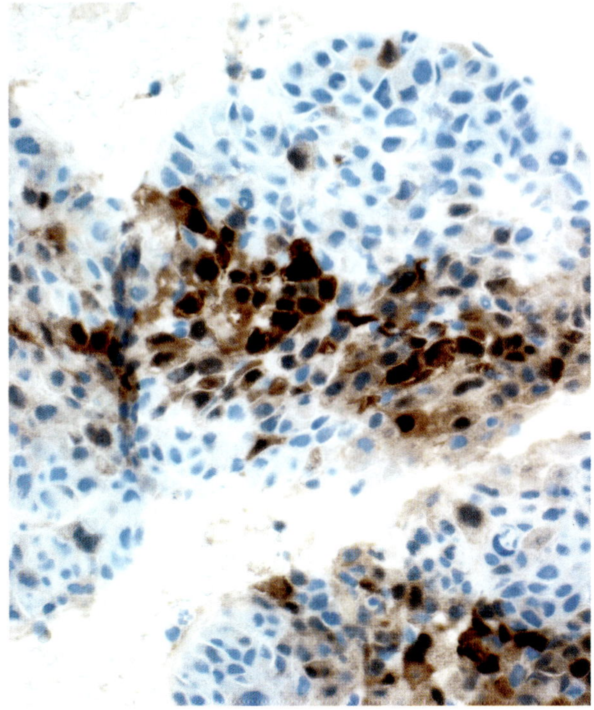

Figure 10-22

HEPATOID CARCINOMA: ARGINASE

An arginase immunostain shows patchy nuclear and cytoplasmic staining.

and endoscopy findings are known at the time of sign-out and are negative. When this is the case, this information can be incorporated into the report, narrowing the differential diagnosis.

Metastatic Hepatoid Carcinomas

Hepatoid carcinomas can arise from a number of extrahepatic organs and metastasize to the liver, creating a diagnostic challenge (fig. 10-21). The most common primary sites for hepatoid carcinomas are the esophagus, stomach, and pancreas, but they also arise from other organs including the lung (43), kidney (44), ampulla of Vater (45), colon (46), gallbladder (47), endometrium (48), and ovary (49). These carcinomas vary in how "hepatoid" they appear on H&E, but in many cases, they have focal areas that are essentially indistinguishable from hepatocellular carcinoma. Their hepatoid nature extends to immunohistochemical findings (50), and they can be positive for HepPar 1, arginase 1, glypican 3, and albumin in situ hybridization and can have a canalicular staining pattern on pCEA or CD10 (fig. 10-22).

Currently, no panel of stains can completely separate a hepatoid carcinoma metastatic to the liver from a primary hepatocellular carcinoma. However, there are several useful clues that can lead to the correct diagnosis. First, many metastatic hepatoid carcinomas have at least some areas that do not look like hepatocellular carcinoma morphologically. For example, there might be focal gland formation. Second, hepatoid carcinomas can have immunostain patterns that are unusual for hepatocellular carcinoma. For example, strong and diffuse staining for CDX2 can suggest a gastrointestinal origin for a hepatoid tumor (fig. 10-23). While about 5 percent of hepatocellular carcinomas are CDX2 positive, the staining in these cases is typically focal or patchy. Third, the presence of advanced fibrosis in the background liver favors a primary liver tumor. Fourth, the microscopic slides of prior surgical resections of tumors from other sites should be re-reviewed. A re-review of the pathology report is often insufficient, as there may have been focal areas of hepatoid differentiation

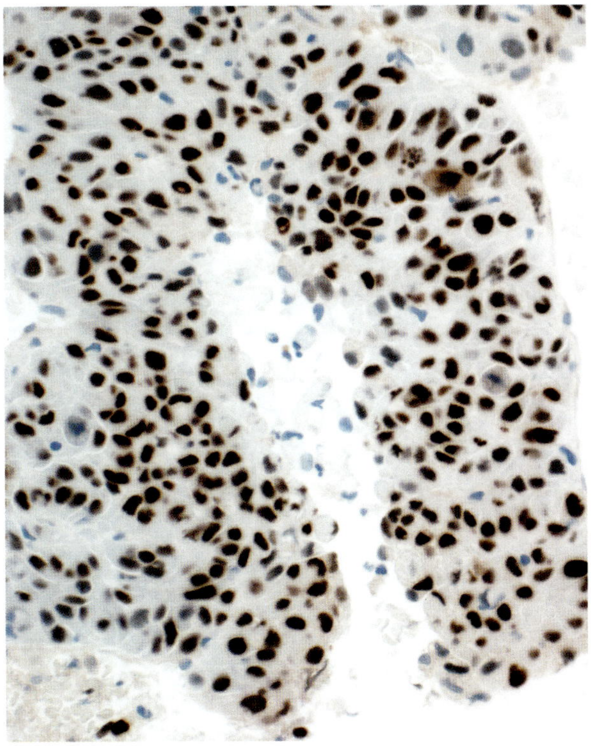

Figure 10-23

HEPATOID CARCINOMA: CDX 2 STAIN

The strong and diffuse nuclear staining is an important clue that this is not primary hepatocellular carcinoma.

that were not mentioned in the original report. Finally, other tumors evident by endoscopic findings or imaging findings can be sampled to exclude a metastatic hepatoid carcinoma.

General Approach to Carcinomas

After hepatocellular carcinoma and cholangiocarcinoma have been excluded, additional stains are often needed to identify potential sites of origin. One useful approach is to perform CK7 and CK20 immunostains, and based on these results (Table 10-3), the clinical findings, and the H&E morphology, perform another set of more focused immunostains (Table 10-4). The CK7/20 profile of tumors is useful, but is intended to be used as a broad guideline and not as a doctrinal position, since there are many exceptions.

HISTOLOGIC GRADING

Carcinomas metastatic to the liver are commonly graded as well, moderately, or poorly differentiated. In general, the grading guidelines of the tumor primary are followed. When the primary is not known, then more general grading guidelines can be used, based on the degree of nuclear pleomorphism, nuclear to cytoplasmic ratio, and evidence of glandular or other differentiation. Neuroendocrine tumors can be graded using the World Health Organization (WHO) guidelines, using either mitotic counts or Ki-67 index (Table 10-5).

Table 10-5

2017 WORLD HEALTH ORGANIZATION (WHO) GRADING SYSTEM FOR NEUROENDOCRINE TUMORS (NET)

Grade	Ki-67 (%)	Mitotic Count (per 10 high-power fields)
NETG1	<3	<2
NETG2	3-20	2-20
NETG3	>20	>20

SITES OF ORIGIN FOR METASTATIC DISEASE

Adrenal Tumors

Both pheochromocytomas and adrenal cortical carcinomas can metastasize to the liver. Adrenal cortical carcinomas can also involve the liver by direct extension. Both of these tumors are sufficiently rare, however, that many pathologists do not encounter them in their careers. Adrenal cortical carcinoma can closely mimic hepatocellular carcinoma, as the tumor cells tend to have abundant eosinophilic cytoplasm, and the neoplasm can grow with a trabecular architecture (fig. 10-24). Immunostains can help clarify the diagnosis when needed (Table 10-4). Pheochromocytomas have the morphology of neuroendocrine tumors, although they often show more nuclear pleomorphism and the nucleoli can be more prominent than typical neuroendocrine tumors. They can also have hyaline globules. Pheochromocytomas are positive for chromogranin and synaptophysin and most are negative for cytokeratins. An S-100 protein stain occasionally highlights sustentacular cells but most metastatic deposits are negative.

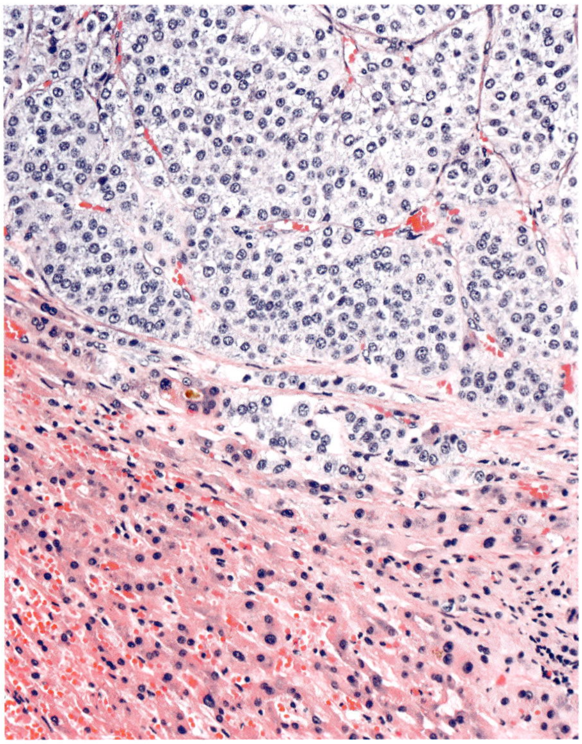

Figure 10-24

ADRENAL CARCINOMA: METASTATIC TO LIVER

This adrenal cortical carcinoma involved the liver by direct extension. The cytology mimics hepatocellular carcinoma, while the growth pattern mimics the macrotrabecular growth pattern that can be seen in some hepatocellular carcinomas.

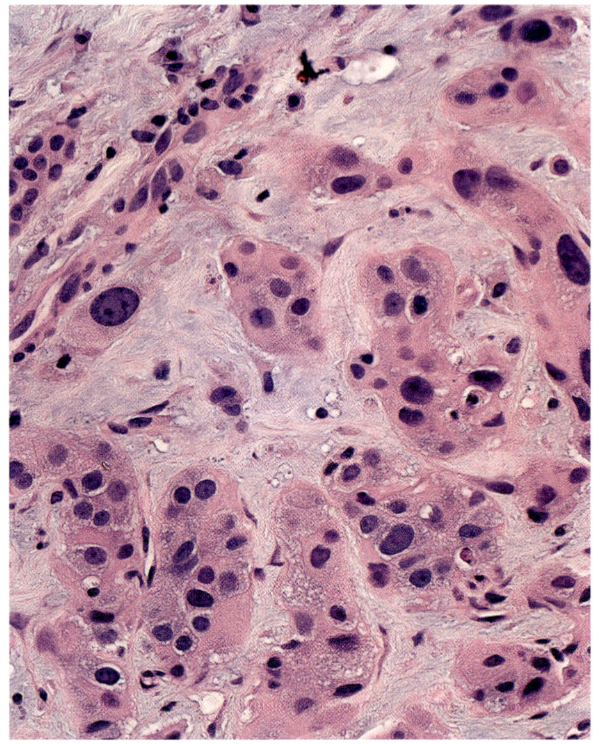

Figure 10-25

BREAST CARCINOMA: METASTATIC TO LIVER

This poorly differentiated carcinoma was positive for mammaglobin and gross cystic disease fluid protein (GCDFP15).

Breast Adenocarcinoma

Breast carcinomas have variable morphology (fig. 10-25), depending on their degree of differentiation and whether the primary tumor is lobular or ductal. They are usually CK7 positive, CK19 negative, and CK20 negative. A typical immunostain panel to evaluate for metastatic breast carcinoma includes ER, gross cystic disease fluid protein-15 (GCDFP-15), and mammaglobin. Progesterone receptor (PR) expression is generally not as useful because it has poor sensitivity and specificity (36).

None of the markers of breast differentiation are perfect and a panel approach is the most robust approach. ER positivity is seen in about 70 percent of breast ductal carcinomas and almost all breast lobular carcinomas, but it is not very specific and can be seen in a number of other tumors. As one example, about two thirds of hilar cholangiocarcinomas are ER positive (51). Mammaglobin and GCDFP-15 are more specific markers of breast carcinoma, and cholangiocarcinomas are typically negative (52,53). Both mammaglobin and GCDFP-15 are cytoplasmic stains and both typically show a patchy staining pattern. In general, GCDFP-15 shows more positive cells than mammaglobin in any given case, but there are many exceptions. Negative staining with these markers does not rule out a breast primary, as mammaglobin is expressed in about 50 to 75 of breast cancers and GCDFP-15 in 25 to 75 percent (54,55). In particular, basal-like breast carcinomas and triple negative breast carcinomas are likely to be negative for both of these markers (56).

Most of the available data are from primary tumors, and there is a paucity of data on how these stains perform in metastatic disease to the liver. Also, the staining frequency, even in primary breast carcinoma, is significantly

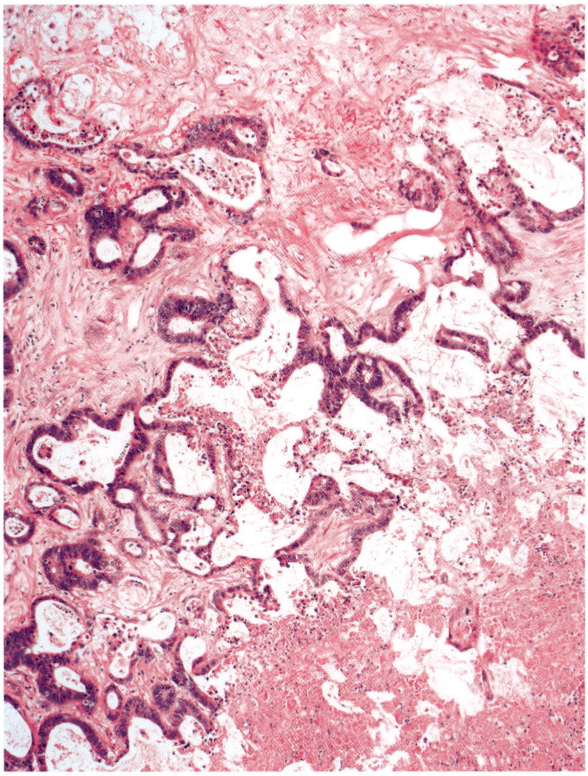

Figure 10-26

COLON CARCINOMA: METASTATIC TO LIVER

The tumor has large glands distended by mucin with dirty necrosis.

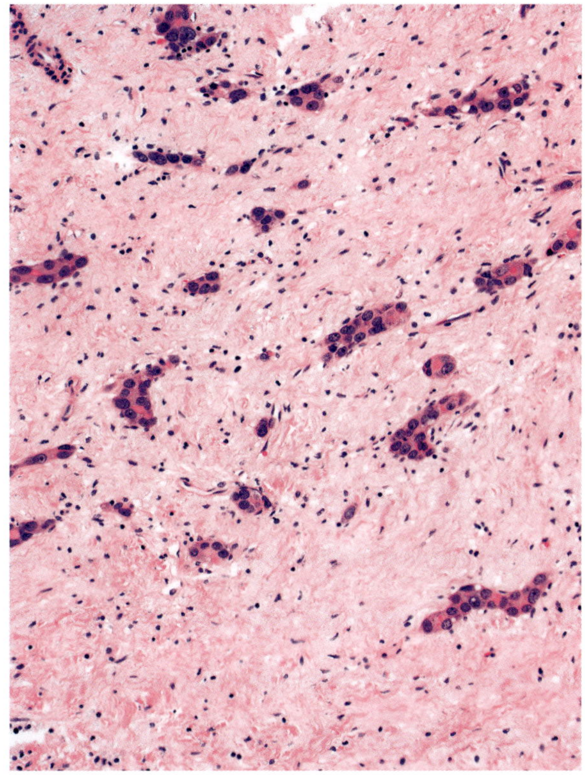

Figure 10-27

COLON CARCINOMA: METASTATIC TO LIVER

This treated colon carcinoma has small, dispersed glands embedded in fibrotic background.

influenced by the specific antibodies used in studies and by the antibody detection methods (55). GATA3 is a nuclear stain and is positive in 90 percent of breast carcinomas, but is not as specific as GCDFP-15 or mammaglobin (55). About 50 percent of breast carcinomas are S-100 protein positive, an important diagnostic pitfall in poorly differentiated neoplasms, as they can mimic melanoma (57).

Colorectal Adenocarcinoma

Colorectal adenocarcinoma is one of the most common carcinomas to metastasize to the liver. In fact, synchronous metastatic colon carcinoma to the liver is found in 15 to 25 percent of individuals at clinical presentation (58). Histologically, metastatic disease is classically characterized by tall columnar cells forming glands that are often large and distended, with abundant dirty necrosis inside the glandular lumens (fig. 10-26). However, the cell morphology and the gland morphology vary considerably and many cases do not have the classic pattern. In most cases, there is little desmoplastic response but some treated tumors can show extensive fibrosis-like changes (fig. 10-27).

The interface of the adenocarcinoma with the non-neoplastic liver can have a number of different patterns, but usually there is a broad pushing border (fig. 10-28), a pseudocapsule (also called desmoplastic) (fig. 10-29), or an infiltrative border (also called replacement pattern) (fig. 10-30). The pushing and pseudocapsule patterns are seen in about one third of cases each, with an infiltrative pattern in 10 percent, and a mixed pattern in 20 percent. Several studies of resected specimens found that an infiltrative border indicates a worse prognosis compared to a pseudocapsule, while a pushing border and a mixed pattern indicates an intermediate prognosis (59–61).

A resection-free margin is universally agreed to be an important prognostic indicator for resected metastatic tumors. However, the

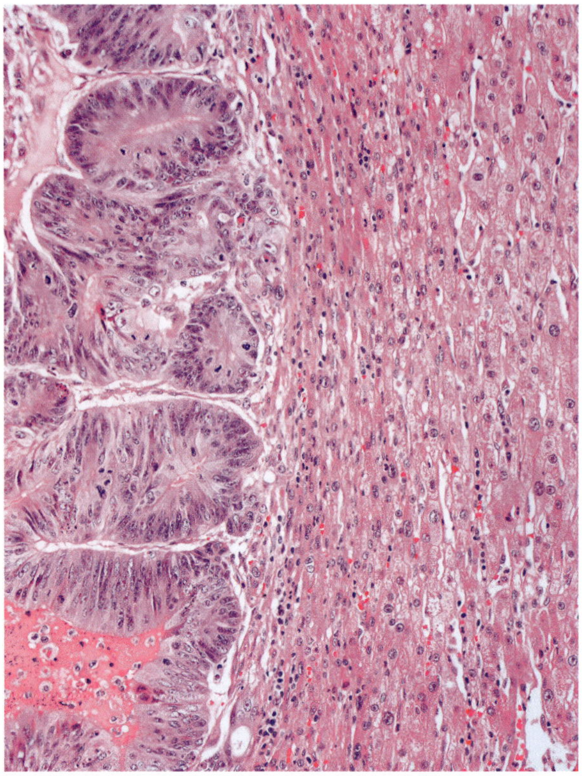

Figure 10-28

COLON CARCINOMA, METASTATIC TO LIVER: PUSHING BORDER

There is a broad pushing interface. A layer of compressed hepatocytes can be seen adjacent to the tumor.

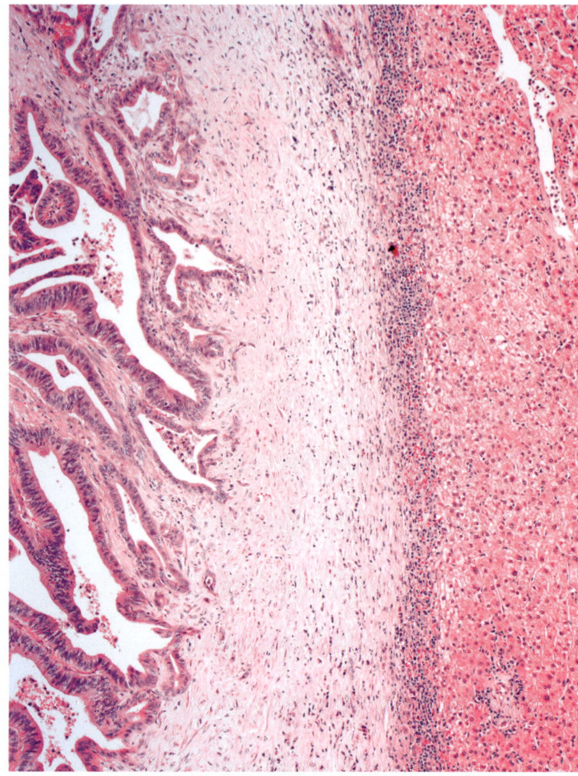

Figure 10-29

COLON CARCINOMA, METASTATIC TO LIVER: CAPSULE BORDER

This colon carcinoma has a dense fibrous pseudocapsule.

optimal length of the resection-free margin remains controversial. One study found a margin of 1 mm was adequate (62), while another study found a margin of 5 mm or less gave a worse prognosis (63). Molecular studies suggest a margin of 5 mm is adequate, as mutant specific DNA is not detectable beyond 4 mm (64).

Most colon carcinomas are CK20 positive, CK7 negative, and CDX2 positive, with the exception of right-sided colon cancers, which also tend to have a higher frequency of microsatellite instability due to defective DNA mismatch repair (MSI-high tumors). These MSI-high adenocarcinomas often show reduced expression of CK20 and CDX2, as well as increased expression of CK7 (40–42). In some cases, evaluating DNA mismatch repair in these tumors by immunostaining for MLH1, MSH2, PMS2, and MSH6 can support a likely colon primary, as microsatellite instability is more common in colon carcinomas. MSI-high status in isolation, however, is not diagnostic of colon carcinoma, since it occurs, albeit rarely, in other carcinomas, including cholangiocarcinoma (65–67). In contrast to colon carcinomas, cholangiocarcinomas are commonly strongly and diffusely positive for CK7 and CK19, with patchy or no staining for CDX2 (68). As an exception, hilar cholangiocarcinomas are often CDX2 positive and are commonly positive for CK20 (31,32,69). Also of note, TTF1 nuclear staining is seen in 4 percent of colorectal carcinomas (70).

KRAS mutations are found in 30 to 50 percent of resected colorectal metastases, a mutation frequency similar to that found in primary tumors. As is true for primary tumors, *KRAS* mutations are a predictor of worse prognosis (71–73). *BRAF* mutations in colorectal metastases are less common than in primary tumors, found in 2 to 4 percent of cases, and also indicate a worse prognosis (71,74).

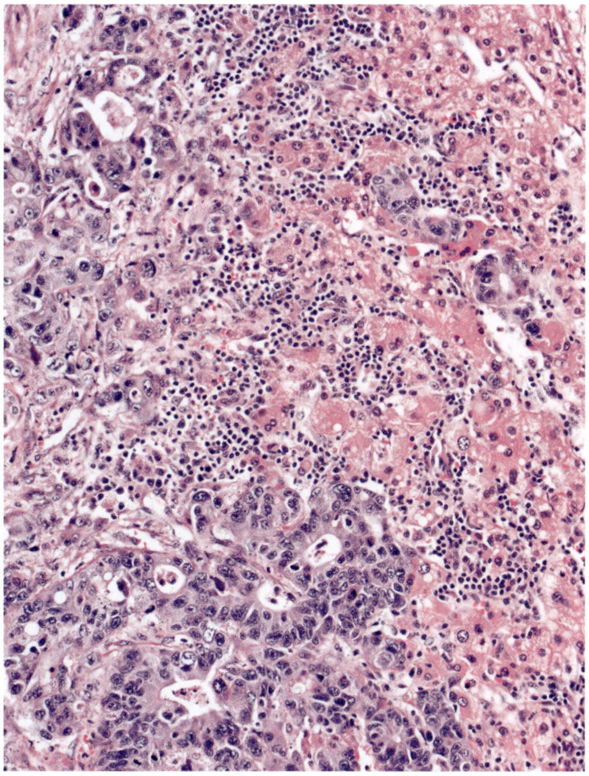

Figure 10-30

COLON CARCINOMA, METASTATIC TO LIVER: INFILTRATIVE BORDER

The tumor has an infiltrative border.

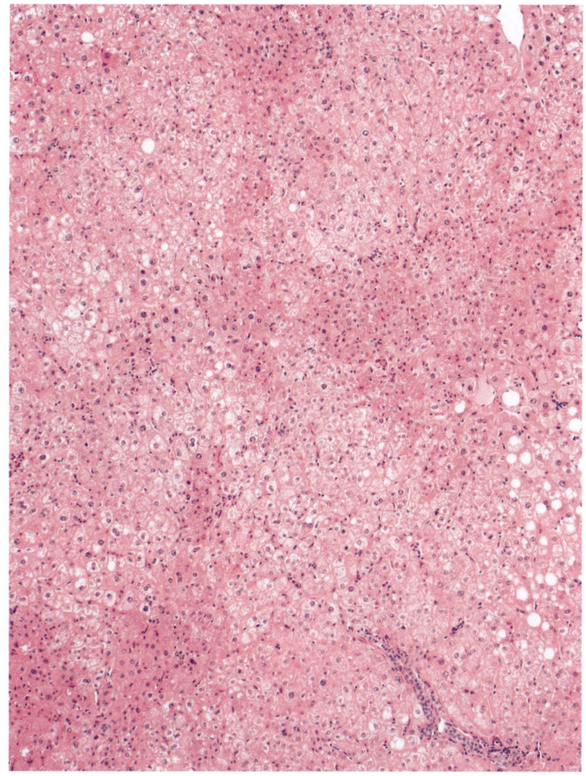

Figure 10-31

BACKGROUND LIVER FOLLOWING TREATMENT WITH OXALIPLATIN

The zone 3 hepatocytes show atrophy and there are sinusoidal congestive changes.

The background liver, when available, should be evaluated for chronic liver disease including chronic hepatitis, fatty liver disease, and fibrosis. In addition, chemotherapy can lead to vascular injury of the sinusoids, called sinusoidal obstructive syndrome (fig. 10-31). The findings in sinusoidal obstructive syndrome appear to be most strongly associated with oxaliplatin use. The background liver can show marked sinusoidal dilatation and congestion, and in some cases, nodular regenerative hyperplasia (75–77). The sinusoidal dilatation and congestion are in a zone 3 distribution and often are associated with mild atrophy of the zone 3 hepatocytes. In some cases, the zone 3 congestion will interconnect, forming a pattern sometimes called "bridging congestion." These chemotherapy related changes are not associated with significant inflammation, duct injury, or obstructive-type biliary changes. In more advanced cases, however, the central veins can show partial or complete obliteration by loose and finely reticulated collagen.

A second drug-induced pattern of injury can be seen with irinotecan, and possibly with oxaliplatin, in which the background liver shows moderate or marked fatty liver disease, sometimes with active steatohepatitis (76). This pattern of injury is often denoted as CASH, for chemotherapy-associated steatohepatitis. Nevertheless, in some cases the fatty liver disease appears to be better explained by the body mass index than by irinotecan exposure (77). In most cases, there probably is a synergistic effect, with both obesity and chemotherapy contributing to the fatty liver disease (78).

Germ Cell Tumors

Germ cell tumors are rare but can metastasize to the liver (fig. 10-32A). The histologic findings can be very challenging, as the morphology can

Figure 10-32

CHORIOCARCINOMA: METASTATIC TO LIVER

A: This CK7-positive choriocarcinoma initially mimicked an undifferentiated carcinoma.

B: An immunostain for human chorionic gonadotropin (HCG) is diffusely positive.

C: Focal staining is seen with glypican 3.

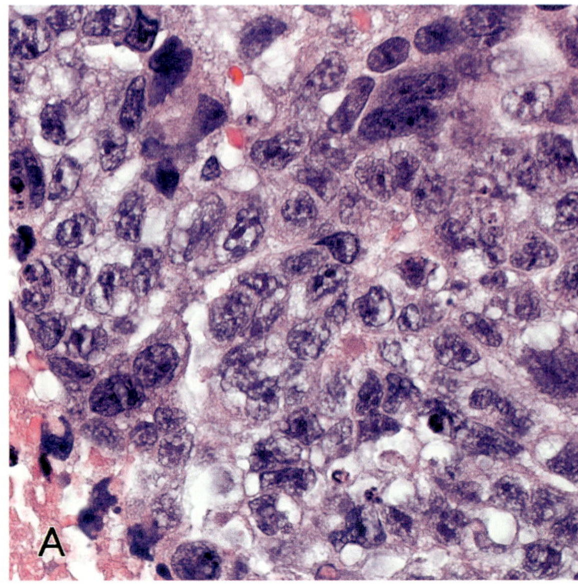

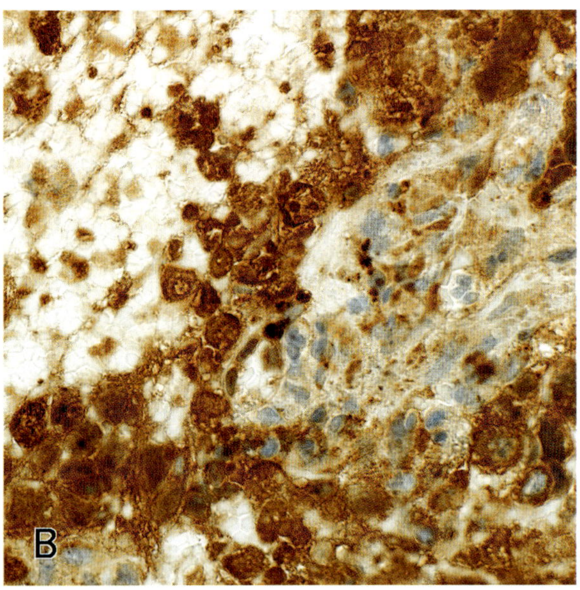

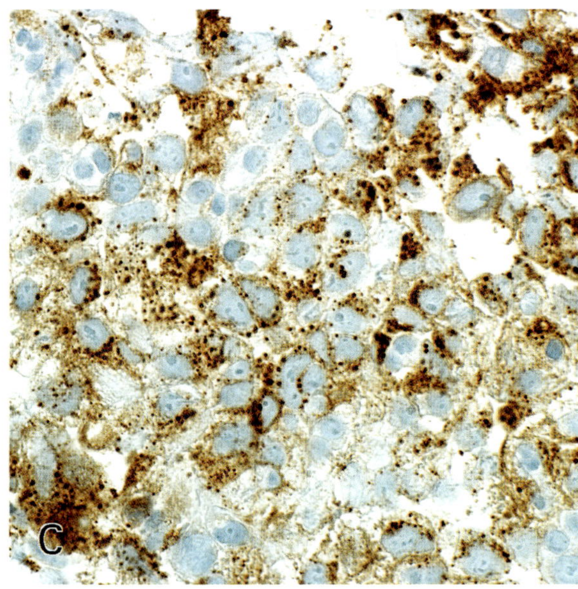

be variable, depending on the germ cell tumor subtype. Low molecular keratin stains are positive in most nonseminoma germ cell tumors. EMA is negative in most germ cell tumors, although a few percent of each subtype are positive, with embryonal carcinomas reaching about 10 percent. SALL4 is a sensitive but not specific marker of germ cell tumors, being positive in almost all seminomas, embryonal carcinomas, yolk sac tumors, and about 70 percent of choriocarcinomas. SALL4 is also positive in hepatocellular carcinomas and thus should not be used as a single marker (79). One reasonable panel to separate a germ cell tumor from a carcinoma is SALL4 and EMA, as germ cell tumors are SALL4 positive and EMA negative and most carcinomas are EMA positive and SALL4 negative. OCT4 is a useful addition if the differential includes embryonal carcinoma or seminoma.

For subtyping germ cell tumors, one useful approach is to classify them into tumors that are OCT4 positive (seminoma, embryonal) and those that are OCT4 negative (yolk sac tumor, choriocarcinoma, and spermatocytic tumor). C-KIT and CD30 can then be used to separate OCT4 positive seminoma (C-KIT positive, CD30 negative) from

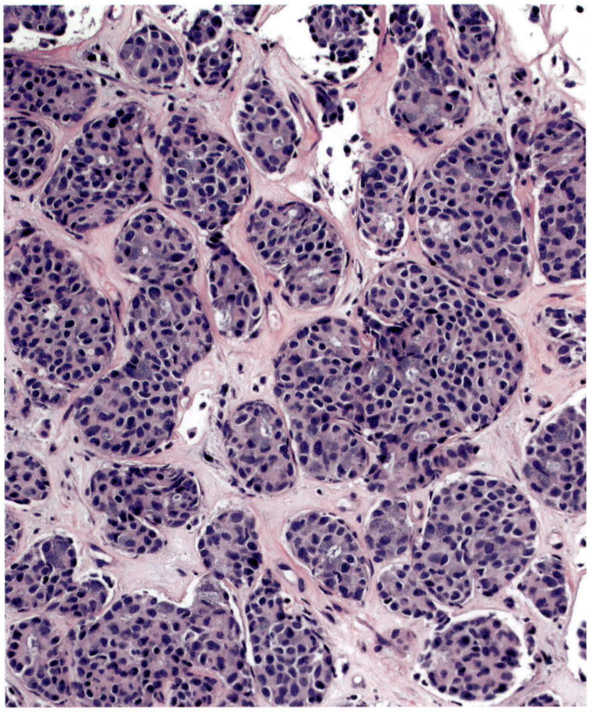

Figure 10-33

LUNG ADENOCARCINOMA: METASTATIC TO LIVER

Gland formation is seen, but the histologic findings are otherwise nondescript.

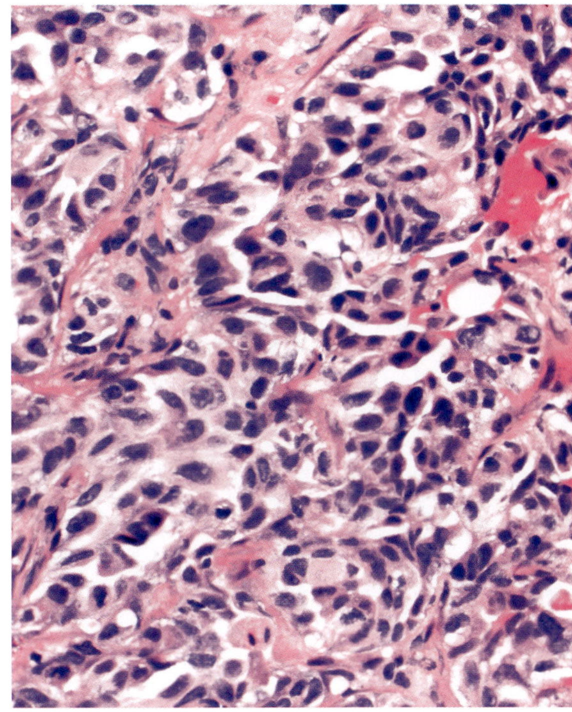

Figure 10-34

LUNG ADENOCARCINOMA: METASTATIC TO LIVER

The tumor is poorly differentiated, but there was a history of lung adenocarcinoma and the tumor is positive for napsin and TTF1.

OCT4 positive embryonal carcinoma (C-KIT negative, CD30 positive). Immunostains for glypican 3, alpha-fetoprotein (AFP), and human chorionic gonadotropin (HCG) are then used to further separate the OCT4-negative tumors, as yolk sac tumors are positive for glypican 3 and AFP, but negative for HCG, whereas choriocarcinomas are HCG positive (fig. 10-32B) but AFP negative, and show variable staining for glypican 3 (fig. 10-32C).

Lung Adenocarcinoma

Primary lung carcinoma is one of the more frequent carcinomas to metastasize to the liver (fig. 10-33). When the clinical findings and the chest imaging findings are consistent with a lung primary, the liver metastases are often not biopsied. In other cases, the clinical and imaging findings are more complicated and other carcinomas are in the differential, including intrahepatic cholangiocarcinoma.

Metastatic lung adenocarcinomas typically do not have the dense desmoplastic response found with many cholangiocarcinomas. Gland formation can be inconspicuous in poorly differentiated tumor deposits (fig. 10-34). Immunostains are helpful, as metastatic lung adenocarcinoma is typically positive for TTF1 (nuclear) and/or napsin-A, while intrahepatic cholangiocarcinomas are negative. However, an important caveat is that about one third of extrahepatic cholangiocarcinomas and gallbladder adenocarcinomas are positive for nuclear TTF1 and about 10 percent are napsin-A positive (36). Cytoplasmic staining for TTF1 is common in hepatocellular carcinomas (80). Nuclear staining is found in about 4 percent of colorectal carcinomas (70).

Neuroendocrine Tumors/Carcinomas

About 5 percent of metastatic neuroendocrine tumors to the liver are hormonally active and can lead to the carcinoid syndrome. The most common secreted hormones are serotonin and kallikrein, which have vasoactive properties. Components of the carcinoid syndrome include rapid heartbeat, asthma-like breathing

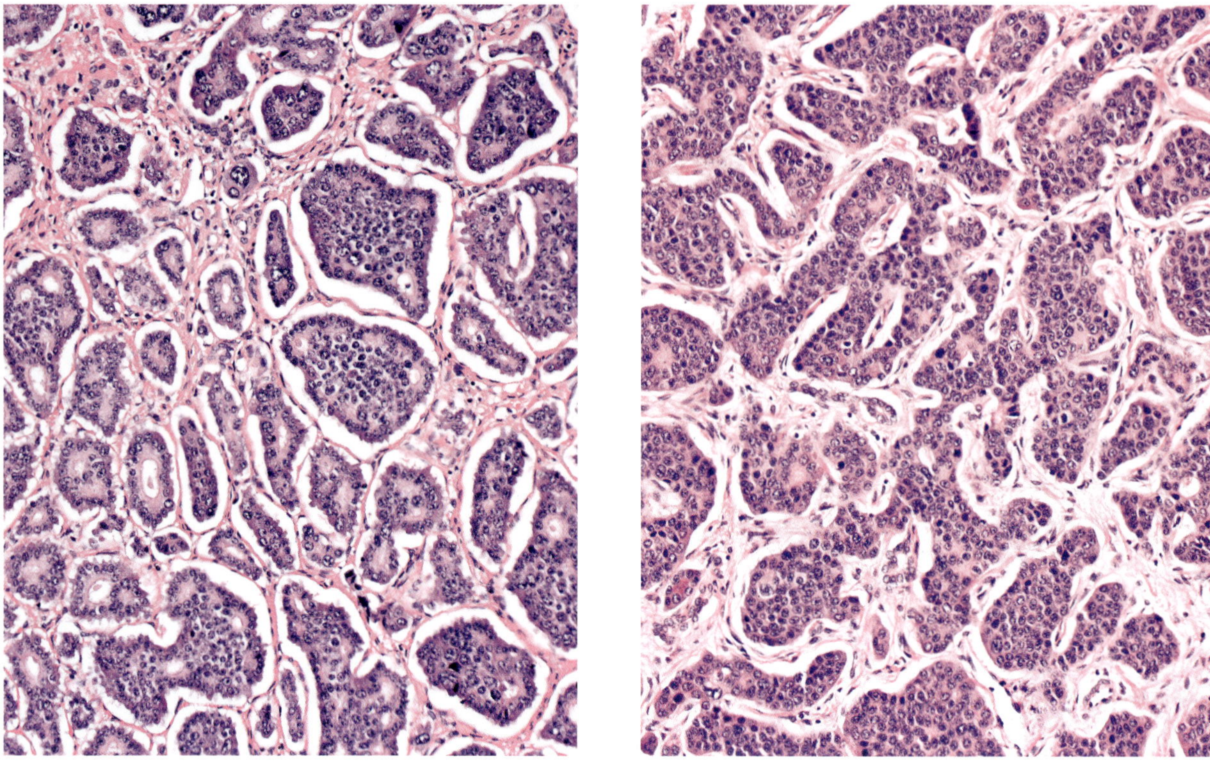

Figure 10-35

NEUROENDOCRINE TUMOR: METASTATIC TO LIVER

Left: This tumor has a mixed nested and pseudoglandular growth pattern.
Right: The tumor has a trabecular growth pattern.

difficulty, diarrhea, and varying degrees of skin flushing. Diarrhea and skin flushing are the most common symptoms. The skin flushing can last from a few minutes to hours and is most prominent on the head and upper chest. The flushing can be triggered by a number of disparate activities, although many cases will have no obvious trigger. Triggers, when identified, range from exercising to stress. The diagnosis of carcinoid syndrome is confirmed by measuring the urine levels of 5-hydroxyindoleacetic acid (5-HIAA), a degradation product of serotonin.

Most neuroendocrine tumors associated with the carcinoid syndrome arise in the gastrointestinal tract. In the primary tumor, the vasoactive hormones serotonin and kallikrein are secreted into the portal blood flow, but the hormones are degraded by the liver. However, when tumors metastasize to the liver, the hormones largely escape liver metabolism and cause symptoms when they reach the systemic circulation.

The morphologic findings in metastatic neuroendocrine tumors are essentially the same as in primary tumors. Growth patterns vary from nested, to trabeculae, to solid sheets of cells (fig. 10-35). Cytologic atypia ranges from minimal in well-differentiated neuroendocrine tumors to striking in poorly differentiated non-small cell neuroendocrine carcinomas. Neuroendocrine tumors that secrete insulin can be surrounded by a rim of hepatocytes with macrovesicular steatosis, even if there is no fatty liver disease in the background liver (81).

Immunostains for both CK7 and CK20 can be negative in metastatic neuroendocrine tumors, depending on the site of origin (Table 10-6), as can other broad spectrum keratins such as Oscar or CKAE1/AE3. CAM5.2 is positive in most cases, as are CK17 and CK19 (82). Tumor differentiation plays a role in the sensitivity of neuroendocrine markers: the sensitivity for chromogranin drops as tumors become less

Table 10-6

IMMUNOHISTOCHEMICAL STAINING PATTERNS (NUMBERS DENOTING PERCENTAGE OF POSITIVE CASES) FOR NON-SMALL CELL NEUROENDOCRINE TUMORS AND CARCINOMAS[a]

Tumor Primary	CK7	CK20	TTF1	CDX2	Islet-1	PAX8	PDX1
Lung	60	<5	40	<5	10	10	10
Pancreas	50	30	<5	<5	90	80	60
Stomach	10	20	<5	<5	10	10	70
Duodenum/jejunum	10	20	<5	<5	90	90	70
Ileum	10	20	<5	90	10	<5	<5
Appendix	10	20	<5	100	10	20	<5
Appendix: goblet cell carcinoid	70	100	insufficient data	insufficient data	insufficient data	insufficient data	insufficient data
Colon	10	40	<5	70	10	20	<5
Rectum	10	40	<5	20	90	80	20

[a]While there are many exceptions, this can be a useful starting point.

well differentiated (83). Many tumors are also positive for CD56, but overall this stain is less useful than chromogranin and synaptophysin, because CD56 is positive in so many non-neuroendocrine carcinomas. Cases initially diagnosed as neuroendocrine carcinoma based solely on CD56 positivity, without compatible morphology, often turn out to have a different diagnosis upon further workup and clinical follow-up. Neuroendocrine tumors are distinguished from neuroendocrine carcinomas based on cytologic atypia; they are graded by Ki-67 or mitotic count according to the WHO criteria (Table 10-5).

The site of tumor origin can be suggested by additional immunostains (Table 10-6): TTF1 staining suggests a lung primary (except for small cell carcinomas, which are often TTF1 positive regardless of site of origin) and CDX2 suggests an appendix, colon, or pancreas primary. Islet-1 and PAX8 are sensitive markers for a pancreas primary, but data on specificity are mixed (84–86). One study reported Islet-1 staining in 90 percent of pancreatic neuroendocrine tumors, 89 percent of duodenal neuroendocrine tumors, 100 percent of rectal neuroendocrine tumors, 38 percent of colonic neuroendocrine tumors, 14 percent of neuroendocrine tumors of the appendix, and 6 percent of ileal neuroendocrine tumors (87). PAX8 is also positive in other gut primaries, including approximately 80 percent of rectal neuroendocrine tumors (85,88). Overall, PAX8 and Islet-1 do not have strong pancreas specificity, but still can be clinically useful, as ileal neuroendocrine tumors are negative in most cases (88). One study found that about 80 percent of well-differentiated rectal neuroendocrine tumors are prostate-specific acid phosphatase (PSAP) positive (89), but the ability of this marker to suggest a rectal primary has not been further established. Follow-up studies have shown that the majority of neuroendocrine tumors (about 85 percent) with no primary site identified on imaging studies arise in the small bowel, in particular the ileum, an observation that can help target surgical exploration (90).

Rarely, neuroendocrine tumors thought to be primary to the liver have been reported, including well-differentiated neuroendocrine tumors, neuroendocrine carcinomas, and small cell carcinomas (91–94). However, because there is no marker or histologic finding that indicates a hepatic primary, the conclusion is based on excluding origin from another site, primarily by imaging studies and endoscopy. Neither imaging studies nor endoscopy can completely exclude another primary site because primary tumors are sometimes below the size detection capabilities of these modalities. For these reasons, neuroendocrine tumors primary to the liver remain controversial and challenging to document.

Some neuroendocrine carcinomas can mimic hepatocellular carcinoma on H&E stains and some can even be HepPar1 (up to 10 percent) and rarely AFP positive (95), but arginase is

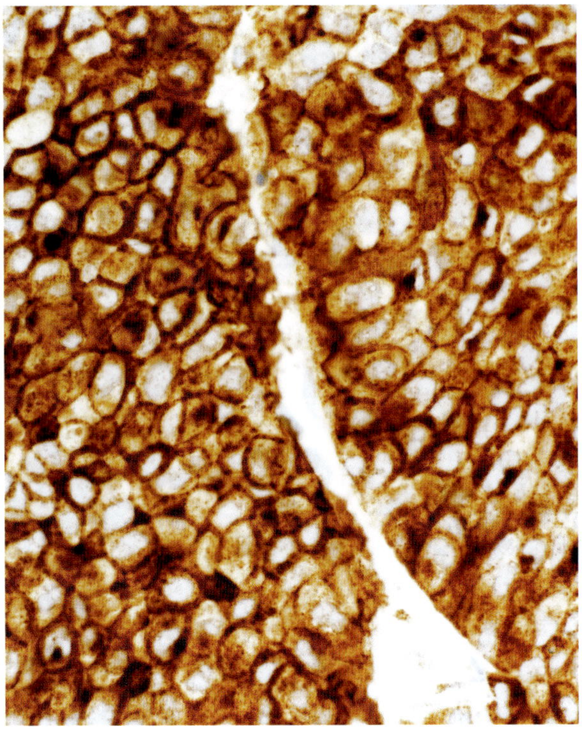

Figure 10-36

NEUROENDOCRINE CARCINOMA: METASTATIC TO LIVER

A glypican 3 immunostain is strongly positive.

typically negative. Glypican 3 is also commonly positive in Merkel cell carcinoma (96) and occasionally in other neuroendocrine carcinomas (fig. 10-36). Other important diagnostic pitfalls revolve around aberrant expression of neuroendocrine markers in non-neuroendocrine tumors. For example, some melanomas are synaptophysin positive (97), especially those with epithelioid morphology, where up to a third of cases can show synaptophysin staining (98). Adrenal cortical carcinomas are often synaptophysin positive. Another important diagnostic pitfall is treated prostate carcinomas, where biopsies of liver metastases can show extensive neuroendocrine differentiation (99). Some angiosarcomas are strongly positive for synaptophysin (fig. 10-37). Pancreatic acinar cell carcinomas often show patchy staining for synaptophysin or chromogranin and are easily mistaken for neuroendocrine carcinomas. Thus, the diagnosis of metastatic neuroendocrine tumors should be confirmed both by positive staining for chromogranin and/or synaptophysin and by negative staining for other markers, chosen based on the H&E morphology. Most diagnostic misclassifications come from relying on too small of a panel of stains or not carefully correlating the immunohistochemical findings with the morphology.

Individuals with neuroendocrine tumors metastatic to the liver may be candidates for liver transplantation. The major selection criteria are based on the 2007 Milan Criteria and the 2012 European Neuroendocrine Tumor Society guidelines (100,101). These guidelines select for patients with well-differentiated neuroendocrine tumors (WHO grades 1 and 2) with diffuse hepatic metastases (but less than 50 percent of hepatic parenchyma replaced by tumor) that are refractory to standard surgical or medical therapies and in whom the primary neuroendocrine tumor has been removed, with stable disease for 6 months. The primary neuroendocrine tumor should be in sites drained by the portal vein circulation.

Small Cell Carcinoma

Small cell carcinomas that are metastatic to the liver look and stain essentially the same as they do in any other organ (fig. 10-38). Tumor cells are small to medium sized, with minimal cytoplasm. They have hyperchromatic nuclei with smudgy chromatin, indistinct nucleoli, and nuclear molding. Mitotic activity is brisk and apoptotic cells are numerous. Ki-67 staining is greater than 90 percent. The tumor cells grow in sheets, ribbons, and clusters and can be associated with a dense desmoplastic response. In most cases, distinct mass lesions are evident on imaging studies, but rarely small cell carcinoma can present with hepatomegaly and acute liver failure, with no mass lesions (102,103). With this presentation, the sinusoids show diffuse and striking involvement by the small cell carcinoma.

Most small cell carcinomas are positive for chromogranin or synaptophysin. Small cell carcinomas are frequently TTF1 positive regardless of the site of origin (104,105), but small cell carcinomas of the lung have a higher frequency of staining compared to non-lung primaries. Sometimes the biopsy or aspirate can "lose" the small cell carcinoma, leaving behind loose connective tissue and fibrosis with only rare

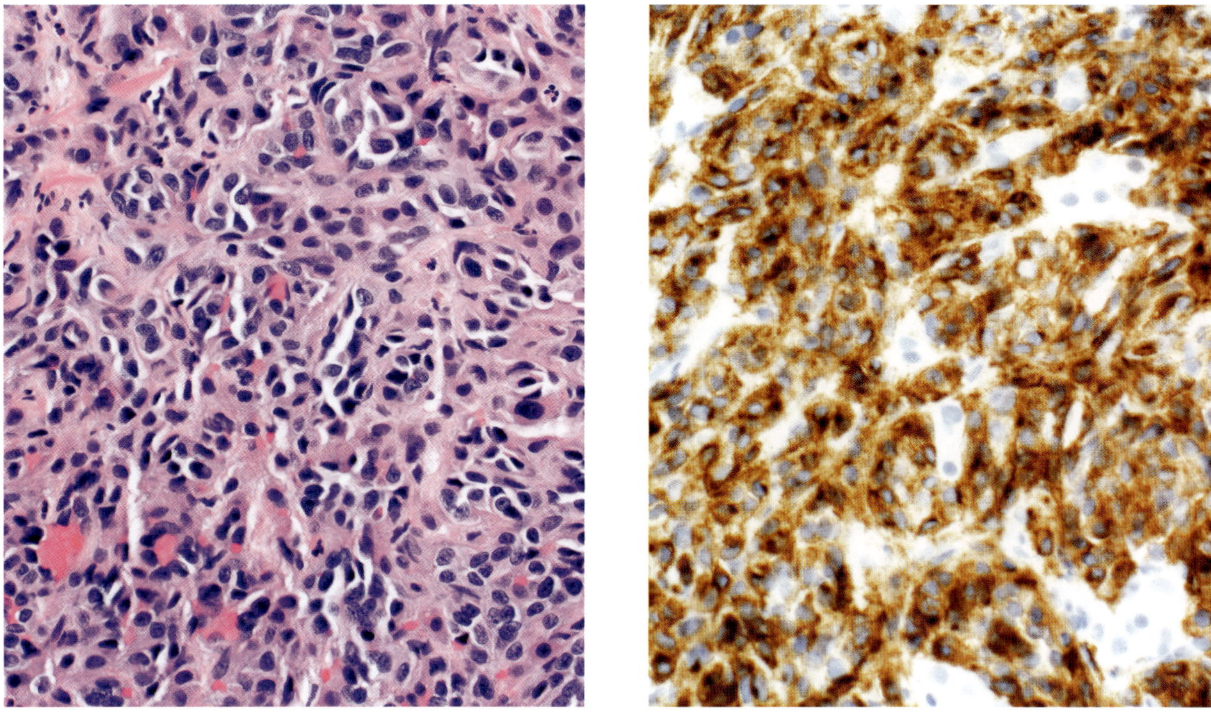

Figure 10-37

ANGIOSARCOMA: METASTATIC TO LIVER

Left: The angiosarcoma has a solid growth pattern with scattered slit-like openings. Right: The angiosarcoma is strongly synaptophysin positive.

tumor cells on the H&E-stained slide (fig. 10-39). If this pattern is seen on a biopsy, immunostains for chromogranin or synaptophysin are very helpful in identifying the tumor.

Small cell carcinomas metastatic to the liver arise from many organs, although lung and gastrointestinal tract are the most common. Colonic adenomas and carcinomas can also be associated with a small cell carcinoma component. In this setting, it is frequently the small cell component that metastasizes to the liver (fig. 10-40). Finally, small cell carcinomas can be part of combined primary tumors of the liver (see chapter 3).

Paraganglioma

Paragangliomas, both extra-adrenal and pheochromocytomas, can closely resemble ordinary neuroendocrine tumors (fig. 10-41) and are synaptophysin and chromogranin positive. A major difference is that essentially all epithelial neuroendocrine tumors are CAM5.2 positive, while paragangliomas are generally negative. S-100 protein immunostains

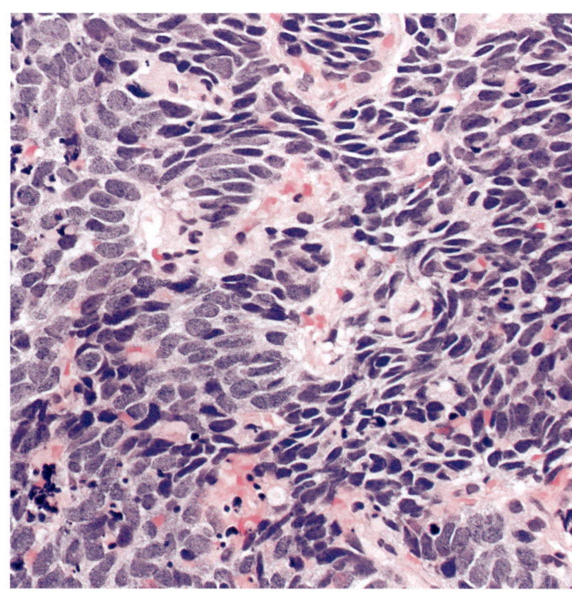

Figure 10-38

SMALL CELL CARCINOMA: METASTATIC TO LIVER

The typical cytologic findings are seen: scant cytoplasm, nuclear molding, and smudgy chromatin.

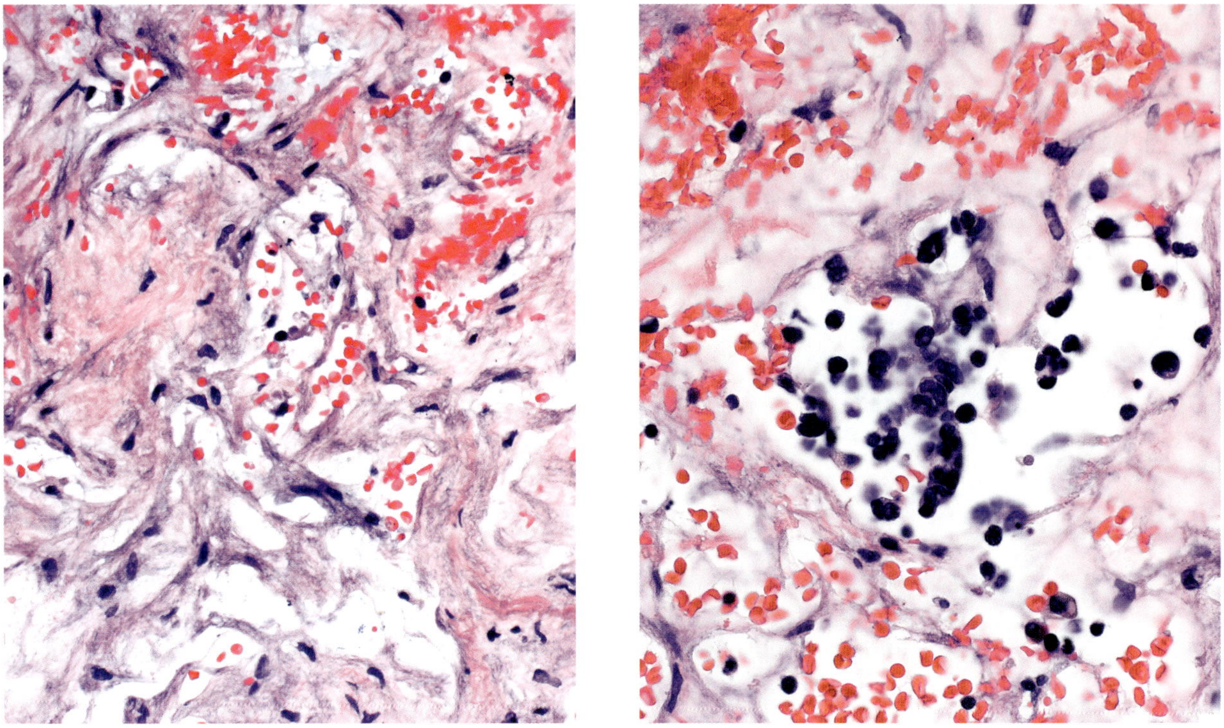

Figure 10-39

SMALL CELL CARCINOMA: METASTATIC TO LIVER

Left: Most of the tumor cells were lost during the aspiration and the specimen is largely acellular, with admixed loose connective tissue and fibrosis.

Right: Only rare scattered tumor cells are seen.

occasionally highlight sustentacular cells, but most cases are negative.

Pancreatic Carcinoma

Pancreatic ductal adenocarcinomas are usually gland forming (fig. 10-42), but can be poorly differentiated carcinomas, growing in sheets or, rarely, diffusely infiltrating the sinusoids (fig. 10-43). Their immunostain profile shows sufficient overlap with biliary and upper gastrointestinal primaries that a prioritized differential can be the best approach for the surgical pathology report. They are typically CK7 positive and variably positive for CDX2 and CK20. DPC4 staining is lost in about 50 percent of pancreatic ductal adenocarcinomas, but the loss is not specific for a pancreatic origin, and is found in about the same number of cholangiocarcinomas and about one third of carcinomas arising in the ampulla of Vater (57).

Pancreatic acinar cell carcinomas grow with acinar formation (fig. 10-44) or as broad sheets, with subtle or nonexistent acinar structures (fig. 10-45, left). The H&E findings can resemble those of neuroendocrine tumors, and both tumors can be synaptophysin and/or chromogranin positive, forming an important diagnostic pitfall. Prominent nucleoli, distinctly granular cytoplasm, and acinar-type structures favor acinar cell carcinoma. Additional stains can solidify the diagnosis, as acinar cell carcinomas are positive for trypsin (fig. 10-45, right) and chymotrypsin. About one third of acinar cell carcinomas show scattered cells that are positive for synaptophysin and/or chromogranin; if more than 30 percent of the cells are positive, the tumor is classified as mixed acinar-endocrine carcinoma. About 5 percent of acinar cell carcinomas are AFP positive by immunohistochemistry and have elevated serum AFP levels. In addition, about 60 percent of acinar cell carcinomas are glypican 3 positive (106). Rare acinar carcinomas primary to the liver have also been reported (107,108). Acinar cell carcinomas of the pancreas

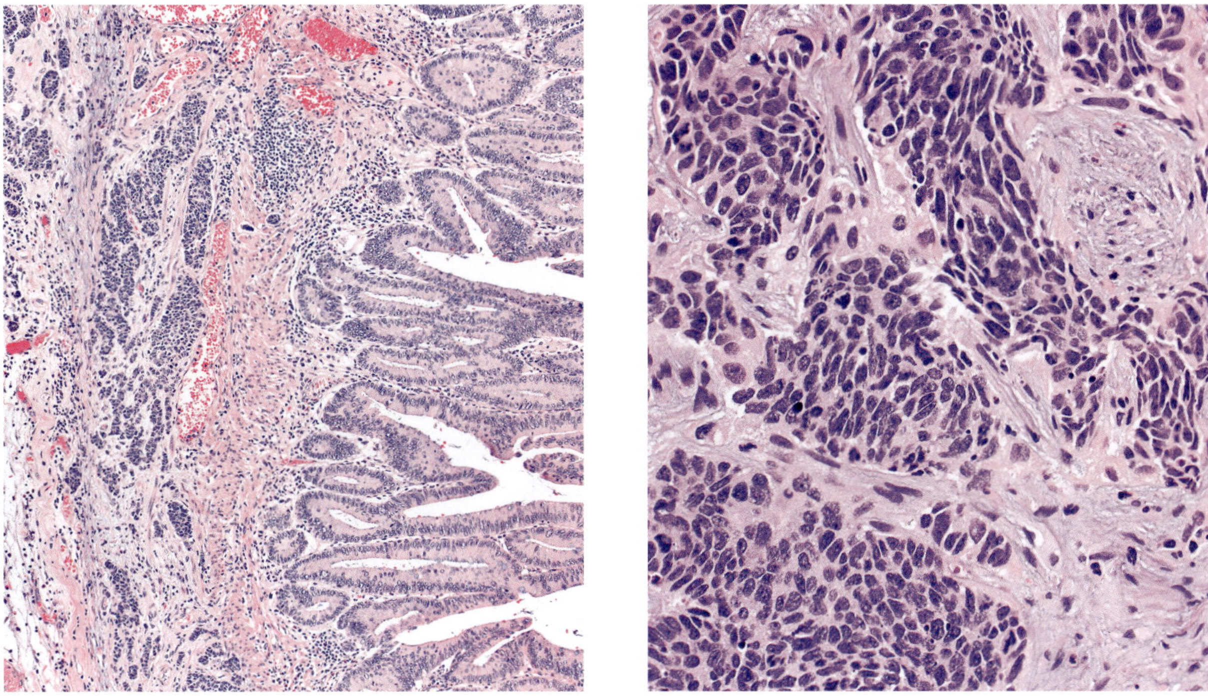

Figure 10-40

COLONIC TUBULAR ADENOMA WITH SMALL CELL COMPONENT

Left: The small cell component is directly below the adenoma.
Right: The small cell carcinoma component metastasized to the liver.

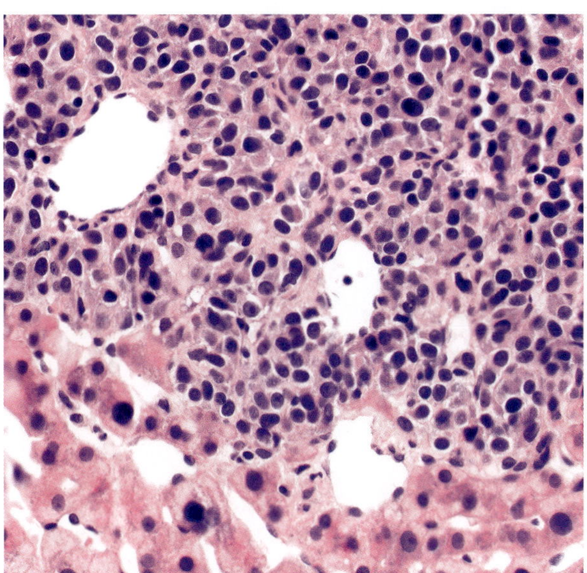

Figure 10-41

METASTATIC PARAGANGLIOMA

This metastatic paraganglioma is positive for synaptophysin and chromogranin but negative for CAM5.2.

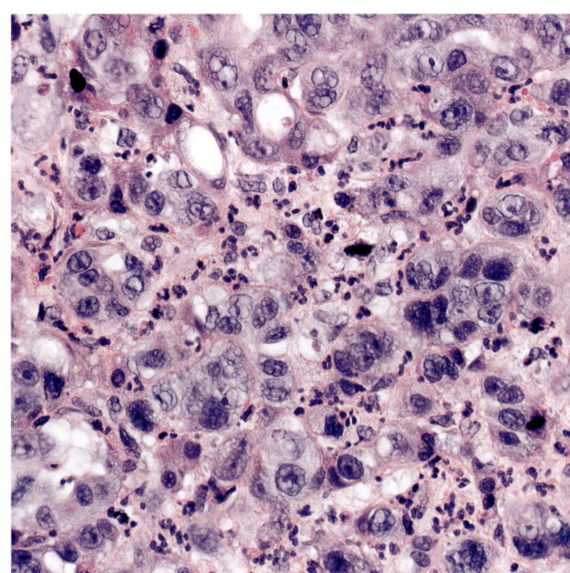

Figure 10-42

PANCREAS DUCTAL ADENOCARCINOMA: METASTATIC TO THE LIVER

Occasional glands are present in this metastatic ductal adenocarcinoma, which also has a brisk neutrophilic infiltrate.

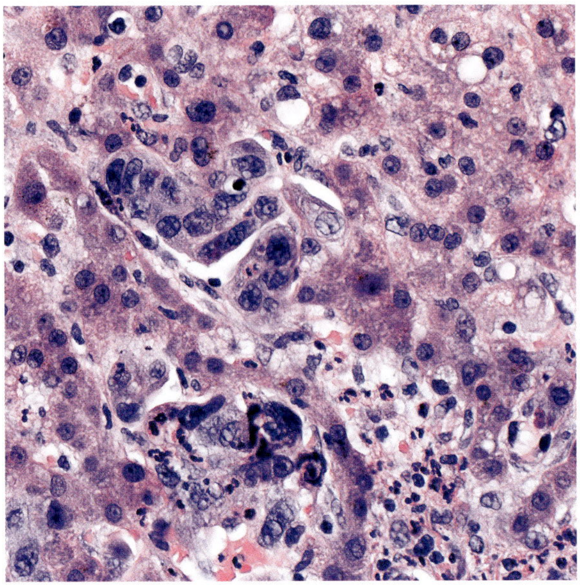

Figure 10-43

PANCREAS DUCTAL ADENOCARCINOMA: METASTATIC TO THE LIVER

This poorly differentiated pancreas carcinoma extensively permeated the liver sinusoids.

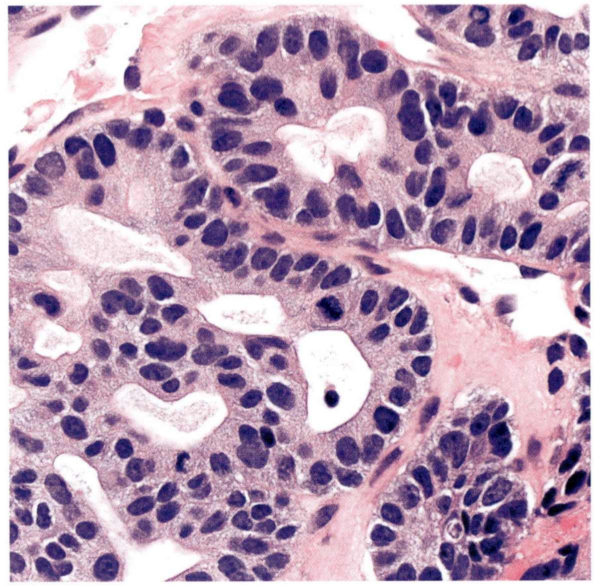

Figure 10-44

PANCREAS ACINAR CELL CARCINOMA: METASTATIC TO LIVER

Gland-like acinar growth is seen.

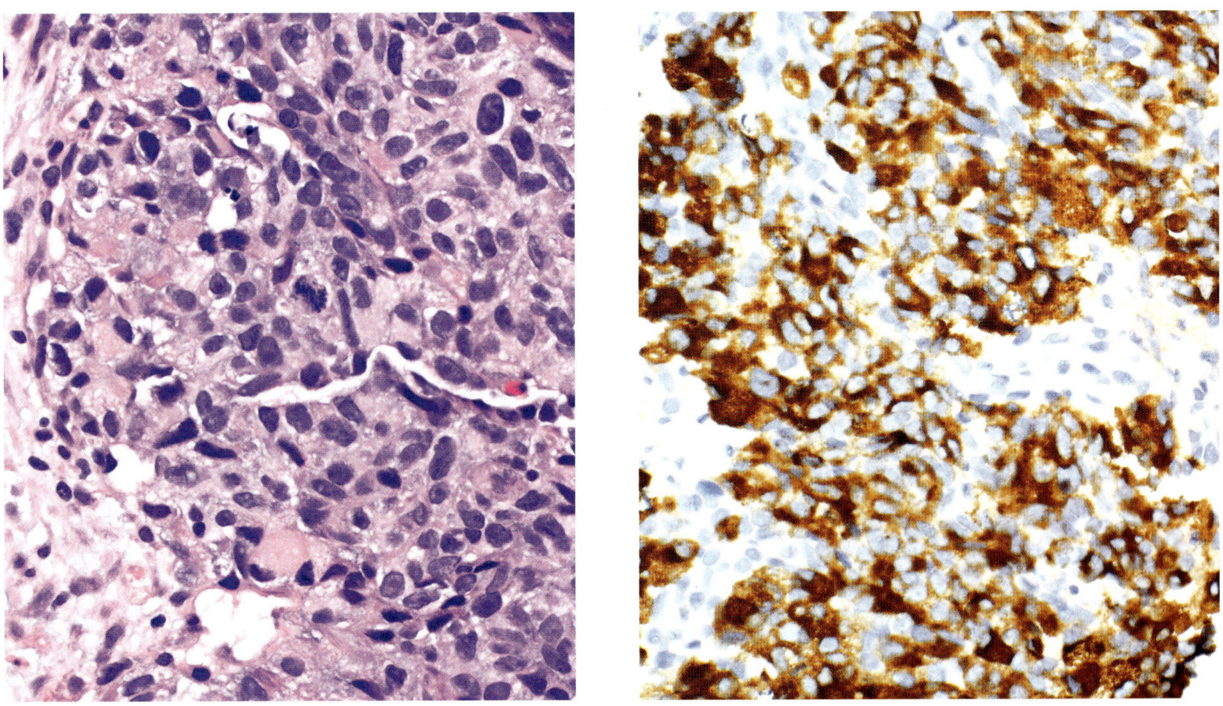

Figure 10-45

PANCREAS ACINAR CELL CARCINOMA: METASTATIC TO LIVER

Left: This case has a solid growth pattern.
Right: An immunostain for trypsin is strongly positive.

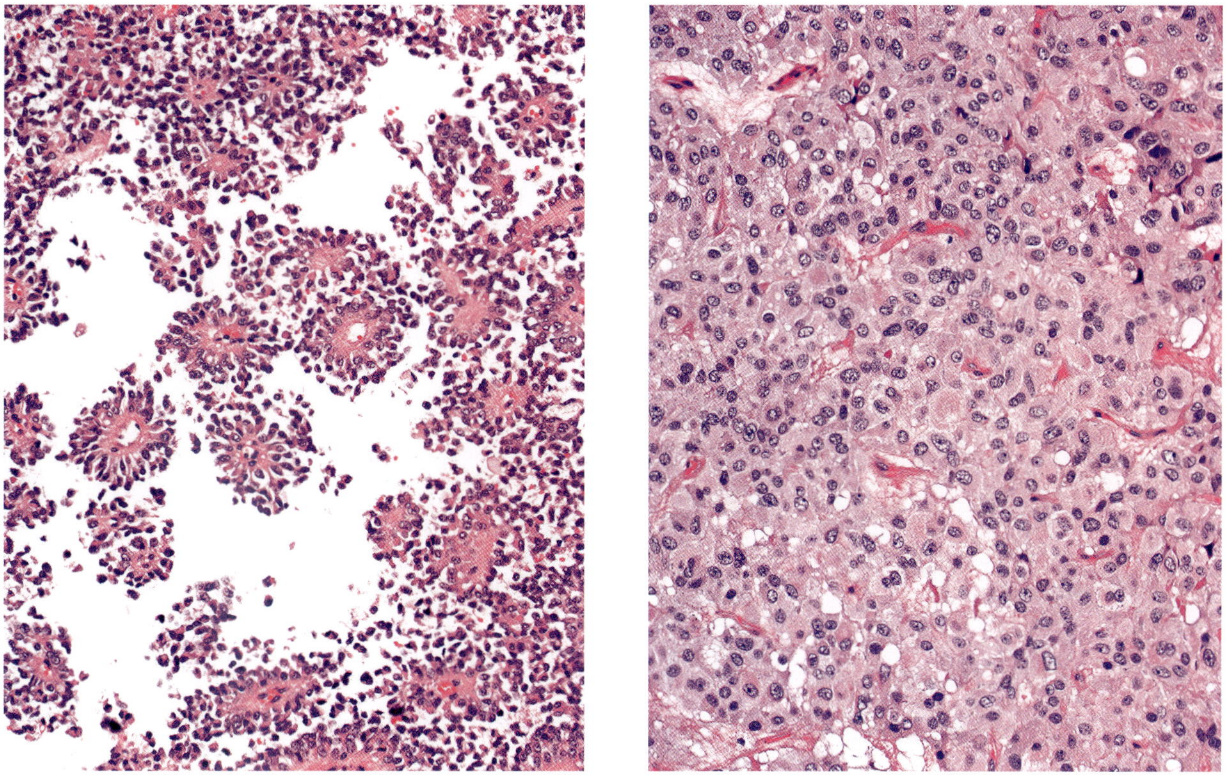

Figure 10-46

PANCREAS SOLID PSEUDOPAPILLARY NEOPLASM

Left: In this area, the cells are discohesive, with residual tumor cells around fibrosis cores, forming pseudopapillary structures. Right: The tumor has a solid growth pattern.

can be aggressive and a significant number of cases have liver metastases at presentation. Thus, a pancreatic primary has to be carefully excluded before entertaining a diagnosis of a primary acinar cell carcinoma of the liver.

Pancreatic solid pseudopapillary neoplasms that metastasize to the liver can grow in solid sheets or with a pseudopapillary architecture (fig. 10-46). The tumor cells are polygonal, with abundant amphophilic to eosinophilic cytoplasm, finely distributed chromatin, and inconspicuous nucleoli. In some cases the tumors cells have cytoplasmic vacuolization, mimicking the fat that can be seen in some hepatocellular carcinomas (see fig. 10-10). While not present in all cases, other clues to the diagnosis include periodic acid–Schiff (PAS)-positive cytoplasmic hyaline globules (which are positive for alpha-1-antitrypsin) and nuclear longitudinal grooves. The stroma surrounding the vessels can become densely hyalinized. Pseudopapillae form in areas secondary to degenerative changes. In some metastatic deposits, there are high-grade areas with sarcomatoid differentiation. Immunostains are positive for CD10, CD56, and progesterone. Beta-catenin is positive for nuclear staining. Keratin staining is variable, with most tumors staining for CKAE1/AE3 and CAM5.2, but negative for CK7. Rare solid pseudopapillary neoplasms thought to be primary to the liver have also been reported (109,110).

Pancreatoblastomas are rare tumors in general and thus are rarely encountered as biopsies of metastatic disease to the liver. They have a mixed differentiation pattern, with areas of acinar, neuroendocrine, and squamous differentiation. Finding the areas of squamous differentiation is the key to recognizing this tumor (fig. 10-47). Pancreatoblastomas are positive for keratins and show variable staining for markers of neuroendocrine (synaptophysin, chromogranin) and acinar (trypsin) differentiation.

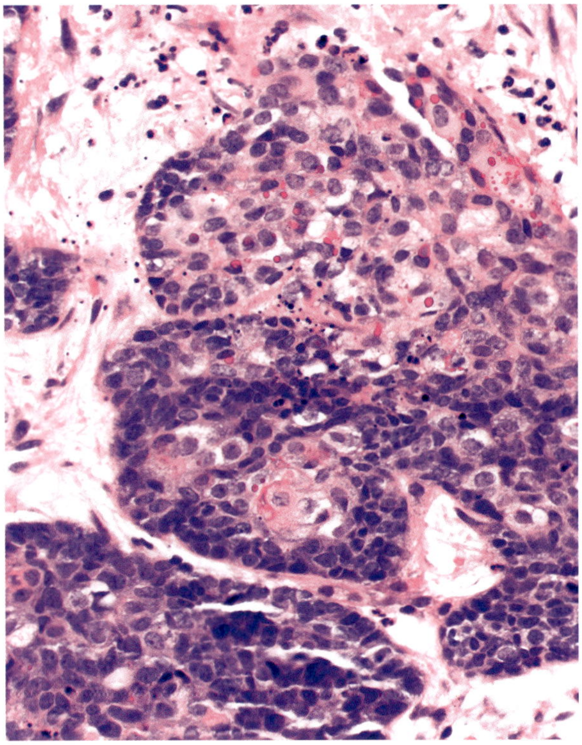

Figure 10-47

PANCREATOBLASTOMA: METASTATIC TO LIVER

The tumor shows focal squamous differentiation.

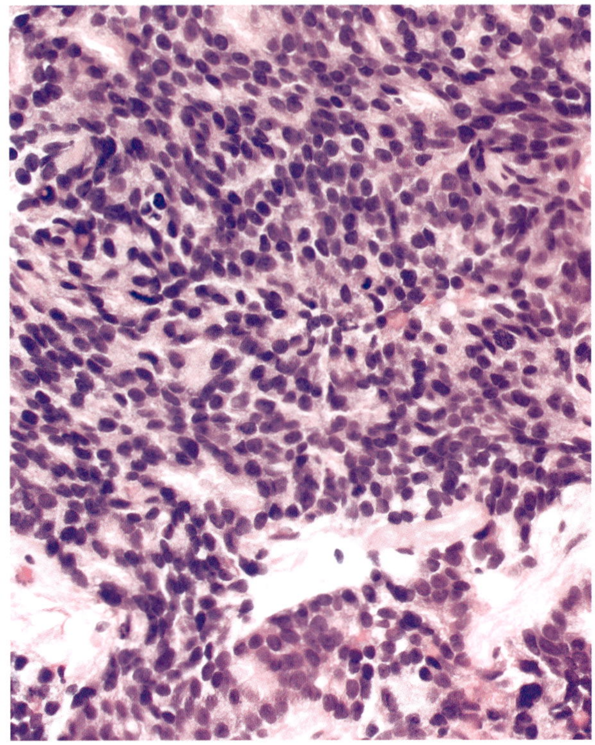

Figure 10-48

PROSTATE ADENOCARCINOMA: METASTATIC TO LIVER

The tumor is poorly differentiated with inconspicuous glands. The diagnosis was confirmed by strong PSA staining.

Prostate Adenocarcinoma

Prostate adenocarcinomas are typically gland forming, even in metastatic deposits, but occasionally grow as sheets of poorly differentiated cells with only vague or nonexistent gland formation (fig. 10-48). Immunostains for CK7 and CK20 are generally negative in lower Gleason grade lesions, but both stains show an increasing frequency of positivity as the tumors become less well differentiated, approaching 50 percent in high-grade tumors. Even in these cases, however, the keratin staining is typically focal and not diffuse (111). Immunostains for prostate-specific antigen (PSA) and prostate-specific acid phosphatase (PSAP) are typically positive. Nuclear staining with ERG can also be found in prostate carcinoma, where it correlates, albeit imperfectly, with the *TMPRSS2-ERG* gene fusion (112). The sensitivity of ERG as a broad marker of prostate carcinoma is low, at about 50 percent, although the frequency of staining increases with increasing Gleason grade (113).

Treated prostate adenocarcinomas, especially following androgen deprivation therapy, can show neuroendocrine differentiation, with positivity for chromogranin and synaptophysin, thereby mimicking neuroendocrine carcinomas (114). Immunostains for PSA and PSAP often show weaker and patchier staining in this setting. Nonetheless, some degree of positive staining for PSA or PSAP, along with an appropriate clinical history, is useful in making a firm diagnosis. Additional histologic findings that suggest the correct diagnosis include residual gland formation and nuclear cytology that is not a good fit for typical neuroendocrine neoplasms, with more nuclear pleomorphism, coarser chromatin, and more prominent nucleoli than found in usual neuroendocrine tumors, and even most neuroendocrine carcinomas.

Renal Carcinoma

Clear cell carcinomas and chromophobe carcinomas both metastasize to the liver. Clear

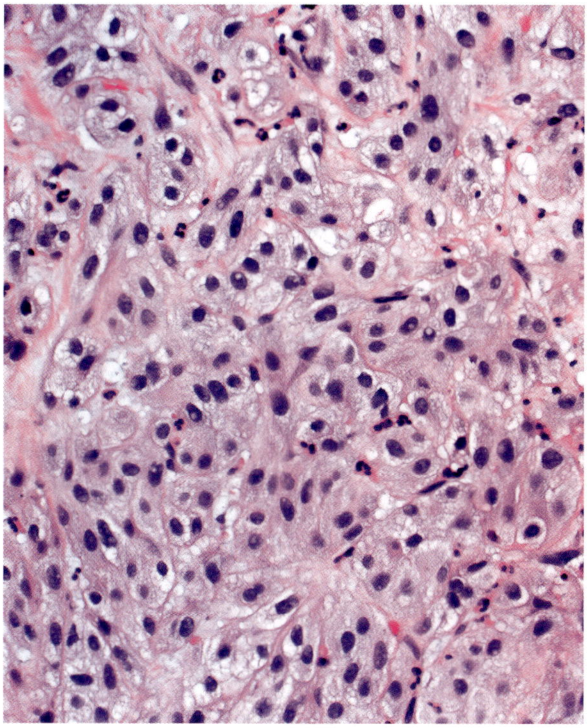

Figure 10-49

CLEAR CELL RENAL CARCINOMA: METASTATIC TO THE LIVER

The tumor cells have abundant clear cytoplasm. HepPar1 and arginase stains were negative, ruling out clear cell hepatocellular carcinoma.

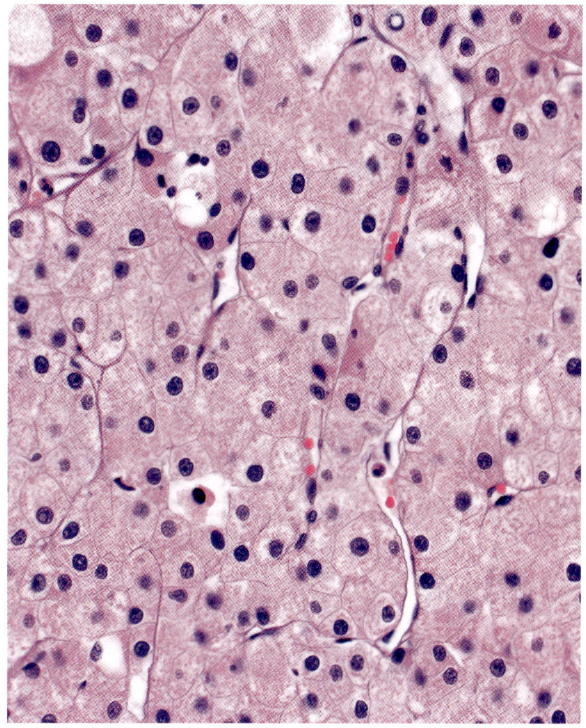

Figure 10-50

CHROMOPHOBE RENAL CELL CARCINOMA: METASTATIC TO THE LIVER

This tumor looks a lot like well-differentiated hepatocellular carcinoma.

cell carcinomas can mimic clear cell hepatocellular carcinoma (fig. 10-49), but negative stains for HepPar1 and arginase, along with positive staining for PAX8, clarify the diagnosis. Chromophobe renal carcinomas can be particularly challenging mimics of well differentiated hepatocellular carcinoma, growing in thickened trabeculae and composed of tumor cells with abundant eosinophilic cytoplasm (fig. 10-50). Chromophobe carcinomas are HepPar1 and arginase negative, but PAX8 positive (fig. 10-51).

Transitional Cell Carcinoma and Squamous Cell Carcinoma

Rarely, squamous cell carcinomas are primary to the liver, either as a cholangiocarcinoma with squamous differentiation (115) or as a pure squamous cell carcinoma (116,117). However, most squamous carcinomas in the liver are metastatic (fig. 10-52). In fact, autopsy studies identify squamous cell carcinomas as one of the most common histologic types to metastasize to the liver, where cervical cancer is a common primary. However, the primary sites for squamous cell carcinomas are often evident from clinical findings and imaging studies. For these reasons, squamous cell carcinomas are less commonly encountered as biopsy material. When biopsied, the tumor cells tend to have abundant cytoplasm with well-defined cell borders.

Urothelial carcinomas also metastasize to the liver. When they are well or moderately differentiated, the morphologic findings are fairly straightforward, but poorly differentiated malignancies may be more difficult to recognize. Immunohistochemistry helps with the correct diagnosis. Both urothelial and squamous carcinomas are positive for CK5/6, p63, and p40. GATA3 stains many different tumors, but suggests a urothelial origin in malignancies with squamous differentiation (118,119). Uroplakin III positivity can also suggest a urothelial origin, but is less sensitive than GATA3 (118).

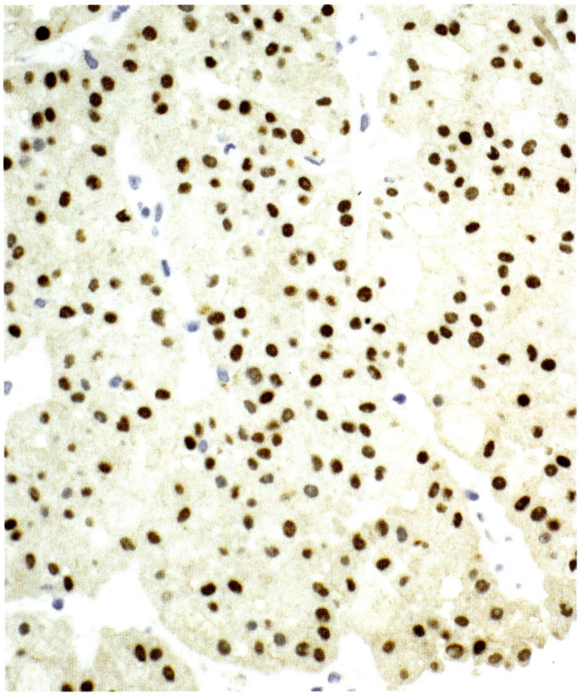

Figure 10-51

CHROMOPHOBE RENAL CELL CARCINOMA: PAX8

The tumor is strongly and diffusely positive.

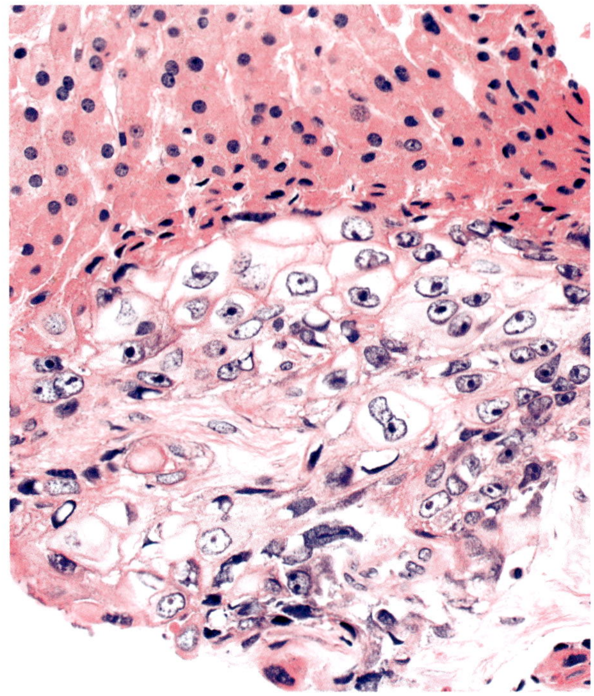

Figure 10-52

SQUAMOUS CELL CARCINOMA: METASTATIC TO THE LIVER

The tumor cells show eosinophilic, glassy cytoplasm and were strongly positive for p40.

METASTATIC SARCOMAS

Gastrointestinal Stromal Tumors and Leiomyosarcomas

The most common metastatic sarcomas to the liver are gastrointestinal stromal tumors (GISTs) and uterine leiomyosarcomas (120). Imaging and clinical findings, when available, often help clarify the differential diagnosis and focus subsequent choices of immunostains.

GISTs are typically spindled in their growth but also can show an epithelioid, myxoid, or a poorly differentiated pattern (fig. 10-53). They are positive for CD117 and DOG1 and negative for desmin (less than 1 percent positive). Immunostains for CD34 (positive in 70 percent of cases) and smooth muscle actin (positive in 30 percent) are not as sensitive or specific. In contrast, metastatic leiomyosarcomas (fig. 10-54) are positive for desmin (nearly 100 percent of cases) and smooth muscle actin, while negative for CD117 and DOG1.

Rare primary leiomyosarcomas of the liver arise from the smooth muscle layers of the inferior vena cava as it courses through the liver, and from there extend into the hepatic parenchyma, and in some cases into the heart. Because of the rarity of this tumor, little is known about risk factors. Initial imaging studies may show a solid mass consistent with a malignancy or may be mistaken for a liver abscess or tumor thrombus (121). In patients with acquired immunodeficiency syndrome (AIDS), the neoplasms can be Epstein-Barr virus (EBV) related (122). Long-term survival is possible with complete resection, but recurrent disease with a prolonged clinical course is common. For patients undergoing resection, the overall 5-year disease-free survival rate is 30 percent, while the 5-year total survival rate is 67 percent (123).

Desmoplastic Small Round Cell Tumor

This rare tumor affects predominately boys and young men. The tumor often grows as angulated nests in a dense desmoplastic background (fig. 10-55) and can mimic neuroendocrine

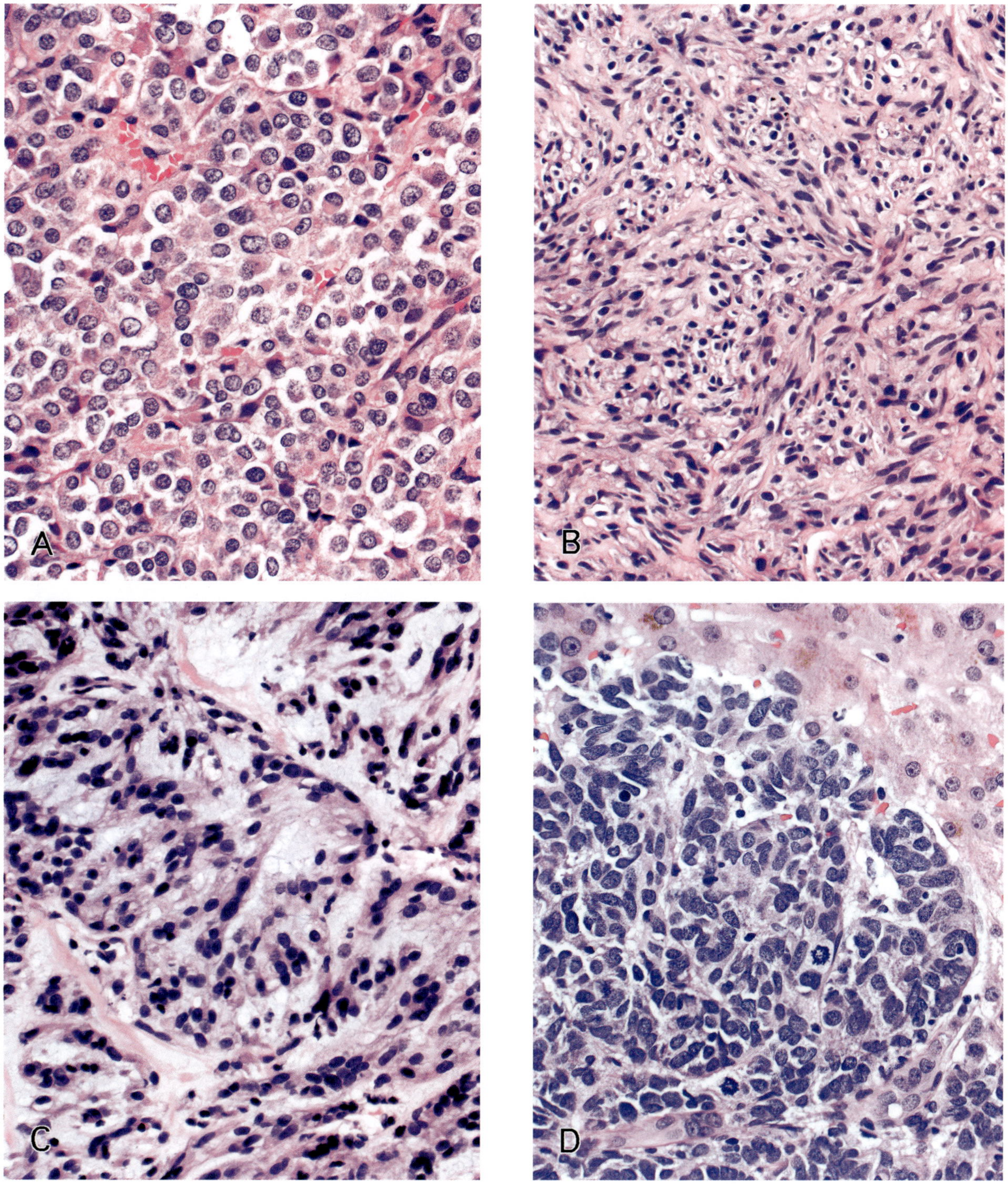

Figure 10-53

GASTROINTESTINAL STROMAL TUMOR (GIST): METASTATIC TO LIVER

A: The tumor has an epithelioid growth pattern.
B: This tumor shows a spindle cell growth pattern.
C: Extensive myxoid changes are seen.
D: This poorly differentiated GIST focally mimicked a neuroendocrine carcinoma.

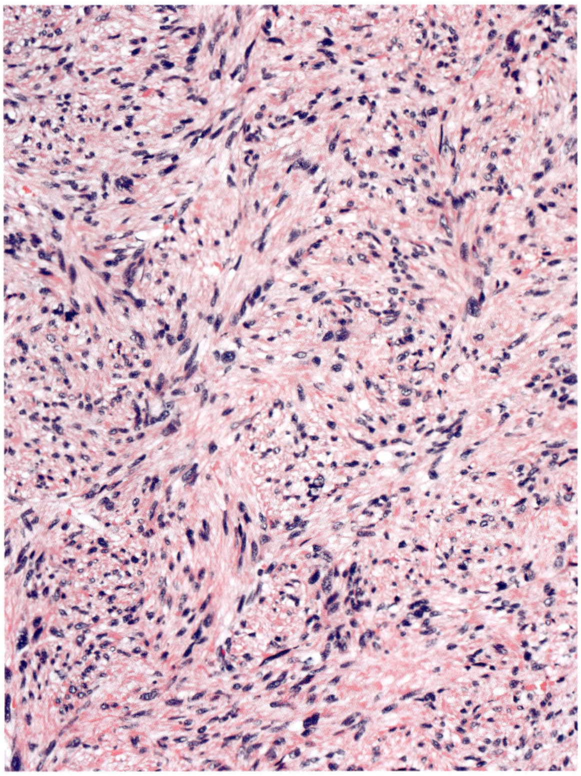

Figure 10-54

LEIOMYOSARCOMA: METASTATIC TO LIVER

The tumor shows fascicles of spindled cells.

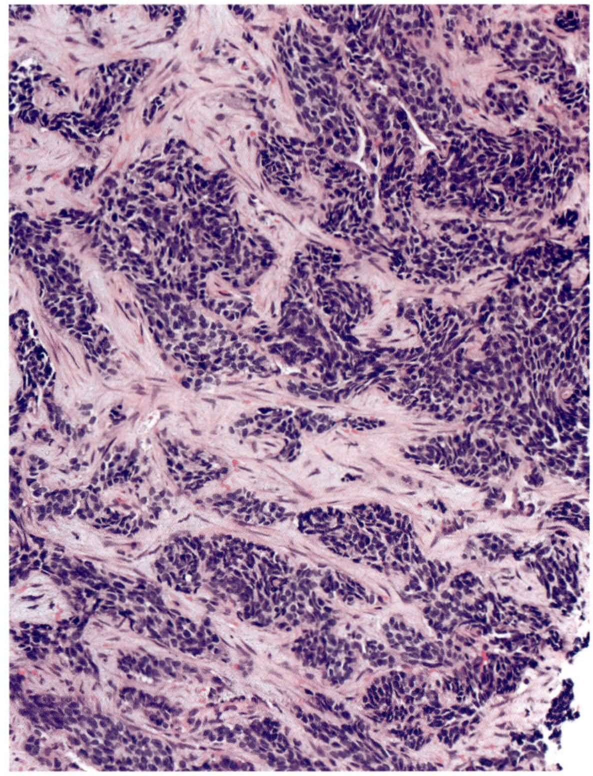

Figure 10-55

DESMOPLASTIC SMALL ROUND CELL TUMOR: METASTATIC TO LIVER

The tumor is growing in cords with a dense desmoplastic response.

carcinoma and cholangiocarcinoma. In some cases, there are metaplastic-type changes, with tubules, signet ring-like cells, rhabdoid-like cells, or squamous metaplasia. Cystic degeneration can occur. The tumor cells tend to have scant cytoplasm and the histology can suggest lymphoma. Mitotic figures are typically numerous.

Immunohistochemistry shows trilineage differentiation, with positive staining for markers of epithelial differentiation (pankeratins [fig. 10-56] and EMA); positive staining for mesenchymal markers (vimentin and desmin [fig. 10-57]), which is classically dot-like; and positive staining for markers of neuroendocrine differentiation (neuron-specific enolase [NSE]). WT1 is also positive and molecular studies show an *EWS-WT1* fusion.

Melanoma

Melanomas are challenging to diagnose because the tumor cells have a variety of morphologies, ranging from spindle cells to epithelioid cells (fig. 10-58) to rhabdoid cells (fig. 10-59). Pigment is present in some cases (fig. 10-60), but most cases are pigment negative. Melanomas are also challenging to recognize because of aberrant immunohistochemical findings. Occasional melanomas show focal positivity for cytokeratins, and some are synaptophysin positive and can be mistaken for neuroendocrine tumors (97), especially when they show epithelioid morphology (98). They may have unusual presentations, such as diffuse sinusoidal tumor infiltrates with elevated liver enzymes and other clinical findings that mimic acute hepatitis (fig. 10-61).

With a positive history of melanoma, a single stain can often confirm a diagnosis. In contrast, a panel approach is needed to fully exclude melanoma because of varying staining patterns, including cases that are S-100 protein negative. A useful staining panel includes S-100

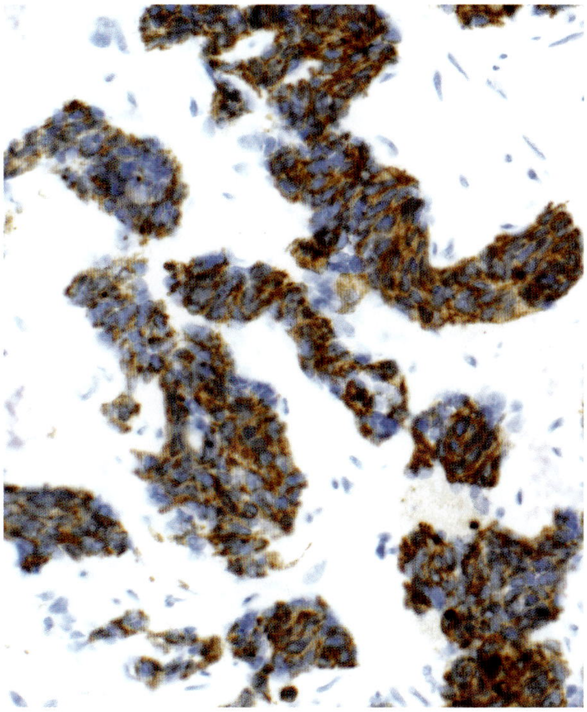

Figure 10-56

DESMOPLASTIC SMALL ROUND CELL TUMOR: METASTATIC TO LIVER

The tumor is diffusely positive for CKAE1/AE3.

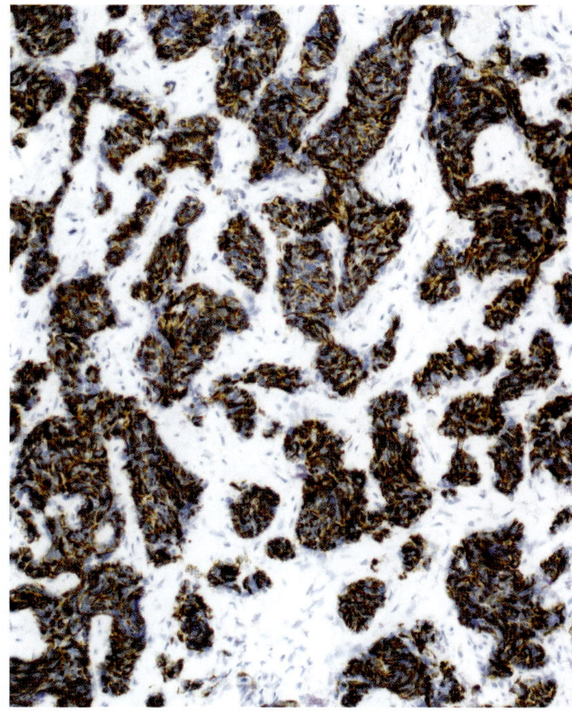

Figure 10-57

DESMOPLASTIC SMALL ROUND CELL TUMOR: METASTATIC TO LIVER

The tumor is diffusely desmin positive.

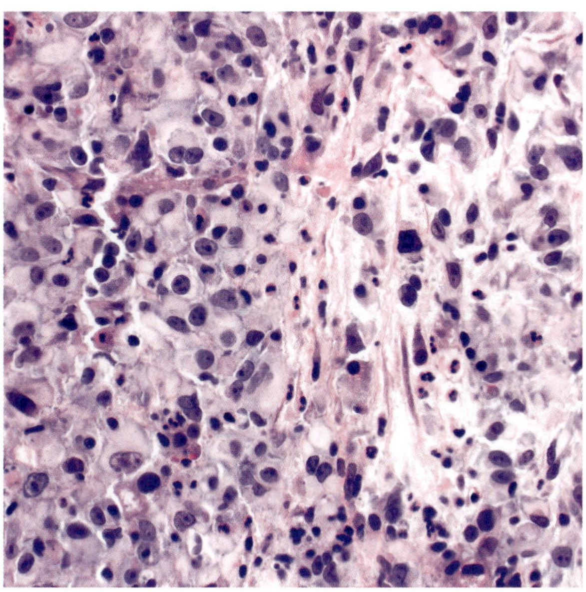

Figure 10-58

METASTATIC MELANOMA: EPITHELIOID

The tumor cells mimic an epithelial malignancy.

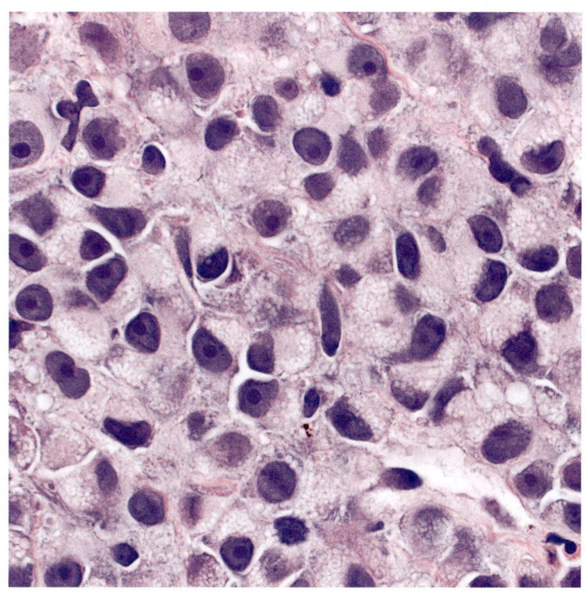

Figure 10-59

MELANOMA, RHABDOID: METASTATIC TO LIVER

This metastatic ocular melanoma has a rhabdoid growth pattern.

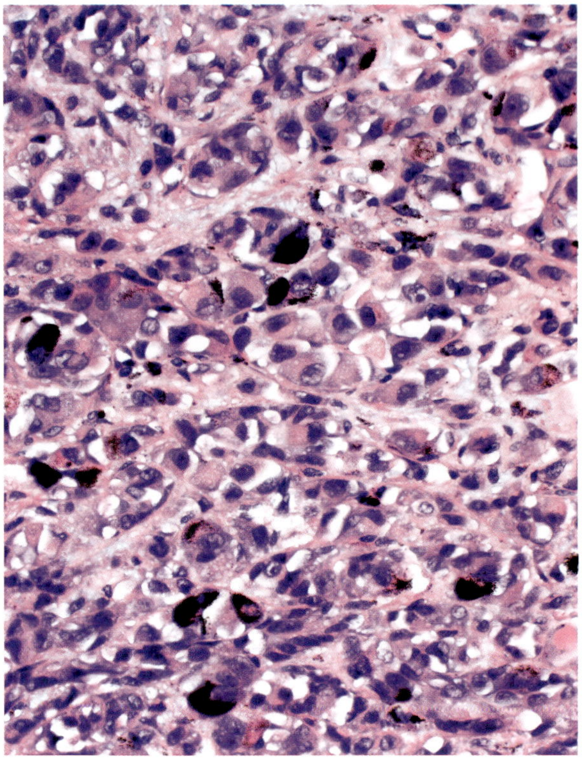

Figure 10-60

MELANOMA: METASTATIC TO LIVER

When present, pigment is an important clue to the possibility of melanoma.

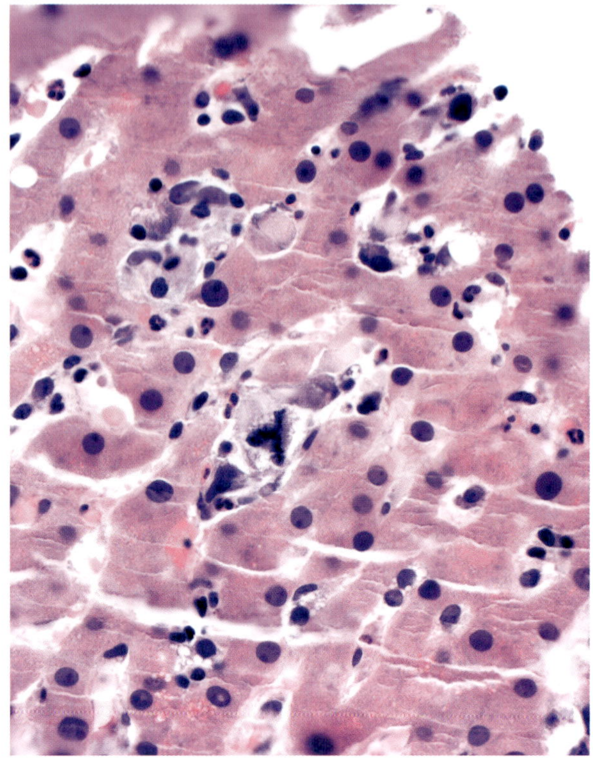

Figure 10-61

METASTATIC MELANOMA: SINUSOIDAL PATTERN

This melanoma presented with acute liver failure and showed diffuse sinusoidal infiltration.

protein, melan-A, and HMB-45, supplemented with SOX10 if needed. Spindle cell melanomas tend to be S-100 protein and SOX10 positive, but negative for the other markers.

ULTRASTRUCTURAL FINDINGS

Ultrastructural examination is not a typical part of the evaluation of adult malignancies.

CYTOLOGIC FINDINGS

The cytology findings correlate broadly with the morphology of the metastatic malignancy and provide important clues to the diagnosis. The approach is essentially the same as for needle biopsies. Metastatic tumors tend to fall into one of the following three categories on aspirates. First, tumors in which the primary site can be identified with a high degree of confidence based on morphology and immunohistochemical stains; colonic adenocarcinoma is one example. Second, tumors in which the specific lineage is identified, but a primary site is not clear; examples include lymphoma, sarcoma, melanoma, neuroendocrine tumors, and squamous cell carcinoma. Third, undifferentiated neoplasms where the available material can be classified as malignant, but does not permit further subclassification.

MOLECULAR GENETIC FINDINGS

Molecular methods can be very useful in confirming a diagnosis, subclassifying selected tumors, and guiding therapy (Table 10-7). In most cases, the primary tumor is used for molecular testing to guide therapy, but in certain cases, the metastatic liver deposits are appropriate material to test.

Molecular testing is less commonly available than immunohistochemical stains and less useful as the primary tool for determining the origin of metastatic tumors, at least currently. However, there is considerable clinical and

Table 10-7

COMMONLY USED MOLECULAR TESTS

Tumor	Reason for Test	Molecular Test
	Primarily Treatment	
Breast carcinoma	Treatment	*HER2* amplification
Cholangiocarcinoma	Treatment	*FGFR2* rearrangement
Colon carcinoma	Treatment/prognosis	*BRAF*
		KRAS
		MSI testing
		HER2
Gastric carcinoma	Treatment	*HER2*
GIST[a]	Treatment	*KIT* gene sequencing
		PDGFRA sequencing
Melanoma	Treatment	*BRAF*
Lung carcinoma	Treatment	*ALK* (2p23) rearrangement
		EGFR mutations
		RET rearrangement
		ROS1 rearrangement
Squamous cell, others	Treatment	*FGFR1* Amplification
	Primarily Diagnosis	
Bile duct brushings	Diagnosis	Aneuploidy
Fibrolamellar carcinoma	Diagnosis	*PRKACA* rearrangement
Xp11 translocation renal carcinoma	Diagnosis	*TFE3* rearrangement
Alveolar rhabdomyosarcoma	Diagnosis	13q14 (*FOXO1* or *FKHR*) rearrangement
Alveolar soft part sarcoma	Diagnosis	*TFE3* rearrangement
Epithelioid hemangioendothelioma	Diagnosis	*WWTR1-CAMTA1* gene rearrangements
Ewing sarcoma (EWS)/primitive neuroectodermal tumors	Diagnosis	*EWSR1* gene rearrangements
Germ cell tumor	Diagnosis	Isochromosome 12p
Granulosa cell tumor	Diagnosis	*FOXL2*, codon 402C>G
Liposarcoma	Diagnosis	*MDM2* amplification
Synovial sarcoma	Diagnosis	SS18 (*SYT*) rearrangements, t(X;18)(p11.2;q11.2)
	Primarily Prognosis	
Neuroblastoma	prognosis	*MYCN* amplification

[a]GIST = gastrointestinal stromal tumor.

commercial interest in developing molecular methods to identify the site of origin for metastatic disease of epithelial origin (124–128). In the majority of cases, a primary tumor site is confidently identified through the combination of clinical findings, laboratory tests, imaging studies, histology, and immunohistochemical studies. Yet, there remains a subset of cases that is not easily classified using these methods, most showing poorly differentiated or undifferentiated histologic features. Molecular testing for primary site identification can sometimes be helpful in this subset of cases.

Some authors argue for a wider role for molecular testing, in the belief that its performance is significantly superior to traditional methods of using the combined findings from clinical examination, laboratory tests, imaging studies, and histology. In this rapidly evolving area, the appropriate role for molecular testing in metastatic disease has not been fully resolved. There are individuals who advocate for both ends of the spectrum, from extensive molecular testing to little or no molecular testing; it seems most likely that the role in the near future will best focus on those cases where no primary is evident after usual evaluation.

PROGNOSIS AND TREATMENT

Liver metastases are a strong indicator of advanced stage disease and most individuals die from their disease; there is a very low cure rate. Even with single metastatic tumors, the median survival period is approximately 5 months (129). Some patients benefit from cryotherapy, arterial chemoembolization, and other regional therapies, extending survival to approximately 30 months (130). Select patients with isolated or small numbers of colon carcinoma metastases are candidates for metastasectomy, with 5- and 10-year survival rates that approach 40 percent and 20 percent, respectively, (131); lung, breast, and other carcinomas can also benefit from metastasectomy in the right clinical setting.

REFERENCES

1. Disibio G, French SW. Metastatic patterns of cancers: results from a large autopsy study. Arch Pathol Lab Med 2008;132:931-939.
2. Su WT, Rutigliano DN, Gholizadeh M, Jarnagin WR, Blumgart LH, La Quaglia MP. Hepatic metastasectomy in children. Cancer 2007;109:2089-2092.
3. Budczies J, von Winterfeld M, Klauschen F, et al. The landscape of metastatic progression patterns across major human cancers. Oncotarget 2015;6:570-583.
4. Seymour K, Charnley RM. Evidence that metastasis is less common in cirrhotic than normal liver: a systematic review of post-mortem case-control studies. Br J Surg 1999;86:1237-1242.
5. Lazaridis G, Pentheroudakis G, Fountzilas G, Pavlidis N. Liver metastases from cancer of unknown primary (CUPL): a retrospective analysis of presentation, management and prognosis in 49 patients and systematic review of the literature. Cancer Treat Rev 2008;34:693-700.
6. Pimiento JM, Teso D, Malkan A, Dudrick SJ, Palesty JA. Cancer of unknown primary origin: a decade of experience in a community-based hospital. Am J Surg 2007;194:833-837; discussion 837-838.
7. Rich NE, Sanders C, Hughes RS, et al. Malignant infiltration of the liver presenting as acute liver failure. Clin Gastroenterol Hepatol 2015;13:1025-1028.
8. Allison KH, Fligner CL, Parks WT. Radiographically occult, diffuse intrasinusoidal hepatic metastases from primary breast carcinomas: a clinicopathologic study of 3 autopsy cases. Arch Pathol Lab Med 2004;128:1418-1423.
9. Fusasaki T, Narita R, Hiura M, et al. Acute hepatic failure secondary to extensive hepatic replacement by metastatic amelanotic melanoma: an autopsy case report. Clin J Gastroenterol 2010;3:327-331.
10. Kaplan GG, Medlicott S, Culleton B, Laupland KB. Acute hepatic failure and multi-system organ failure secondary to replacement of the liver with metastatic melanoma. BMC Cancer 2005;5:67.
11. Alexopoulou A, Koskinas J, Deutsch M, Delladetsima J, Kountouras D, Dourakis SP. Acute liver failure as the initial manifestation of hepatic infiltration by a solid tumor: report of 5 cases and review of the literature. Tumori 2006;92:354-357.
12. McGuire BM, Cherwitz DL, Rabe KM, Ho SB. Small-cell carcinoma of the lung manifesting as acute hepatic failure. Mayo Clin Proc 1997;72:133-139.
13. Athanasakis E, Mouloudi E, Prinianakis G, Kostaki M, Tzardi M, Georgopoulos D. Metastatic liver disease and fulminant hepatic failure: presentation of a case and review of the literature. Eur J Gastroenterol Hepatol 2003;15:1235-1240.
14. Simone C, Murphy M, Shifrin R, Zuluaga Toro T, Reisman D. Rapid liver enlargement and hepatic failure secondary to radiographic occult tumor invasion: two case reports and review of the literature. J Med Case Rep 2012;6:402.
15. Matsueda K, Yamamoto H, Yoshida Y, Notohara K. Hepatoid carcinoma of the pancreas producing protein induced by vitamin K absence or antagonist II (PIVKA-II) and alpha-fetoprotein (AFP). J Gastroenterol 2006;41:1011-1019.
16. Rao P, Lahat G, Arnold C, et al. Angiosarcoma: a tissue microarray study with diagnostic implications. Am J Dermatopathol 2013;35:432-437.
17. Makhlouf HR, Ishak KG, Goodman ZD. Epithelioid hemangioendothelioma of the liver: a clinicopathologic study of 137 cases. Cancer 1999;85:562-582.
18. Gustmann C, Altmannsberger M, Osborn M, Griesser H, Feller AC. Cytokeratin expression and vimentin content in large cell anaplastic lymphomas and other non-Hodgkin's lymphomas. Am J Pathol 1991;138:1413-1422.
19. Otis CN, Powell JL, Barbuto D, Carcangiu ML. Intermediate filamentous proteins in adult granulosa cell tumors. An immunohistochemical study of 25 cases. Am J Surg Pathol 1992;16:962-968.
20. Suster S, Moran CA, Dominguez-Malagon H, Quevedo-Blanco P. Germ cell tumors of the mediastinum and testis: a comparative immunohistochemical study of 120 cases. Hum Pathol 1998;29:737-742.

21. Sing Y, Ramdial PK, Ramburan A, Sewram V. Cytokeratin expression in gastrointestinal stromal tumors: morphology, meaning, and mimicry. Indian J Pathol Microbiol 2014;57:209-216.
22. Iwata J, Fletcher CD. Immunohistochemical detection of cytokeratin and epithelial membrane antigen in leiomyosarcoma: a systematic study of 100 cases. Pathol Int 2000;50:7-14.
23. Lagana S, Hsiao S, Bao F, et al. HepPar-1 and Arginase-1 Immunohistochemistry in Adenocarcinoma of the Small Intestine and Ampullary Region. Arch Pathol Lab Med 2015;139:791-795.
24. Fornelli A, Bondi A, Jovine E, Eusebi V. Intrahepatic cholangiocarcinoma resembling a thyroid follicular neoplasm. Virchows Arch 2010;456:339-342.
25. Chablé-Montero F, Shah B S A, Montante-Montes de Oca D, Angeles-Angeles A, Henson DE, Albores-Saavedra J. Thyroid-like cholangiocarcinoma of the liver: an unusual morphologic variant with follicular, trabecular and insular patterns. Ann Hepatol 2012;11:961-965.
26. Estrella JS, Othman ML, Taggart MW, et al. Intrabiliary growth of liver metastases: clinicopathologic features, prevalence, and outcome. Am J Surg Pathol 2013;37:1571-1579.
27. Riopel MA, Klimstra DS, Godellas CV, Blumgart LH, Westra WH. Intrabiliary growth of metastatic colonic adenocarcinoma: a pattern of intrahepatic spread easily confused with primary neoplasia of the biliary tract. Am J Surg Pathol 1997;21:1030-1036.
28. Chiu CT, Chiang JM, Yeh TS, et al. Clinicopathological analysis of colorectal cancer liver metastasis and intrahepatic cholangiocarcinoma: are they just apples and oranges? Dig Liver Dis 2008;40:749-754.
29. Shimonishi T, Miyazaki K, Nakanuma Y. Cytokeratin profile relates to histological subtypes and intrahepatic location of intrahepatic cholangiocarcinoma and primary sites of metastatic adenocarcinoma of liver. Histopathology 2000;37:55-63.
30. Maeda T, Kajiyama K, Adachi E, Takenaka K, Sugimachi K, Tsuneyoshi M. The expression of cytokeratins 7, 19, and 20 in primary and metastatic carcinomas of the liver. Mod Pathol 1996;9: 901-909.
31. Jinawath A, Akiyama Y, Yuasa Y, Pairojkul C. Expression of phosphorylated ERK1/2 and homeodomain protein CDX2 in cholangiocarcinoma. J Cancer Res Clin Oncol 2006;132:805-810.
32. Chu PG, Schwarz RE, Lau SK, Yen Y, Weiss LM. Immunohistochemical staining in the diagnosis of pancreatobiliary and ampulla of Vater adenocarcinoma: application of CDX2, CK17, MUC1, and MUC2. Am J Surg Pathol 2005;29:359-367.
33. Ferrone CR, Ting DT, Shahid M, et al. The ability to diagnose intrahepatic cholangiocarcinoma definitively using novel branched DNA-enhanced albumin RNA in situ hybridization technology. Ann Surg Oncol 2016;23:290-296.
34. Padden J, Ahrens M, Kalsch J, et al. Immunohistochemical markers distinguishing cholangiocellular carcinoma from pancreatic ductal adenocarcinoma discovered by proteomic analysis of microdissected cells. Mol Cell Proteomics 2016;15:1072-1082.
35. Lok T, Chen L, Lin F, Wang HL. Immunohistochemical distinction between intrahepatic cholangiocarcinoma and pancreatic ductal adenocarcinoma. Hum Pathol 2014;45:394-400.
36. Surrey LF, Frank R, Zhang PJ, Furth EE. TTF-1 and Napsin-A are expressed in a subset of cholangiocarcinomas arising from the gallbladder and hepatic ducts: continued caveats for utilization of immunohistochemistry panels. Am J Surg Pathol 2014;38:224-227.
37. Ryu HS, Lee K, Shin E, et al. Comparative analysis of immunohistochemical markers for differential diagnosis of hepatocelluar carcinoma and cholangiocarcinoma. Tumori 2012;98:478-484.
38. Radwan NA, Ahmed NS. The diagnostic value of arginase-1 immunostaining in differentiating hepatocellular carcinoma from metastatic carcinoma and cholangiocarcinoma as compared to HepPar-1. Diagn Pathol 2012;7:149.
39. Fan Z, van de Rijn M, Montgomery K, Rouse RV. Hep par 1 antibody stain for the differential diagnosis of hepatocellular carcinoma: 676 tumors tested using tissue microarrays and conventional tissue sections. Mod Pathol 2003;16:137-144.
40. Hinoi T, Tani M, Lucas PC, et al. Loss of CDX2 expression and microsatellite instability are prominent features of large cell minimally differentiated carcinomas of the colon. Am J Pathol 2001;159:2239-2248.
41. McGregor DK, Wu TT, Rashid A, Luthra R, Hamilton SR. Reduced expression of cytokeratin 20 in colorectal carcinomas with high levels of microsatellite instability. Am J Surg Pathol 2004;28:712-718.
42. Gurzu S, Jung I. Aberrant pattern of the cytokeratin 7/cytokeratin 20 immunophenotype in colorectal adenocarcinomas with BRAF mutations. Pathol Res Pract 2012;208:163-166.
43. Haninger DM, Kloecker GH, Bousamra Ii M, Nowacki MR, Slone SP. Hepatoid adenocarcinoma of the lung: report of five cases and review of the literature. Mod Pathol 2014;27:535-542.
44. Shim J, Go H, Lim YS, Moon KC, Ro JY, Cho YM. Hepatoid differentiation in renal cell carcinoma: a rare histologic pattern with clinical significance. Ann Diagn Pathol 2014;18:363-368.

45. Gardiner GW, Lajoie G, Keith R. Hepatoid adenocarcinoma of the papilla of Vater. Histopathology 1992;20:541-544.
46. Chen Y, Schaeffer DF, Yoshida EM. Hepatoid adenocarcinoma of the colon in a patient with inflammatory bowel disease. World J Gastroenterol 2014;20:12657-12661.
47. Maitra A, Murakata LA, Albores-Saavedra J. Immunoreactivity for hepatocyte paraffin 1 antibody in hepatoid adenocarcinomas of the gastrointestinal tract. Am J Clin Pathol 2001;115:689-694.
48. Wu QY, Wan XY, Xie X, Lu BJ. Endometrial hepatoid adenocarcinoma: a rare cause of elevated serum alpha-fetoprotein. J Obstet Gynaecol Res 2014;40:873-877.
49. Wang L, Zhong Y, Sun L, Zhou H, Chen W, Zhang X. Clinical and pathological features of hepatoid carcinoma of the ovary. World J Surg Oncol 2013;11:29.
50. Chandan VS, Shah SS, Torbenson MS, Wu TT. Arginase-1 Is frequently positive in hepatoid adenocarcinomas. Hum Pathol 2016;55:11-16.
51. Fan ZJ, Wu Y, Wang ZJ. [Expression of estrogen receptor and progesterone receptor in hilar cholangiocarcinoma and their clinical significances]. Zhonghua Yi Xue Za Zhi 2005;85:2651-2653. [Chinese]
52. Yang Z. The utility of villin and mammaglobin in the differential diagnosis between intrahepatic cholangiocarcinoma and breast cancer. Appl Immunohistochem Mol Morphol 2015;23:19-25.
53. Akasofu M, Kawahara E, Kurumaya H, Nakanishi I. Immunohistochemical detection of breast specific antigens and cytokeratins in metastatic breast carcinoma in the liver. Acta Pathol Jpn 1993;43:736-744.
54. Bhargava R, Beriwal S, Dabbs DJ. Mammaglobin vs GCDFP-15: an immunohistologic validation survey for sensitivity and specificity. Am J Clin Pathol 2007;127:103-113.
55. Gown AM, Fulton RS, Kandalaft PL. Markers of metastatic carcinoma of breast origin. Histopathology 2016;68:86-95.
56. Lewis GH, Subhawong AP, Nassar H, et al. Relationship between molecular subtype of invasive breast carcinoma and expression of gross cystic disease fluid protein 15 and mammaglobin. Am J Clin Pathol 2011;135:587-591.
57. Matsushima S, Mori M, Adachi Y, Matsukuma A, Sugimachi K. S100 protein positive human breast carcinomas: an immunohistochemical study. J Surg Oncol 1994;55:108-113.
58. Adam R, de Gramont A, Figueras J, et al. Managing synchronous liver metastases from colorectal cancer: a multidisciplinary international consensus. Cancer Treat Rev 2015;41:729-741.
59. Nielsen K, Rolff HC, Eefsen RL, Vainer B. The morphological growth patterns of colorectal liver metastases are prognostic for overall survival. Mod Pathol 2014;27:1641-1648.
60. Eefsen RL, Vermeulen PB, Christensen IJ, et al. Growth pattern of colorectal liver metastasis as a marker of recurrence risk. Clin Exp Metastasis 2015;32:369-381.
61. Pinheiro RS, Herman P, Lupinacci RM, et al. Tumor growth pattern as predictor of colorectal liver metastasis recurrence. Am J Surg 2014;207:493-498.
62. Hamady ZZ, Lodge JP, Welsh FK, et al. One-millimeter cancer-free margin is curative for colorectal liver metastases: a propensity score case-match approach. Ann Surg 2014;259:543-548.
63. Nuzzo G, Giuliante F, Ardito F, et al. Influence of surgical margin on type of recurrence after liver resection for colorectal metastases: a single-center experience. Surgery 2008;143:384-393.
64. Holdhoff M, Schmidt K, Diehl F, et al. Detection of tumor DNA at the margins of colorectal cancer liver metastasis. Clin Cancer Res 2011;17:3551-3557.
65. Liu D, Momoi H, Li L, Ishikawa Y, Fukumoto M. Microsatellite instability in thorotrast-induced human intrahepatic cholangiocarcinoma. Int J Cancer 2002;102:366-371.
66. Limpaiboon T, Krissadarak K, Sripa B, Jearanaikoon P, Bhuhisawasdi V, Chau-in S, et al. Microsatellite alterations in liver fluke related cholangiocarcinoma are associated with poor prognosis. Cancer Lett 2002;181:215-222.
67. Liengswangwong U, Karalak A, Morishita Y, et al. Immunohistochemical expression of mismatch repair genes: a screening tool for predicting mutator phenotype in liver fluke infection-associated intrahepatic cholangiocarcinoma. World J Gastroenterol 2006;12:3740-3745.
68. Geller SA, Dhall D, Alsabeh R. Application of immunohistochemistry to liver and gastrointestinal neoplasms: liver, stomach, colon, and pancreas. Arch Pathol Lab Med 2008;132:490-499.
69. Rullier A, Le Bail B, Fawaz R, Blanc JF, Saric J, Bioulac-Sage P. Cytokeratin 7 and 20 expression in cholangiocarcinomas varies along the biliary tract but still differs from that in colorectal carcinoma metastasis. Am J Surg Pathol 2000;24:870-876.
70. Dettmer M, Kim TE, Jung CK, Jung ES, Lee KY, Kang CS. Thyroid transcription factor-1 expression in colorectal adenocarcinomas. Pathol Res Pract 2011;207:686-690.
71. Karagkounis G, Torbenson MS, Daniel HD, et al. Incidence and prognostic impact of KRAS and BRAF mutation in patients undergoing liver surgery for colorectal metastases. Cancer 2013; 119:4137-4144.

72. Schirripa M, Bergamo F, Cremolini C, et al. BRAF and RAS mutations as prognostic factors in metastatic colorectal cancer patients undergoing liver resection. Br J Cancer 2015;112:1921-1928.
73. Kemeny NE, Chou JF, Capanu M, et al. KRAS mutation influences recurrence patterns in patients undergoing hepatic resection of colorectal metastases. Cancer 2014;120:3965-3971.
74. Teng HW, Huang YC, Lin JK, et al. BRAF mutation is a prognostic biomarker for colorectal liver metastasectomy. J Surg Oncol 2012;106:123-129.
75. Morris-Stiff G, White AD, Gomez D, et al. Nodular regenerative hyperplasia (NRH) complicating oxaliplatin chemotherapy in patients undergoing resection of colorectal liver metastases. Eur J Surg Oncol 2014;40:1016-1020.
76. Vauthey JN, Pawlik TM, Ribero D, et al. Chemotherapy regimen predicts steatohepatitis and an increase in 90-day mortality after surgery for hepatic colorectal metastases. J Clin Oncol 2006;24:2065-2072.
77. Ryan P, Nanji S, Pollett A, et al. Chemotherapy-induced liver injury in metastatic colorectal cancer: semiquantitative histologic analysis of 334 resected liver specimens shows that vascular injury but not steatohepatitis is associated with preoperative chemotherapy. Am J Surg Pathol 2010;34:784-791.
78. Fernandez FG, Ritter J, Goodwin JW, Linehan DC, Hawkins WG, Strasberg SM. Effect of steatohepatitis associated with irinotecan or oxaliplatin pretreatment on resectability of hepatic colorectal metastases. J Am Coll Surg 2005;200:845-853.
79. Gonzalez-Roibon N, Katz B, Chaux A, et al. Immunohistochemical expression of SALL4 in hepatocellular carcinoma, a potential pitfall in the differential diagnosis of yolk sac tumors. Hum Pathol 2013;44:1293-1299.
80. Lei JY, Bourne PA, diSant'Agnese PA, Huang J. Cytoplasmic staining of TTF-1 in the differential diagnosis of hepatocellular carcinoma vs cholangiocarcinoma and metastatic carcinoma of the liver. Am J Clin Pathol 2006;125:519-525.
81. Atwell TD, Lloyd RV, Nagorney DM, Fidler JL, Andrews JC, Reading CC. Peritumoral steatosis associated with insulinomas: appearance at imaging. Abdom Imaging 2008;33:571-574.
82. Erickson LA, Lloyd RV. Practical markers used in the diagnosis of endocrine tumors. Adv Anat Pathol 2004;11:175-189.
83. Helpap B, Kollermann J. Immunohistochemical analysis of the proliferative activity of neuroendocrine tumors from various organs. Are there indications for a neuroendocrine tumor-carcinoma sequence? Virchows Arch 2001;438:86-91.
84. Schmitt AM, Riniker F, Anlauf M, et al. Islet 1 (Isl1) expression is a reliable marker for pancreatic endocrine tumors and their metastases. Am J Surg Pathol 2008;32:420-425.
85. Koo J, Mertens RB, Mirocha JM, Wang HL, Dhall D. Value of Islet 1 and PAX8 in identifying metastatic neuroendocrine tumors of pancreatic origin. Mod Pathol 2012;25:893-901.
86. Sangoi AR, Ohgami RS, Pai RK, Beck AH, McKenney JK, Pai RK. PAX8 expression reliably distinguishes pancreatic well-differentiated neuroendocrine tumors from ileal and pulmonary well-differentiated neuroendocrine tumors and pancreatic acinar cell carcinoma. Mod Pathol 2011;24:412-424.
87. Graham RP, Shrestha B, Caron BL, et al. Islet-1 is a sensitive but not entirely specific marker for pancreatic neuroendocrine neoplasms and their metastases. Am J Surg Pathol 2013;37:399-405.
88. Long KB, Srivastava A, Hirsch MS, Hornick JL. PAX8 expression in well-differentiated pancreatic endocrine tumors: correlation with clinicopathologic features and comparison with gastrointestinal and pulmonary carcinoid tumors. Am J Surg Pathol 2010;34:723-729.
89. Federspiel BH, Burke AP, Sobin LH, Shekitka KM. Rectal and colonic carcinoids. A clinicopathologic study of 84 cases. Cancer 1990;65:135-140.
90. Bergsland EK, Nakakura EK. Neuroendocrine tumors of unknown primary: is the primary site really not known? JAMA Surg 2014;149:889-890.
91. Donadon M, Torzilli G, Palmisano A, et al. Liver resection for primary hepatic neuroendocrine tumours: report of three cases and review of the literature. Eur J Surg Oncol 2006;32:325-328.
92. Yalav O, Ulku A, Akcam TA, Demiryurek H, Doran F. Primary hepatic neuroendocrine tumor: five cases with different preoperative diagnoses. Turk J Gastroenterol 2012;23:272-278.
93. Shastri A, Msaouel P, Montagna C, et al. Primary hepatic small cell carcinoma: two case reports, molecular characterization and pooled analysis of known clinical data. Anticancer Res 2016;36:271-277.
94. Huang YQ, Xu F, Yang JM, Huang B. Primary hepatic neuroendocrine carcinoma: clinical analysis of 11 cases. Hepatobiliary Pancreat Dis Int 2010;9:44-48.
95. Zhu X, Yong H, Zhang L, et al. Pure alpha-fetoprotein-producing neuroendocrine carcinoma of the pancreas: a case report. BMC Gastroenterol 2015;15:16.
96. He H, Fang W, Liu X, Weiss LM, Chu PG. Frequent expression of glypican-3 in Merkel cell carcinoma: an immunohistochemical study of 55 cases. Appl Immunohistochem Mol Morphol 2009;17:40-46.

97. Eyden B, Pandit D, Banerjee SS. Malignant melanoma with neuroendocrine differentiation: clinical, histological, immunohistochemical and ultrastructural features of three cases. Histopathology 2005;47:402-409.
98. Romano RC, Carter JM, Folpe AL. Aberrant intermediate filament and synaptophysin expression is a frequent event in malignant melanoma: an immunohistochemical study of 73 cases. Mod Pathol 2015;28:1033-1042.
99. Pouessel D, Gallet B, Bibeau F, et al. Liver metastases in prostate carcinoma: clinical characteristics and outcome. BJU Int 2007;99:807-811.
100. Mazzaferro V, Pulvirenti A, Coppa J. Neuroendocrine tumors metastatic to the liver: how to select patients for liver transplantation? J Hepatol 2007;47:460-466.
101. Pavel M, Baudin E, Couvelard A, et al. ENETS Consensus Guidelines for the management of patients with liver and other distant metastases from neuroendocrine neoplasms of foregut, midgut, hindgut, and unknown primary. Neuroendocrinology 2012;95:157-176.
102. Lo AA, Lo EC, Li H, et al. Unique morphologic and clinical features of liver predominant/primary small cell carcinoma—autopsy and biopsy case series. Ann Diagn Pathol 2014;18:151-156.
103. Sato K, Takeyama Y, Tanaka T, Fukui Y, Gonda H, Suzuki R. Fulminant hepatic failure and hepatomegaly caused by diffuse liver metastases from small cell lung carcinoma: 2 autopsy cases. Respir Investig 2013;51:98-102.
104. Kaufmann O, Dietel M. Expression of thyroid transcription factor-1 in pulmonary and extrapulmonary small cell carcinomas and other neuroendocrine carcinomas of various primary sites. Histopathology 2000;36:415-420.
105. Ordonez NG. Value of thyroid transcription factor-1 immunostaining in distinguishing small cell lung carcinomas from other small cell carcinomas. Am J Surg Pathol 2000;24:1217-1223.
106. Mounajjed T, Zhang L, Wu TT. Glypican-3 expression in gastrointestinal and pancreatic epithelial neoplasms. Hum Pathol 2013;44:542-550.
107. Wildgruber M, Rummeny EJ, Gaa J. Primary acinar cell carcinoma of the liver. Rofo 2013; 185:572-57.
108. Agaimy A, Kaiser A, Becker K, et al. Pancreatic-type acinar cell carcinoma of the liver: a clinicopathologic study of four patients. Mod Pathol 2011;24:1620-1626.
109. Thai E, Dalla Valle R, Silini EM. Primary solid papillary tumor of the liver. Pathol Res Pract 2012;208:250-253.
110. Kim YI, Kim ST, Lee GK, Choi BI. Papillary cystic tumor of the liver. A case report with ultrastructural observation. Cancer 1990;65:2740-2746.
111. Goldstein NS. Immunophenotypic characterization of 225 prostate adenocarcinomas with intermediate or high Gleason scores. Am J Clin Pathol 2002;117:471-477.
112. Sung JY, Jeon HG, Jeong BC, et al. Correlation of ERG immunohistochemistry with molecular detection of TMPRSS2-ERG gene fusion. J Clin Pathol 2015;69:586-592.
113. Font-Tello A, Juanpere N, de Muga S, et al. Association of ERG and TMPRSS2-ERG with grade, stage, and prognosis of prostate cancer is dependent on their expression levels. Prostate 2015;75:1216-1226.
114. Hirano D, Okada Y, Minei S, Takimoto Y, Nemoto N. Neuroendocrine differentiation in hormone refractory prostate cancer following androgen deprivation therapy. Eur Urol 2004;45:586-592; discussion 592.
115. Maeda T, Takenaka K, Taguchi K, et al. Adenosquamous carcinoma of the liver: clinicopathologic characteristics and cytokeratin profile. Cancer 1997;80:364-371.
116. Roediger WE, Dymock RB. Primary squamous carcinoma of the liver: clinical and histopathological features. Aust N Z J Surg 1991;61:720-722.
117. Zhang XF, Du ZQ, Liu XM, Lv Y. Primary squamous cell carcinoma of liver: case series and review of literatures. Medicine (Baltimore) 2015;94:e868.
118. Chang A, Amin A, Gabrielson E, et al. Utility of GATA3 immunohistochemistry in differentiating urothelial carcinoma from prostate adenocarcinoma and squamous cell carcinomas of the uterine cervix, anus, and lung. Am J Surg Pathol 2012;36:1472-1476.
119. Epstein JI, Egevad L, Humphrey PA, Montironi R, Members of the ISUP Immunohistochemistry in Diagnostic Urologic Pathology Group. Best practices recommendations in the application of immunohistochemistry in the prostate: report from the International Society of Urologic Pathology consensus conference. Am J Surg Pathol 2014;38:e6-e19.
120. Stavrou GA, Flemming P, Oldhafer KJ. Liver resection for metastasis due to malignant mesenchymal tumours. HPB (Oxford) 2006;8:110-113.
121. Gates LK, Jr., Cameron AJ, Nagorney DM, Goellner JR, Farley DR. Primary leiomyosarcoma of the liver mimicking liver abscess. Am J Gastroenterol 1995;90:649-652.
122. Chelimilla H, Badipatla K, Ihimoyan A, Niazi M. A rare occurrence of primary hepatic leiomyosarcoma associated with Epstein Barr virus infection in an AIDS patient. Case Rep Gastrointest Med 2013;2013:691862.

123. Wachtel H, Jackson BM, Bartlett EK, et al. Resection of primary leiomyosarcoma of the inferior vena cava (IVC) with reconstruction: a case series and review of the literature. J Surg Oncol 2015;111:328-333.
124. Handorf CR, Kulkarni A, Grenert JP, et al. A multicenter study directly comparing the diagnostic accuracy of gene expression profiling and immunohistochemistry for primary site identification in metastatic tumors. Am J Surg Pathol 2013;37:1067-1075.
125. Maxwell JE, Sherman SK, Stashek KM, O'Dorisio TM, Bellizzi AM, Howe JR. A practical method to determine the site of unknown primary in metastatic neuroendocrine tumors. Surgery 2014;156:1359-65; discussion 65-66.
126. Sherman SK, Maxwell JE, Carr JC, et al. Gene expression accurately distinguishes liver metastases of small bowel and pancreas neuroendocrine tumors. Clin Exp Metastasis 2014;31:935-944.
127. Kulkarni A, Pillai R, Ezekiel AM, Henner WD, Handorf CR. Comparison of histopathology to gene expression profiling for the diagnosis of metastatic cancer. Diagn Pathol 2012;7:110.
128. Lal A, Panos R, Marjanovic M, et al. A gene expression profile test to resolve head & neck squamous versus lung squamous cancers. Diagn Pathol 2013;8:44.
129. Riihimaki M, Thomsen H, Hemminki A, Sundquist K, Hemminki K. Comparison of survival of patients with metastases from known versus unknown primaries: survival in metastatic cancer. BMC Cancer 2013;13:36.
130. Yan TD, Padang R, Morris DL. Longterm results and prognostic indicators after cryotherapy and hepatic arterial chemotherapy with or without resection for colorectal liver metastases in 224 patients: longterm survival can be achieved in patients with multiple bilateral liver metastases. J Am Coll Surg 2006;202:100-111.
131. Frankel TL, D'Angelica MI. Hepatic resection for colorectal metastases. J Surg Oncol 2014;109:1-107.

11 LYMPHOID-HEMATOPOIETIC TUMORS AND TUMOR-LIKE LESIONS

The liver is often secondarily involved in lymphoid and hematopoietic neoplasms that originate from other organs. This involvement may already be observed at the initial presentation, but becomes more obvious at advanced stages. Intrahepatic infiltration by malignant lymphoma, leukemia, and Langerhans cell histiocytosis belongs to this category. Although much rarer, hematolymphoid neoplasms may also primarily develop in the liver, and examples include low- and high-grade malignant lymphomas, myeloid sarcoma, and plasmacytoma. This chapter describes the clinical and pathologic features of the primary and secondary liver lesions of hematolymphoid neoplasms. Since a comprehensive review of the morphologic features, immunophenotypes, and underlying molecular abnormalities of each entity is beyond the scope of this chapter, readers interested in these neoplasms may refer to the Armed Forces Institute of Pathology (AFIP) Atlas of Tumor Pathology Fascicles on Tumors of the Lymph Nodes and Spleen (1) or Tumors of the Bone Marrow (2) and the World Health Organization (WHO) Classification of Tumours of Haematopoietic and Lymphoid Tissues (3). Tumor-like lesions that need to be discriminated from true hematolymphoid neoplasms are also discussed at the end of this chapter.

PRIMARY HEPATIC LYMPHOMA

Primary hepatic lymphoma is a malignant lymphoid neoplasm that is confined to the liver or perihepatic nodal sites without distant involvement at presentation (4). Distant lymphadenopathy, splenomegaly, and bone marrow involvement are not observed for at least 6 months after the onset of hepatic disease, except for hepatosplenic T-cell lymphoma, which commonly affects the spleen and bone marrow at initial presentation (5). Primary hepatic lymphoma is rare and accounts for 0.4 percent of extranodal non-Hodgkin lymphomas (4,6).

Lymphoid neoplasms originating in the liver need to be discriminated from those with secondary hepatic involvement because their clinical management and prognoses differ distinctly (5). Patients with primary hepatic lymphoma have a better prognosis than those with secondary hepatic involvement, with the latter presentation indicating a more advanced stage. Three major histologic types of primary hepatic lymphomas with distinct clinicopathologic features are described below.

Diffuse Large B-Cell Lymphoma

Definition. *Diffuse large B-cell lymphoma* is a primary hepatic, high-grade lymphoma consisting of large pleomorphic neoplastic cells with a B-cell immunophenotype that have a diffuse growth pattern.

General and Clinical Features. This most common histologic type of primary hepatic lymphoma accounts for over 90 percent of cases. Men are more commonly affected, with a male to female ratio of 2 to 1 (7). Most patients are adults (median age, 53 years) with pediatric cases rarely reported (7).

Patients present with right upper quadrant pain, abdominal discomfort, jaundice, or B symptoms such as fever and weight loss. A rare, but critical presentation is acute liver failure (8,9). Some patients (about 20 percent) have a history of infection with hepatitis C virus (HCV) and human immunodeficiency virus (HIV) (4,10). Other patients have chronic hepatitis B but its association with hepatic lymphoma is less obvious; it currently remains unclear whether hepatitis B virus (HBV) infection is a predisposing factor (4,7,11).

Imaging findings include a solitary, discrete nodule/mass (60 percent), multiple lesions (35 to 40 percent), and diffuse infiltration (about 5 percent), with the last presentation indicating a poor prognosis (5,12). Tumors are typically

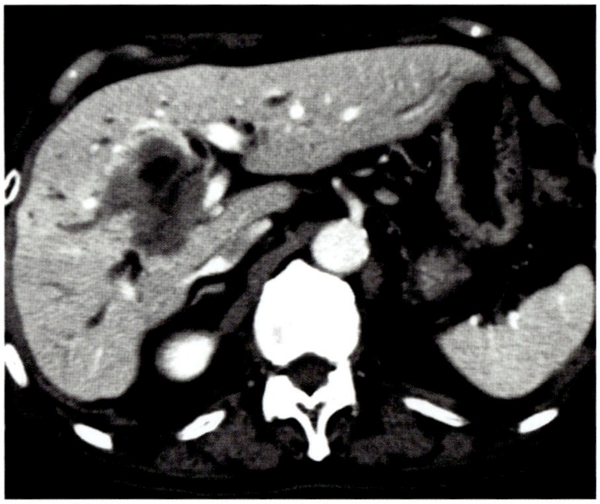

Figure 11-1

PRIMARY HEPATIC LYMPHOMA (DIFFUSE LARGE B-CELL LYMPHOMA)

An enhanced computerized tomography (CT) scan shows a mass lesion involving the liver parenchyma and intrahepatic large bile duct. Entrapped bile ducts are dilated.

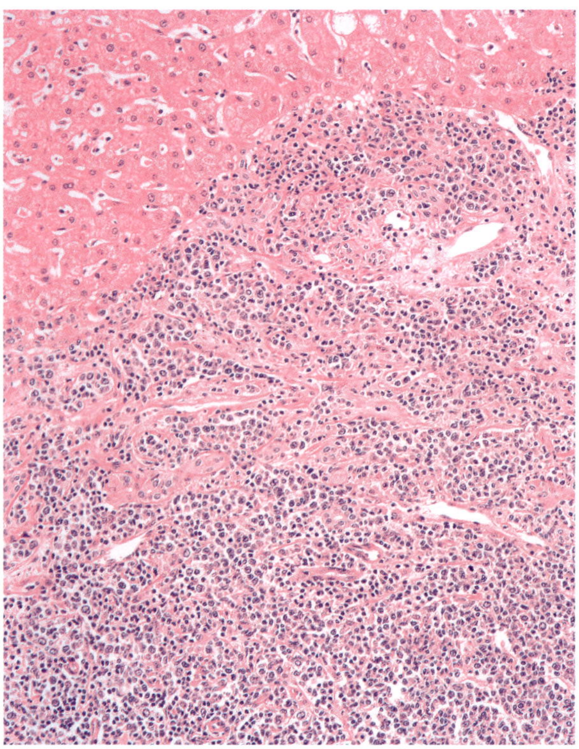

Figure 11-2

PRIMARY HEPATIC LYMPHOMA (DIFFUSE LARGE B-CELL LYMPHOMA)

A well-circumscribed nodular lesion consisting of large atypical lymphocytes is observed.

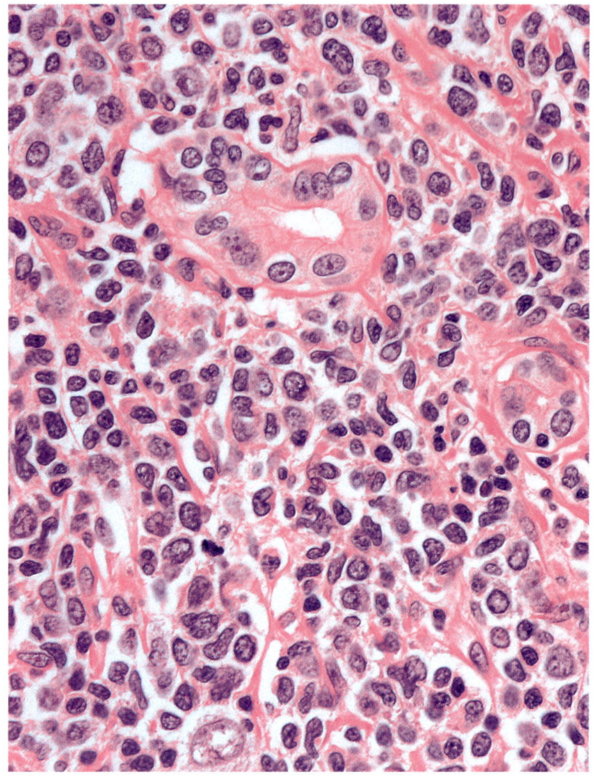

Figure 11-3

PRIMARY HEPATIC LYMPHOMA (DIFFUSE LARGE B-CELL LYMPHOMA)

Pleomorphic tumor cells have large irregularly shaped nuclei.

located in the liver parenchyma, while rare examples are periductal mass lesions that resemble biliary neoplasms (fig. 11-1). Treatment responses and prognoses vary widely, and the International Prognostic Index (IPI) has been used to predict clinical behavior (13).

Microscopic Findings. The histologic features are similar to those of diffuse large B-cell lymphomas that develop at other anatomic sites. Hepatic lesions consist of large atypical lymphoid cells arranged in a sheet fashion (fig. 11-2). Cells are variably pleomorphic and have enlarged plump nuclei, with or without distinct nucleoli (fig. 11-3). Mitotic figures are easily identified. Some cases may have numerous apoptotic bodies with a starry sky appearance resembling Burkitt lymphoma (fig. 11-4). A biopsy diagnosis may be challenging because of crush artefacts or small sample sizes (fig. 11-5). Tumors are typically well circumscribed grossly,

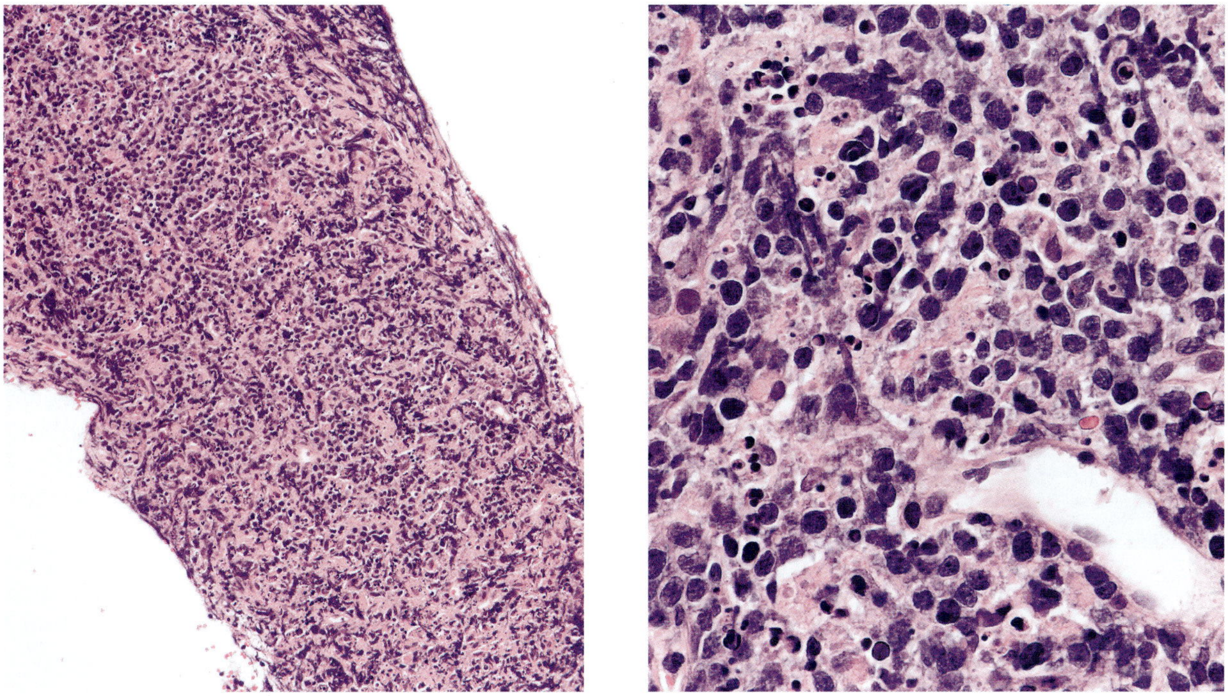

Figure 11-4

PRIMARY HEPATIC LYMPHOMA (DIFFUSE LARGE B-CELL LYMPHOMA)

Left: In this needle biopsy sample, atypical lymphocytes are arranged in a diffuse manner. Right: A high-power view reveals many apoptotic bodies, giving a starry-sky appearance.

however, microscopic extension along portal tracts and sinusoids is sometimes observed.

Immunohistochemical Findings. Immunohistochemistry shows that the cells express CD20, CD79a, and other B-cell markers (fig. 11-6).

Cytologic Findings. Large lymphoid cells are arranged individually, with no obvious cell-cell connection (fig. 11-7). Under low-power magnification, this appearance contrasts well with carcinomas, in which neoplastic cells are more cohesive. The lymphoma cells have a high nuclear to cytoplasmic ratio, discrete cell borders, large vesicular nuclei, and frequent apoptotic nuclear debris (fig. 11-8). The presence of "lymphoglandular bodies" (cytoplasmic fragments of lymphocytes) in the background indicates that the lesion has originated from lymphocytes.

Extranodal Marginal Zone Lymphoma

Definition. *Extranodal marginal zone lymphoma* is a low-grade B-cell lymphoma composed of variably differentiated, heterogeneous B lymphocytes, including monocytoid cells, small lymphocytes, and scattered immunoblasts. The

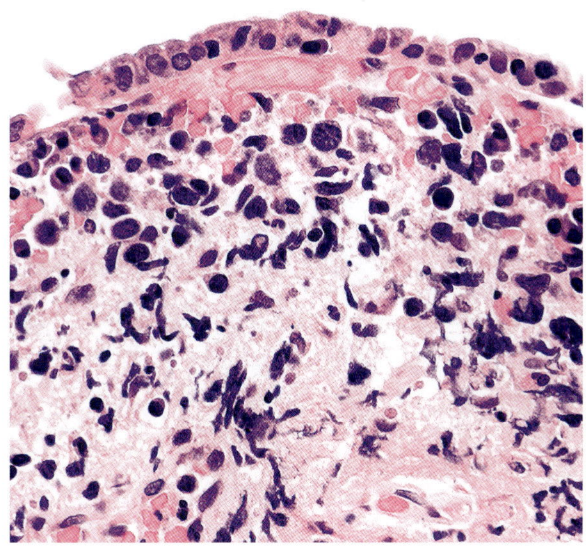

Figure 11-5

PRIMARY HEPATIC LYMPHOMA (DIFFUSE LARGE B-CELL LYMPHOMA)

The large bile duct was involved in the tumor mass. Intrabiliary biopsy confirmed tumor cells in the subepithelial stroma.

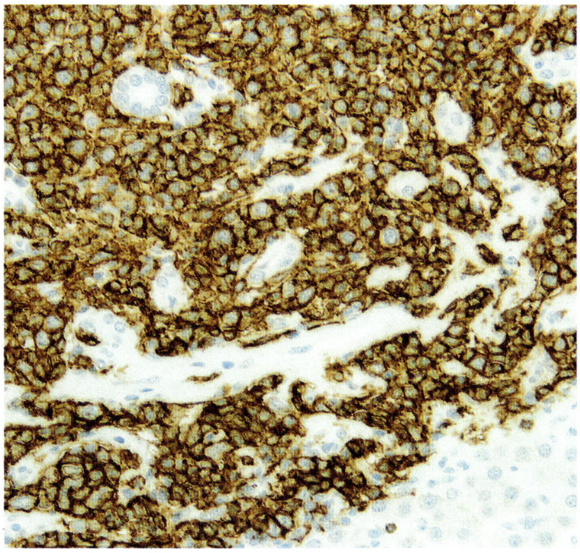

Figure 11-6

PRIMARY HEPATIC LYMPHOMA (DIFFUSE LARGE B-CELL LYMPHOMA)

Tumor cells are diffusely positive for the CD20 immunostain.

cells proliferate in the marginal zone of reactive lymphoid follicles and extend into the interfollicular region (3).

General and Clinical Features. This histologic type accounts for 3 percent of primary hepatic lymphomas (7). Since other types of low-grade lymphoma, such as follicular lymphoma and mantle cell lymphoma, develop far less frequently in the liver, this is the most common form of low-grade B-cell lymphoma originating at this anatomic site.

Similar to other organs, primary hepatic marginal zone B-cell lymphoma is expected to develop from mucosa-associated lymphoid tissue (MALT), and is often referred to as *MALT lymphoma* (14). Men and women are equally affected, with a median age of 61 years (15). Approximately 30 percent of patients have a history of chronic hepatitis B, chronic hepatitis C, or primary biliary cirrhosis (16–19). Solitary liver masses form in 80 percent of patients; the rest have multiple lesions (15).

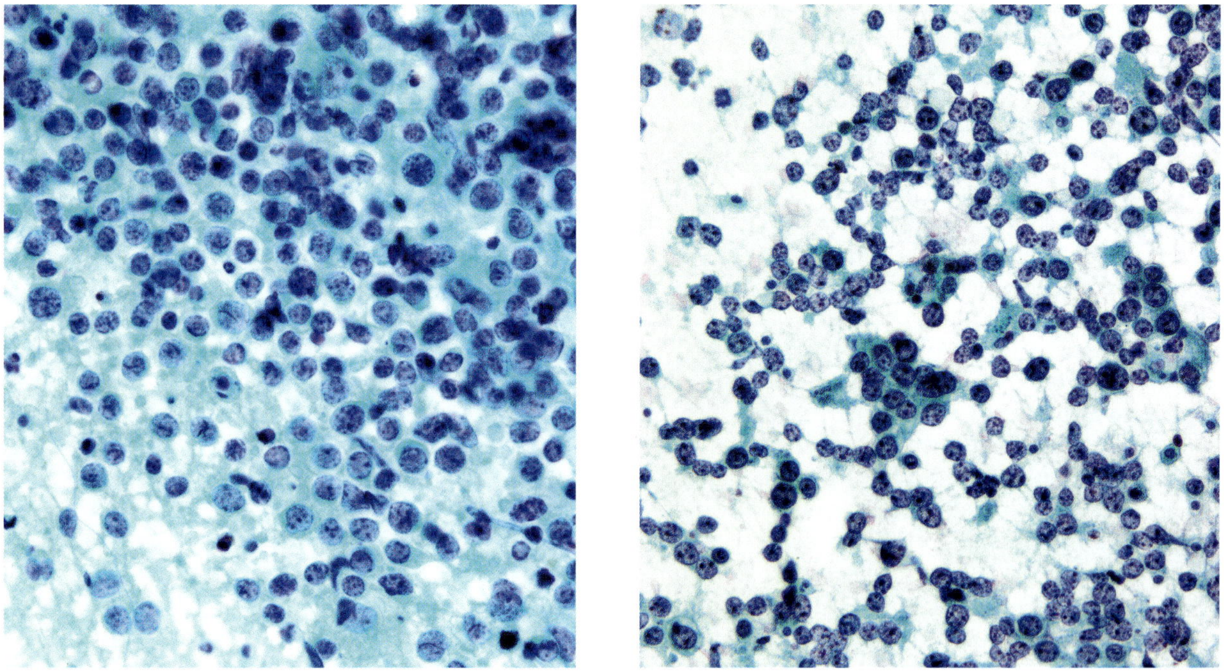

Figure 11-7

PRIMARY HEPATIC LYMPHOMA (DIFFUSE LARGE B-CELL LYMPHOMA)

Left: This aspiration sample reveals discohesive, large lymphoid cells with mildly pleomorphic nuclei and coarse chromatin.

Right: Although some cells are aggregated, cell-cell connections are not conspicuous. Atypical cells are more than two-fold larger than background reactive small lymphocytes.

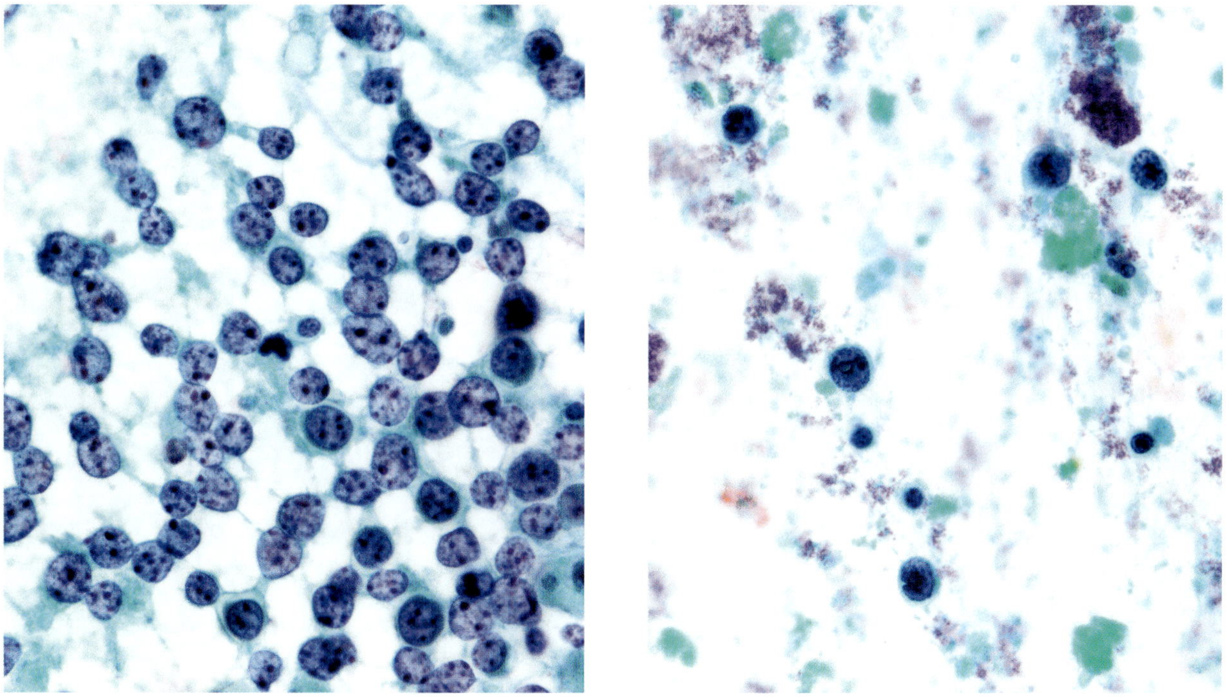

Figure 11-8

PRIMARY HEPATIC LYMPHOMA (DIFFUSE LARGE B-CELL LYMPHOMA

Left: Tumor cells have vesicular nuclei and multiple distinct nucleoli.
Right: A biliary brushing cytology sample reveals a few atypical lymphoid cells.

Patients are typically treated with chemotherapy and/or surgical resection. Although follow-up periods have been less than several years in previous studies, most documented patients are alive at the time of reporting (15,20).

Microscopic Findings. Nodular lesions consist of small to medium-sized atypical lymphocytes that diffusely proliferate around reactive lymphoid follicles, external to a preserved mantle zone (fig. 11-9) (21). The lymphoma cells have hyperchromatic nuclei with slightly irregular nuclear membranes (centrocyte-like morphology) (fig. 11-10). In some cells, the cytoplasm becomes pale, leading to a monocytoid appearance. Large cells resembling immunoblasts are also present, but do not predominate. Plasmacytic differentiation is sometimes observed.

Lymphoepithelial lesions are found in small bile ducts, the architecture of which is significantly distorted due to the infiltration of atypical lymphocytes (fig. 11-11). This hallmark finding often becomes more obvious on immunostaining for cytokeratins (fig. 11-12).

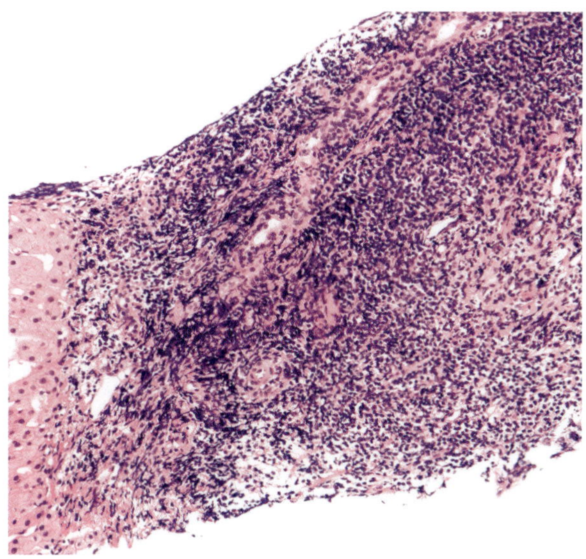

Figure 11-9

PRIMARY HEPATIC LYMPHOMA (EXTRANODAL MARGINAL ZONE LYMPHOMA)

Liver needle biopsy shows a well-circumscribed lesion consisting of small lymphocytes. Small bile ducts are also involved.

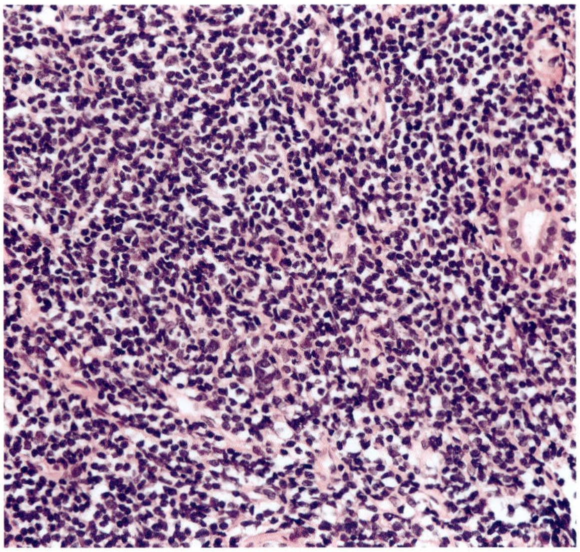

Figure 11-10

PRIMARY HEPATIC LYMPHOMA (EXTRANODAL MARGINAL ZONE LYMPHOMA)

The tumor cells are arranged in a diffuse pattern, giving a monotonous appearance.

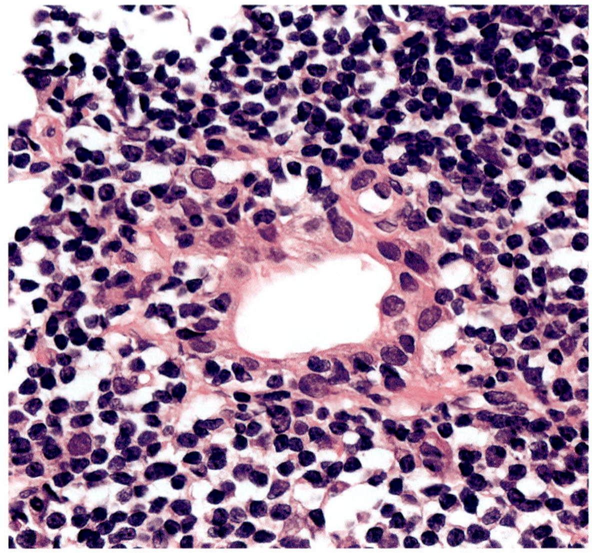

Figure 11-11

PRIMARY HEPATIC LYMPHOMA (EXTRANODAL MARGINAL ZONE LYMPHOMA)

Atypical lymphocytes infiltrate the epithelial layer of the bile duct (lymphoepithelial lesion).

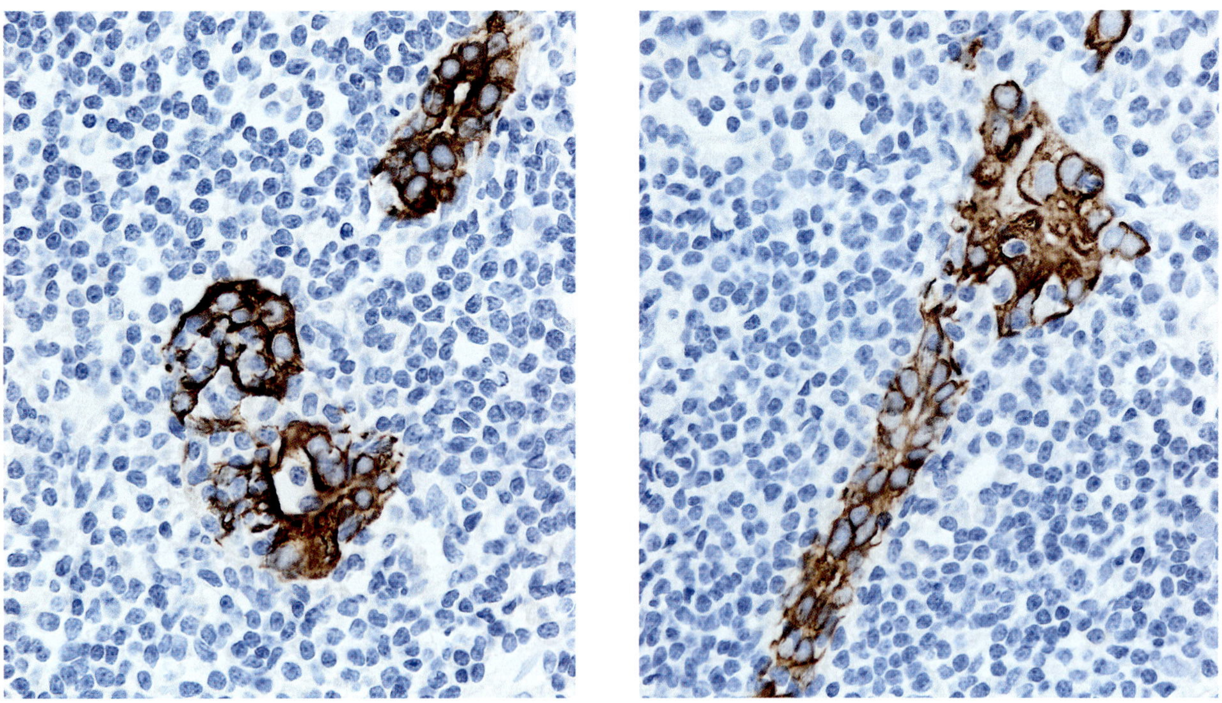

Figure 11-12

PRIMARY HEPATIC LYMPHOMA (EXTRANODAL MARGINAL ZONE LYMPHOMA)

Left: CAM5.2 immunostaining reveals a lymphoepithelial lesion that was not obvious on hematoxylin and eosin (H&E)-stained sections.

Right: CAM5.2 immunostaining highlights the epithelial layer disrupted by lymphocytic infiltration.

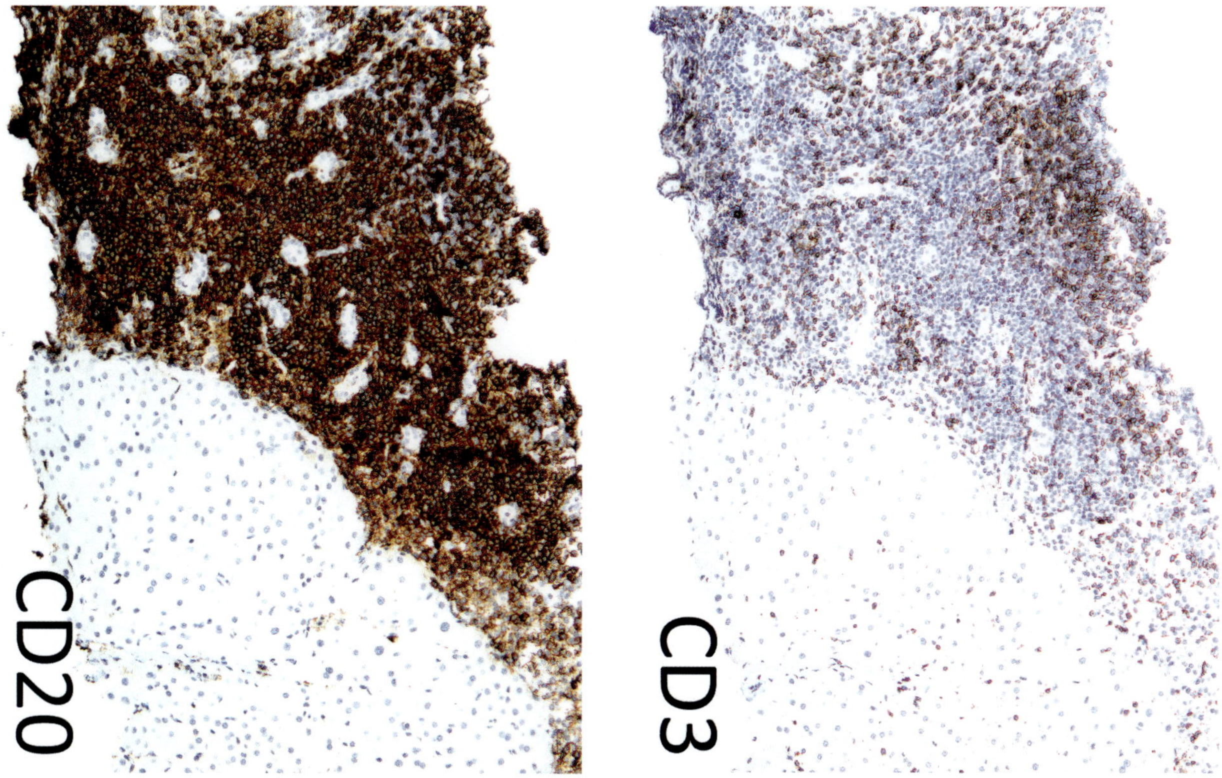

Figure 11-13

PRIMARY HEPATIC LYMPHOMA (EXTRANODAL MARGINAL ZONE LYMPHOMA)

The lesion consists of a large number of CD20-positive B lymphocytes (left) and markedly smaller number of CD3-positive T lymphocytes (right). The B-cell predominant appearance assists in differentiating marginal zone lymphoma from hepatic pseudolymphoma (see also figure 11-53).

Proliferating lymphocytes are immunoreactive to CD20 and CD79a (fig. 11-13, left), and negative for CD3, CD5, and CD10 (fig. 11-13, right).

Cytologic Findings. Aspiration samples contain small to medium-sized lymphoid cells that are slightly larger and more monotonous in appearance than reactive lymphocytes (fig. 11-15). Occasional immunoblasts and plasma cells coexist. Although cellular atypia is milder than that in diffuse large B-cell lymphoma, the nuclei appear to be hyperchromatic and slightly irregular in shape (fig. 11-16). Nucleoli are inconspicuous. Atypical lymphocytes intermingled with epithelial cells, representing a lymphoepithelial lesion, may be observed. The differentiation between marginal zone lymphoma and reactive lymphoid lesions is generally challenging on pure cytologic grounds, requiring additional histologic, flow cytometric, and gene rearrangement studies.

Molecular Genetic Findings. Among genetic alterations identified in marginal zone lymphomas at various anatomic sites, t(14;18)(q32;q21) is supposedly the most common in hepatic lymphomas, being detected in 4 out of 4 cases examined (20,22). In contrast, t(11;18)(q21;q21) is more frequently detected in gastric and pulmonary extranodal marginal zone lymphomas (22).

Differential Diagnosis. An important, sometimes challenging differential diagnosis is hepatic pseudolymphoma (reactive lymphoid hyperplasia), another condition presenting with single or multiple lymphoid nodules in the liver parenchyma (see below). The presence of a lymphoepithelial lesion, B-cell-predominant cellular population, and more monotonous histologic appearance (fig. 11-10) suggest extranodal marginal zone lymphoma over pseudolymphoma. In situ hybridization for light chains and a gene

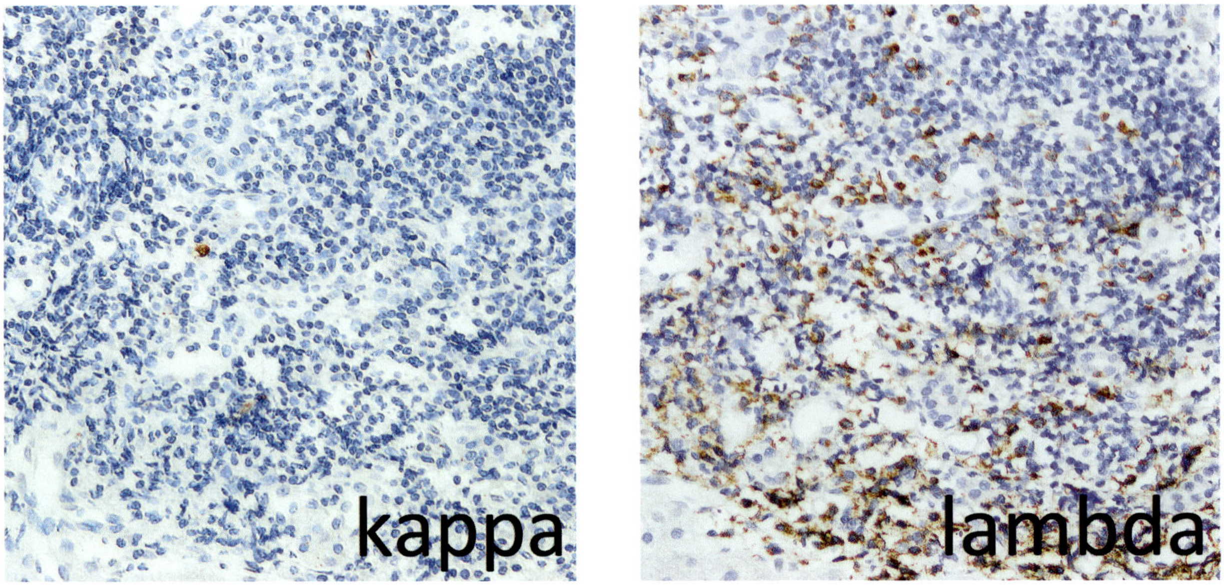

Figure 11-14

PRIMARY HEPATIC LYMPHOMA (EXTRANODAL MARGINAL ZONE LYMPHOMA)

In situ hybridization for kappa (left) and lambda (right) chains suggests that proliferating lymphocytes are clonal.

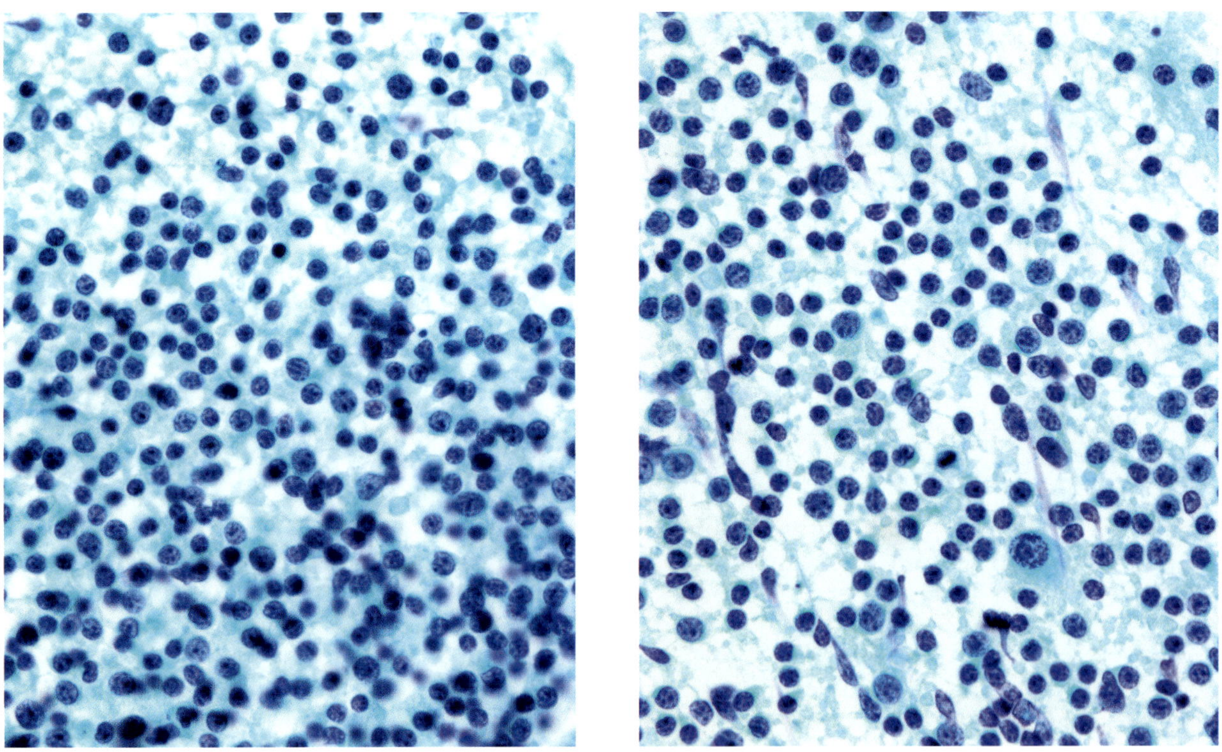

Figure 11-15

PRIMARY HEPATIC LYMPHOMA (EXTRANODAL MARGINAL ZONE LYMPHOMA)

Left: The aspiration sample contains small atypical lymphocytes that are slightly irregular in size.
Right: The cells have mildly hyperchromatic nuclei and coarse chromatin.

rearrangement analysis are useful for proving monoclonality in these lymphomas (fig. 11-14). Fluorescent in situ hybridization (FISH) for chromosomal translocations helps differentiate marginal zone lymphoma from reactive processes.

Hepatosplenic T-Cell Lymphoma

Definition. *Hepatosplenic T-cell lymphoma* is a rare primary hepatosplenic lymphoma defined as an extranodal neoplasm derived from cytotoxic T cells, histologically demonstrating widespread sinusoidal infiltration in the liver, spleen, and bone marrow (23). Although tumor cells are typically of the $\gamma\delta$ T-cell phenotype, cases of the $\alpha\beta$ subtype have also been described. In a recent study on 28 cases, the $\gamma\delta$ receptor was expressed in 20 cases (74 percent), the $\alpha\beta$ receptor in 5 (19 percent), and neither (double negative) in 2 (7 percent) (24).

Clinical Features. Hepatosplenic T-cell lymphomas develop in three different populations: healthy individuals with no prior history of autoimmune diseases or immunodeficiency (72 percent), immunocompromised individuals (e.g., post-transplantation, primary malignancies, and autoimmune diseases on treatment) (18 percent), and patients with inflammatory bowel disease treated with immunomodulators and/or tumor necrosis factor-alpha (TNF-α) inhibitors (10 percent) (25). Men are more commonly affected, with a male to female ratio of 2.5 to 1.0 and a median age of approximately 35 years; the $\alpha\beta$ variant predominantly affects women (26).

This neoplasm typically shows a rapidly progressive course, with the mean time of diagnosis to death approximately 2 years (26–28). Poor prognostic factors are elevated bilirubin levels at presentation and $\alpha\beta$ T-cell receptor expression (24).

Microscopic Findings. The liver is enlarged, with extensive intrasinusoidal infiltration by atypical lymphocytes arranged in cords or small nests (fig. 11-17, left). The cells have medium-sized hyperchromatic nuclei with irregular nuclear membranes and inconspicuous nucleoli (fig. 11-17, right). Portal tracts may also be involved to a milder degree (23). The architecture of liver cell plates is distorted, whereas hepatocyte necrosis is not conspicuous overall.

Immunohistochemical Findings. The neoplastic cells are positive for CD3 and typically negative for CD4, CD5, and CD8. The T-cell restricted intracellular antigen (TIA-1) is generally expressed, while granzyme B and perforin (proteins released by cytotoxic T cells) are not, suggesting that cells are cytotoxically inactive (23). Immunostaining for $\alpha\beta$ and $\gamma\delta$ chains assists in the subtyping of the neoplastic cells (fig. 11-18).

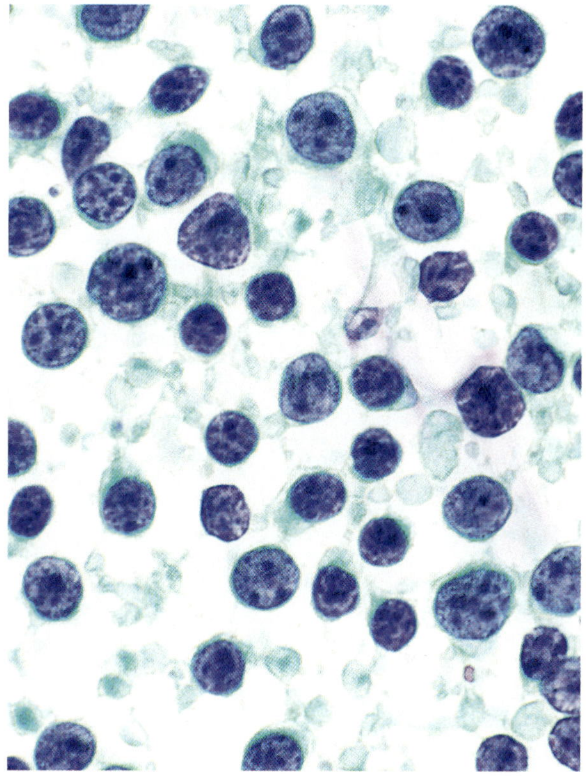

Figure 11-16

PRIMARY HEPATIC LYMPHOMA (EXTRANODAL MARGINAL ZONE LYMPHOMA)

At high magnification, the tumor cells appear to have slightly irregular nuclear size and coarse chromatin.

Molecular Genetic Findings. Cytogenetic and a FISH analyses reveal isochromosome 7q (42 percent) or trisomy 8 (33 percent), with the latter indicating a poor prognosis (24).

SECONDARY HEPATIC INVOLVEMENT IN MALIGNANT LYMPHOMA

This category is defined as hepatic involvement by systemic or multiorgan malignant lymphomas. The primary site may be either nodal or extranodal, but may be impossible to specify in cases with extensive systemic involvement.

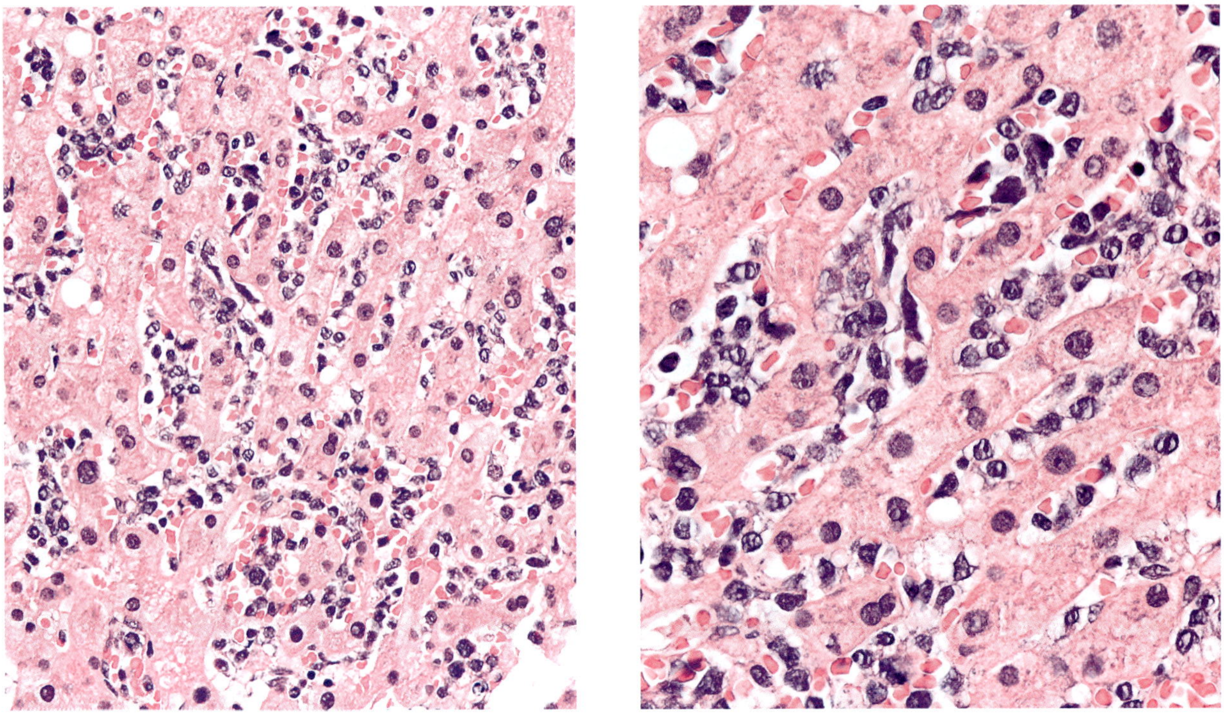

Figure 11-17

PRIMARY HEPATIC LYMPHOMA (HEPATOSPLENIC T-CELL LYMPHOMA)

Left: Atypical lymphocytes are aggregated in sinusoids. Despite extensive infiltration, hepatocyte injury is not conspicuous.

Right: Cells have enlarged vesicular nuclei with irregular nuclear membranes.

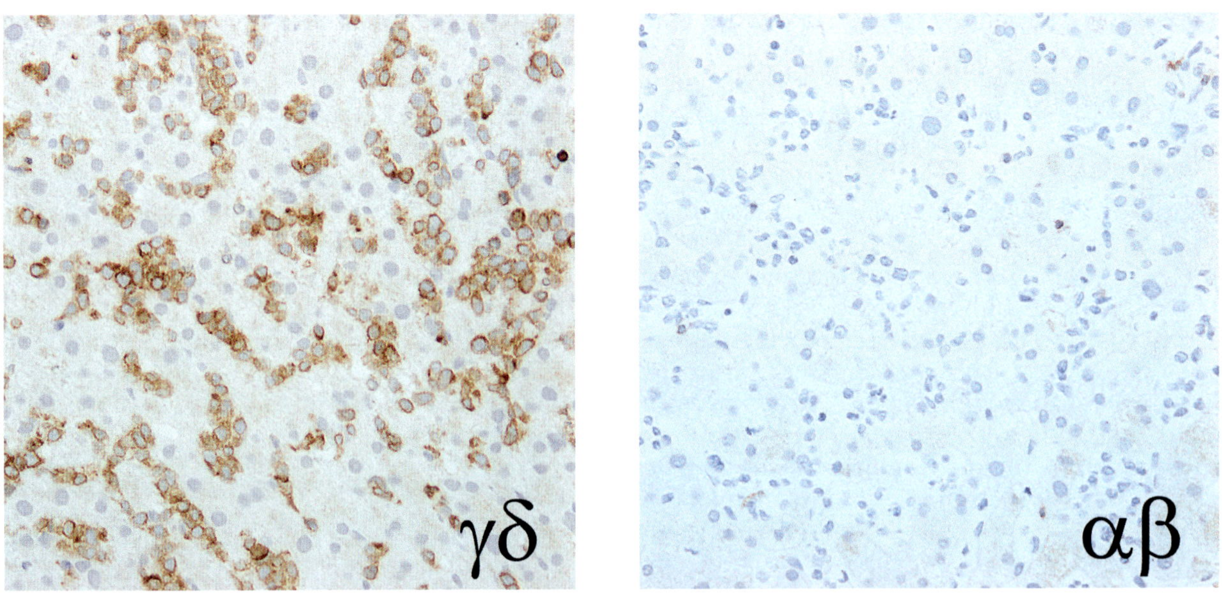

Figure 11-18

PRIMARY HEPATIC LYMPHOMA (HEPATOSPLENIC T-CELL LYMPHOMA)

On immunostaining, the γδ receptor is expressed, while the αβ receptor is negative.

Table 11-1

HISTOLOGIC PATTERNS OF INTRAHEPATIC INFILTRATION IN INDIVIDUAL HEMATOLYMPHOID NEOPLASMS

	Histologic Patterns of Infiltration
Primary hepatic lymphomas	
Diffuse large B-cell lymphoma	Generally nodular, rarely diffuse infiltrative
Extranodal marginal zone lymphoma	Nodular lesions involving portal tracts
Hepatosplenic T-cell lymphoma	Extensive sinusoidal infiltration
Secondary hepatic involvement in lymphomas	
Diffuse large B-cell lymphoma	Predominantly nodular (70%) or portal (30%) infiltration
Intravascular large B-cell lymphoma	Sinusoidal infiltration
Marginal zone lymphoma	Portal involvement, with minor sinusoidal or nodular infiltration
Mantle cell lymphoma	Mixed portal and nodular infiltration
Other low-grade B-cell lymphomas	Predominantly portal involvement
T-cell lymphoma	Mixed sinusoidal and portal infiltration
NK-cell lymphoma	Mixed sinusoidal and portal infiltration
Adult T-cell leukemia/lymphoma	Predominantly portal involvement with sinusoidal infiltration
Myeloid neoplasms	
Leukemic infiltration	Mixed sinusoidal and portal infiltration
Myeloid sarcoma	Nodular lesions with adjacent sinusoidal infiltration
Plasma cell neoplasms	
Plasma cell myeloma	Generally portal or sinusoidal infiltration
Plasmacytoma	Nodular lesions

Secondary liver involvement by extrahepatic or systemic malignant lymphomas is common, with a reported prevalence ranging between 15 and 27 percent at disease onset and exceeding 50 percent at autopsy (5). It occurs irrespective of histologic type (e.g., B-cell, T-cell, and Hodgkin lymphomas).

Secondary hepatic involvement by malignant lymphomas is generally diagnosed by needle biopsies or at autopsy. Most patients are clinically suspected to have malignant lymphoma or are already diagnosed by tissue samples taken from other sites. In some cases, however, elevated liver enzymes or symptomatic intrahepatic infiltration by lymphoma may be the first sign of a previously undiagnosed lymphoma.

Various histologic patterns of tumor infiltration occur, and are classified as portal infiltrates, nodular aggregates in the parenchyma, sinusoidal infiltration, and mixed patterns (29). Although not entirely specific, individual histologic types of malignant lymphoma tend to show certain patterns of tumor infiltration (Table 11-1).

B-Cell Lymphomas

Diffuse large B-cell lymphomas typically consist of multiple nodular aggregates of tumor cells inside the liver parenchyma (fig. 11-19) (29). Portal infiltrates (30 percent) and sinusoidal infiltration of atypical lymphocytes (10 percent) may also be present (figs. 11-20, 11-21) (29). Although the diagnosis is generally straightforward, some cases with abundant reactive T cells (e.g., *T-cell rich B-cell lymphoma*) pose a diagnostic challenge.

One rare subtype is *intravascular large B-cell lymphoma*, which is characterized by the presence of tumor cells inside small blood vessels without extravascular infiltration. This uncommon form of B-cell neoplasm is disseminated widely at presentation, commonly affecting the central nervous system and skin and rarely, the liver (30). The affected hepatic parenchyma grossly shows subtle changes, while a histologic examination discloses the widespread intrasinusoidal infiltration of large lymphoma cells that are positive for B-cell markers (fig. 11-22) (31–33). *Burkitt lymphoma* also commonly shows a nodular pattern of tumor proliferation, as well as subcapsular infiltration, possibly due to direct spread from the visceral peritoneum (34).

In low-grade B-cell lymphomas, including *small lymphocytic lymphoma*, *marginal zone lymphoma*, and *mantle cell lymphoma*, the portal infiltration pattern becomes more dominant (29). Similar to primary hepatic marginal zone lymphomas, lymphoepithelial lesions may be

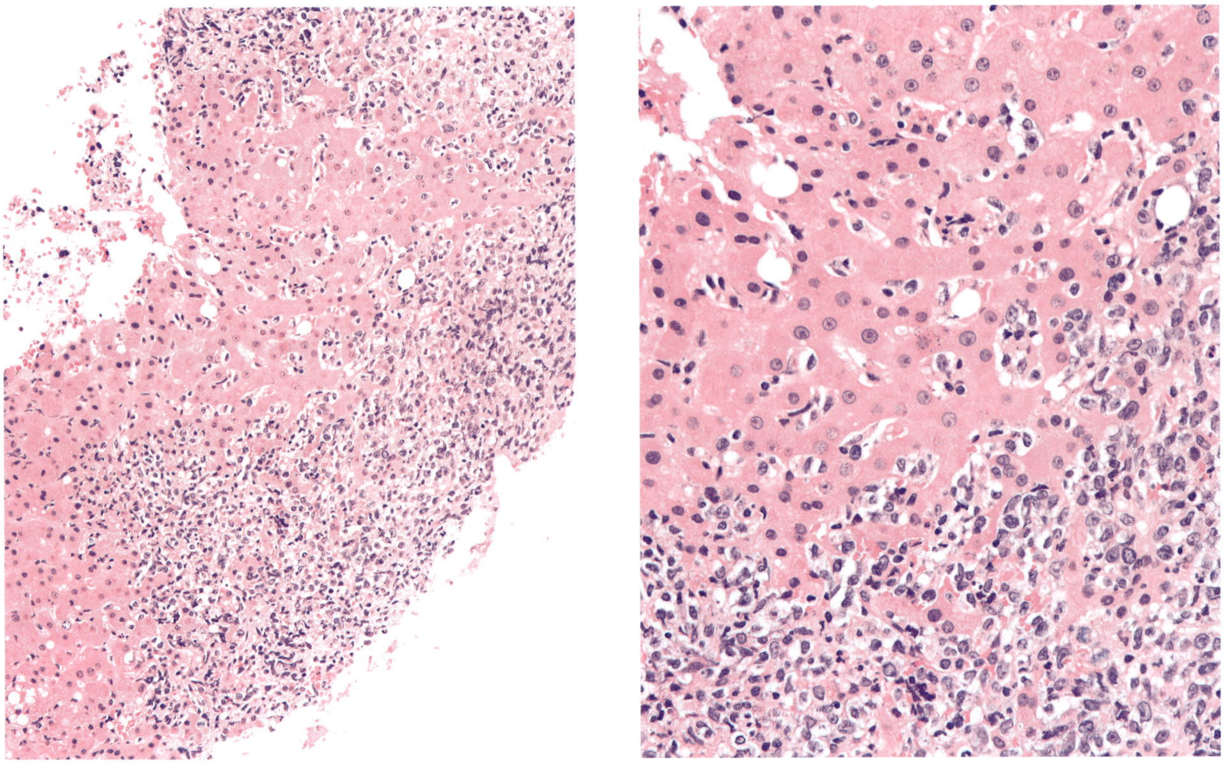

Figure 11-19

SECONDARY LIVER INVOLVEMENT IN DIFFUSE LARGE B-CELL LYMPHOMA

Left: The tumor exhibits predominantly parenchymal involvement.
Right: Intrasinusoidal infiltration is observed.

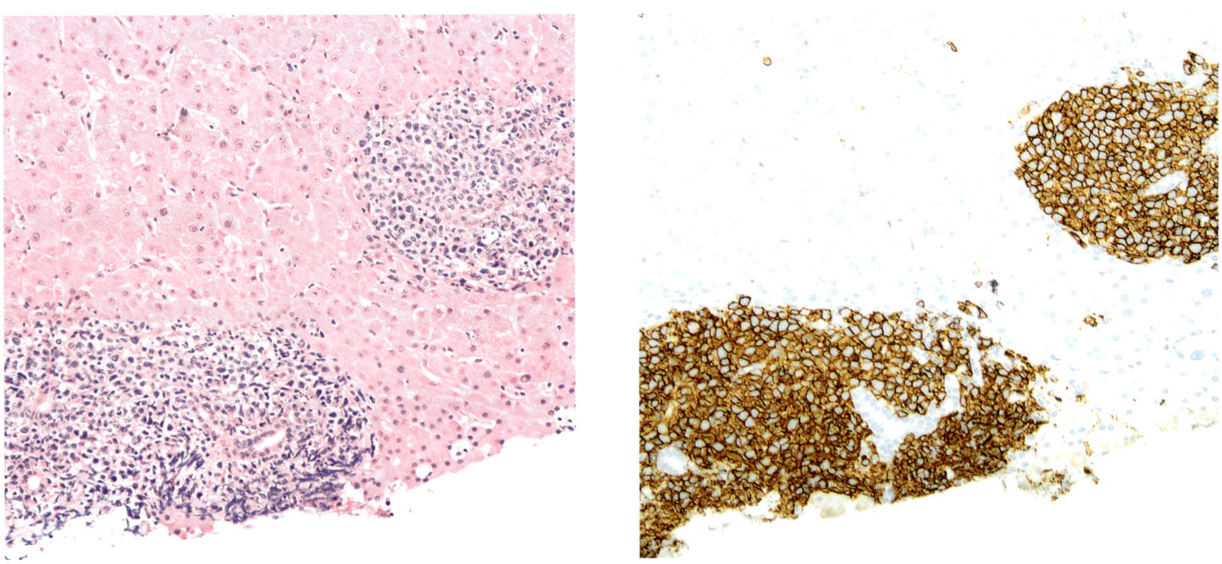

Figure 11-20

SECONDARY LIVER INVOLVEMENT IN DIFFUSE LARGE B-CELL LYMPHOMA

The nodular infiltration of lymphoma cells is observed in the portal tracts. (left: H&E stain; right: CD20 immunostain.)

observed in secondary liver involvement by extrahepatic marginal zone lymphomas.

T-Cell or NK-Cell Lymphomas

These lymphomas typically show widespread sinusoidal infiltration, with or without additional portal or parenchymal involvement (fig. 11-23) (29). Kupffer cells are focally hypertrophic, and may cause hemophagocytosis or a granulomatous reaction. Viral infections (e.g., Epstein-Barr virus [EBV]) may also show a predominant sinusoidal infiltration of T cells, and poses a differential diagnosis challenge. Differentiation is difficult based on morphologic features alone, and may require clonality analyses by T-cell receptor-γ rearrangements.

Unlike other T-cell lymphomas, *adult T-cell leukemia/lymphoma,* caused by human T-cell leukemia virus, predominantly shows portal involvement, with milder sinusoidal infiltration (fig. 11-24). Sometimes this is associated with zonal hepatocyte loss and subsequent fibrosis, possibly due to vascular obliteration with tumor infiltration (figs. 11-25, 11-26) (35,36).

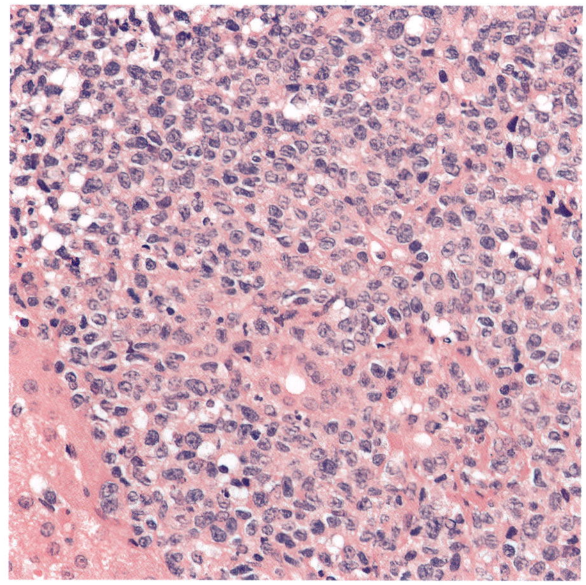

Figure 11-21

SECONDARY LIVER INVOLVEMENT IN DIFFUSE LARGE B-CELL LYMPHOMA

Large neoplastic lymphocytes are arranged in a diffuse manner.

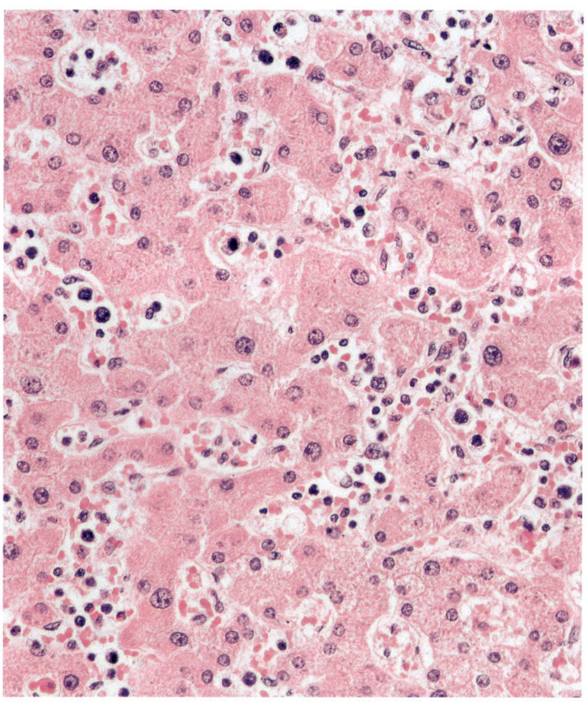

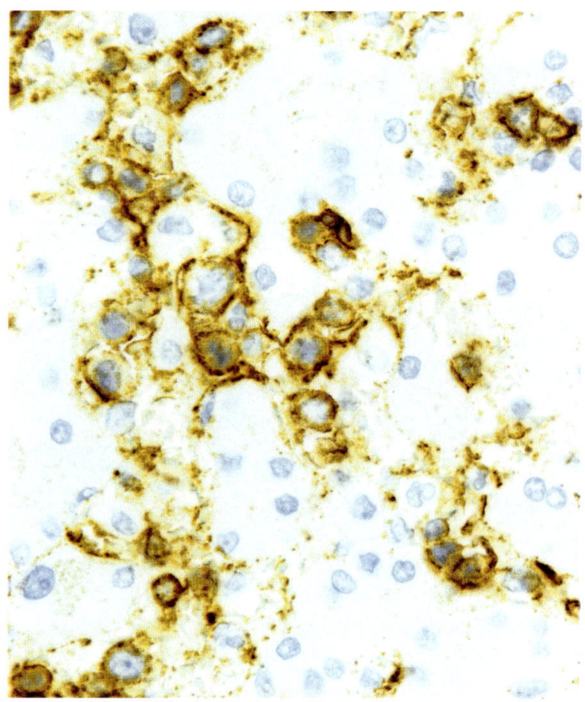

Figure 11-22

SECONDARY LIVER INVOLVEMENT IN INTRAVASCULAR LYMPHOMA

Left: Large atypical lymphocytes are observed in sinusoids.
Right: Large atypical lymphocytes in sinusoids are immunoreactive to CD20.

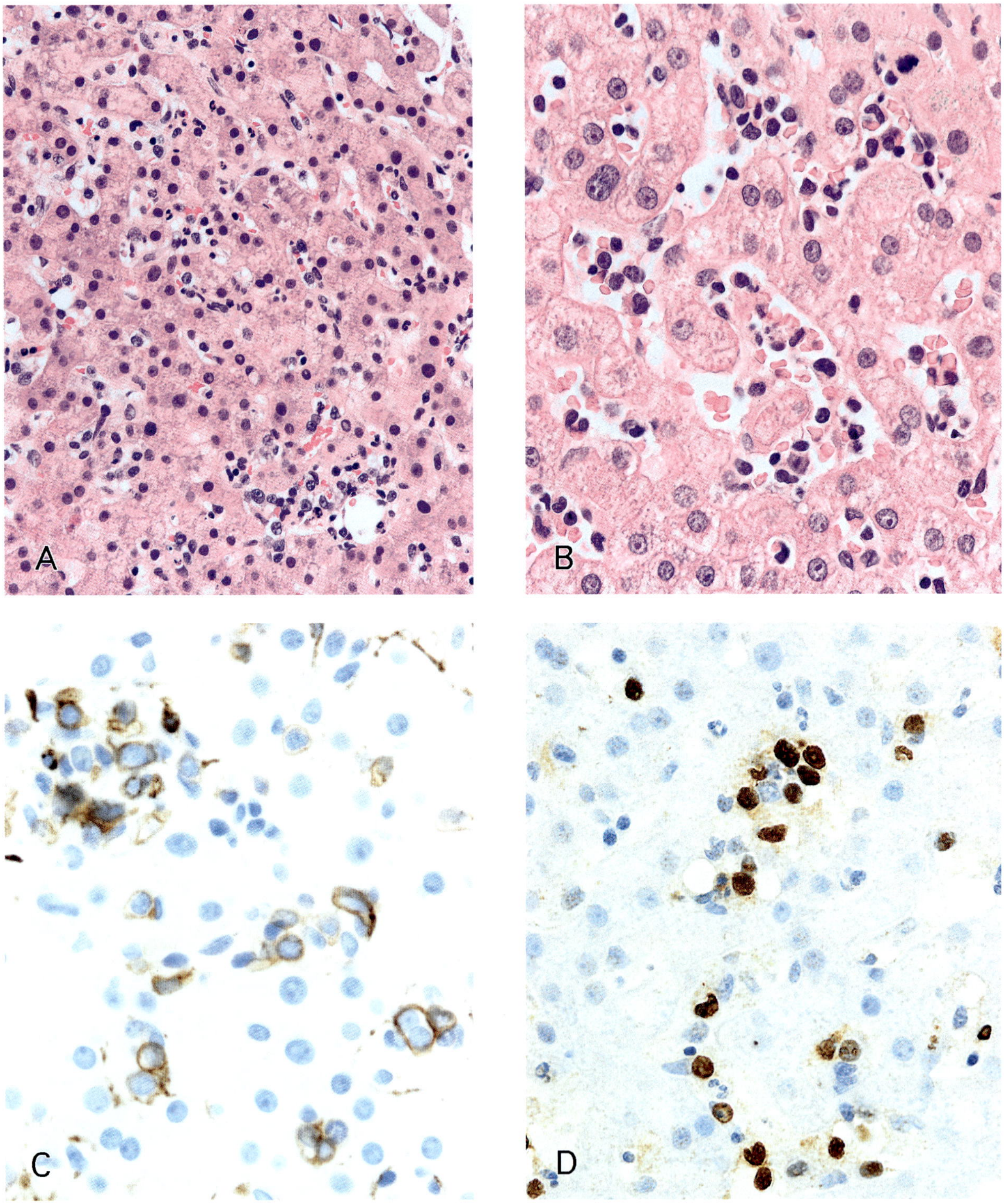

Figure 11-23

SECONDARY LIVER INVOLVEMENT IN NK-CELL LYMPHOMA

A,B: Several atypical lymphocytes associated with apoptotic bodies are mainly observed inside sinusoids.
C: They are immunoreactive to CD56.
D: EBER is also positive.

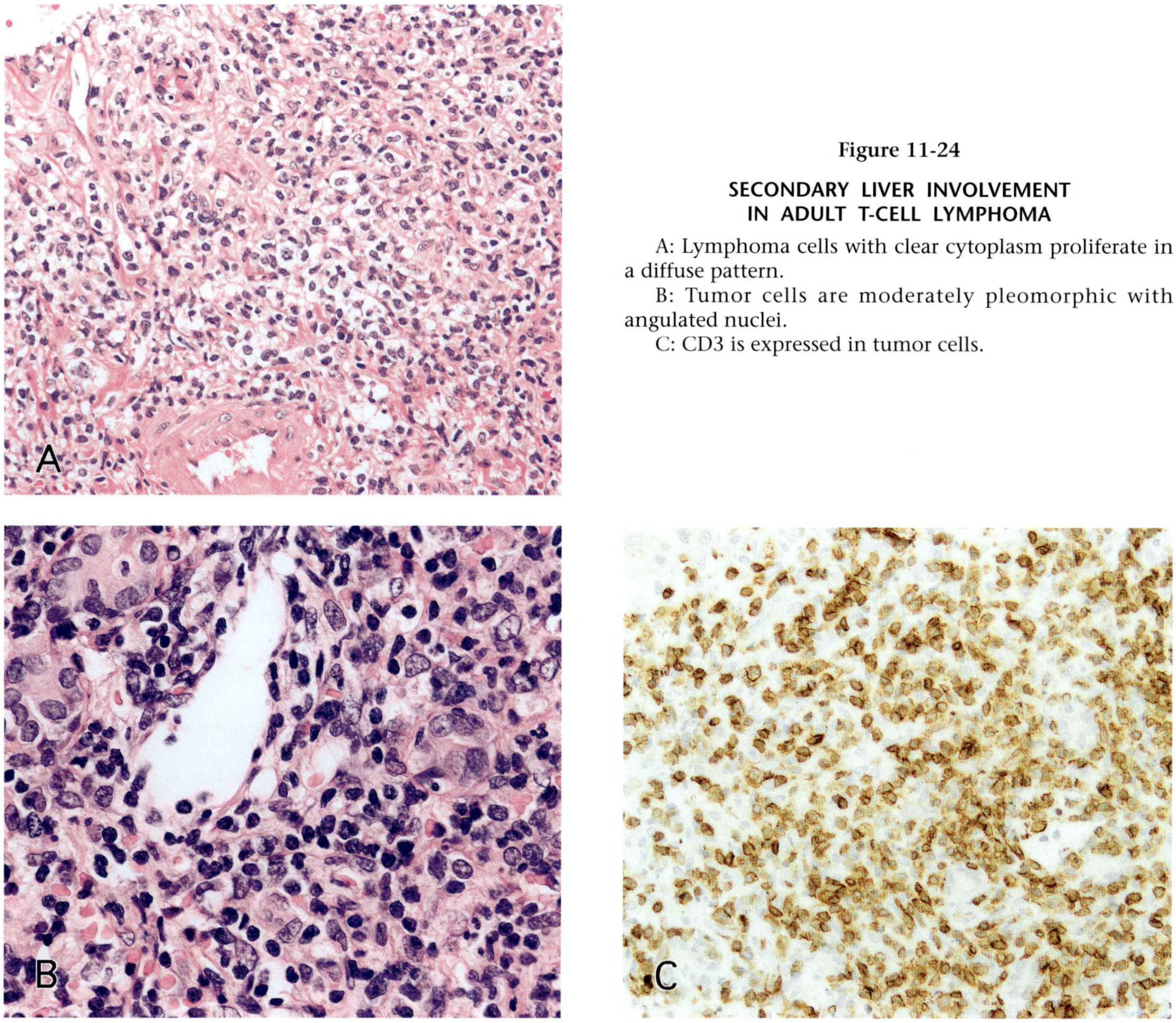

Figure 11-24

SECONDARY LIVER INVOLVEMENT IN ADULT T-CELL LYMPHOMA

A: Lymphoma cells with clear cytoplasm proliferate in a diffuse pattern.

B: Tumor cells are moderately pleomorphic with angulated nuclei.

C: CD3 is expressed in tumor cells.

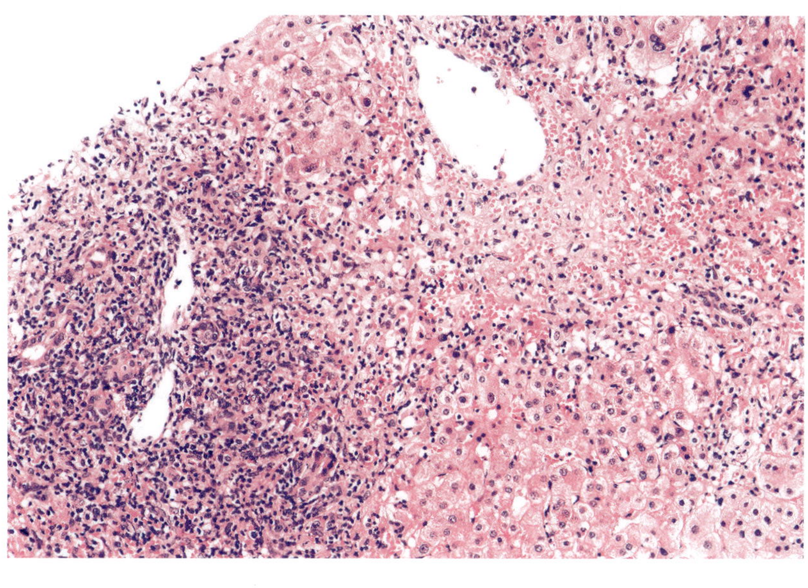

Figure 11-25

SECONDARY LIVER INVOLVEMENT IN ADULT T-CELL LYMPHOMA

The portal tract is infiltrated by lymphoma cells (lower left), while the perivenular area shows zonal cell loss and stromal collapse (upper right).

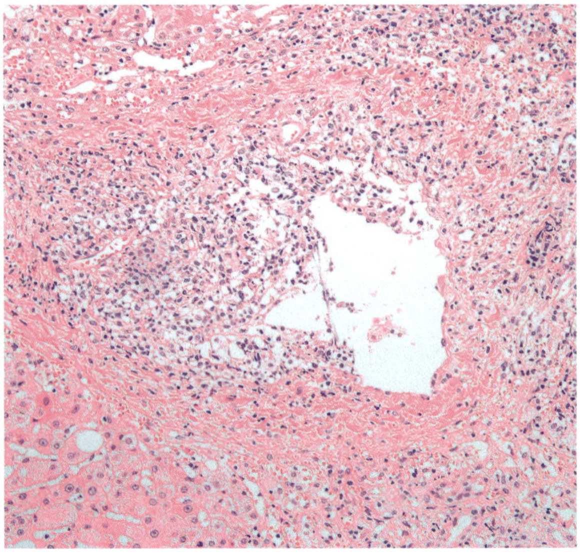

Figure 11-26

SECONDARY LIVER INVOLVEMENT IN ADULT T-CELL LYMPHOMA

A small vein is partially obliterated by tumor infiltration.

Hodgkin Lymphoma

Liver deposits in *Hodgkin lymphoma* markedly vary in size and number. Some cases show numerous small or minute nodules; others show large masses or a combination of these (34). Patients with hepatic involvement often also have splenic involvement (37).

Histologically, Hodgkin lymphoma typically shows the portal infiltration pattern of involvement (fig. 11-27) (29). Intrahepatic small portal tracts are enlarged with mixed inflammatory infiltrates that include lymphocytes, plasma cells, and neutrophils (fig. 11-28). The recognition of large atypical lymphocytes with irregular nuclei against the background of a mixed inflammatory infiltrate is a diagnostic clue (fig. 11-29). Classic Reed-Sternberg cells are identified in 20 percent of cases (29). Immunostaining for CD30, CD15, and PAX5 or EBV-encoded RNA (EBER) in situ hybridization contributes to establishing the nature of atypical lymphocytes (fig. 11-30).

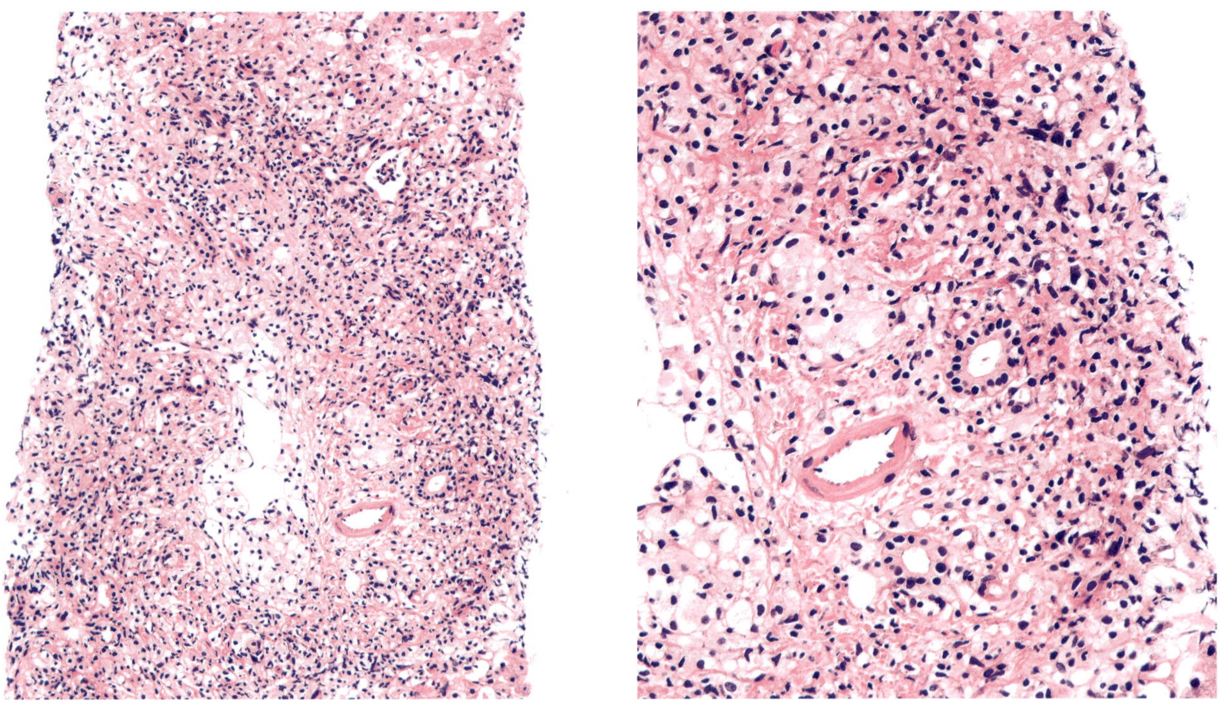

Figure 11-27

SECONDARY LIVER INVOLVEMENT IN HODGKIN LYMPHOMA

Left: The portal tract is enlarged with a ductular reaction and mild inflammatory infiltration. The paucicellular appearance may be mistaken for a reactive process.

Right: The portal infiltrate consists of lymphocytes and occasional neutrophils. A few large atypical cells are also observed.

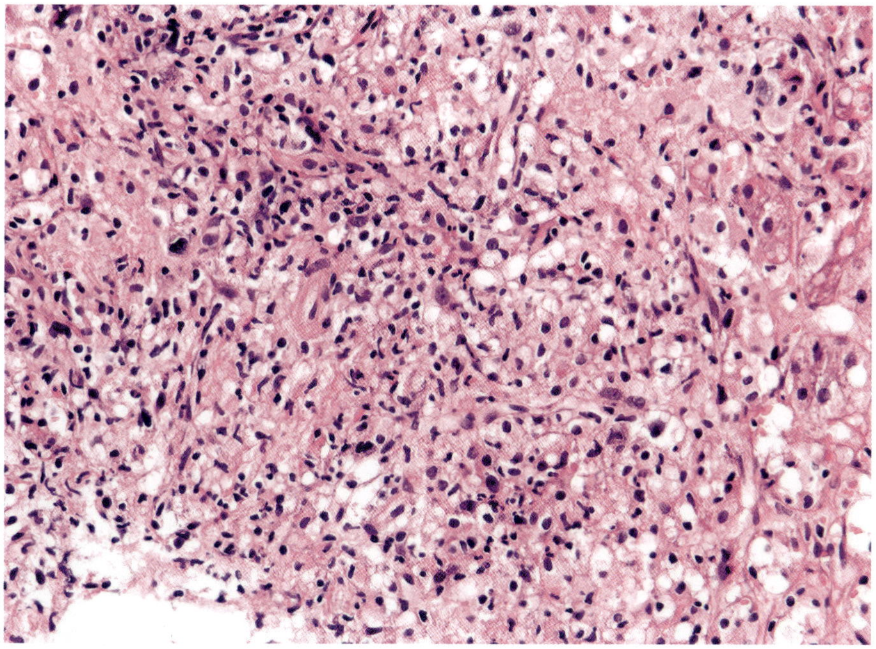

Figure 11-28

SECONDARY LIVER INVOLVEMENT IN HODGKIN LYMPHOMA

A few large atypical lymphocytes are present against the background of a mixed inflammatory infiltrate.

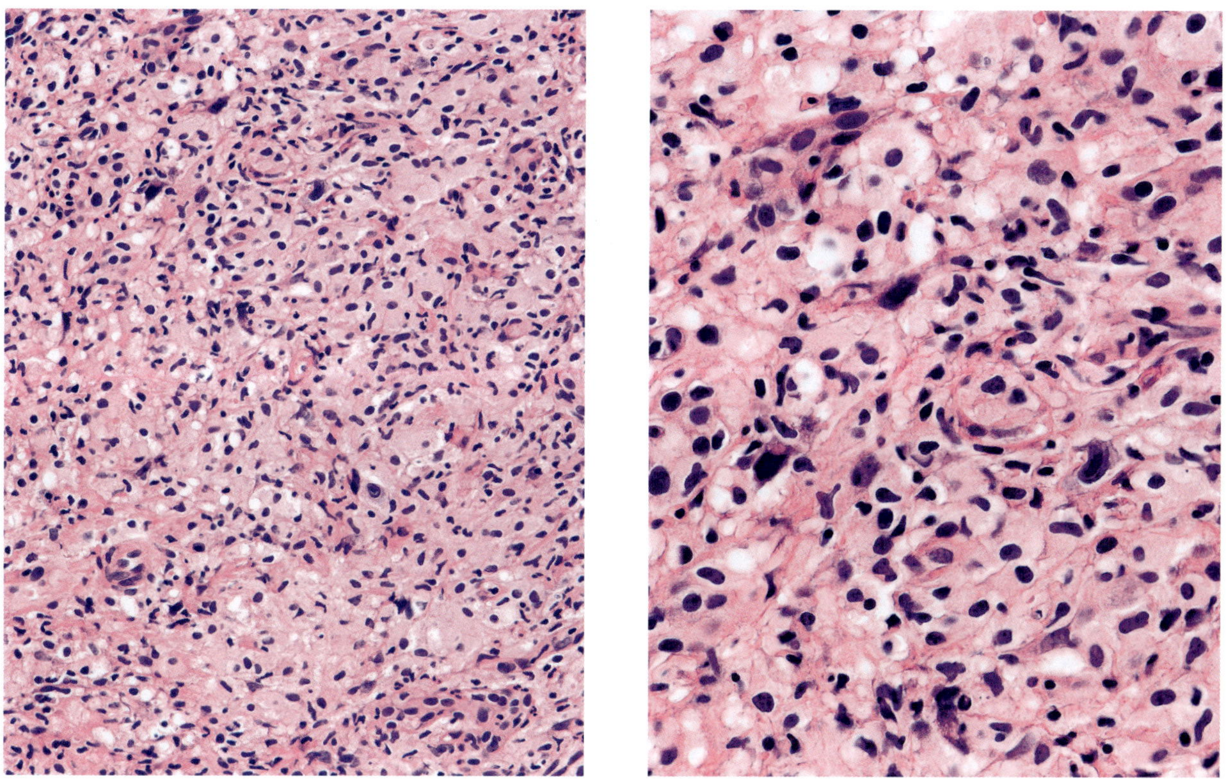

Figure 11-29

SECONDARY LIVER INVOLVEMENT IN HODGKIN LYMPHOMA

Left: Aggregated macrophages give a somewhat granulomatous appearance. Some large atypical lymphocytes are also present.

Right: Large atypical lymphocytes have distinct nucleoli.

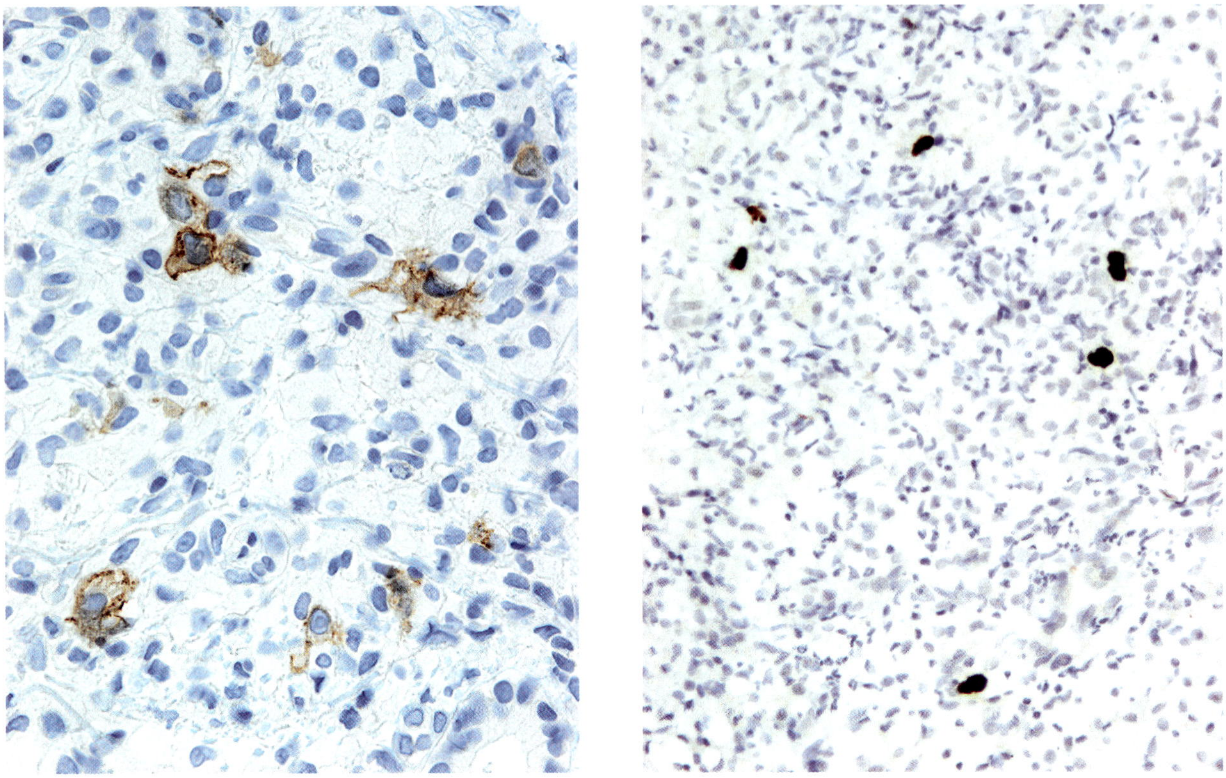

Figure 11-30

SECONDARY LIVER INVOLVEMENT IN HODGKIN LYMPHOMA

Left: CD30 is expressed in the tumor cells (immunostain).
Right: Epstein-Barr virus encoded RNA (EBER) in situ hybridization highlights scattered tumor cells.

Hodgkin lymphoma is also known to induce a granulomatous reaction, peliosis hepatis, and severe bile duct injury (e.g., ductopenia) (34). These changes occur in either isolation or in association with intrahepatic tumor infiltration. Therefore, Hodgkin lymphoma should be included in the differential diagnosis of unexplained granulomatous hepatitis or vanishing bile duct syndrome (38).

POST-TRANSPLANT LYMPHOPROLIFERATIVE DISORDER

Post-transplant lymphoproliferative disorder (PTLD) is a spectrum of lymphoproliferative disorders that develop in patients who have been immunosuppressed following liver, kidney, heart, lung, or bone marrow transplantation. Although most PTLDs are composed predominantly of B lymphocytes or plasma cells, T-cell and Hodgkin lymphomas that develop in a post-transplant setting are also included in this category (3).

Most of PTLDs are driven by EBV infection, although up to 30 percent are EBV negative and their etiology remains largely unknown (39). One of the risk factors for PTLD is EBV seronegativity at the time of transplantation; therefore, the incidence of PTLD is higher in children (40). Since the intensity of the immunosuppressive regimen is another risk factor, the incidence of PTLD is the lowest (about 1 percent) in patients with kidney transplantation, intermediate (1 to 2 percent) in those with liver or heart transplantation, and the highest (over 5 percent) in those receiving lung or intestinal allografts (39). Although PLTD occurs in various organs, including the lymph node, tonsil, gastrointestinal tract, and lung, the liver is the most frequently affected site for liver transplant patients.

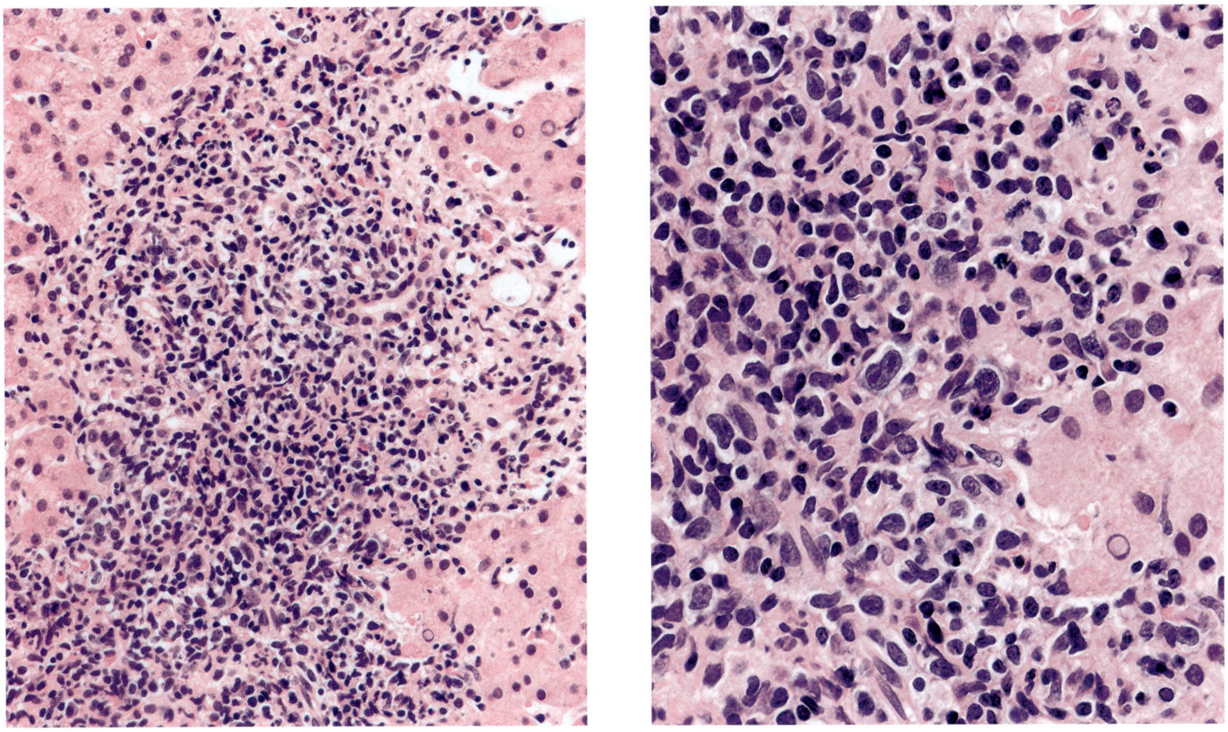

Figure 11-31

POST-TRANSPLANT LYMPHOPROLIFERATIVE DISORDER (AN EARLY LESION)

Left: The portal tract is enlarged with infiltration by a polymorphic inflammatory infiltrate. Right: A high-magnification view reveals occasional large atypical lymphocytes.

Histologic Types

According to their morphologic appearance, PTLDs are classified into four categories by their degree of malignancy: 1) early lesions, 2) polymorphic PTLD, 3) monomorphic PTLD, and 4) classic Hodgkin lymphoma-type.

Early Lesions. The hepatic lobular architecture is well preserved, and portal tracts are enlarged with a mixed cellular infiltrate including many plasma cells and occasional bland-looking immunoblasts (fig. 11-31). EBER in situ hybridization marks occasional lymphocytes, particularly large immunoblasts (fig. 11-32). B cells and T cells are both abundantly present and are generally polyclonal. When an early lesion occurs in liver allografts, its discrimination from rejection or other inflammatory conditions (e.g., recurrent viral hepatitis) may be challenging. Features favoring PTLD include the presence of a large number of plasmacytoid cells and immunoblasts, frequent mitotic figures, and sparse eosinophils (34).

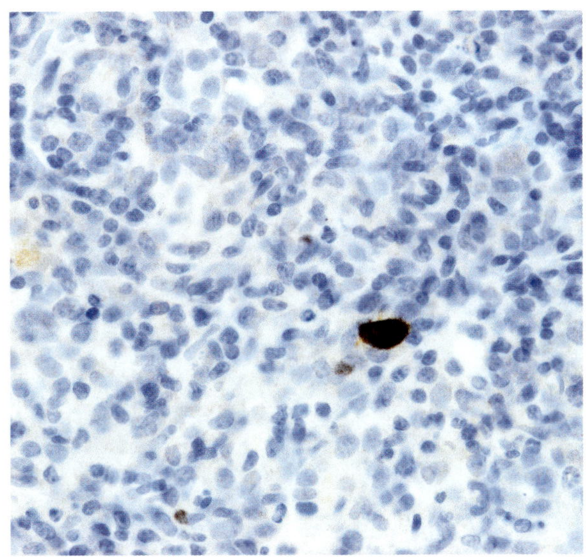

Figure 11-32

POST-TRANSPLANT LYMPHOPROLIFERATIVE DISORDER (AN EARLY LESION)

A single large lymphocyte is positive for EBER in situ hybridization.

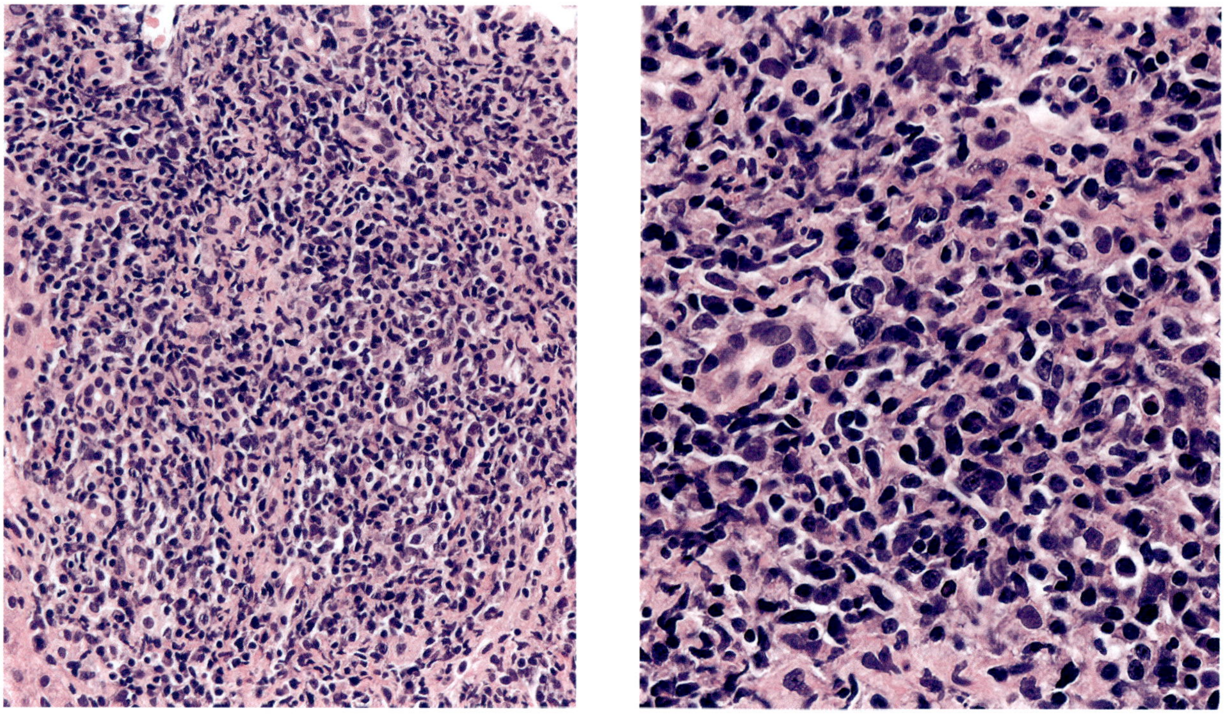

Figure 11-33

POLYMORPHIC POST-TRANSPLANT LYMPHOPROLIFERATIVE DISORDER

Left: An atypical lymphoid infiltrate is observed in a portal tract and spills over the adjacent parenchyma. Right: The infiltrating cells are polymorphic and more atypical than early lesions.

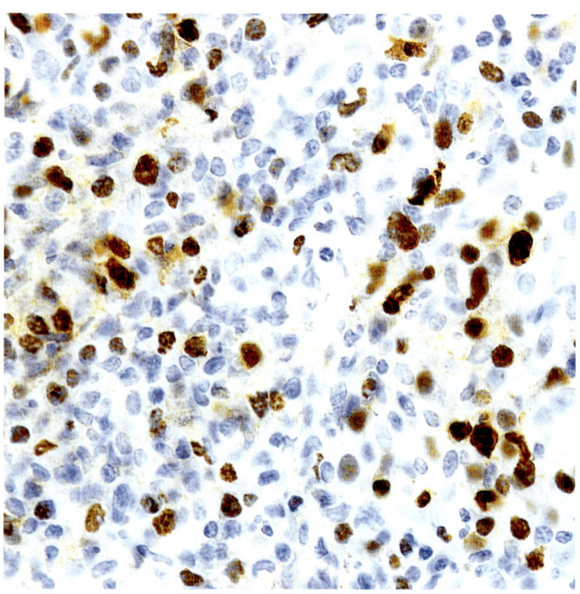

Figure 11-34

POLYMORPHIC POST-TRANSPLANT LYMPHOPROLIFERATIVE DISORDER

EBER in situ hybridization reveals many positive cells.

Polymorphic PTLD. This more destructive form effaces the portal tract architecture, with or without parenchymal involvement. Although infiltrating lymphocytes show variable cellular maturation, atypical large lymphocytes are easily identified (fig. 11-33). The number of EBER-positive atypical lymphocytes is larger than that in early lesions (fig. 11-34). Mitotic figures and necrosis may be present. The monoclonality of the infiltrating lymphocytes is proven in most cases by in situ hybridization for light chains or a gene rearrangement analysis.

Monomorphic PTLD. These lesions are morphologically indistinguishable from malignant lymphomas that develop in immunocompetent patients. Most monomorphic PTLDs have a B-cell phenotype. Diffuse large B-cell lymphoma and Burkitt lymphoma are two common histologic types, both typically presenting with nodular liver lesions. Indolent B-cell lymphomas (e.g., follicular lymphoma and extranodal marginal zone lymphoma) in allograft recipients are not considered to be a type of PLTD.

Up to 15 percent of monomorphic PTLDs originate from T cells or NK cells, and present slightly later than B-cell PTLDs. T-cell PTLDs often develop in extranodal sites; the liver is involved in 18 percent of cases and is the fifth most commonly affected organ following bone marrow, spleen, peripheral blood, and skin (41). Two common histologic types are peripheral T-cell lymphoma, not otherwise specified, and hepatosplenic T-cell lymphoma (41,42). EBV positivity in T-cell post-transplant neoplasms is approximately 35 percent, which is markedly lower than that in B-cell PTLDs (41). The positive incidence also varies among histologic types: 50 percent in peripheral T-cell lymphoma, not otherwise specified and less than 10 percent in hepatosplenic T-cell lymphoma (41).

Classic Hodgkin Lymphoma. This is the least common form of PTLD, and needs to be diagnosed based on the morphologic criteria used in nontransplant patients.

LEUKEMIC INFILTRATION AND MYELOID SARCOMA

Definition. Myeloid neoplasms involve the liver in two distinct manners: diffuse intrasinusoidal infiltration or mass-forming lesions (*myeloid sarcoma*). The former is more common and occurs exclusively in leukemic patients. The latter, defined as liver nodules/masses effacing the hepatic lobular architecture, is a rare manifestation and develops either in isolation or in association with bone marrow involvement (43). Myeloid sarcoma is also called *granulocytic sarcoma* or *chloroma*.

General and Clinical Features. One study, in which autopsy specimens were mainly examined, confirmed intrahepatic tumor infiltration in 60 to 70 percent of acute leukemias and over 80 percent of chronic leukemias, in incidences higher than for malignant lymphomas (50 to 60 percent) (44). Hepatic involvement in acute leukemias is not systematically evaluated in everyday practice; in patients with leukemia who have unexplained hepatomegaly or liver dysfunction biopsies are considered to exclude the possibility of concomitant liver disease. Other liver pathologies that potentially occur in isolation or in association with leukemic cell infiltration include ischemic necrosis due to sinusoidal infiltration of tumor cells, nodular regenerative hyperplasia, and venous outflow block (45–48). Extramedullary hematopoiesis is a common histologic finding in patients with bone marrow disease. In patients with bone marrow transplantation, liver dysfunction may trigger the diagnosis of relapse.

Myeloid sarcoma may develop de novo with no obvious bone marrow involvement, or it may occur before, concurrent with, or after the diagnosis of acute myeloid leukemia or other myeloproliferative disorders (49). Although myeloid sarcoma occurs in any organ, hepatic involvement is rare. Patients present with various abdominal symptoms, most frequently jaundice (50–52). Myeloid sarcoma in the liver forms discrete masses, the imaging features of which are similar to those of malignant lymphoma (5).

Microscopic Findings. Hepatic involvement in acute leukemias is characterized by the diffuse, nondestructive infiltration of leukemic cells into portal tracts and sinusoids (44). Sinusoidal infiltration is typically predominant in *acute myeloid leukemias* (fig. 11-35), while portal tract infiltrates may become more obvious in *lymphoblastic leukemias* (fig. 11-36) (34). In *chronic myelogenous leukemia*, more than 50 percent of patients have hepatomegaly at initial presentation, and sinusoidal infiltration by leukemic cells becomes obvious in acute blastic crisis (34,44). *Chronic lymphocytic leukemia* causes liver dysfunction, generally in the late stage, and the hepatic infiltrate is observed mainly in portal tracts (34,44). In *hairy cell leukemia*, sinusoidal infiltration by leukemic cells is a common finding, and there is often diffuse or patchy sinusoidal dilatation mimicking peliosis hepatis or hemangioma (53,54). Discrete liver nodules consisting of solid tumor cell aggregates are another rare manifestation of this indolent form of leukemia (55,56).

Myeloid sarcoma histologically consists of myeloid blasts arranged in sheets and effacing the hepatic lobular architecture, sometimes associated with the infiltration of neoplastic cells into nearby sinusoids (49,52). Tumors with a myelomonocytic or pure monocytic morphology are common in this presentation. The tumor cells are positive for CD68/KP1, myeloperoxidase, CD117, CD99, and CD34 (57). The expression of CD68/PG-M1, CD168, and CD14 suggests monocytic differentiation (58–61).

Figure 11-35

LEUKEMIC INFILTRATION (ACUTE MYELOID LEUKEMIA)

A: Intrasinusoidal cellularity is increased.

B: Infiltrating cells are moderately pleomorphic with irregularly shaped nuclei.

C: They are positive for myeloperoxidase.

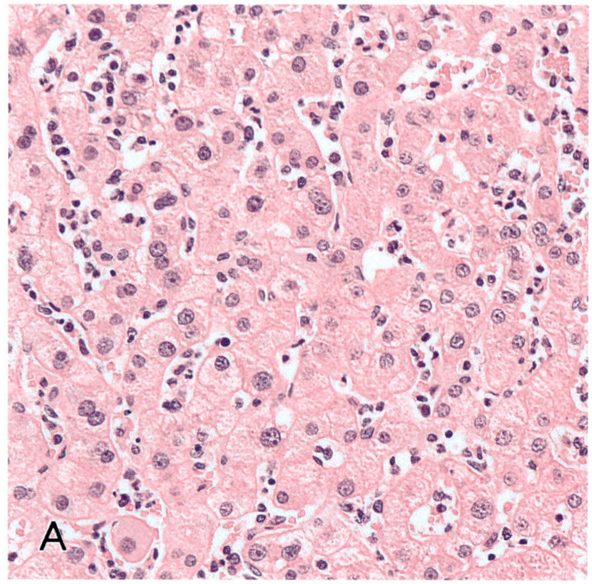

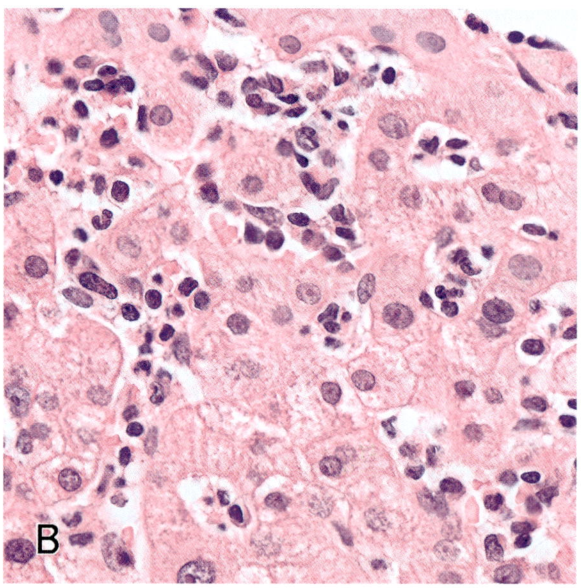

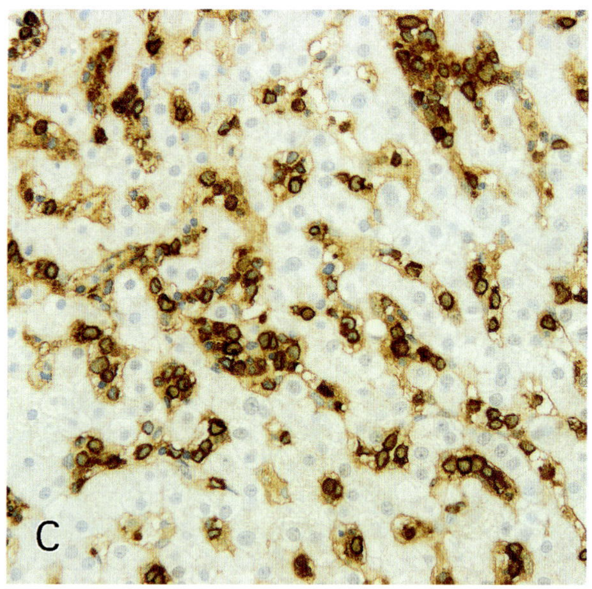

PLASMA CELL NEOPLASMS

Definition. One of the two hepatic manifestations of plasma cell neoplasms is intrahepatic involvement in *plasma cell myeloma* (also called *multiple myeloma*) derived from bone marrow, while the other is *mass-forming plasmacytoma* that primarily develops in the liver without bone marrow disease.

General and Clinical Features. Although hepatic involvement in plasma cell myeloma is less common than in leukemias, autopsy series have shown that 64 percent of patients with multiple myeloma have extraosseous disease, with the liver being the third most commonly affected site (29 percent), following the spleen (31 percent) and kidneys (31 percent) (62). Another liver histology review (mainly based on postmortem specimens) of 33 patients with myeloma also confirmed infiltration by myeloma cells in 32 percent of patients (44). These studies suggest that subclinical liver involvement may be more frequent than expected (44). Extraosseous disease is more common in younger patients and in those with more aggressive subtypes of

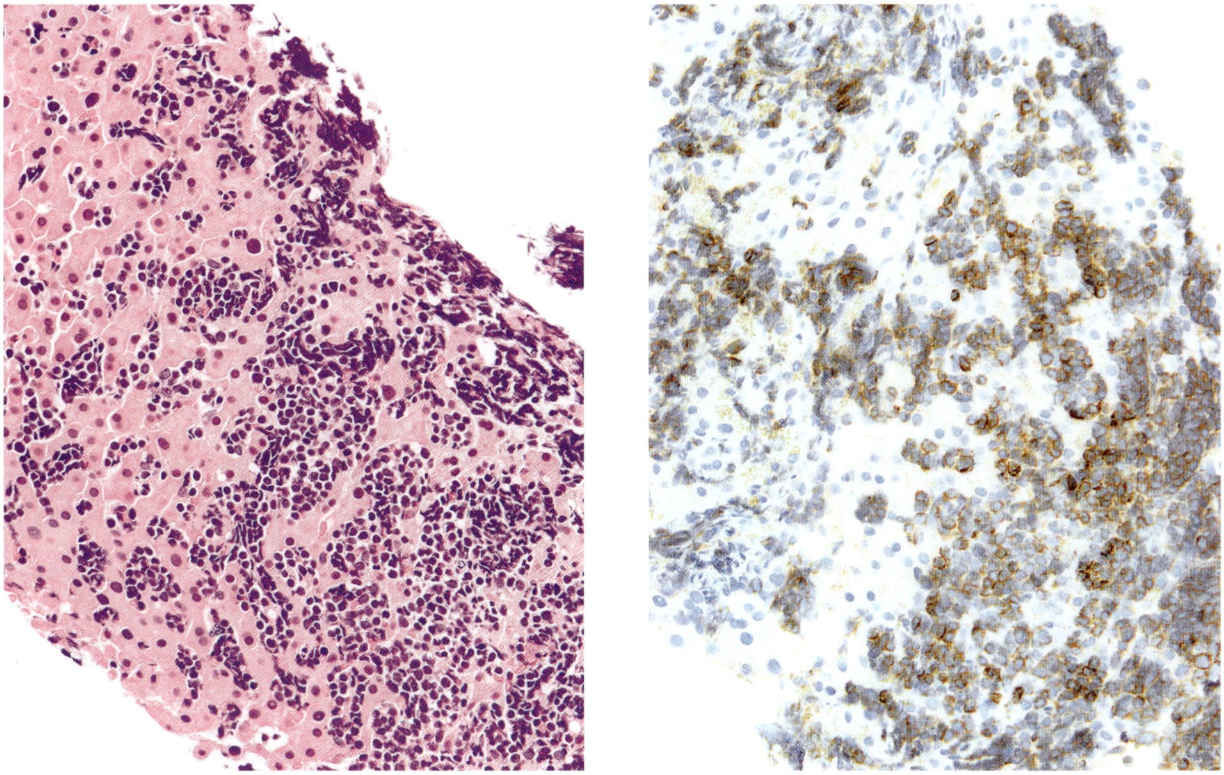

Figure 11-36

LEUKEMIC INFILTRATION (B-LYMPHOBLASTIC LEUKEMIA)

Left: Atypical mononuclear cells with a high nuclear to cytoplasmic ratio extensively infiltrate along sinusoids. Right: CD20 is positive.

myeloma (e.g., nonsecretory myeloma) (63). Approximately 50 percent of patients with hepatic involvement have discrete masses detectable on imaging, while the rest show diffuse or patchy microscopic infiltration (62).

Isolated plasmacytoma without bone marrow involvement may also develop in the liver (64–66). Primary hepatic plasmacytoma is rare, and may progress to classic systemic plasma cell myeloma. Generally, a solitary discrete mass or nodule is seen in the liver on imaging.

Microscopic Findings. The infiltration of monotypic plasma cells is observed in sinusoids or portal tracts, and may aggregate in nodules (fig. 11-37) (44). Tumors are composed of mature-looking, slightly atypical plasma cells arranged in isolated cells, small aggregates, or rarely, sheets (fig. 11-38). The cells are immunoreactive to CD79a and CD138. The lack of CD20 expression is important for differentiation from B-cell lymphomas with prominent plasmacytic differentiation. Immunohistochemistry for immunoglobulin heavy chains and in situ hybridization for light chains are useful for confirming the monoclonal nature (fig. 11-37A–C). Another pathology potentially involving the liver in patients with myeloma is amyloidosis, in which amyloid deposition is observed in the walls of blood vessels or along the space of Disse (67,68).

LANGERHANS CELL HISTIOCYTOSIS

Definition. *Langerhans cell histiocytosis* is a rare disorder characterized by the clonal proliferation of Langerhans cell histiocytes that infiltrate various tissues and organs. Synonyms include *histiocytosis X, Langerhans cell granulomatosis, eosinophilic granuloma* (solitary lesion), *Hand-Schüller-Christian disease* (multiple lesions), and *Letterer-Siwe disease* (disseminated disease or visceral involvement) (3,69).

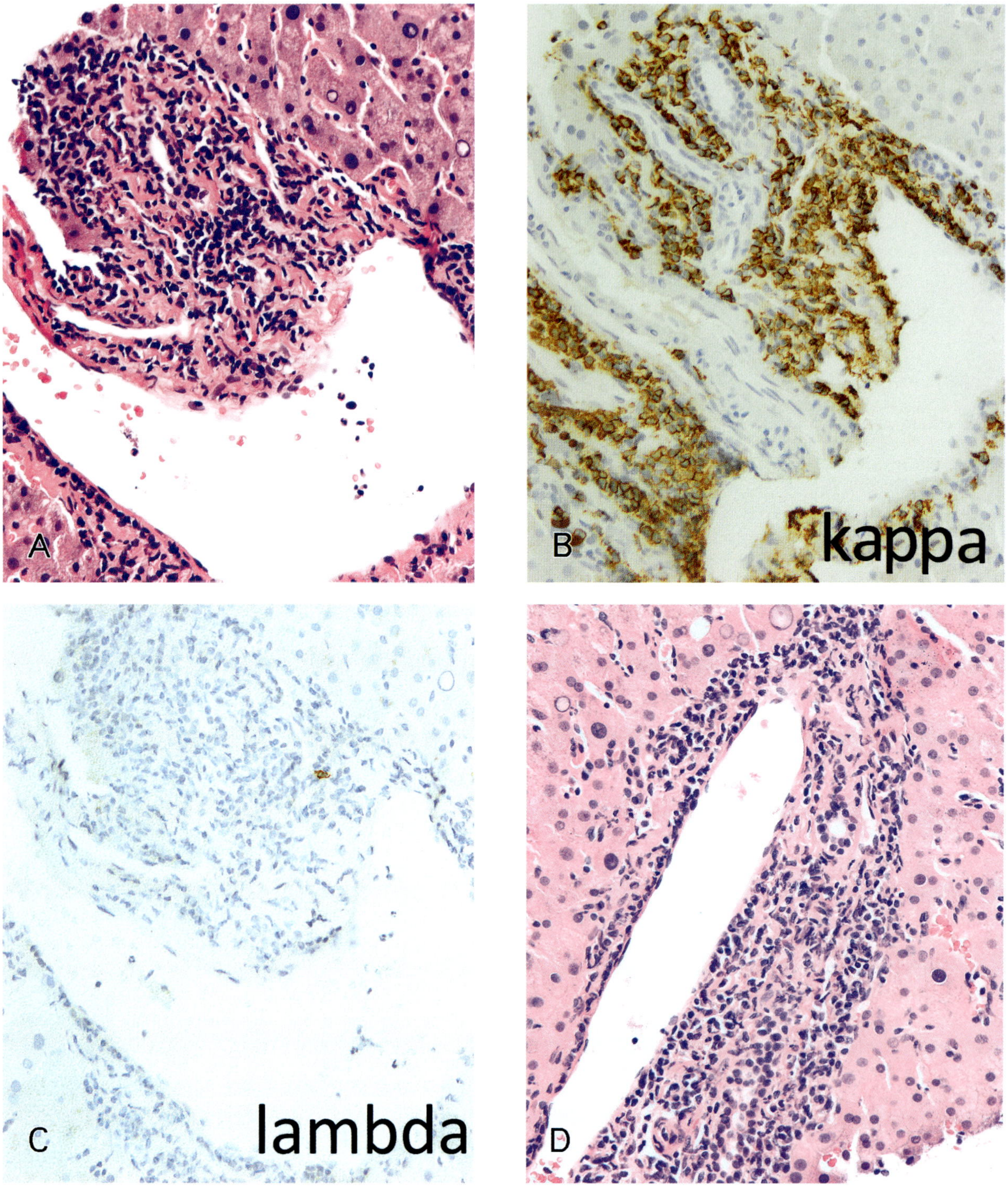

Figure 11-37

LIVER INVOLVEMENT IN PLASMA CELL MYELOMA

A: The portal tract is mildly infiltrated by mononuclear cells.
B: The cells are diffusely positive for the kappa chain on in situ hybridization.
C: The lambda chain is not expressed.
D: Myeloma cells are mainly present in the portal tract.

General and Clinical Features. Langerhans cell histiocytosis most commonly affects bone, and sometimes involves extraskeletal organs (e.g., skin, lungs, and lymph nodes). Although hepatic involvement has been reported in up to 15 percent of patients with multisystemic involvement (70,71), Langerhans cell histiocytosis confined to the liver is unusual.

The typical liver manifestation is sclerosing cholangiopathy (71,72). According to a study by Kaplan et al. (73), in which 94 cases of hepatobiliary Langerhans cell histiocytosis were examined (9 of their own cases and 84 cases reported in the literature), patients' ages ranged between 7 days and 62 years, with a median of 18 months, and a 2 to 1 female predominance. Common clinical presentations were hepatosplenomegaly, jaundice, liver dysfunction, and ascites.

Gross Findings. Hepatobiliary Langerhans cell histiocytosis presents with demarcated liver nodules and/or periductal infiltrative lesions (fig. 11-39), with the latter leading to the imaging features of sclerosing cholangitis or cystic dilatation of the bile duct (74). The degree of fibrosis in the background liver varies, and some patients may already have liver cirrhosis at initial presentation (73).

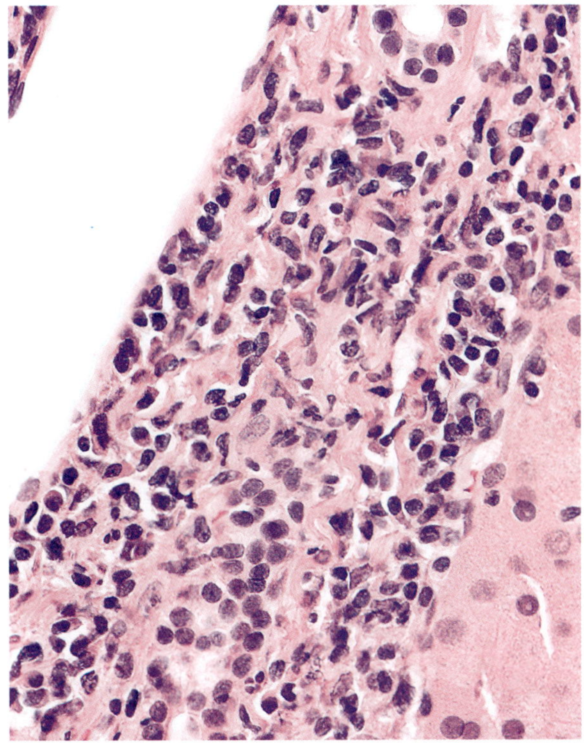

Figure 11-38

LIVER INVOLVEMENT IN PLASMA CELL MYELOMA

Infiltrating cells show only mild cellular atypia. Some have a plasmacytoid appearance.

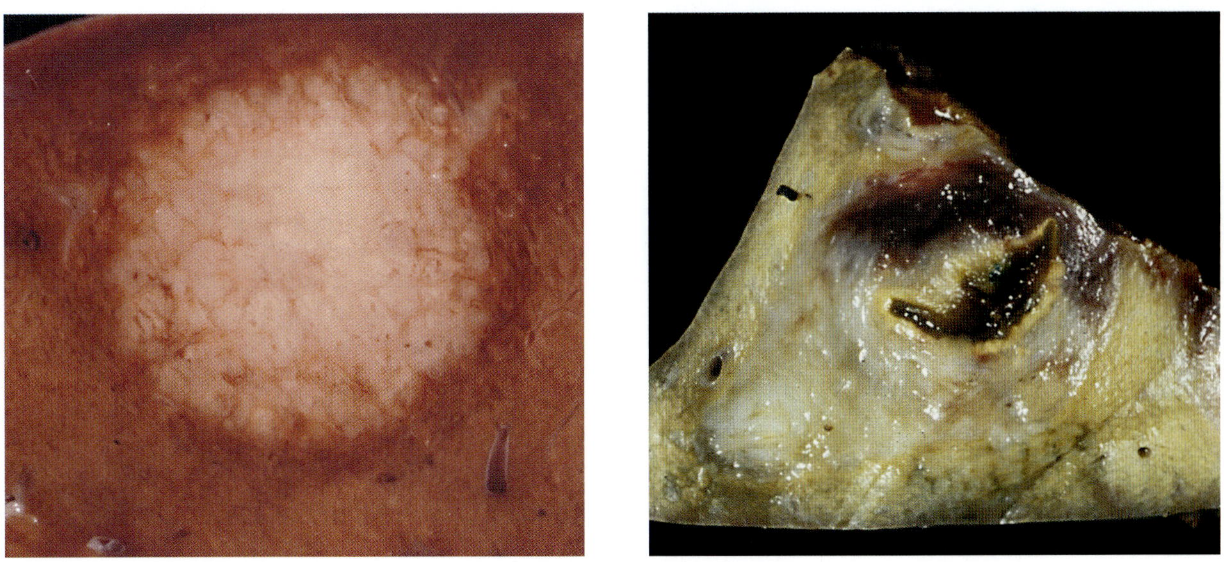

Figure 11-39

LANGERHANS CELL HISTIOCYTOSIS

Left: The section shows a nodular, light tan lesion.
Right: The large portal area contains a dilated necrotic bile duct with surrounding fibrosis.

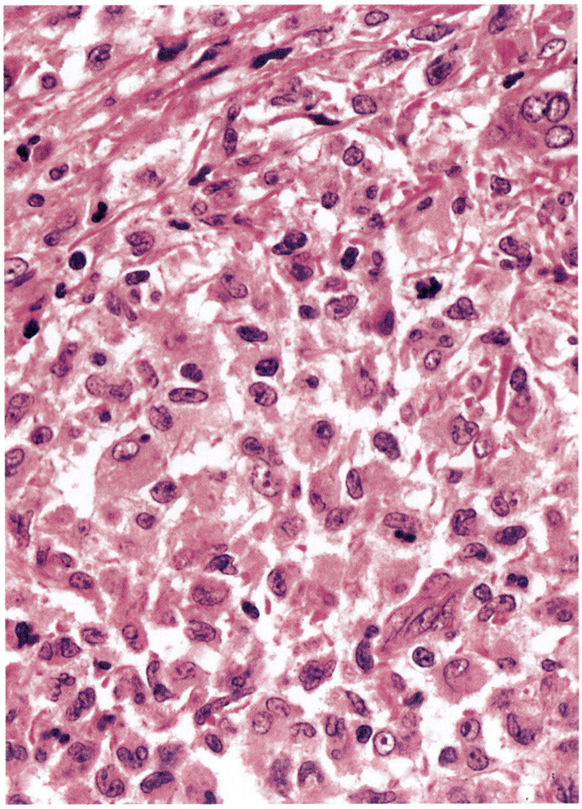

Figure 11-40

LANGERHANS CELL HISTIOCYTOSIS

Langerhans cells have ill-defined outlines, eosinophilic cytoplasm, and vesicular nuclei.

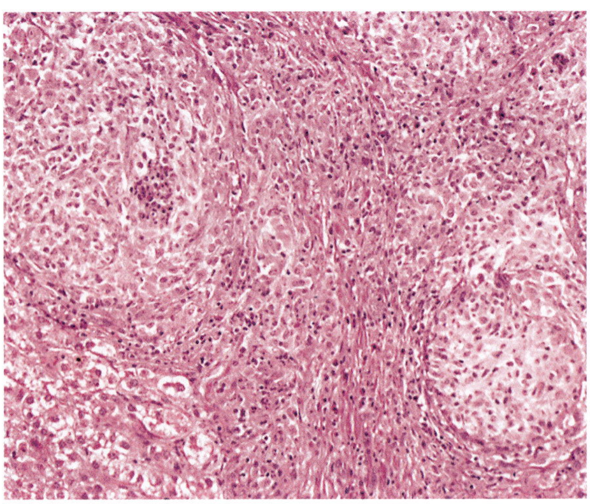

Figure 11-41

LANGERHANS CELL HISTIOCYTOSIS

Two focal, granulomatous aggregates of Langerhans cells.

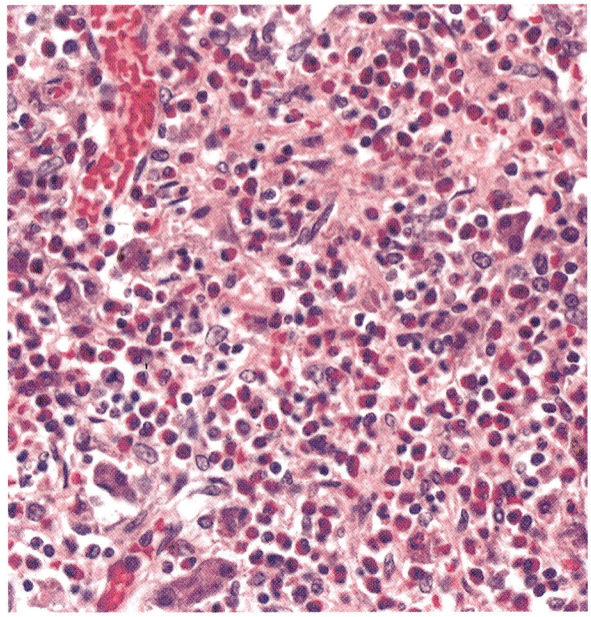

Figure 11-42

LANGERHANS CELL HISTIOCYTOSIS

Numerous eosinophils are noted in the infiltrate.

Microscopic Findings. A hallmark histologic finding is the infiltration by Langerhans cell histiocytes that typically have abundant pink cytoplasm, coffee-bean shaped or contorted nuclei, and inconspicuous nucleoli (fig. 11-40). They are always accompanied by variable numbers of eosinophils, lymphocytes, and neutrophils. Multinucleated giant cells may coexist. The number of diagnostic histiocytes varies. Nested aggregates of Langerhans cells potentially give a granulomatous appearance (fig. 11-41), while extensive background inflammatory infiltrates may mask the diagnostic cells (fig. 11-42) (69,75). Portal tracts and periportal areas are primarily affected in most cases, leading to the proposed progression model that Langerhans cells initially infiltrate portal connective tissue and then involve the liver parenchyma or sinusoids (73).

Small bile ducts are damaged by the periductal or intraepithelial infiltration of Langerhans cells (fig. 11-43). These changes may be accompanied by periductal concentric fibrosis and bile duct destruction, the histologic features of which may be potentially mistaken for primary sclerosing cholangitis (PSC), particularly on needle biopsies (fig. 11-44).

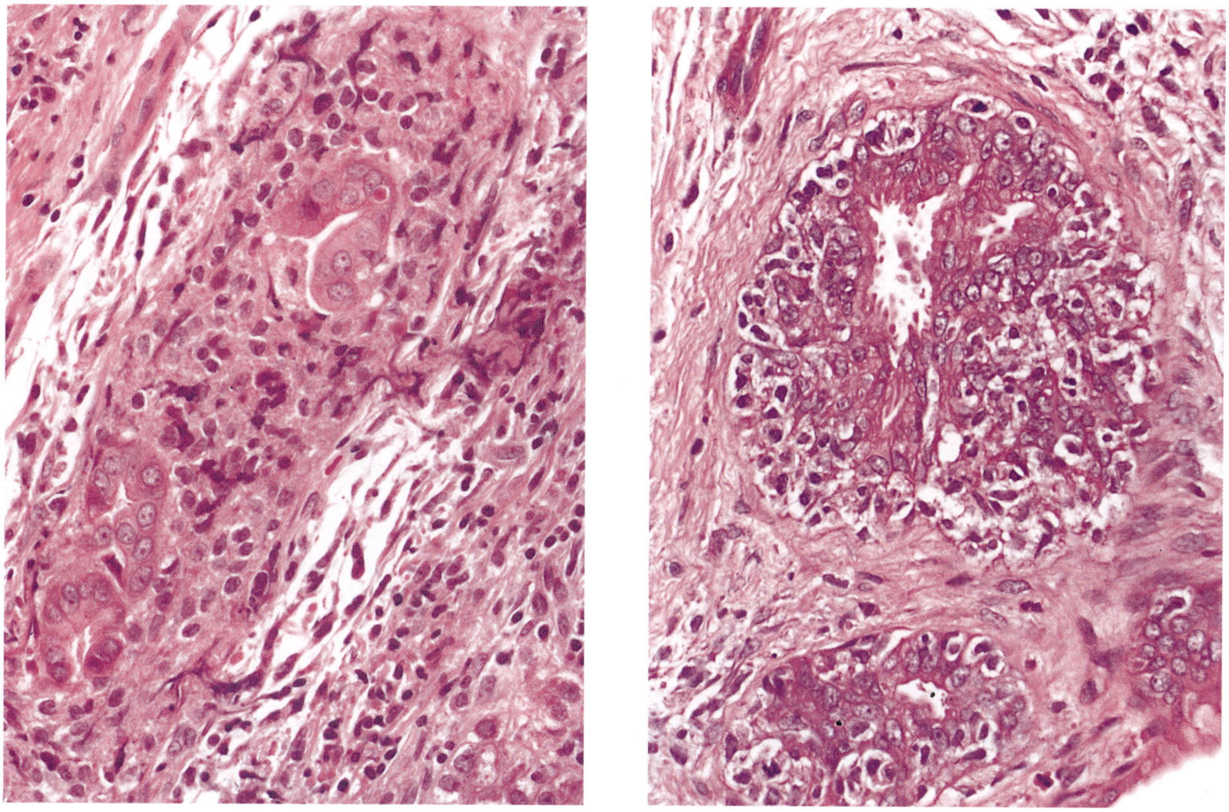

Figure 11-43

LANGERHANS CELL HISTIOCYTOSIS

The bile ducts are surrounded and infiltrated by Langerhans cells.

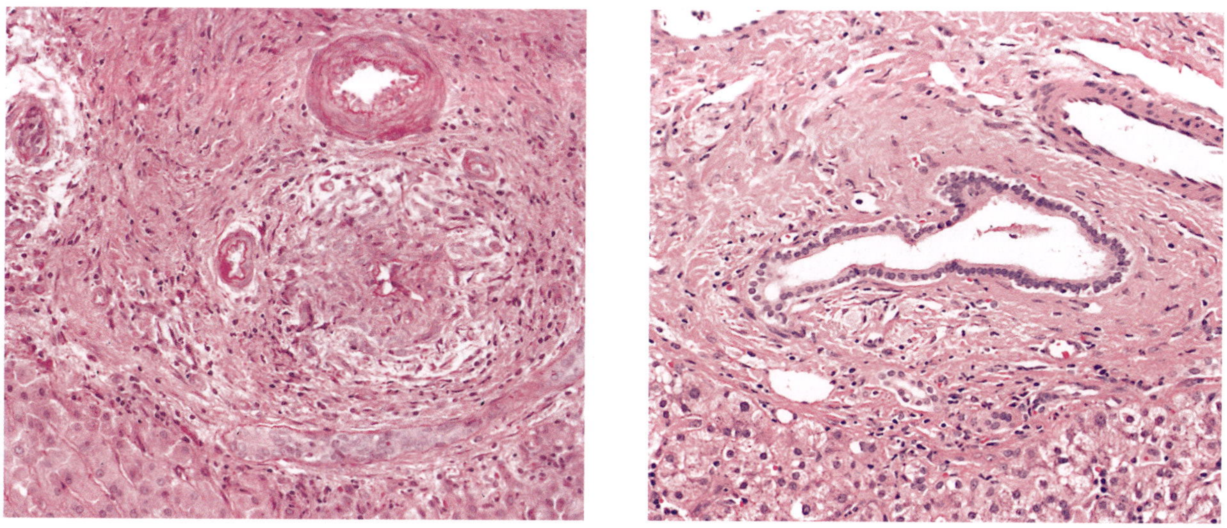

Figure 11-44

LANGERHANS CELL HISTIOCYTOSIS

Left: A destroyed bile duct is located adjacent to an artery in a portal area.
Right: There is periductal fibrosis.

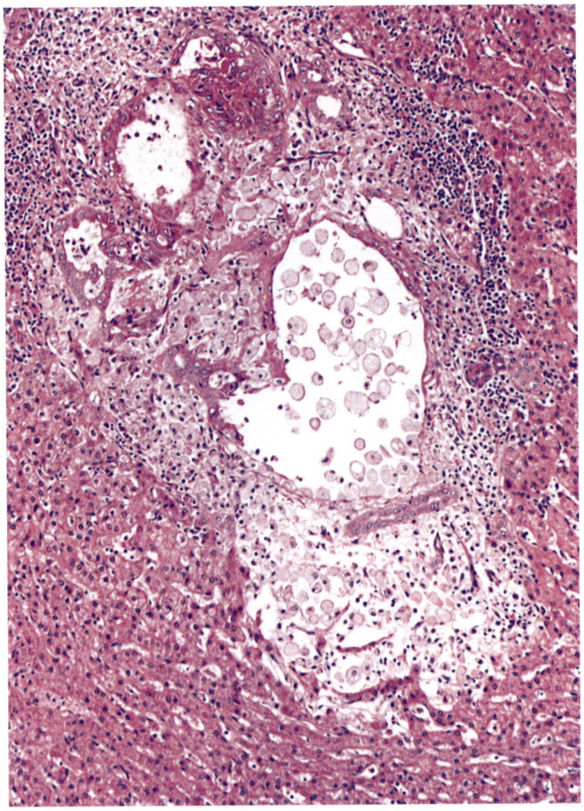

Figure 11-45

LANGERHANS CELL HISTIOCYTOSIS

A ruptured bile duct contains and is surrounded by pseudoxanthomatous cells. The portal area is also infiltrated by inflammatory cells, and some Langerhans cells were detected by CD1a immunostaining (not shown).

Large bile ducts involved by Langerhans cell histiocytosis show cystic dilatation or rupture with periductal xanthogranulomatous inflammation (fig. 11-45). Liver tissue located separately from the lesions often shows the features of secondary sclerosing cholangitis such as a ductular reaction, copper-associated protein deposition, and biliary-type fibrosis. Even after successful treatment, liver fibrosis may progress to biliary cirrhosis because of irreversible bile duct injury.

Immunohistochemical Findings. Immunostaining assists in confirming the nature of the Langerhans cells. Cells are positive for S-100 protein, CD1a, and CD207 (langerin) (fig. 11-46) (76,77). The latter two are more specific for Langerhans cells because Kupffer cells may be immunoreactive to S-100 protein. Typical Birbeck granules may be found ultrastructurally in Langerhans cells.

Differential Diagnosis. Since Langerhans cell histiocytosis is a well-known cause of secondary sclerosing cholangitis, a differential diagnosis includes other forms of sclerosing cholangitis such as PSC and immunodeficiency-related cholangiopathy (78). Thus, the possibility of Langerhans cell histiocytosis needs to be excluded in children with suspected sclerosing cholangitis. Liver biopsies with additional immunohistochemistry are useful in this aspect; however, the diagnostic features of Langerhans cell histiocytosis may not be observed in biopsy specimens taken from the peripheral liver parenchyma. Imaging studies (e.g., bone and lungs) and physical examination (e.g., skin) for the extrahepatic manifestations of Langerhans cell histiocytosis assist in confirming or excluding this condition (71).

Treatment and Prognosis. Patients with multisystem Langerhans cell histiocytosis represent a heterogeneous group with respect to disease severity and outcome (79). Despite systemic therapy, approximately 20 percent of patients with multisystem involvement have a progressive disease course (80). Hepatic involvement is a known risk factor: the 3-year survival rate is 96.7 percent in patients without and 51.8 percent in those with liver involvement (81). Liver transplantation is considered for patients with liver cirrhosis and end-stage liver disease due to secondary sclerosing cholangitis, with two thirds of patients expected to achieve long-term survival (82,83). Disease recurrence in the liver allograft occurs in up to 30 percent of patients (84,85).

TUMOR-LIKE LESIONS

Hepatic Pseudolymphoma

Definition. *Hepatic pseudolymphoma* is a form of idiopathic reactive lymphoid proliferation manifesting in liver nodules (86). This condition is also called *reactive lymphoid hyperplasia of the liver.*

General and Clinical Features. Sharifi et al. (87) reported three cases of hepatic pseudolymphoma in 1999, and several dozen cases have since been reported. This condition was originally considered to be extremely rare,

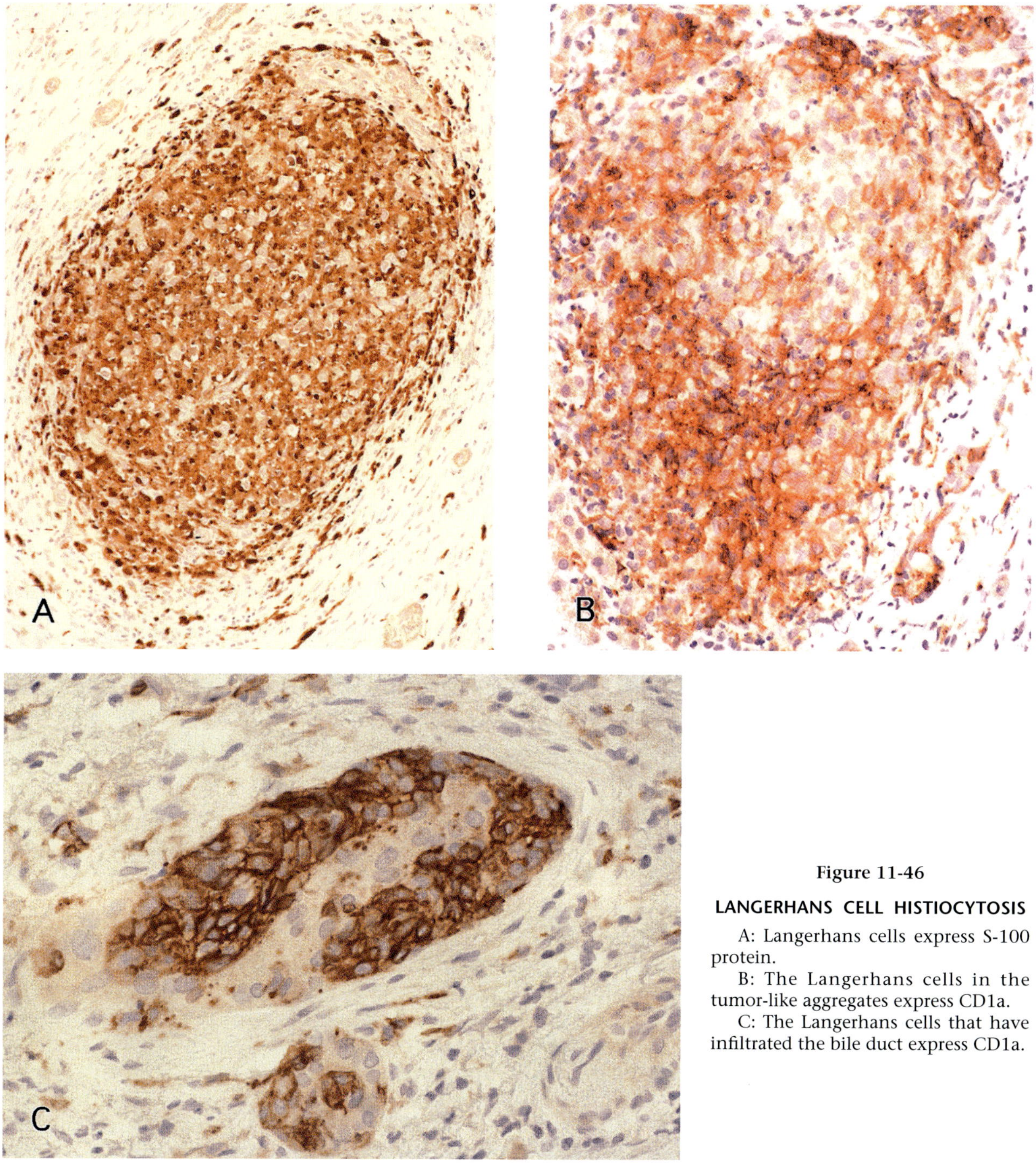

Figure 11-46

LANGERHANS CELL HISTIOCYTOSIS

A: Langerhans cells express S-100 protein.

B: The Langerhans cells in the tumor-like aggregates express CD1a.

C: The Langerhans cells that have infiltrated the bile duct express CD1a.

but has been increasingly detected because of recent advances in imaging techniques. This is a benign condition with no known risk of malignant transformation. Tumors may regress spontaneously without treatment.

Patients are generally adults older than 30 years, with rare pediatric cases also described (88). Women are more commonly affected than men, with a male to female ratio of 1 to 4. Patients are typically asymptomatic, and imaging studies incidentally disclose single (80 percent) or multiple (20 percent) liver nodules (86,89). Liver tumors range from less than 1.0 cm to 5.5 cm in diameter (mean, 1.7 cm).

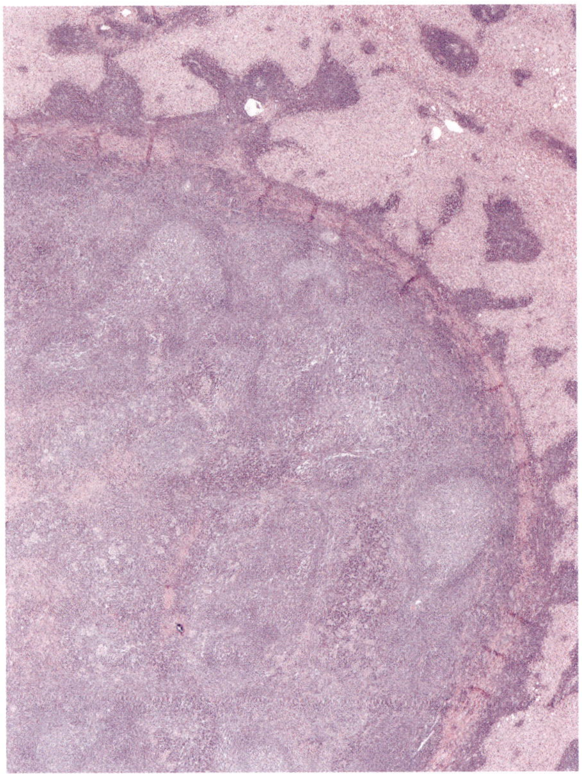

Figure 11-47

HEPATIC PSEUDOLYMPHOMA

A lymphoid nodule is observed in the liver parenchyma. The lymphoid process extends into the adjacent liver tissue along portal tracts.

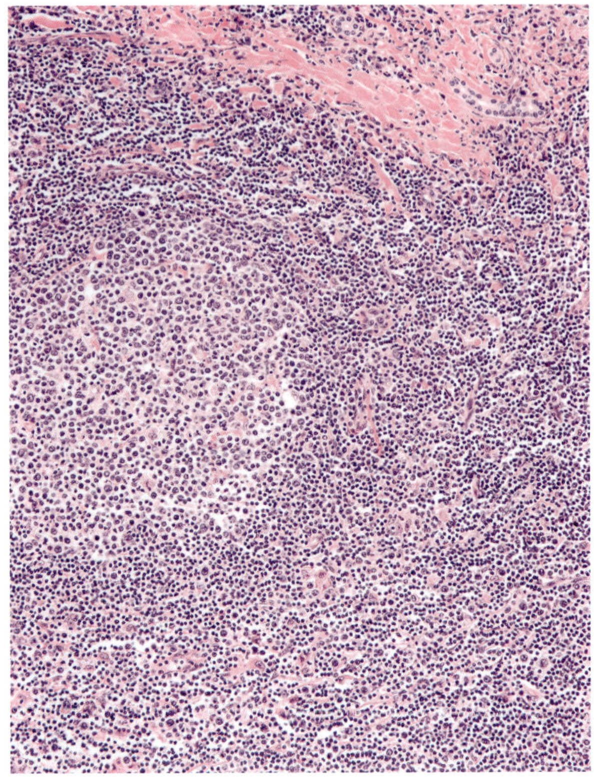

Figure 11-48

HEPATIC PSEUDOLYMPHOMA

The nodule consists of lymphoid follicles and interfollicular lymphoid tissue.

In 27 percent of cases, pseudolymphoma develops in patients with chronic liver disease (e.g., primary biliary cholangitis, chronic viral hepatitis, and non-alcoholic steatohepatitis) (86,89,90). One fourth of patients have extrahepatic autoimmune diseases (e.g., Sjögren syndrome and Hashimoto thyroiditis), while another fourth have a history of malignancy including gastric, colon, and renal cell cancers (86). Although the frequent association with autoimmune and malignant diseases is of interest, it may merely be because those patients often undergo abdominal imaging studies, and, thus, have more chance of being diagnosed.

Microscopic Findings. The liver nodules are fairly well-circumscribed and located inside the liver parenchyma, with no direct involvement in large portal tracts (fig. 11-47). The lesions consist of densely arranged lymphocytes forming occasional lymphoid follicles (fig. 11-48) (86,87). The cells are mature looking, with no atypical features such as nuclear enlargement or pleomorphism (fig. 11-49).

Lymphoid follicles are surrounded by a mantle zone and contain tingible body macrophages, in keeping with a reactive pattern. Fibrosis and plasmacytic infiltration are focally noted (fig. 11-50). Several histiocytes and immunoblasts are present in interfollicular areas, and small non-necrotizing granulomas may also be observed (fig. 11-51). Intrahepatic small bile ducts entrapped within the nodules are slightly attenuated; however, the lining epithelium is intact with no classic features of lymphoepithelial lesions (fig. 11-52). The lymphocytic infiltrate often spills over the adjacent liver parenchyma along the portal tracts (fig. 11-47) (86).

Immunohistochemical Findings. Immunostaining reveals a zonal distribution of T cells in the interfollicular area and B cells are

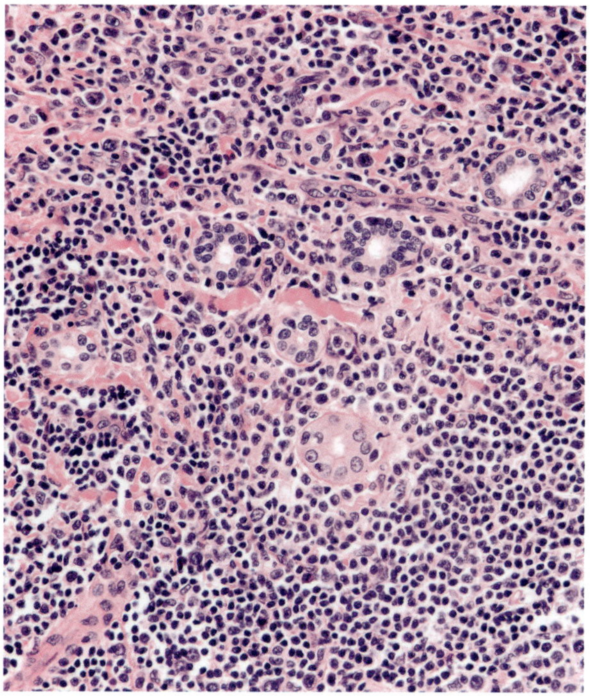

Figure 11-49

HEPATIC PSEUDOLYMPHOMA

Infiltrating cells are mainly small mature lymphocytes with no atypical features. Several eosinophils are also present in this field.

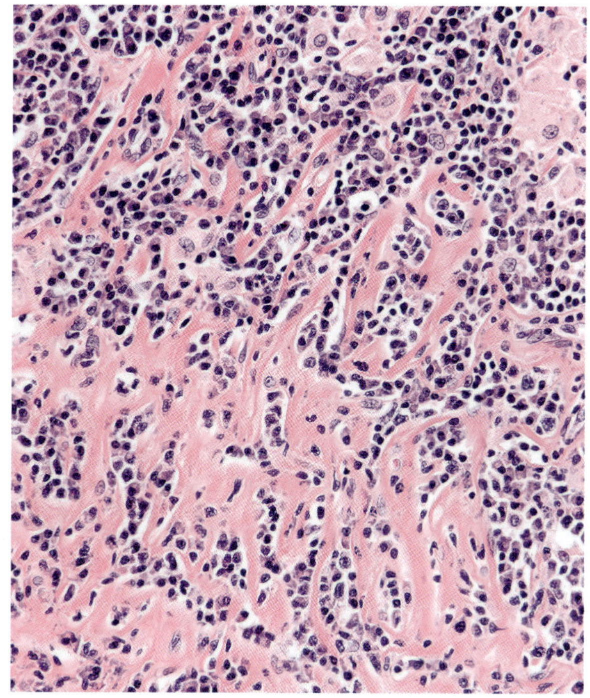

Figure 11-50

HEPATIC PSEUDOLYMPHOMA

Plasmacytic differentiation and fibrosis are focally observed.

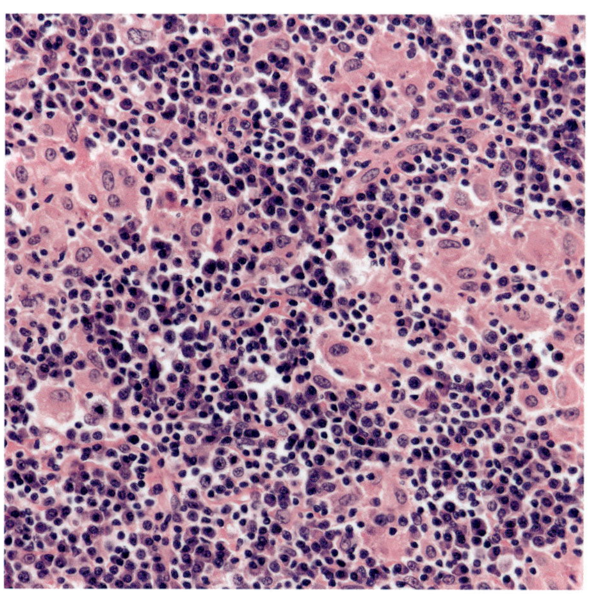

Figure 11-51

HEPATIC PSEUDOLYMPHOMA

A granulomatous reaction is observed in the interfollicular area.

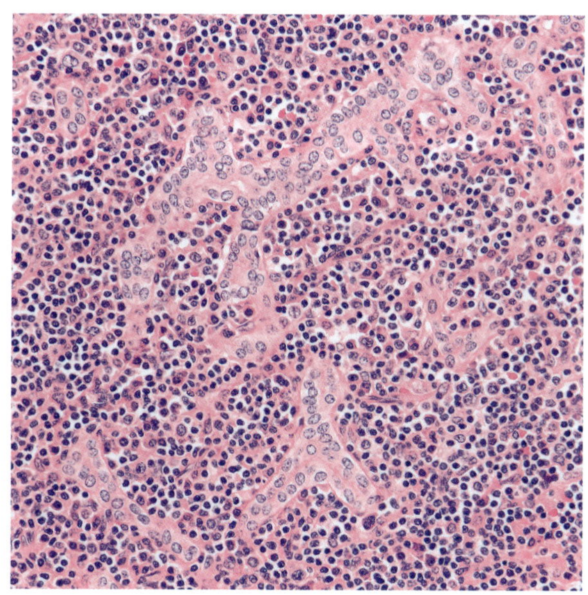

Figure 11-52

HEPATIC PSEUDOLYMPHOMA

Entrapped bile ducts are irregular in shape, however, intraepithelial lymphocytic infiltration is rare.

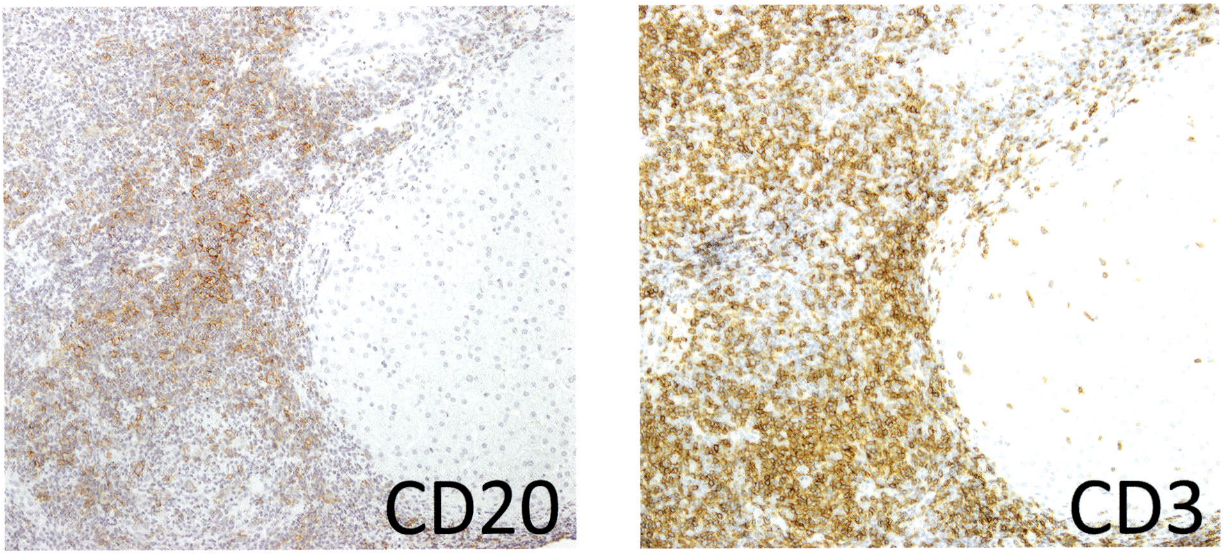

Figure 11-53

HEPATIC PSEUDOLYMPHOMA

Immunostaining confirms a T-cell predominant inflammatory infiltrate. The appearance differs distinctly from marginal zone lymphoma, in which B cells are typically predominant (see also figure 11-13) (left: CD20 immunostain; right: CD3 immunostain).

predominantly present in follicles. Similar to other reactive lymphoid lesions, T cells are generally dominant or almost equal in density to B cells (fig. 11-53). Immunostaining for CK7 shows entrapped bile ducts, particularly at the periphery of nodules. IgG4-positive plasma cells are rare or only focally aggregated. The polyclonal nature of infiltrating lymphocytes may be proven by in situ hybridization for light chains or a gene rearrangement analysis (86,87).

Differential Diagnosis. A main entity in the differential diagnosis is MALT lymphoma (Table 11-2). Differentiation is particularly challenging in needle biopsy samples because the pattern of infiltration into adjacent liver parenchyma under low-power magnification may be similar in both conditions. MALT lymphoma consists of more monotonous cellular components. Severe duct injuries with intraepithelial lymphocytic infiltration also suggest that this lymphoma is more likely; however, diagnostic changes may not be found in biopsy specimens. Immunostaining and in situ hybridization are useful for proving a B-cell predominant cellular population, with light chain restriction supporting the diagnosis of MALT lymphoma (see figs. 11-13, 11-14).

Follicular Cholangitis

Definition. *Follicular cholangitis* is a rare form of idiopathic inflammatory cholangiopathy characterized by dense lymphocytic infiltration accompanied by many lymphoid follicles along large bile ducts. Infiltrating lymphocytes are polyclonal in nature.

General and Clinical Features. This condition commonly manifests as mass lesions around perihilar or intrahepatic large bile ducts; rarely, more diffuse bile duct strictures reminiscent of PSC are seen (91). Patients most frequently present with jaundice. No association with particular serologic abnormalities or extrahepatic autoimmune diseases is known. A histologic examination of surgically resected specimens is currently essential for establishing the diagnosis; therefore, this condition is supposedly underdiagnosed, and some cases may have been labeled as PSC or simply a benign bile duct stricture of uncertain nature.

Gross and Microscopic Findings. Gross examination reveals a whitish, ill-defined nodule surrounding the large bile duct (fig. 11-54). A hallmark histologic feature is a duct-centered massive lymphocytic infiltration associated

Table 11-2

CLINICOPATHOLOGIC FEATURES OF HEPATIC PSEUDOLYMPHOMA, MARGINAL ZONE LYMPHOMA, FOLLICULAR CHOLANGITIS, AND IGG4-RELATED INFLAMMATORY PSEUDOTUMOR

	Hepatic Pseudolymphoma	Marginal Zone Lymphoma	Follicular Cholangitis	IgG4-Related Inflammatory Pseudotumor
Age	>30 years	>40 years	>40 years	>50 years
Gender (M/F)	1/4	1/1	1/1	4/1
Serologic features	Potentially autoimmune abnormalities	None	None	IgG4 elevation (~80%), ANA (~40%)
Potentially associated liver lesions	Chronic liver diseases in ~30% (e.g., viral hepatitis, PBC[a], NASH)	Chronic liver diseases in ~30% (e.g., viral hepatitis, PBC)	None	IgG4-related sclerosing cholangitis
Other organ lesions	Autoimmune diseases (~25%), malignancy (~25%)	None	None	IgG4-related disease (e.g., autoimmune pancreatitis, sialadenitis, retroperitoneal fibrosis)
Location and shape	Nodular lesions in the liver parenchyma	Nodular lesions in the liver parenchyma	Periductal mass lesions around large bile ducts	Periductal mass lesions around large bile ducts
Histologic features	Aggregated mature lymphocytes with reactive lymphoid follicles	Proliferation of atypical small lymphocytes; B-cell predominant population; lymphoepithelial lesion; proven monoclonality	Lymphocytic cholangitis rich in lymphoid follicles; a fibrotic rim beneath the epithelial lining; polyclonal lymphocytes	Sclerosing inflammation with lymphoplasmacytic filtration and occasional eosinophils; storiform fibrosis; obliterative phlebitis; many IgG4-positive plasma cells

[a]PBC = primary biliary cholangiocarcinoma; NASH = nonalcoholic steatohepatitis; ANA = antinuclear antibody.

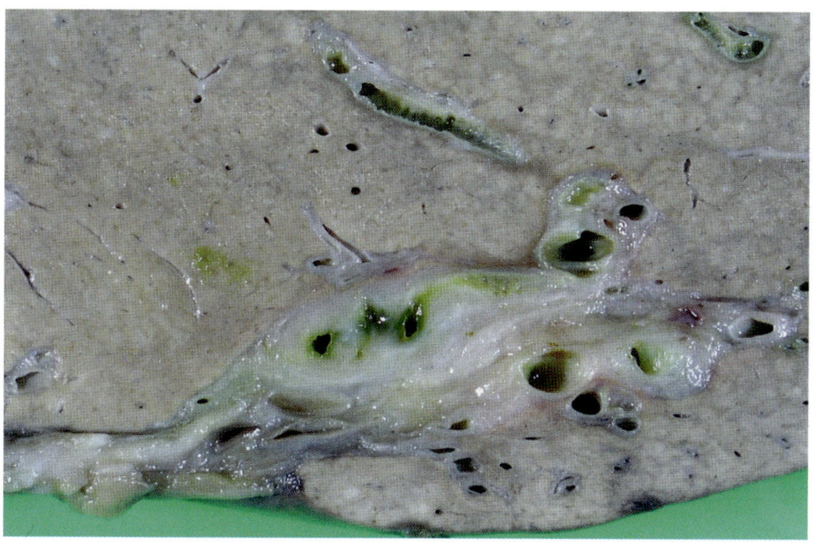

Figure 11-54

FOLLICULAR CHOLANGITIS

An ill-defined, fibrotic nodule is observed around the large bile duct. The upstream bile ducts are dilated.

with many lymphoid follicles and fibrotic rims in the subepithelial area of the affected ducts (fig. 11-55) (91–93). Germinal centers are well circumscribed and surrounded by a mantle zone; they contain mitotically active lymphocytes and tingible body macrophages. Plasma cells and eosinophils are also present, but do not dominate (fig. 11-56). The epithelial

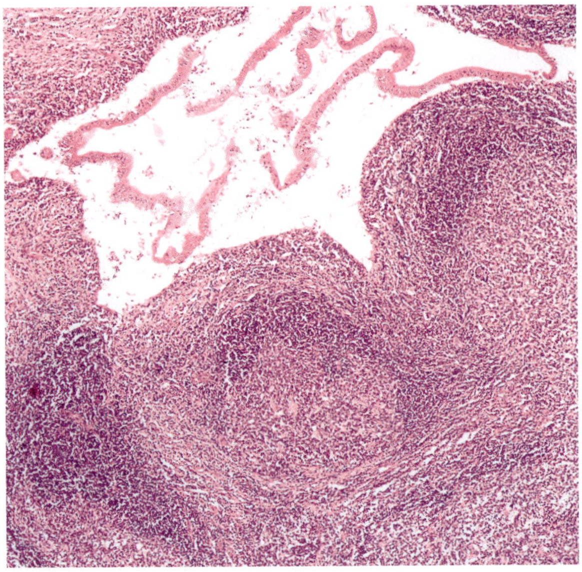

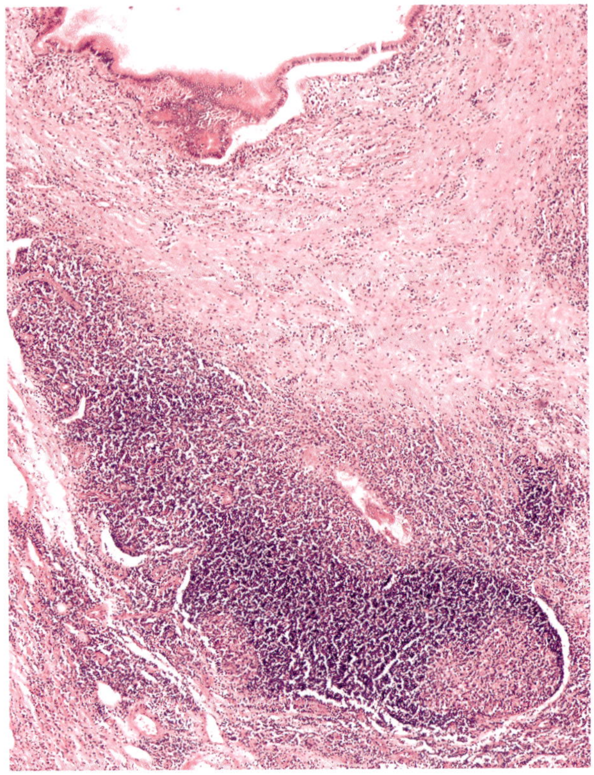

Figure 11-55

FOLLICULAR CHOLANGITIS

Above: The affected bile duct is heavily infiltrated by lymphocytes with lymphoid follicles.

Right: A fibrous rim beneath the duct epithelium is occasionally observed in this condition.

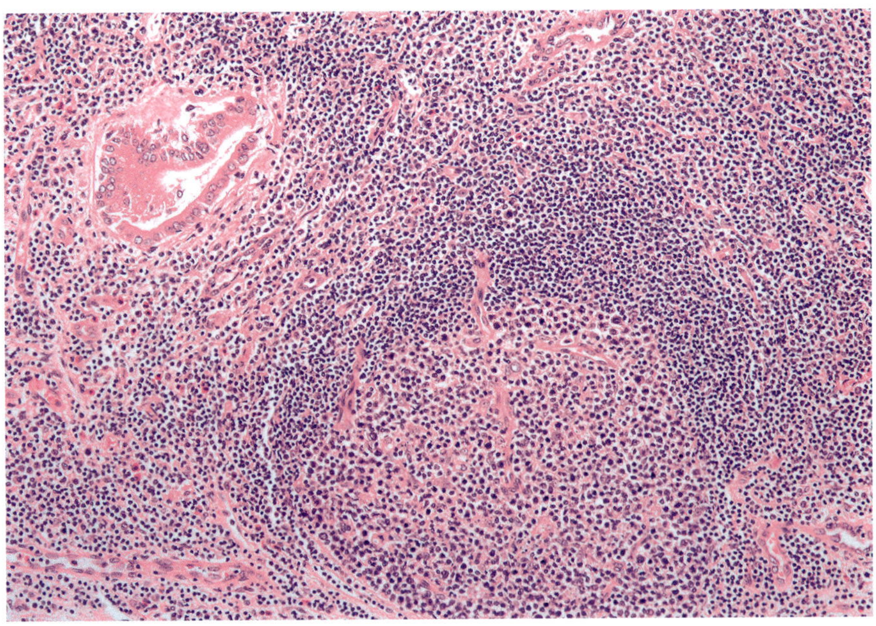

Figure 11-56

FOLLICULAR CHOLANGITIS

No atypical features are observed in lymphoid follicles and the interfollicular area.

lining of the affected bile ducts is intact, with no features of a lymphoepithelial lesion. Overall, fibrosis is mild (fig. 11-57). A similar inflammatory process rich in lymphoid follicles is known to occur in the pancreas and gallbladder, and is referred to as follicular pancreatitis and follicular cholecystitis, respectively (91).

Differential Diagnosis. Follicular cholangitis needs to be discriminated from PSC, IgG4-related inflammatory pseudotumors, and hepatic pseudolymphoma (Table 11-2) (94,95). PSC affects the biliary tree more diffusely. Fibro-obliterative changes in bile ducts (e.g., periductal concentric fibrosis and bile duct loss) are observed in PSC, but not in follicular cholangitis. Epithelial ulceration and xanthogranulomatous inflammation are features suggesting PSC over follicular cholangitis. A caveat is that some of the affected bile ducts may have lymphoid follicles and a subepithelial fibrous rim in otherwise typical PSC.

IgG4-related inflammatory pseudotumor also involves large bile ducts, but is more fibrotic in its microscopic appearance than follicular cholangitis. Histologic evidence of obliterative phlebitis, storiform fibrosis, and a large number of IgG4-positive plasma cells, coupled with a high IgG4/IgG plasma cell ratio, supports the diagnosis of IgG4-related inflammatory pseudotumor (see also chapter 9). Follicular cholangitis and hepatic pseudolymphoma have similar cellular components. The latter, however, generally affects the liver parenchyma with no large duct involvement (86).

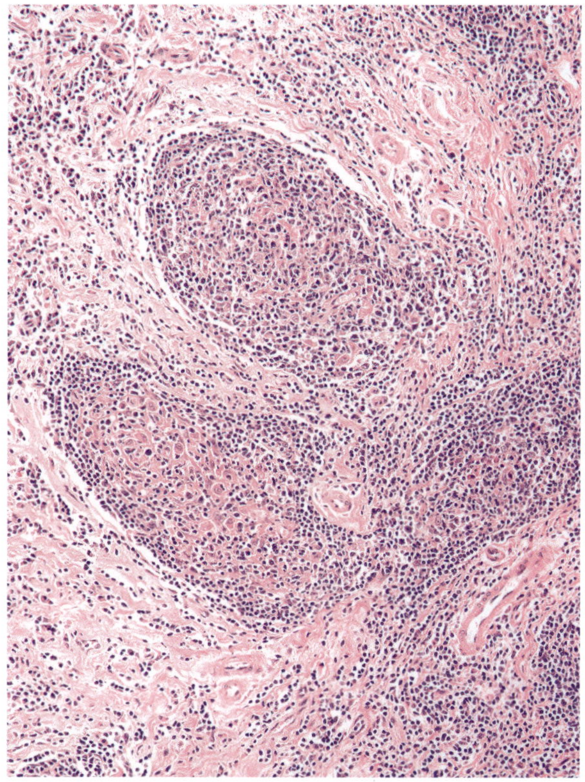

Figure 11-57

FOLLICULAR CHOLANGITIS

Fibrosis may be focally present, as here.

Extramedullary Hematopoiesis

Extramedullary hematopoiesis is a common finding in liver specimens of patients with bone marrow diseases such as chronic myeloproliferative disorders, anaplastic anemia, and extensive bone metastasis of malignancy (96). A few megakaryocytes of unknown significance may also be incidentally found in liver biopsies from patients with no known bone marrow failure.

Histologically, erythroid and myeloid precursors or megakaryocytes of variable proportions are observed in sinusoids and the space of Disse (fig. 11-58) (34). The portal tracts may also be involved in extensive cases. Although a diagnosis is generally straightforward, intrasinusoidal immature hematopoietic cells arranged in cords or nests may be mistaken for leukemic infiltration, particularly in the absence of megakaryocytes (fig. 11-58D). Although mitotic figures are occasionally present, cellular atypia and pleomorphism are not. A diagnostic clue is to identify mixed cellular lineages by morphologic or immunohistochemical analysis (fig. 11-59). Commonly used immunohistochemical markers are myeloperoxidase and CD33 for granulocytic lineages, and factor VIII and CD61 for megakaryocytes.

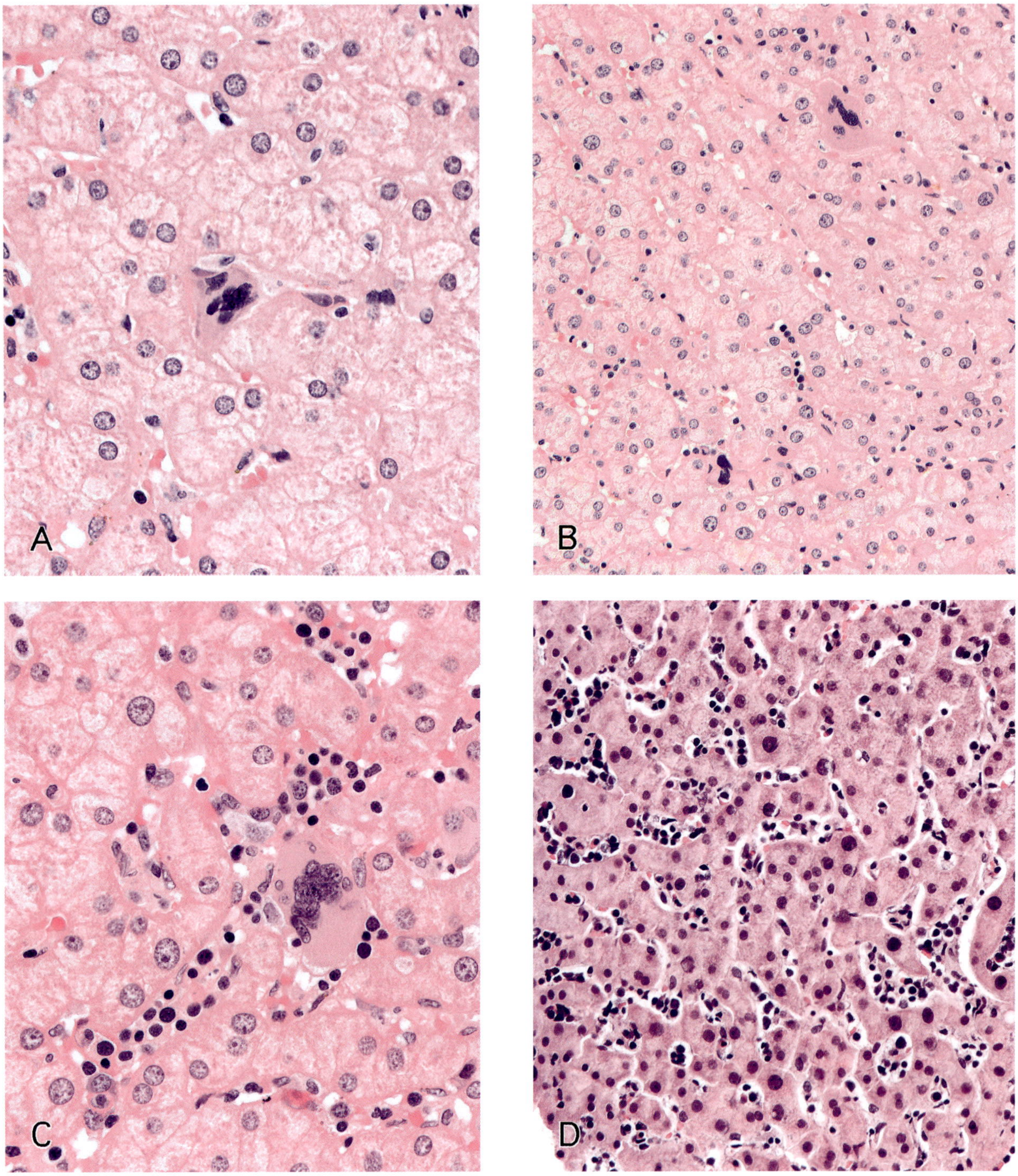

Figure 11-58

EXTRAMEDULLARY HEMATOPOIESIS

A: Isolated megakaryocytes are present in the sinusoids.

B: In addition to megakaryocytes, myeloid or erythroid precursors are present in the sinusoids.

C: Hematopoietic precursors are aggregated.

D: Extensive extramedullary hematopoiesis may be mistaken for the sinusoidal infiltration of hematolymphoid neoplasms, particularly in the absence of megakaryocytes.

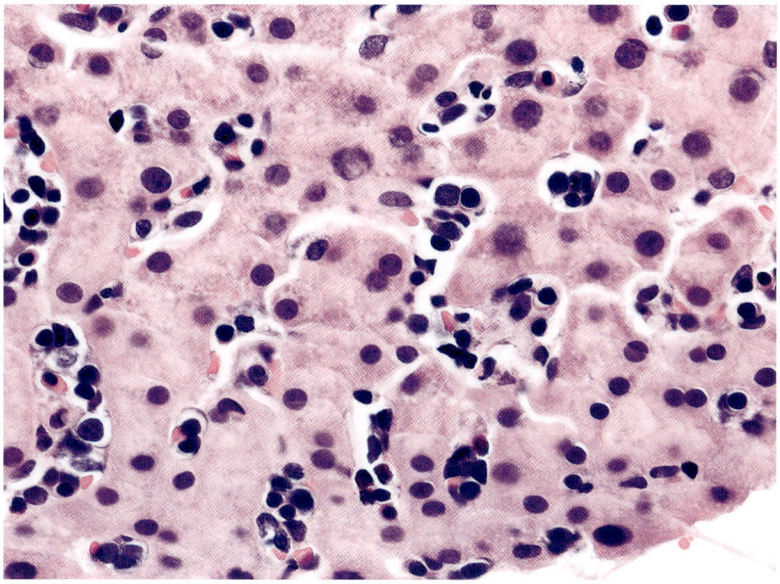

Figure 11-59

EXTRAMEDULLARY HEMATOPOIESIS

Under high magnification, some cells appear to have eosinophilic cytoplasm, suggesting granulocytic differentiation.

REFERENCES

1. Medeiros LJ, O'Malley DP, Caraway NP, Vega F, Elenitoba-Johnson KS, Lim, MS. Tumors of the lymph nodes and spleen. AFIP Atlas of Tumor Pathology, 4th Series, Fascicle, 25. Washington, DC: American Registry of Pathology; 2017.
2. Foucar K, Kroft S, McKenna RW, Peterson LC. Tumors of the bone marrow. AFIP Atlas of Tumor Pathology, 4th Series, Fascicle 24. Washington, DC: American Registry of Pathology; 2016.
3. Swerdlow SH, Campo E, Harris NL, Jaffe ES, Pileri SA, Stein H, et al. World Health Organization classification of tumours of haematopoietic and lymphoid tissues, 4th ed. Lyon: IARC; 2008.
4. Noronha V, Shafi NQ, Obando JA, Kummar S. Primary non-Hodgkin's lymphoma of the liver. Crit Rev Oncol Hematol 2005;53:199-207.
5. Tomasian A, Sandrasegaran K, Elsayes KM, Shanbhogue A, Shaaban A, Menias CO. Hematologic malignancies of the liver: spectrum of disease. Radiographics 2015;35:71-86.
6. Freeman C, Berg JW, Cutler SJ. Occurrence and prognosis of extranodal lymphomas. Cancer 1972;29:252-260.
7. Lei KI. Primary non-Hodgkin's lymphoma of the liver. Leuk Lymphoma 1998;29:293-299.
8. Salo J, Nomdedeu B, Bruguera M, et al. Acute liver failure due to non-Hodgkin's lymphoma. Am J Gastroenterol 1993;88:774-776.
9. Cameron AM, Truty J, Truell J, et al. Fulminant hepatic failure from primary hepatic lymphoma: successful treatment with orthotopic liver transplantation and chemotherapy. Transplantation 2005;80:993-996.
10. Bronowicki JP, Bineau C, Feugier P, et al. Primary lymphoma of the liver: clinical-pathological features and relationship with HCV infection in French patients. Hepatology 2003;37:781-787.
11. Aozasa K, Mishima K, Ohsawa M. Primary malignant lymphoma of the liver. Leuk Lymphoma 1993;10:353-357.
12. Emile JF, Azoulay D, Gornet JM, et al. Primary non-Hodgkin's lymphomas of the liver with nodular and diffuse infiltration patterns have different prognoses. Ann Oncol 2001;12:1005-1010.
13. [No authors listed] A predictive model for aggressive non-Hodgkin's lymphoma. The International Non-Hodgkin's Lymphoma Prognostic Factors Project. N Engl J Med 1993;329:987-994.
14. Isaacson PG, Chott A, Nakamura S, Muller-Hermelink HK, Harris NL, Swerdlow SH. Extranodal marginal zone lymphoma of mucosa-associated lymphoid tissue (MALT lymphoma). In: Swerdlow SH, Campo E, Harris NL, et al., eds. World Health Organization classification of tumours of haematopoietic and lymphoid tissues, 4th ed. Lyon: IARC; 2008:214-217.
15. Doi H, Horiike N, Hiraoka A, et al. Primary hepatic marginal zone B cell lymphoma of mucosa-associated lymphoid tissue type: case report and review of the literature. Int J Hematol 2008;88:418-423.

16. Prabhu RM, Medeiros LJ, Kumar D, et al. Primary hepatic low-grade B-cell lymphoma of mucosa-associated lymphoid tissue (MALT) associated with primary biliary cirrhosis. Mod Pathol 1998;11:404-410.
17. Ascoli V, Lo Coco F, Artini M, Levrero M, Martelli M, Negro F. Extranodal lymphomas associated with hepatitis C virus infection. Am J Clin Pathol 1998;109:600-609.
18. Ye MQ, Suriawinata A, Black C, Min AD, Strauchen J, Thung SN. Primary hepatic marginal zone B-cell lymphoma of mucosa-associated lymphoid tissue type in a patient with primary biliary cirrhosis. Arch Pathol Lab Med 2000;124:604-608.
19. Takeshima F, Kunisaki M, Aritomi T, et al. Hepatic mucosa-associated lymphoid tissue lymphoma and hepatocellular carcinoma in a patient with hepatitis B virus infection. J Clin Gastroenterol 2004;38:823-826.
20. Kiesewetter B, Mullauer L, Streubel B, et al. Primary mucosa-associated lymphoid tissue (MALT) lymphoma of the liver: clinical, molecular, and microbiological aspects. Ann Hematol 2012;91: 1817-1818.
21. Isaacson PG, Banks PM, Best PV, McLure SP, Muller-Hermelink HK, Wyatt JI. Primary low-grade hepatic B-cell lymphoma of mucosa-associated lymphoid tissue (MALT)-type. Am J Surg Pathol 1995;19:571-575.
22. Streubel B, Simonitsch-Klupp I, Müllauer L, et al. Variable frequencies of MALT lymphoma-associated genetic aberrations in MALT lymphomas of different sites. Leukemia 2004;18:1722-1726.
23. Gaulard P, Jaffe ES, Krenacs L, Macon WR. Hepatosplenic T-cell lymphoma. In: Swerdlow SH, Campo E, Harris NL, et al., eds. World Health Organization classification of tumours of haematopoietic and lymphoid tissues, 4th ed. Lyon: IARC; 2008:292-293.
24. Yabe M, Medeiros LJ, Tang G, et al. Prognostic factors of hepatosplenic T-cell lymphoma: clinicopathologic study of 28 cases. Am J Surg Pathol 2016;40:676-688.
25. Thai A, Prindiville T. Hepatosplenic T-cell lymphoma and inflammatory bowel disease. J Crohns Colitis 2010;4:511-522.
26. Macon WR, Levy NB, Kurtin PJ, et al. Hepatosplenic alphabeta T-cell lymphomas: a report of 14 cases and comparison with hepatosplenic gammadelta T-cell lymphomas. Am J Surg Pathol 2001;25:285-296.
27. Weidmann E. Hepatosplenic T cell lymphoma. A review on 45 cases since the first report describing the disease as a distinct lymphoma entity in 1990. Leukemia 2000;14:991-997.
28. Belhadj K, Reyes F, Farcet JP, et al. Hepatosplenic gammadelta T-cell lymphoma is a rare clinicopathologic entity with poor outcome: report on a series of 21 patients. Blood 2003;102:4261-4269.
29. Baumhoer D, Tzankov A, Dirnhofer S, Tornillo L, Terracciano LM. Patterns of liver infiltration in lymphoproliferative disease. Histopathology 2008;53:81-90.
30. Lui PC, Wong GK, Poon WS, Tse GM. Intravascular lymphomatosis. J Clin Pathol 2003;56:468-470.
31. Shiraki K, Sugimoto K, Deguchi M, Ito N, Masuda C, Takei Y. Hepatic intravascular large B cell lymphoma. Intern Med 2007;46:1761-1762.
32. Higurashi T, Takahashi H, Inamori M, et al. Intravascular lymphoma: usefulness of liver biopsy in the clinical setting. Intern Med 2009;48:2155-2156.
33. Sekiguchi N, Joshita S, Yoshida T, et al. Liver dysfunction and thrombocytopenia diagnosed as intravascular large B-cell lymphoma using a timely and accurate transjugular liver biopsy. Intern Med 2013;52:1903-1908.
34. Goodman ZD, Luigi MT, Wee A. Tumours and tumour-like lesions of the liver. In: Burt A, Portmann B, Ferrell L, eds. MacSween's pathology of the liver, 6th ed. Edinburgh: Elsevier; 2012:761-851.
35. Ohshima K. Pathological features of diseases associated with human T-cell leukemia virus type I. Cancer Sci 2007;98:772-778.
36. Kawano H, Wakahashi K, Ebara S, et al. Unusual hepatic involvement with significant fibrosis in adult T cell leukemia. Ann Hematol 2014;93:897-898.
37. Rappaport H, Berard CW, Butler JJ, Dorfman RF, Lukes RJ, Thomas LB. Report of the Committee on Histopathological Criteria Contributing to Staging of Hodgkin's Disease. Cancer Res 1971;31:1864-1965.
38. Hubscher SG, Lumley MA, Elias E. Vanishing bile duct syndrome: a possible mechanism for intrahepatic cholestasis in Hodgkin's lymphoma. Hepatology 1993;17:70-77.
39. Swerdlow SH, Webber SA, Chadburn A, Ferry JA. Post-transplant lymphoproliferative disorders. In: Swerdlow SH, Campo E, Harris NL, et al., eds. World Health Organization classification of tumours of haematopoietic and lymphoid tissues, 4th ed. Lyon: IARC; 2008:343-349.
40. Webber SA, Naftel DC, Fricker FJ, et al. Lymphoproliferative disorders after paediatric heart transplantation: a multi-institutional study. Lancet 2006;367:233-239.
41. Swerdlow SH. T-cell and NK-cell posttransplantation lymphoproliferative disorders. Am J Clin Pathol 2007;127:887-895.
42. Lundell R, Elenitoba-Johnson KS, Lim MS. T-cell posttransplant lymphoproliferative disorder occurring in a pediatric solid-organ transplant patient. Am J Surg Pathol 2004;28:967-973.

43. Pileri SA, Orazi A, Falini B. Myeloid sarcoma. In: Swerdlow SH, Campo E, Harris NL, Jaffe ES, et al., eds. World Health Organization classification of tumours of haematopoietic and lymphoid tissues. Lyon: IARC; 2008:140-141.
44. Walz-Mattmüller R, Horny HP, Ruck P, Kaiserling E. Incidence and pattern of liver involvement in haematological malignancies. Pathol Res Pract 1998;194:781-789.
45. Shehab TM, Kaminski MS, Lok AS. Acute liver failure due to hepatic involvement by hematologic malignancy. Dig Dis Sci 1997;42:1400-1405.
46. Pieri G, Theocharidou E, Burroughs AK. Liver in haematological disorders. Best Pract Res Clin Gastroenterol 2013;27:513-530.
47. Costa F, Choy CG, Seiter K, Hann L, Thung SN, Michaeli J. Hepatic outflow obstruction and liver failure due to leukemic cell infiltration in chronic lymphocytic leukemia. Leuk Lymphoma 1998;30:403-410.
48. Picardi M, Muretto P, Luciano L. Budd-Chiari syndrome in chronic myeloid leukemia. Haematologica 2000;85:429.
49. Norsworthy KJ, Bhatnagar B, Singh ZN, Gojo I. Myeloid sarcoma of the hepatobiliary system: a case series and review of the literature. Acta Haematol 2016;135:241-251.
50. Piccaluga PP, Ascani S, Agostinelli C, et al. Myeloid sarcoma of liver: an unusual cause of jaundice. Report of three cases and review of literature. Histopathology 2007;50:802-805.
51. Lee JY, Lee WS, Jung MK, et al. Acute myeloid leukemia presenting as obstructive jaundice caused by granulocytic sarcoma. Gut Liver 2007;1:182-185.
52. Wandroo FA, Murray J, Mutimer D, Hubscher S. Acute myeloid leukaemia presenting as cholestatic hepatitis. J Clin Pathol 2004;57:544-545.
53. Zafrani ES, Degos F, Guigui B, et al. The hepatic sinusoid in hairy cell leukemia: an ultrastructural study of 12 cases. Hum Pathol 1987;18:801-807.
54. Nanba K, Soban EJ, Bowling MC, Berard CW. Splenic pseudosinuses and hepatic angiomatous lesions. Distinctive features of hairy cell leukemia. Am J Clin Pathol 1977;67:415-426.
55. Sahar N, Schiby G, Davidson T, Kneller A, Apter S, Farfel Z. Hairy cell leukemia presenting as multiple discrete hepatic lesions. World J Gastroenterol 2009;15:4453-4456.
56. Al-Za'abi AM, Boerner SL, Geddie W. Hairy cell leukemia presenting as a discrete liver mass: diagnosis by fine needle aspiration biopsy. Diagn Cytopathol 2008;36:128-132.
57. Pileri SA, Ascani S, Cox MC, et al. Myeloid sarcoma: clinico-pathologic, phenotypic and cytogenetic analysis of 92 adult patients. Leukemia 2007;21:340-350.
58. Chang CC, Eshoa C, Kampalath B, Shidham VB, Perkins S. Immunophenotypic profile of myeloid cells in granulocytic sarcoma by immunohistochemistry. Correlation with blast differentiation in bone marrow. Am J Clin Pathol 2000;114:807-811.
59. Garcia C, Gardner D, Reichard KK. CD163: a specific immunohistochemical marker for acute myeloid leukemia with monocytic differentiation. Appl Immunohistochem Mol Morphol 2008;16:417-421.
60. Klco JM, Kulkarni S, Kreisel FH, Nguyen TD, Hassan A, Frater JL. Immunohistochemical analysis of monocytic leukemias: usefulness of CD14 and Kruppel-like factor 4, a novel monocyte marker. Am J Clin Pathol 2011;135:720-730.
61. Rollins-Raval MA, Roth CG. The value of immunohistochemistry for CD14, CD123, CD33, myeloperoxidase and CD68R in the diagnosis of acute and chronic myelomonocytic leukaemias. Histopathology 2012;60:933-942.
62. Oshima K, Kanda Y, Nannya Y, et al. Clinical and pathologic findings in 52 consecutively autopsied cases with multiple myeloma. Am J Hematol 2001;67:1-5.
63. Varettoni M, Corso A, Pica G, Mangiacavalli S, Pascutto C, Lazzarino M. Incidence, presenting features and outcome of extramedullary disease in multiple myeloma: a longitudinal study on 1003 consecutive patients. Ann Oncol 2010;21:325-330.
64. Demirhan B, Sökmensüer C, Karakayali H, Güngen Y, Doüan A, Haberal M. Primary extramedullary plasmacytoma of the liver. J Clin Pathol 1997;50:74-76.
65. Weichhold W, Labouyrie E, Merlio JP, Masson B, de Mascarel A. Primary extramedullary plasmacytoma of the liver. A case report. Am J Surg Pathol 1995;19:1197-1202.
66. Lee JY, Won JH, Kim HJ, et al. Solitary extramedullary plasmacytoma of the liver without systemic monoclonal gammopathy. J Korean Med Sci 2007;22:754-757.
67. Buck FS, Koss MN. Hepatic amyloidosis: morphologic differences between systemic AL and AA types. Hum Pathol 1991;22:904-907.
68. Chopra S, Rubinow A, Koff RS, Cohen AS. Hepatic amyloidosis. A histopathologic analysis of primary (AL) and secondary (AA) forms. Am J Pathol 1984;115:186-193.
69. Ishak KG, Goodman ZD, Stocker JT. Tumors of the liver and intrahepatic bile ducts. AFIP Atlas of Tumor Pathology, 4th Series, Fascicle 31. Washington, DC: American Registry of Pathology; 1999.
70. Jaffe R. Liver involvement in the histiocytic disorders of childhood. Pediatr Dev Pathol 2004;7: 214-225.

71. Portmann BC, Roberts EA. Developmental abnormalities and liver disease in childhood. In: Burt A, Portmann B, Ferrell L, eds. MacSween's pathology of the liver, 6th ed. Edinburgh: Elsevier; 2012:101-156.
72. Finn LS, Jaffe R. Langerhans' cell granuloma confined to the bile duct. Pediatr Pathol Lab Med 1997;17:461-468.
73. Kaplan KJ, Goodman ZD, Ishak KG. Liver involvement in Langerhans' cell histiocytosis: a study of nine cases. Mod Pathol 1999;12:370-378.
74. Shi Y, Qiao Z, Xia C, et al. Hepatic involvement of Langerhans cell histiocytosis in children—imaging findings of computed tomography, magnetic resonance imaging and magnetic resonance cholangiopancreatography. Pediatr Radiol 2014;44:713-718.
75. Portmann B, Zen Y. Inflammatory disease of the bile ducts-cholangiopathies: liver biopsy challenge and clinicopathological correlation. Histopathology 2012;60:236-248.
76. Krenacs L, Tiszalvicz L, Krenacs T, Boumsell L. Immunohistochemical detection of CD1A antigen in formalin-fixed and paraffin-embedded tissue sections with monoclonal antibody 010. J Pathol 1993;171:99-104.
77. Romani N, Clausen BE, Stoitzner P. Langerhans cells and more: langerin-expressing dendritic cell subsets in the skin. Immunol Rev 2010;234:120-141.
78. Roberts EA. Primary sclerosing cholangitis in children. J Gastroenterol Hepatol 1999;14:588-593.
79. Donadieu J, Bernard F, van Noesel M, et al. Cladribine and cytarabine in refractory multisystem Langerhans cell histiocytosis: results of an international phase 2 study. Blood 2015; 126:1415-1423.
80. Minkov M. Multisystem Langerhans cell histiocytosis in children: current treatment and future directions. Paediatr Drugs 2011;13:75-86.
81. [No authors listed] A multicentre retrospective survey of Langerhans' cell histiocytosis: 348 cases observed between 1983 and 1993. The French Langerhans' Cell Histiocytosis Study Group. Arch Dis Child 1996;75:17-24.
82. Zandi P, Panis Y, Debray D, Bernard O, Houssin D. Pediatric liver transplantation for Langerhans' cell histiocytosis. Hepatology 1995;21:129-33.
83. Griffiths W, Davies S, Gibbs P, Thillainayagam A, Alexander G. Liver transplantation in an adult with sclerosing cholangitis due to Langerhans cell histiocytosis. J Hepatol 2006;44:829-831.
84. Hadzic N, Pritchard J, Webb D, et al. Recurrence of Langerhans cell histiocytosis in the graft after pediatric liver transplantation. Transplantation 2000;70:815-819.
85. Newell KA, Alonso EM, Kelly SM, Rubin CM, Thistlethwaite JR Jr, Whitington PF. Association between liver transplantation for Langerhans cell histiocytosis, rejection, and development of posttransplant lymphoproliferative disease in children. J Pediatr 1997;131(Pt 1):98-104.
86. Zen Y, Fujii T, Nakanuma Y. Hepatic pseudolymphoma: a clinicopathological study of five cases and review of the literature. Mod Pathol 2010;23:244-250.
87. Sharifi S, Murphy M, Loda M, Pinkus GS, Khettry U. Nodular lymphoid lesion of the liver: an immune-mediated disorder mimicking low-grade malignant lymphoma. Am J Surg Pathol 1999;23:302-308.
88. Snover DC, Filipovich AH, Dehner LP, Krivit W. 'Pseudolymphoma'. A case associated with primary immunodeficiency disease and polyglandular failure syndrome. Arch Pathol Lab Med 1981;105:46-49.
89. Okada T, Mibayashi H, Hasatani K, et al. Pseudolymphoma of the liver associated with primary biliary cirrhosis: a case report and review of literature. World J Gastroenterol 2009;15:4587-4592.
90. Hayashi M, Yonetani N, Hirokawa F, et al. An operative case of hepatic pseudolymphoma difficult to differentiate from primary hepatic marginal zone B-cell lymphoma of mucosa-associated lymphoid tissue. World J Surg Oncol 2011;9:3.
91. Zen Y, Ishikawa A, Ogiso S, Heaton N, Portmann B. Follicular cholangitis and pancreatitis - clinicopathological features and differential diagnosis of an under-recognized entity. Histopathology 2012;60(2):261-269.
92. Aoki T, Kubota K, Oka T, Hasegawa K, Hirai I, Makuuchi M. Follicular cholangitis: another cause of benign biliary stricture. Hepatogastroenterology 2003;50:639-642.
93. Fujita T, Kojima M, Gotohda N, et al. Incidence, clinical presentation and pathological features of benign sclerosing cholangitis of unknown origin masquerading as biliary carcinoma. J Hepatobiliary Pancreat Sci 2010;17:139-146.
94. Zen Y, Nakanuma Y, Portmann B. Immunoglobulin G4-related sclerosing cholangitis: pathologic features and histologic mimics. Semin Diagn Pathol 2012;29:205-211.
95. Zen Y, Kawakami H, Kim JH. IgG4-related sclerosing cholangitis: all we need to know. J Gastroenterol 2016;51:295-312.
96. Brunt EM, Gouw AS, Hubscher SG, et al. Pathology of the liver sinusoids. Histopathology 2014;64:907-920.

12 PATHOLOGIC STAGING OF PRIMARY MALIGNANT NEOPLASMS IN LIVER

The major role of the pathologist is to provide an accurate diagnosis and to precisely stage a cancer. The stratification of staging in liver cancer relates closely to prognosis and recommendation of specific therapeutic options. Several staging systems have been developed, including the most widely used in the United States as well as worldwide, the American Joint Committee on Cancer (AJCC) TNM system (1,2). This system provides detailed pathologic parameters to communicate not only among pathologists, but also among health providers of other disciplines, including oncologists, surgeons, and radiologists.

Like the 7th edition (3), the most current AJCC cancer staging system, the 8th edition, separately stages cancers arising from hepatocytes (1) and intrahepatic bile ducts (2). The separation is based on the significant differences in the clinical, pathologic, tumor biologic, therapeutic, and prognostic aspects of these two entities.

The AJCC TNM staging system assesses pathologic parameters including tumor size and number, vascular invasion, lymph node metastasis, local invasion, and distant metastasis. Since underlying liver disease in primary liver cancer is common, it is recommended that background liver (preferably away from the tumor to avoid histologic changes confounded by adjacent mass effects) be evaluated and reported, especially the degree of fibrosis, as advanced fibrosis (modified Ishak score of 5 to 6) portends a worse prognosis (1). Several scoring systems for liver fibrosis exist and are widely used, such as the Batts-Ludwig system (4), modified Ishak system (5), and METAVIR system (6).

CANCERS ARISING FROM HEPATOCYTES

Table 12-1 shows the current AJCC cancer staging system for cancers arising from hepatocytes, including hepatocellular carcinoma and fibrolamellar carcinoma (1). Table 12-2 compares the current edition with 7th edition (3). The changes in the current edition are in the T category and described below.

Previously not divided, T1 is now subdivided into T1a and T1b. T1a is assigned when there is a solitary tumor 2 cm or smaller, while T1b is assigned when there is a solitary tumor larger than 2 cm, and without vascular invasion. Irrespective of vascular invasion, as long as the tumor is solitary and not greater than 2 cm, it is assigned as T1a. The 7th edition (3) excluded vascular invasion from the T1 category.

Table 12- 1

AJCC TNM STAGING OF PRIMARY LIVER CANCER (HEPATOCELLULAR CARCINOMA AND FIBROLAMELLAR CARCINOMA)[a]

T Category	T Criteria
TX	Primary tumor cannot be assessed
T0	No evidence of primary tumor
T1	Solitary tumor ≤2 cm, or >2 cm without vascular invasion
T1a	Solitary tumor ≤2 cm
T1b	Solitary tumor >2 cm without vascular invasion
T2	Solitary tumor >2 cm with vascular invasion, or multiple tumors, none >5 cm
T3	Multiple tumors, at least one of which is >5 cm
T4	Single tumor or multiple tumors of any size involving a major branch of the portal vein or hepatic vein, or tumor(s) with direct invasion of adjacent organs other than the gallbladder or with perforation of visceral peritoneum
N Category	**N Criteria**
NX	Regional lymph nodes cannot be assessed
N0	No regional lymph node metastasis
N1	Regional lymph node metastasis
M Category	**M Criteria**
M0	No distant metastasis
M1	Distant metastasis

[a]From AJCC Cancer Staging Manual, 8th edition, 2017 (1).

Table 12-2

SUMMARY OF CHANGES OF 2017 AJCC TNM STAGING OF PRIMARY LIVER CANCER[a]

Change	Details of Change
Definition of primary tumor (T)	T1 is now divided into two subcategories: T1a, solitary tumor ≤2 cm and T1b, solitary tumor without vascular invasion, >2 cm
Definition of primary tumor (T)	T2 now includes solitary tumor with vascular invasion >2 cm, or multiple tumors, none >5 cm
Definition of primary tumor (T)	T3a is now categorized as T3
Definition of primary tumor (T)	T3b: Tumors involving a major branch of the portal vein or hepatic vein formerly were categorized as T3b and are now categorized as T4

[a]From AJCC Cancer Staging Manual, 8th Edition, 2017 (1).

Table 12-3

AJCC TNM STAGING OF INTRAHEPATIC BILE DUCT CANCER[a]

T Category	T Criteria
TX	Primary tumor cannot be assessed
T0	No evidence of primary tumor
Tis	Carcinoma in situ (intraductal tumor)
T1	Solitary tumor without vascular invasion, ≤5 cm or >5 cm
T1a	Solitary tumor ≤5 cm without vascular invasion
T1b	Solitary tumor >5 cm without vascular invasion
T2	Solitary tumor with intrahepatic vascular invasion or multiple tumors, with or without vascular invasion
T3	Tumor perforating the visceral peritoneum
T4	Tumor involving local extrahepatic structures by direct invasion
N Category	**N Criteria**
NX	Regional lymph nodes cannot be assessed
N0	No regional lymph node metastasis
N1	Regional lymph node metastasis present
M Category	**M Criteria**
M0	No distant metastasis
M1	Distant metastasis present

[a] From AJCC Cancer Staging Manual, 8th Edition, 2017 (2).

The new T2 category includes solitary tumor with vascular invasion over 2 cm or multiple tumors, none greater than 5 cm. The previous edition did not have size distinction when there is vascular invasion.

The T3 category now only includes multiple tumors, with at least one tumor greater than 5 cm. In the previous edition, T3 was subdivided into T3a and T3b.

The previous T3b category, with single or multiple tumors of any size involving a major branch of the portal vein or hepatic vein, is now re-categorized as T4. Tumor(s) with direct direct invasion of adjacent organs other than the gallbladder or with perforation of visceral peritoneum remain as T4.

The rationale behind these changes are based on cumulative survival data (7). For instance, recent data show that patients with solitary hepatocellular carcinoma (HCC) up to 2 cm have no significant difference in survival when there is or is not vascular invasion, hence, patients with a single tumor 2 cm or smaller, irrespective of microvascular invasion, are now grouped as T1a. Also, patients with solitary HCC larger than 2 cm and microvascular invasion have similar survival rates as those with multiple HCC, 5 cm or larger, so these two groups are categorized together in the current T2 staging. In the current AJCC system, the definition of multiple tumors includes satellitosis, multifocal tumors, and intrahepatic metastases.

CANCERS ARISING FROM INTRAHEPATIC BILE DUCTS

Table 12-3 shows the most current AJCC 8th edition staging system for cancers arising from the intrahepatic bile ducts, including intrahepatic cholangiocarcinoma, combined hepatocellular-cholangiocarcinoma, and primary neuroendocrine tumors of the liver (2). Table 12-4 compares the 8th edition with the 7th edition (3). Newly added primary neuroendocrine tumors of the liver and other changes in the T category are described below.

Previously not divided, the T1 category is now subdivided into T1a and T1b to reflect the prognostic impact of tumor size. Solitary

Table 12-4

SUMMARY OF CHANGES OF 2017 AJCC TNM STAGING OF INTRAHEPATIC BILE DUCTS[a]

Change	Details of Change
Definition of primary tumor (T)	The T1 category is revised to account for the prognostic impact of tumor size (T1a: ≤5 cm vs. T1b: >5 cm)
Definition of primary tumor (T)	The T2 category is modified to reflect the equivalent prognostic value of vascular invasion and tumor multifocality
Definition of primary tumor (T)	The AJCC Cancer Staging manual, 7th edition T4 category describing the tumor growth pattern was eliminated from staging but is still recommended for data collection

[a]From AJCC Cancer Staging Manual, 8th edition, 2017 (2).

tumor without vascular invasion 5 cm or less is assigned as T1a, whereas T1b is assigned when it is greater than 5 cm.

Previously subdivided, the T2 category now lumps solitary tumor with intrahepatic vascular invasion and multiple tumors with or without vascular invasion together as a single category. The rationale behind this is that the prognostic significance of vascular invasion and tumor multifocality appears the same (2).

Previously assigned as T3, tumors involving local extrahepatic structures by direct invasion are now assigned as T4. The previous T4 category (tumor with periductal invasion) is now eliminated from staging, given its uncertain prognostic impact, but is still recommended for data collection.

Like the previous edition, the most current AJCC staging system still includes the rare combined hepatocellular-cholangiocarcinoma as a primary carcinoma of the intrahepatic bile ducts. This is a debatable issue, as neither the cancer cell of origin (8–18), clinical presentation, pathology, tumor biology, therapeutic modalities, or outcome of combined hepatocellular-cholangiocarcinoma are the same as those of cholangiocarcinoma (19,20). A separate staging system may need to be developed for this unique cancer.

The extremely rare primary neuroendocrine tumors of the liver are also included in the most current AJCC staging. The previous edition included a chapter of neuroendocrine tumors of various sites in the digestive system (3) but did not include hepatic primary neuroendocrine tumors, likely due to their extreme rarity. In fact, as no marker or histologic finding thus far indicates a hepatic primary, a diagnosis of primary neuroendocrine tumor of the liver is essentially based on excluding origin from another site, primarily by imaging studies and endoscopy, although neither modality can completely exclude another primary site, limiting their sensitivity. The actual applicability of staging for neuroendocrine tumors primary to the liver may be questionable.

The current 8th edition of AJCC system (2) includes adenocarcinomas arising from intraductal papillary neoplasms of the bile duct and mucinous cystic neoplasms.

REFERENCES

1. Abou-Alfa G, Pawlik T, Shindoh J, Vauthey JN. In: Amin M, Edge S, Greene F, eds. AJCC Cancer Staging Manual, 8th ed. Switzerland: Springer; 2017:287-293.
2. Aloia T, Pawlik T, Taouli B, Rubbia-Brandt L, Vauthey J-N. AJCC Cancer Staging Manual. In: Amin M, Edge S, Greene F, eds, 8th ed. Switzerland: Springer; 2017:295-302.
3. Edge SB, Byrd D, Compton C, Fritz A, Greene F, Trotti A I. AJCC cancer staging handbook: from the AJCC cancer staging manual, 7th ed. New York: Springer; 2010:718.
4. Batts KP, Ludwig J. Chronic hepatitis. An update on terminology and reporting. Am J Surg Pathol 1995;19:1409-1417.
5. Ishak K, Baptista A, Bianchi L, et al. Histological grading and staging of chronic hepatitis. J Hepatol 1995;22:696-699.
6. Bedossa P. Intraobserver and interobserver variations in liver biopsy interpretation in patients with chronic hepatitis C. The French METAVIR Cooperative Study Group. Hepatology 1994;20(Pt 1):15-20.
7. Shindoh J, Andreou A, Aloia TA, et al. Microvascular invasion does not predict long-term survival in hepatocellular carcinoma up to 2 cm: reappraisal of the staging system for solitary tumors. Ann Surg Oncol 2013;20:1223-1229.
8. Theise ND, Saxena R, Portmann BC, et al. The canals of Hering and hepatic stem cells in humans. Hepatology 1999;30:1425-1433.
9. Falkowski O, An HJ, Ianus IA, et al. Regeneration of hepatocyte 'buds' in cirrhosis from intrabiliary stem cells. J Hepatol 2003;39:357-364.
10. Kofman AV, Morgan G, Kirschenbaum A, et al. Dose- and time-dependent oval cell reaction in acetaminophen-induced murine liver injury. Hepatology 2005;41:1252-1261.
11. Kuwahara R, Kofman AV, Landis CS, Swenson ES, Barendswaard E, Theise ND. The hepatic stem cell niche: identification by label-retaining cell assay. Hepatology 2008;47:1994-2002.
12. Theise ND, Yao JL, Harada K, et al. Hepatic 'stem cell' malignancies in adults: four cases. Histopathology 2003;43:263-271.
13. Wu PC, Lai VC, Fang JW, Gerber MA, Lai CL, Lau JY. Hepatocellular carcinoma expressing both hepatocellular and biliary markers also expresses cytokeratin 14, a marker of bipotential progenitor cells. J Hepatol 1999;31:965-966.
14. Kim H, Choi GH, Na DC, et al. Human hepatocellular carcinomas with "Stemness"-related marker expression: keratin 19 expression and a poor prognosis. Hepatology 2011;54:1707-1717.
15. Kim H, Park C, Han KH, et al. Primary liver carcinoma of intermediate (hepatocyte-cholangiocyte) phenotype. J Hepatol 2004;40:298-304.
16. Durnez A, Verslype C, Nevens F, et al. The clinicopathological and prognostic relevance of cytokeratin 7 and 19 expression in hepatocellular carcinoma. A possible progenitor cell origin. Histopathology 2006;49:138-151.
17. Zhang F, Chen XP, Zhang W, et al. Combined hepatocellular cholangiocarcinoma originating from hepatic progenitor cells: immunohistochemical and double-fluorescence immunostaining evidence. Histopathology 2008;52:224-232.
18. Yamashita T, Ji J, Budhu A, et al. EpCAM-positive hepatocellular carcinoma cells are tumor-initiating cells with stem/progenitor cell features. Gastroenterology 2009;136:1012-1024.
19. Wachtel MS, Zhang Y, Xu T, Chiriva-Internati M, Frezza EE. Combined hepatocellular cholangiocarcinomas; analysis of a large database. Clin Med Pathol 2008;1:43-47.
20. Lee JH, Chung GE, Yu SJ, et al. Long-term prognosis of combined hepatocellular and cholangiocarcinoma after curative resection comparison with hepatocellular carcinoma and cholangiocarcinoma. J Clin Gastroenterol 2011;45:69-75.

Index*

*In a series of numbers, those in boldface indicate the main discussion of the entity.

D

E

F

G

H

N

P

R

S

T